GASTROENTEROLOGY AND HEPATOLOGY

The Comprehensive Visual Reference

GASTROENTEROLOGY AND HEPATOLOGY

The Comprehensive Visual Reference

series editor
Mark Feldman, MD
Southland Professor and Vice Chairman
Department of Internal Medicine
University of Texas Southwestern
Medical Center at Dallas
Chief, Medical Service
Veterans Affairs Medical Center
Dallas, Texas

volume 2

Colon, Rectum, and Anus

volume editor
C. Richard Boland, MD
Chief, Division of Gastroenterology
Department of Medicine
University of California, San Diego
La Jolla, California

With 18 contributors

CM
CURRENT MEDICINE
PHILADELPHIA

Current Medicine
400 Market Street
Suite 700
Philadelphia, PA 19106

Managing Editor	*Lori J. Bainbridge*
Development Editor	*Kelly Streeter*
Editorial Assistant	*Jennifer Rosenblum*
Indexer	*Maria Coughlin*
Art Director	*Paul Fennessy*
Design and Layout	*Robert LeBrun*
Illustration Director	*Ann Saydlowski*
Illustrators	*Wieslawa Langenfield, Beth Starkey, Larry Ward, Lisa Weischedel, and Gary Welch*
Typesetting Director	*Colleen Ward*
Production	*David Myers and Lori Holland*

Colon, rectum, and anus/volume editor, C. Richard Boland.
p. cm. – (Gastroenterology and hepatology; v. 2)
Includes biliographical references and index.
ISBN 1-878132-79-2 (hardcover)
1. Colon (Anatomy)—Atlases. 2. Rectum—Atlases. 3.Anus—Atlases. I. Boland, C. Richard, 1947- . II. Series.
[DNLM: 1.Colonic Diseases—atlases. 2. Rectal Diseases—atlases. WI 17 G257 1996 v.2]
RC807.C65 1996
616.3′44—dc20
DNLM/DLC
for Library of Congress 95-32010
CIP

Library of Congress Cataloging-in-Publication Data
ISBN 1-878132-79-2

Printed in Singapore by Imago Productions (FE) Pte Ltd.

10 9 8 7 6 5 4 3 2 1

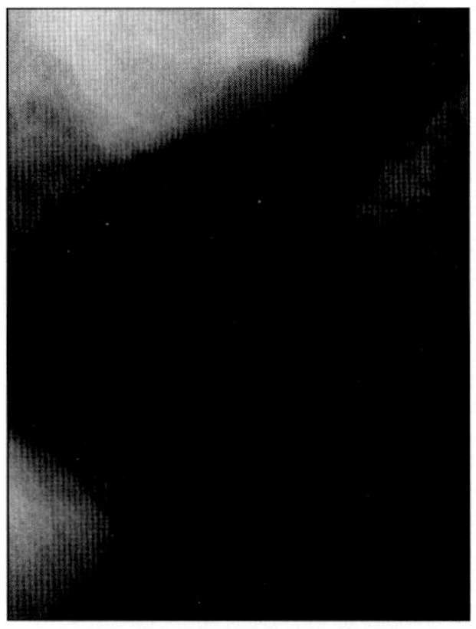

Series Preface

In recent years dramatic developments in the practice of gastroenterology have unfolded, and the specialty has become, more than ever, a visual discipline. Advances in endoscopy, radiology, or a combination of the two, such as endoscopic retrograde cholangiopancreatography and endoscopic ultrasonography, have occurred in the past 2 decades. Because of advanced imaging technology, a gastroenterologist, like a dermatologist, is often able to directly view the pathology of a patient's organs. Moreover, practicing gastroenterologists and hepatologists can frequently diagnose disease from biopsy samples examined microscopically, often aided by an increasing number of special staining techniques. As a result of these advances, gastroenterology has grown as rapidly as any subspecialty of internal medicine.

Gastroenterology and Hepatology: The Comprehensive Visual Reference is an ambitious 8-volume collection of images that pictorially displays the gastrointestinal tract, liver, biliary tree, and pancreas in health and disease, both in children and adults. The series is comprised of 89 chapters containing nearly 4000 images accompanied by legends. The images in this collection include not only traditional photographs but also charts, tables, drawings, algorithms, and diagrams, making this collection much more than an atlas in the conventional sense. Chapters are authored by experts selected by one of the eight volume editors, who carefully reviewed each chapter within their volume.

Disorders of the gastrointestinal tract, liver, biliary tree, and pancreas are common in children and adults. *Helicobacter pylori* gastritis is the most frequent bacterial infection of humans and is a risk factor for peptic ulcer disease and gastric malignancies. Colorectal carcinoma is the second leading cause of cancer mortality in the United States, with nearly 60,000 deaths in 1990. Pancreatic cancer resulted in an additional 25,000 deaths. Liver disease is also an important cause of morbidity and mortality, with more that 25,000 deaths from cirrhosis alone in 1990. Gallstone disease is also common in our society, with increasing reliance on laparoscopic cholecystectomy in symptomatic individuals. Inflammatory bowel diseases (ulcerative colitis, Crohn's disease) are also widespread in all segments of the population; their causes still elude us.

The past few decades have also witnessed striking advances in the therapy of gastrointestinal disorders. Examples include "cure" of peptic ulcer disease by eradicating *H. pylori* with antimicrobial agents, healing of erosive esophagitis with proton pump inhibitor drugs, remission of chronic viral hepatitis B or C with interferon-α2b, and hepatic transplantation for patients with fulminant hepatic failure or end-stage liver disease. Therapeutic endoscopic techniques have proliferated that ameliorate the need for surgical procedures. Endoscopic advances include placement of peroral endoscopic gastrostomy tubes for nutritional support, insertion of stents in the bile duct or esophagus to relieve malignant obstruction, and the use of injection therapy, thermal coagulation, or laser therapy to treat bleeding ulcers and other lesions, including tumors. *Gastroenterology and Hepatology: The Comprehensive Visual Reference* will cover these advances and many others in the field of gastroenterology.

I wish to thank a number of people for their contributions to this series. The dedication and expertise of the other volume editors—Willis Maddrey, Rick Boland, Paul Hyman, Nick LaRusso, Roy Orlando, Larry Schiller, and Phil Toskes—was critical and most appreciated. The nearly 100 contributing authors were both creative and generous with their time and teaching materials. Special thanks to Abe Krieger, President of Current Medicine, for recruiting me for this unique project and to his talented associates at Current Medicine, especially Kelly Streeter who served as developmental editor.

The images contained in this 8-volume collection are available in print as well as in slide format, and the series is soon being formatted for CD-ROM use. All of us who have participated in this ambitious project hope that each of the 8 volumes, as well as the entire collection, will be useful to physicians and health professionals throughout the world involved in the diagnosis and treatment of patients of all ages who suffer from gastrointestinal disorders.

Mark Feldman, MD

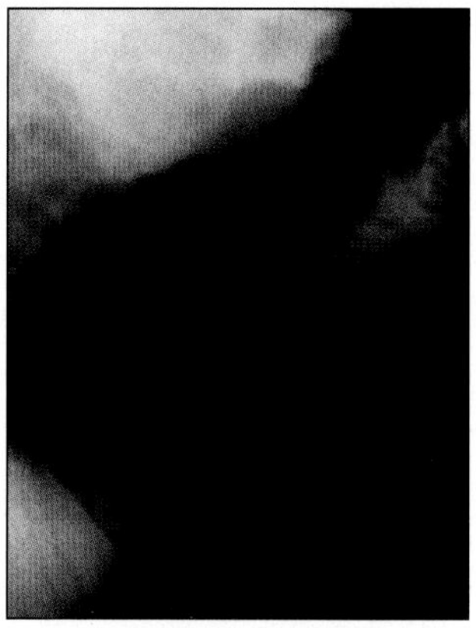

Volume Preface

The distal-most portion of the alimentary tract has long been important to gastroenterologists because of its propensity to develop disease and produce symptoms. This region of the gut has taken on additional importance over the past several decades with the emergence of technologies that permit a sensitive diagnosis of a variety of treatable conditions. The diagnosis and treatment of diseases of the colon, rectum, and anus are dominated by a need for the accurate interpretation of visual images. To begin with, the anatomy and physiology of this region are best communicated with images that range from anatomical drawings to the depiction of wave forms of neuromuscular activity. The introduction of diagnostic and therapeutic colonoscopy over the past 25 years has revolutionized our ability to make a precise diagnosis and administer nonsurgical treatment to life-threatening conditions such as lower gastrointestinal bleeding and colorectal neoplasia. Gastrointestinal bleeding and large intestinal cancer continue to be among the most common problems encountered by the gastroenterologist, and teaching the principles of management of these conditions requires a visual database.

The 11 chapters in this volume include a large collection of the most critical images required for teaching. The chapters on anatomy and physiology, endoscopy, radiology, and pathology provide a framework for understanding the structure and function of normal and diseased colon. Our appreciation of colorectal anatomy has not changed in recent years; however, our understanding of intestinal physiology has been in constant evolution. An understanding of these principles is essential for a proper interpretation of the symptoms and complications of dysmotility, diverticulosis, and gastrointestinal bleeding. In *Colon, Rectum, and Anus*, the figures presented are complementary, and slides from several of the chapters can be combined to enhance lectures.

The diagnosis and management of colorectal neoplasia and inflammatory bowel disease depend on proper interpretations of visual imagery derived from radiologic, pathologic, and endoscopic disciplines. These chapters cover a broad range of disorders. High-quality images of illustrative radiographs and key pathologic lesions are especially valuable for a lecture, and the contributors provided a number of examples especially useful to educators. In particular, the surgical images in the *Colon and Rectal Surgery* chapter, by Frederic Eckhauser, James Knol, and Lisa Colletti, illustrate some of the new operative procedures available for the treatment of colorectal disease, which may have been relatively inaccessible to nonsurgeons.

Each figure is supported by an explanatory caption. The chapters were not written to serve as single, fully prepared lectures, but rather each author has created a comprehensive collection of images that illustrate and supplement any lecture on the colon, rectum, or anus. As such, this collection will be useful for many years as an enduring educational resource. I wish to thank each of the individual authors for an outstanding effort in which the literature was surveyed for images of particular teaching value and for sharing images from their personal collections for this volume.

C. Richard Boland, MD

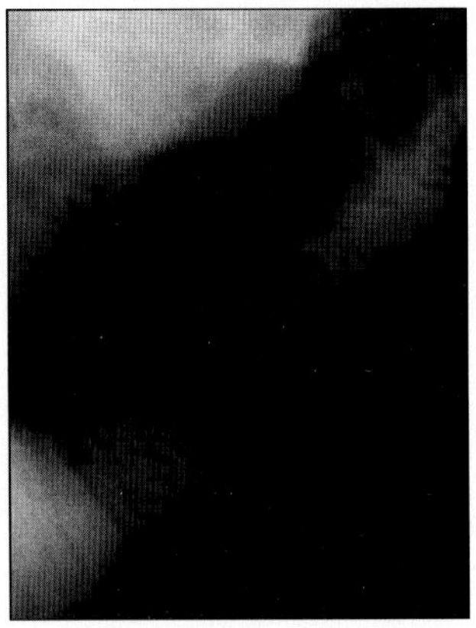

Contributors

Jeffrey L. Barnett, MD
Associate Professor
Department of Internal Medicine
University of Michigan Medical Center
Ann Arbor, Michigan

Carlos Belmonte-Montes, MD
Visiting Fellow
Department of Surgery
University of Minnesota
St. Paul, Minnesota

Robert S. Bresalier, MD
Associate Professor of Medicine
Department of Medicine
University of Michigan School of Medicine
Ann Arbor, Michigan
Director, Gastrointestinal Oncology
Henry Ford Health Sciences Center
Detroit, Michigan

Lisa M. Colletti, MD
Assistant Professor
Department of Surgery
Division of Gastrointestinal Surgery
University of Michigan Medical Center
Ann Arbor, Michigan

Christopher S. Cutler, MD
Fellow in Gastroenterology/Hepatology
Department of Medicine
Indiana University School of Medicine
Indianapolis, Indiana

Frederic E. Eckhauser, MD
Professor, Department of Surgery
Chief, Division of Gastrointestinal Surgery
University of Michigan Medical Center
Ann Arbor, Michigan

Lawrence S. Friedman, MD
Associate Professor of Medicine
Harvard Medical School
Associate Physician
Gastrointestinal Unit
Massachusetts General Hospital
Boston, Massachusetts

Fiona Graeme-Cook, MD
Instructor in Pathology
Harvard Medical School
Assistant in Pathology
Department of Pathology
Massachusetts General Hospital
Boston, Massachusetts

Joel K. Greenson, MD
Assistant Professor
Department of Pathology
University of Michigan Medical Center
Ann Arbor, Michigan

William L. Hasler, MD
Assistant Professor
Department of Internal Medicine
Division of Gastroenterology
University of Michigan Medical Center
Ann Arbor, Michigan

James A. Knoll, MD
Associate Professor
Department of Surgery
Division of Gastrointestinal Surgery
University of Michigan Medical Center
Ann Arbor, Michigan

Timothy T. Nostrant, MD, FACP, FACG
Associate Professor of Medicine
Department of Internal Medicine
University of Michigan Medical Center
Ann Arbor, Michigan

J. Javier Perez-Ramirez, MD
Visiting Fellow
Department of Surgery
University of Minnesota
St. Paul, Minnesota

Douglas K. Rex, MD
Professor, Department of Medicine
Indiana University School of Medicine
Indianapolis, Indiana

David A. Rothenberger, MD
Clinical Professor of Surgery
Chief, Division of Colorectal Surgery
Department of Surgery
University of Minnesota
St. Paul, Minnesota

Robert H. Schapiro, MD
Associate Clinical Professor
Department of Medicine
Harvard University
Chief, Gastrointestinal Endoscopy
Massachusetts General Hospital
Boston, Massachusetts

Edward T. Stewart, MD
Professor, Department of Radiology
Medical College of Wisconsin
Chief, GI Radiology
Froedtert Memorial Lutheran Hospital
Milwaukee, Wisconsin

Arnold Wald, MD
Professor, Department of Medicine
University of Pittsburgh
Division of Gastroenterology and Hepatology
University of Pittsburgh Medical Center
Pittsburgh, Pennsylvania

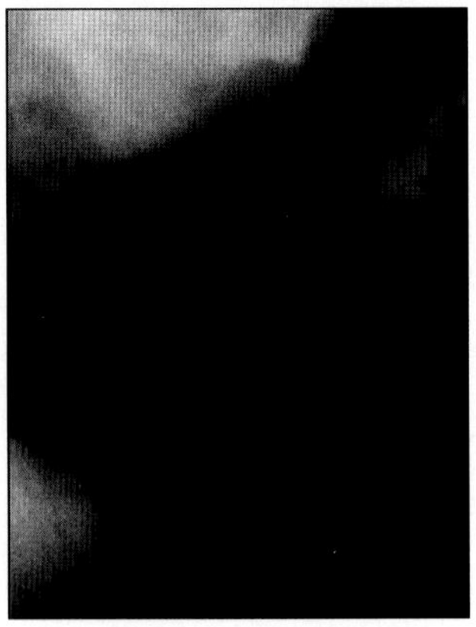

Contents

Chapter 4

Inflammatory Colitides

LAWRENCE S. FRIEDMAN
FIONA GRAEME-COOK
ROBERT H. SCHAPIRO

Chapter 5

Anorectal and Colonic Dysmotility

ARNOLD WALD

Chapter 6

Diseases of the Anus

JEFFREY L. BARNETT

Chapter 7
Lower Gastrointestinal Bleeding

Chapter 8
Colon and Rectal Surgery

Chapter 9
Colonic Diverticulosis

Chapter 10
Radiologic Images

EDWARD T. STEWART

Chapter 11
Pathology of the Colon and Rectum

JOEL K. GREENSON

Chapter 1

Embryology, Anatomy, and Physiology of the Colon, Rectum, and Anus

William L. Hasler

The colon, rectum, and anus have the major role of evacuating solid waste material in an efficient and socially convenient fashion. This evacuation is accomplished by anatomical and histological properties that are specifically designed for the characteristic motor and absorptive properties of the colon. Furthermore, an abundant colonic flora is present presumably for various metabolic activities as well as for suppression of growth of pathogenic organisms that might induce gastrointestinal or systemic disease.

The anatomy of the colon is most remarkable for the arrangement of the smooth muscle layers (*see* Figs. 1-3 to 1-5). For most of the length of the colon, there is a prominent circular muscle layer with the longitudinal layer being restricted to three thin bands. The circular layer forms characteristic constrictions, known as the *haustra*, which give the colon a sacculated appearance. The colon possesses a rich intrinsic innervation contained within the submucosal plexus, which is believed to regulate most of the absorptive and secretory activities, and the myenteric plexus, which controls colonic motor function (*see* Figs. 1-12 and 1-13). Additionally, colonic function is modulated by extrinsic neural influences from the splanchnic and pelvic nerves and possibly from the vagus nerves as well (*see* Figs. 1-11 and 1-29). The mucosa of the colon is quite different from that of the small intestine, with deep parallel crypts instead of prominent villi (*see* Figs. 1-6 to 1-8). This difference most likely pertains to the predominant requirement for the colon to absorb fluids and electrolytes rather than digest and absorb nutrients. Arterial and venous blood to the colon is supplied by the superior and inferior mesenteric vessels, which provide extensive collaterals to ensure adequate perfusion of the colon during periods of rest and activity (*see* Figs. 1-9 and 1-10). Finally the colon possesses an elaborate lymphatic drainage system, which is important for its immunologic activities (*see* Fig. 1-14).

The motor activity of the colon is characterized by several distinct patterns that aid in the mixing of fecal material, as well as its propulsion, to afford efficient extraction of fluid and electrolytes as well as to promote controlled evacuation. Studies of colonic transit demonstrate a slow movement of intracolonic contents from the cecum to the rectum over the course of 1 to 2 days in normal individuals (*see* Figs. 1-15 and 1-16). The time course of propulsion through the distinct regions of the colon is not constant, with most available evidence suggesting that the ascending colon and rectum provide specialized storage capabilities for fecal material. These transit patterns are formed from the concerted actions of several distinct motor patterns and their corresponding myoelectric complexes. Short-duration contractions are stationary motor patterns present over very restricted lengths of colon, which mix the fecal material to extract water (*see* Fig. 1-17). Short-duration contractions are regulated by short spike bursts, electrical phenomena that are tightly controlled by colonic slow wave activity, also known as *electrical control activity* (*see* Figs. 1-18 to 1-21). Electrical control activity is generated in a specific region at the submucosal border of the circular muscle layer. Long-duration contractions, controlled by the myoelectrical correlate, the long spike bursts, may be stationary or propagate for short distances in either an orad or aboral direction (*see* Figs. 1-17, 1-18, and 1-21). Long-duration contractions assist in both mixing and short-distance propulsion of fecal material. High-amplitude propagated contractions, controlled by the myoelectrical correlate, the migrating long spike bursts, propagate in an aboral direction over long lengths of colon and are believed to be responsible for mass movements of feces (*see* Figs. 1-17, 1-18, and 1-21). High-amplitude propagated contractions may precede spontaneous defecation, suggesting an important physiologic role for this motor pattern in fecal evacuation (*see* Figs. 1-23 and 1-24). Finally, studies in dogs demonstrate an organized pattern known as the *colonic migrating motor complex*, with the associated migrating myoelectric complex, which occurs every 40 to 50 minutes (*see* Fig. 1-22). This motor pattern has not been described in humans, although this difference may stem from methodologic issues rather than species differences.

Motor activity of the colon is extensively modified by external influences. Ingestion of a meal results in marked increases in colonic motor activity, which are mediated by cholinergic neural pathways (*see* Figs. 1-25 and 1-26). The colon possesses a peristaltic reflex, a response to an intraluminal bolus that induces an aborally propulsive motor response (*see* Figs. 1-27 and 1-28). Studies in some animal species suggest that vagal input can modify motor activity at least in the proximal colon (*see* Fig. 1-29). Finally, the central nervous system has potent effects on colonic motor activity, with stress inducing significant increases in contractile activity (*see* Fig. 1-30).

A major function of the colon is to dehydrate the fecal bolus to minimize fluid loss with defecation. Of the 1.5 L of fluid that are presented to the colon, only 100 mL are passed into the stool (*see* Fig. 1-31). This process is accomplished by the concerted action of a number of ionic pumps and transporters as well as membrane characteristics that are quite distinct from those of the small intestine (*see* Figs. 1-31 and Table 1-1). Sodium absorption is accomplished via two routes, an electrogenic and an electroneutral pathway, and is responsible for the bulk of water absorption in the colon (*see* Table 1-1 and Table 1-1). The high levels of potassium in the stool are explained by an active secretion of potassium into the colonic lumen, a phenomenon accomplished by the action of a specific potassium channel that may be modulated by intracellular messengers and externally by aldosterone and epinephrine (*see* Fig. 1-33). The absorption of sodium mandates a concurrent absorption of chloride. To dispose of the anion, an active chloride secretion is accomplished by a specific chloride channel, which may be modulated by intracellular messengers (*see* Fig. 1-34).

In addition to its motor and absorptive properties, the colon possesses a luxuriant flora predominantly made up of anaerobic organisms that serve several presumed functions (*see* Fig. 1-35 and Table 1-2). Although the precise importance of the bacterial colonization of the colon is uncertain, studies in germ-free animals show significant alterations in body weight, hydration status, and immune function, suggesting important roles in these areas. Colonic bacteria also reduce stool pH, which presumably drives certain biochemical reactions by changing oxidation-reduction characteristics in the colonic lumen. Finally, it has been proposed that the colonic flora suppresses growth of pathogenic organisms.

The anatomy of the anorectum is quite different from more proximal regions of the colon and is specifically designed for controlled evacuation of the fecal bolus (*see* Figs. 1-36 and 1-37). The longitudinal muscle layer envelops the rectum, in contrast to the proximal colon. The rectal mucosa is smooth and the rectal wall is capacious, owing to the storage function of this region. The circular muscle of the anus forms a prominent internal anal sphincter, which provides a tonic closure at the anus. Additionally, specialized skeletal muscles from the levator ani apparatus provide a muscular sling that aids in maintenance of continence and control of defecation. In contrast to the more proximal colon, the mucosa of the most distal rectum and anus shows a transition to squamous histology (*see* Fig. 1-38). Specific arterial blood to the anus is supplied by the inferior rectal artery (*see* Fig. 1-39), and specific extrinsic innervation to this region is provided by the pudendal nerve (*see* Fig. 1-11).

A number of factors are critical for maintenance of fecal continence. These factors include the dehydrated nature of the stool and a capacious and distensible rectum (*see* Figs. 1-40 and 1-44). The anus provides a constant level of tone, and the puborectalis component of the levator ani muscles remains tonically contracted, thus providing a functional obstruction to stool passage (*see* Figs. 1-40 and 1-41). The external anal sphincter aids continence upon introduction of a fecal bolus into the rectum by voluntarily contracting (*see* Fig. 1-42). Finally, the anal mucosa possesses an elaborate set of nerve endings that are capable of distinguishing solid and liquid material from gas, thus allowing the individual to decide whether rectal evacuation is appropriate (*see* Fig. 1-43).

Defecation involves the coordinated interaction of several muscular structures in and surrounding the anorectum (*see* Fig. 1-45 to 1-48). Passage of the fecal bolus into the rectum induces a reflex relaxation of the internal anal sphincter, known as the *rectoanal inhibitory reflex* (*see* Fig. 1-45). If defecation is not desired, there is contraction of the external sphincter and puborectalis. Upon voluntary defecation, contractions of the diaphragm, rectus abdominis muscles, and the terminal aspects of the levator ani muscles are evoked that provide a propulsive force by increasing intra-abdominal pressure. Associated with this force is an increase in rectal pressure from rectal contraction and relaxation of the internal anal sphincter as well as relaxation of the puborectalis muscle, which allows a straightening of the anorectal angle to allow effortless evacuation of the fecal material.

The anatomic characteristics of the colon, rectum, and anus develop early in fetal life. The colon herniates into the umbilical cord at 5 weeks of gestation but returns, rotating counterclockwise as it reenters the abdominal cavity, to achieve its final position with the cecum in the right lower quadrant at 12 weeks of gestation (*see* Fig. 1-1). The fetal cloaca is divided by caudal migration of tissue to form the urogenital sinus and the rectum during the 6th to the 10th weeks (*see* Fig. 1-2). The anal membrane ruptures at 10 weeks to allow formation of the anal canal.

NORMAL EMBRYONIC DEVELOPMENT

Human colon

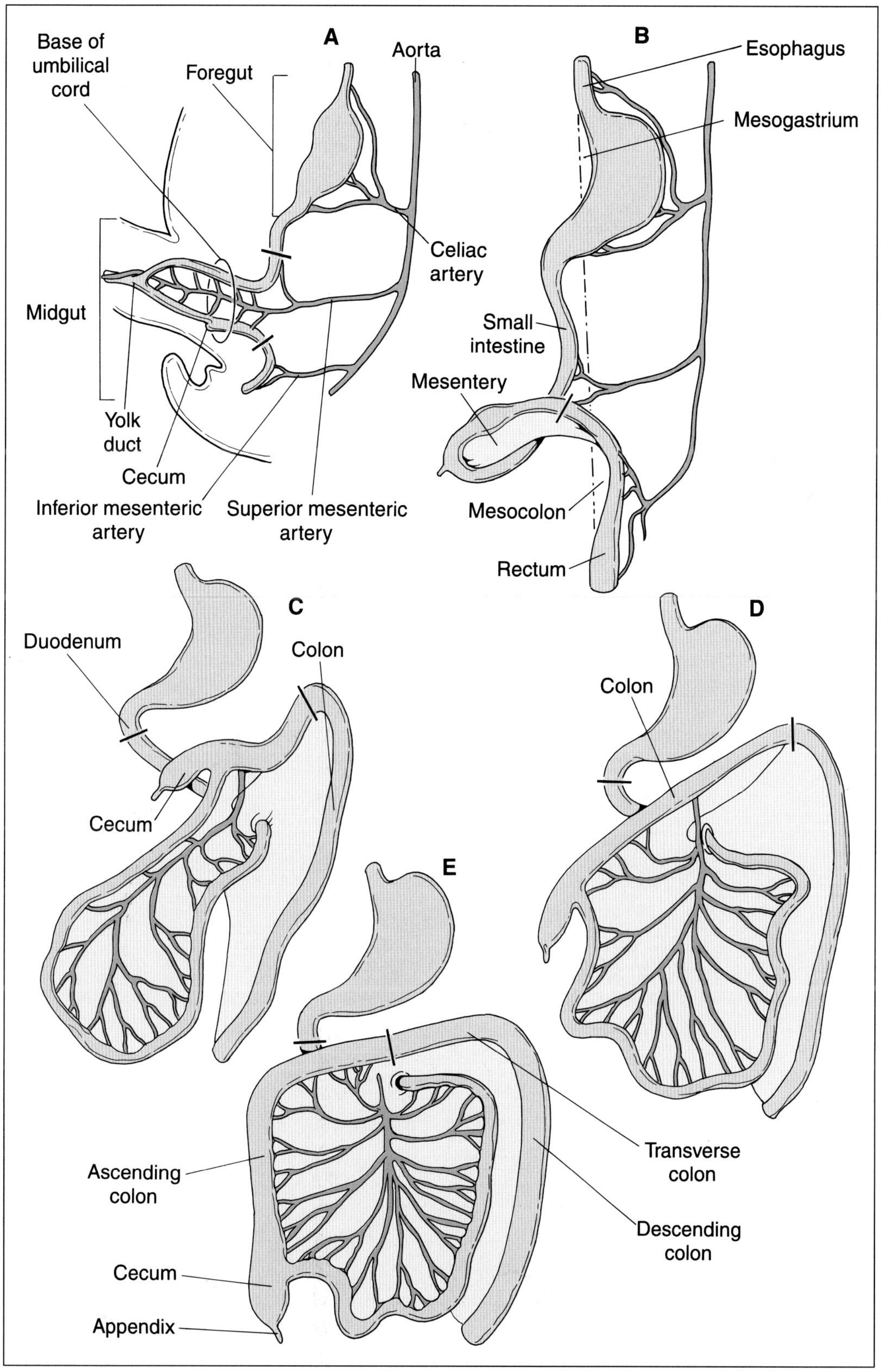

FIGURE 1-1.

The normal embryonic development of the human colon is shown. The proximal colon from the cecum to the region of the splenic flexure is formed from the embryonic midgut, whereas the more distal regions develop from the hindgut. The midgut, supplied by the superior mesenteric artery, is herniated through into the umbilical cord at 5 weeks (**A**). Over the next several weeks, the midgut returns to the intestinal cavity, with the colon undergoing counterclockwise rotation, to achieve its final position with the cecum in the right lower quadrant of the abdomen after 12 weeks of gestation (**B–E**). With this characteristic rotation, the colon comes to reside anterior to the superior mesenteric artery. Over the course of further fetal development, portions of the descending and ascending colon and rectum become posteriorly fixed to become retroperitoneal structures. (*From* Carlson [1]; with permission.)

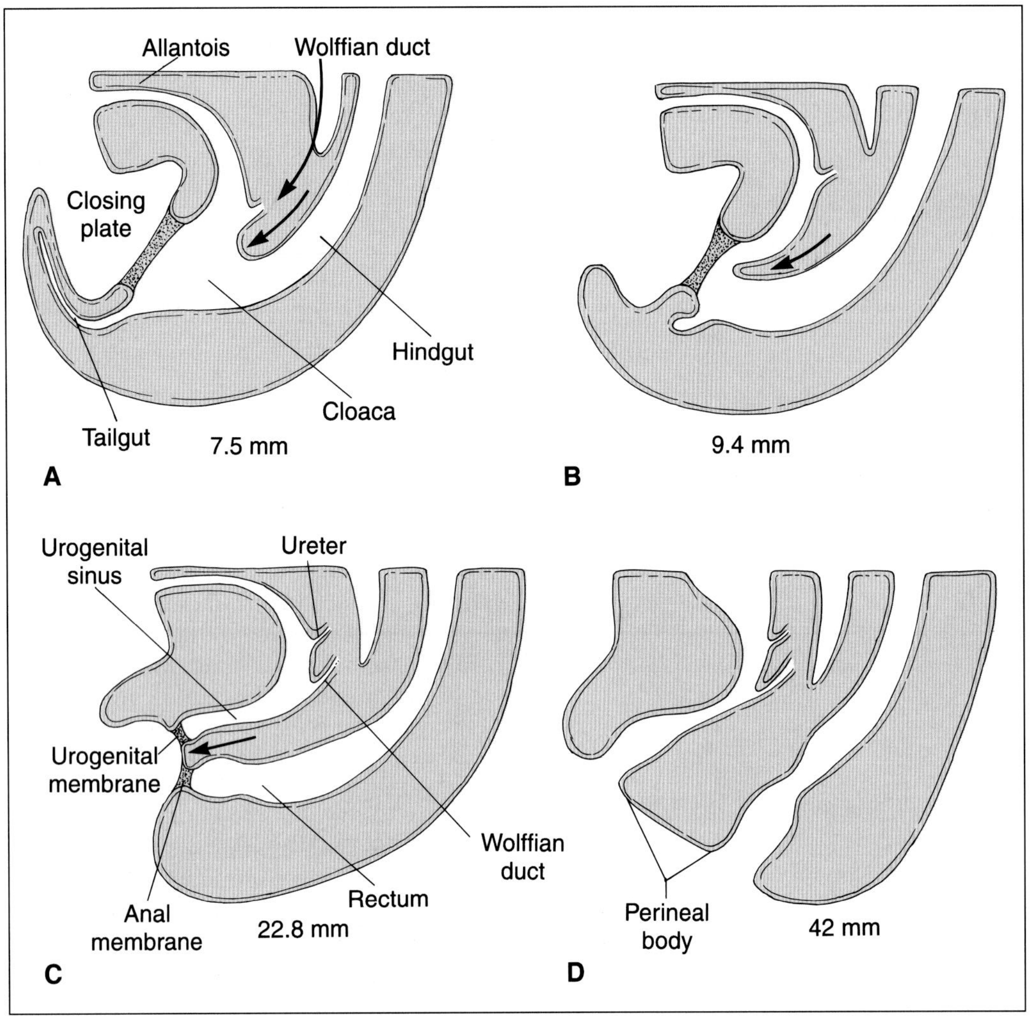

FIGURE 1-2.

The normal embryonic development of the rectoanal region is shown. In the 5th week, the cloaca is formed from the embryonic allantois, hindgut, and tailgut (**A**). Over the next several weeks, there is caudal migration of tissue to separate the allantois, which becomes the urogenital sinus, and the hindgut, which becomes the rectum (**B** and **C**). The fusion of the urorectal septum with the closing plate forms the perineal body. During the 10th gestational week, the urogenital and anal membranes rupture (**D**). (*From* Mulholland [2]; with permission.)

ANATOMY OF THE COLON

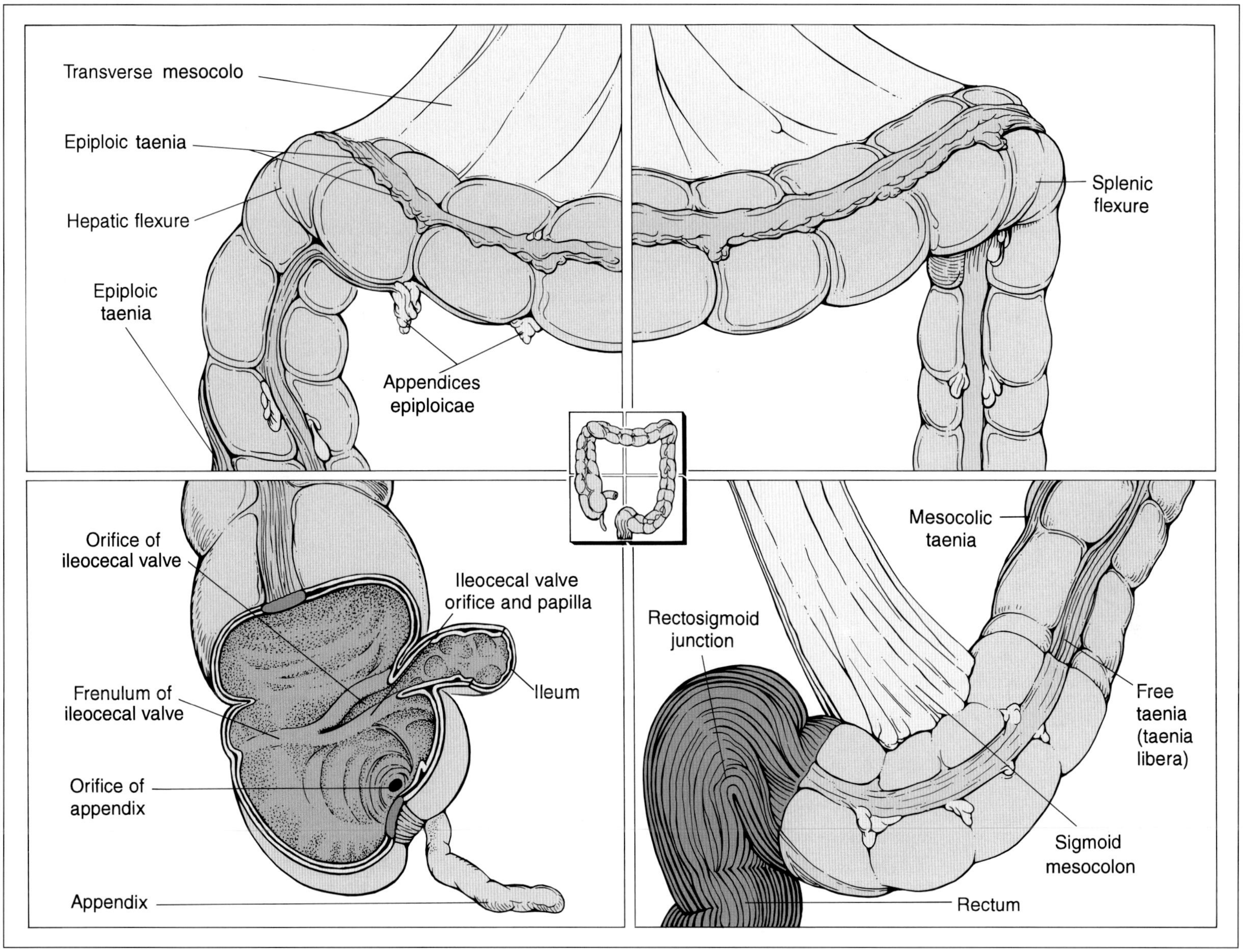

FIGURE 1-3.

The anatomy of the colon is shown. The most proximal region of the colon, the cecum, connects to the distal ileum via the ileocecal valve, a slitlike sphincter that regulates fluid flow from the small intestine into the colon and prevents coloileal reflux. The appendix, an anatomic structure with an unclear physiologic role, joins the cecum via the appendiceal orifice. The ascending, transverse, and descending colonic muscular layers include a circumferential circular layer with three overlying thin strips of longitudinal muscle, the taenia coli (epiploic, libera, and mesocolic), 120° apart. In the rectosigmoid region, the longitudinal muscle merges to envelop the entire circumference of the colon. Overlying the muscle layers of the intraperitoneal portion of the colon is a serosal layer, whereas the retroperitoneal portions of the colon are covered by an adventitial layer. Colonic haustra are defined by the circular muscle folds termed *plicae semilunares coli*. Mesenteric attachment to the intraperitoneal portion of the colon is incomplete, being restricted to the transverse and sigmoid mesocolons. The appendices epiploicae are subserosal fat collections associated with the taenia coli.

LAYERS OF THE COLON

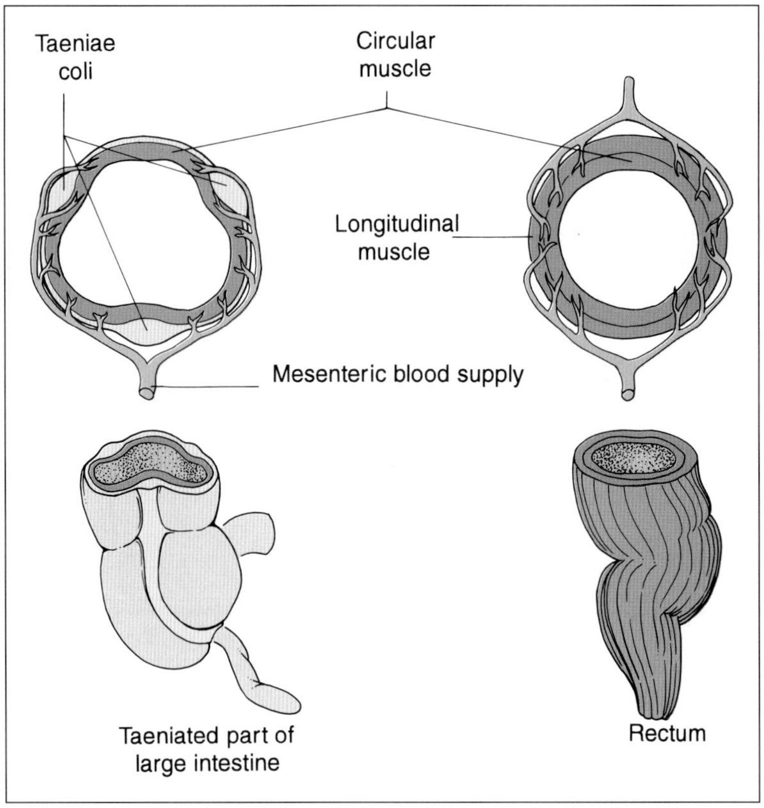

FIGURE 1-4.

The arrangements of the circular and longitudinal muscle layers in the different regions of the colon are shown in this diagram. In the ascending, transverse, and descending colons, the circular muscle is circumferential, whereas the longitudinal muscle is confined to the three taenia coli. The blood supply for these regions of the colon are supplied via the mesenteric attachments that are anatomically associated with one of the taenia coli. In contrast, the longitudinal muscle envelops the entire circumference of the rectum, which is supplied by penetrating blood vessels not contained within a mesenteric attachment. (*Adapted from* Christensen [3]; with permission.)

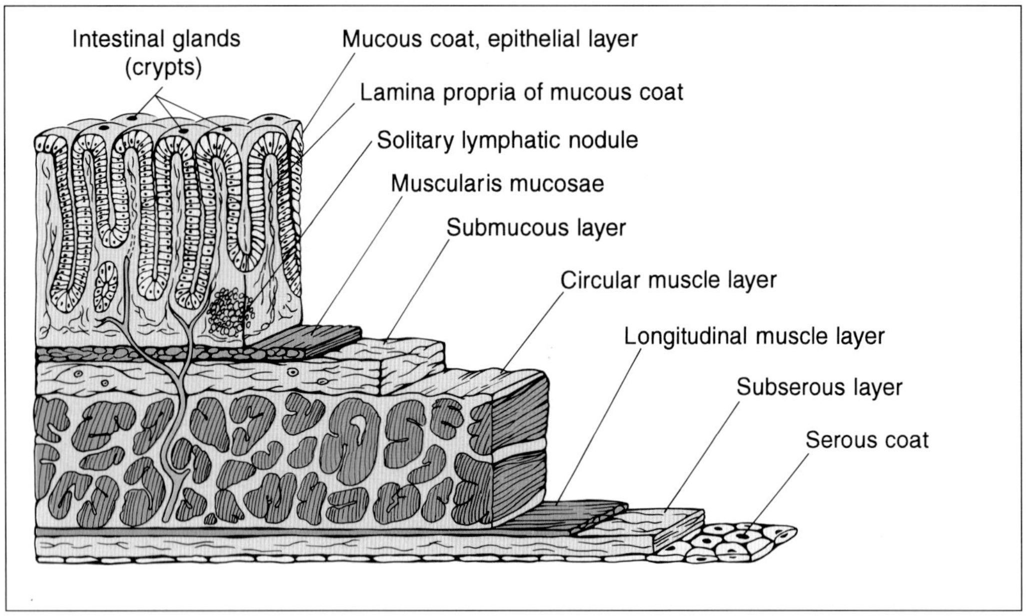

FIGURE 1-5.

The layers of the colonic wall are shown. The colonic mucosa consists of an epithelial layer with distinctive crypts as well as a lamina propria with variable numbers of inflammatory cells. Overlying the epithelial layer is a mucous coat secreted by the colonic epithelial cells. Separating the mucosa from the submucosa is a muscular layer termed the *muscularis mucosae*. The submucosal layer is rich in fibrous and neural tissue. Below the submucosal layer is a thick circumferential circular layer. A much thinner longitudinal muscle layer is continuous in the rectum but is restricted to the taenia coli in the ascending, transverse, and descending colons. Between the longitudinal and circular muscle layers resides a rich layer of neural tissue, the myenteric plexus. The colon is covered by subserosal and serosal layers in the intraperitoneal regions of the colon and by an adventitial layer in the retroperitoneal regions of the colon (rectum and parts of the ascending and descending colon). (*Adapted from* Staubesand [4]; with permission.)

NORMAL COLONIC MUCOSA

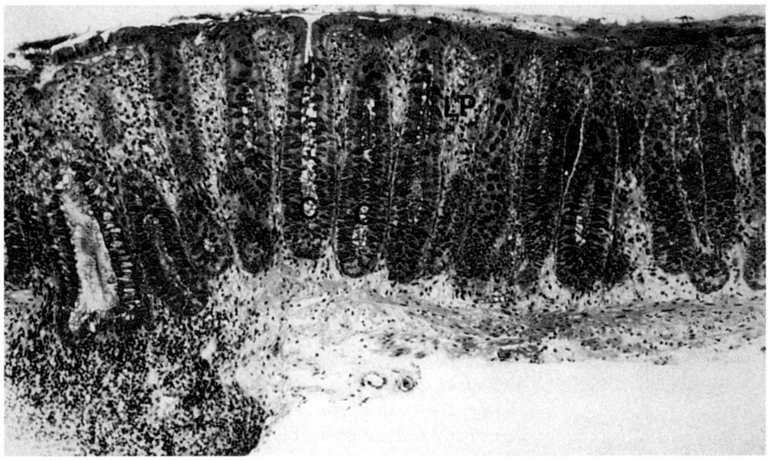

FIGURE 1-6.

Normal colonic mucosa is shown in this biopsy specimen from human colon. The epithelial layer consists of columnar cells and goblet cells that form characteristic crypts oriented in parallel fashion. Beneath the epithelial layer, the lamina propria contains small numbers of inflammatory cells (lymphocytes, plasma cells) as well as stromal elements and supporting tissues. (*From* Mulholland [2]; with permission.)

EPITHELIAL CELLS

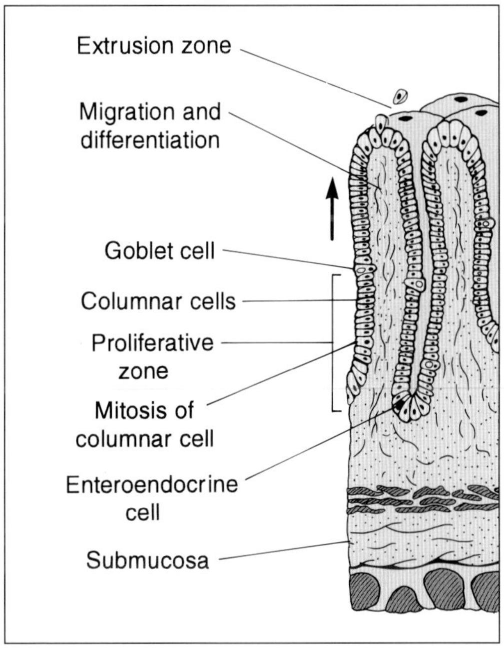

FIGURE 1-7.

The maturation process of colonic epithelial cells is shown in this diagram. At the base of the crypts, relatively immature columnar cells undergo mitosis in a zone of proliferation. Over the course of 3 to 5 days, the columnar cells migrate toward the colonic lumen to a zone of migration and differentiation, during which time the cells become mature epithelial cells. Epithelial cells in the colonic lumen itself slough off in a zone of extrusion and are continually replaced by cells migrating from below. Goblet cells within the epithelial layer secrete a mucous layer that presumably has protective effects for the colonic mucosa. In the bases of the crypts, enteroendocrine cells reside, which serve modulatory roles for the secretory activities of the colonic epithelium. (*Adapted from* Williamson [5]; with permission.)

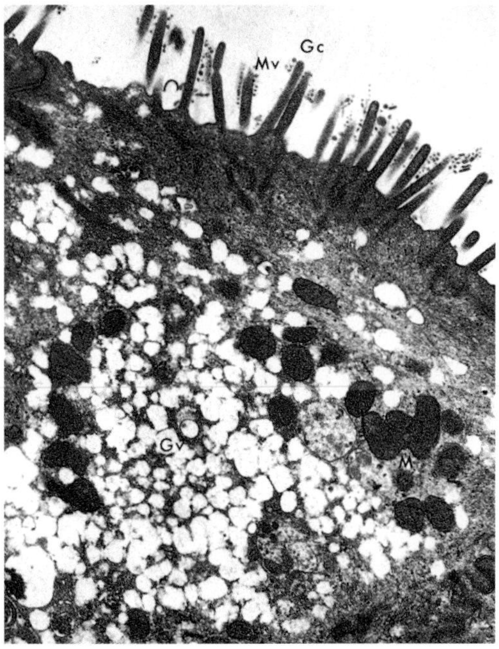

FIGURE 1-8.

An electron micrograph of a human rectal columnar epithelial cell is shown. Microvilli are present on the surface of the epithelial cells, although they are less abundant than in the small intestine. A prominent glycoprotein overlies the microvilli. Numerous membrane-bound vesicles are present near the luminal surface of the epithelial cell. The role of these vesicles is uncertain, but the presence of glycoproteins within the vesicles suggests probable involvement in the secretory activities of the colon. The presence of numerous mitochondria is indicative of significant metabolic activity in this region. (*From* Trier and Winter [6]; with permission.)

ARTERIAL BLOOD SUPPLY

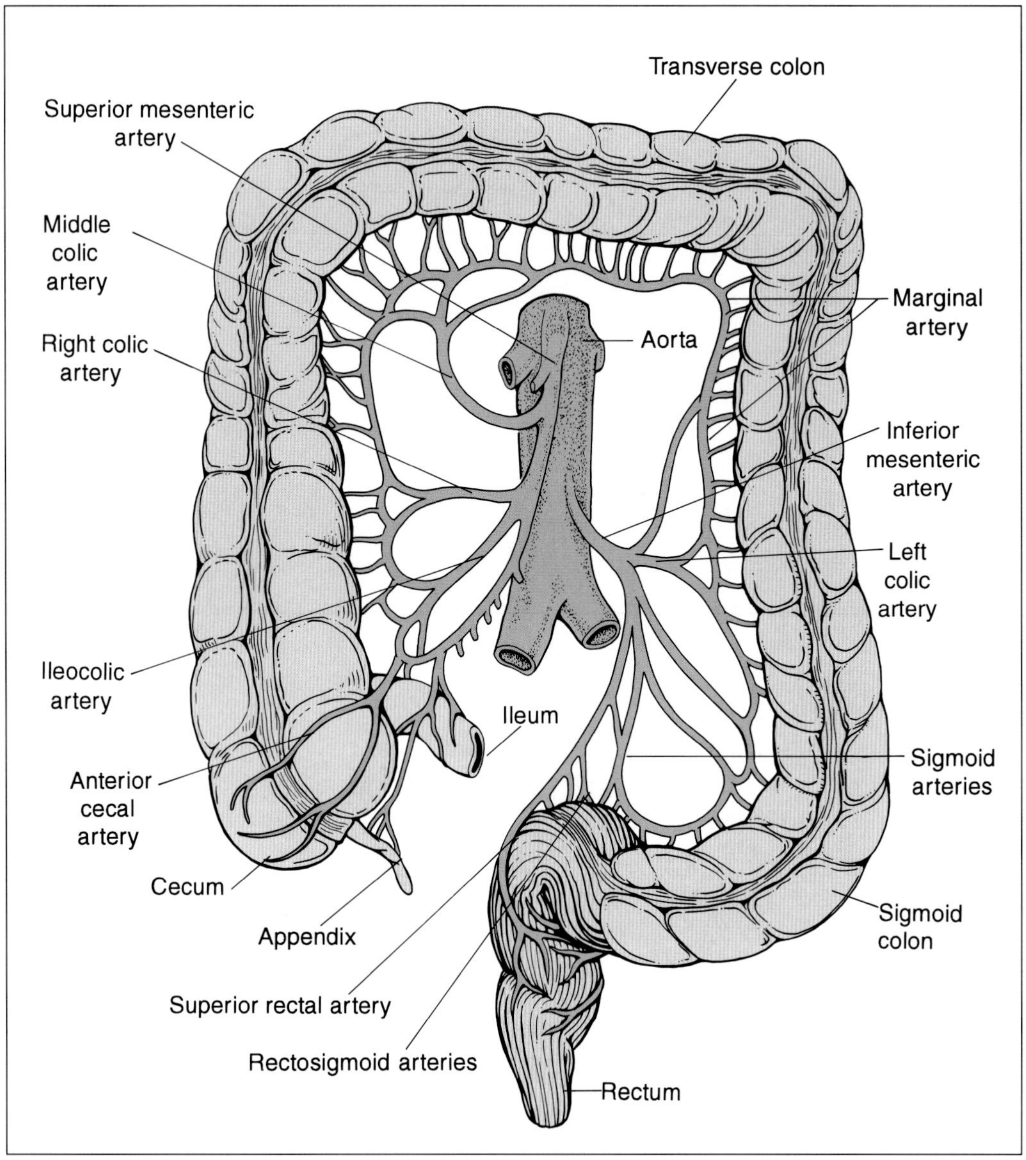

FIGURE 1-9.

The arterial blood supply to the colon is shown. The cecum, ascending colon, and transverse colon receive blood predominantly via the superior mesenteric circulation, which divides into the ileocolic, right colic, and middle colic arteries, whereas the descending and rectosigmoid colons obtain predominantly an inferior mesenteric blood supply, which divides into the left colic, sigmoid, rectosigmoid, and superior rectal arteries. An anastomosis of the two circulations is made via the marginal artery. (*Adapted from* Melloni *et al.* [7]; with permission.)

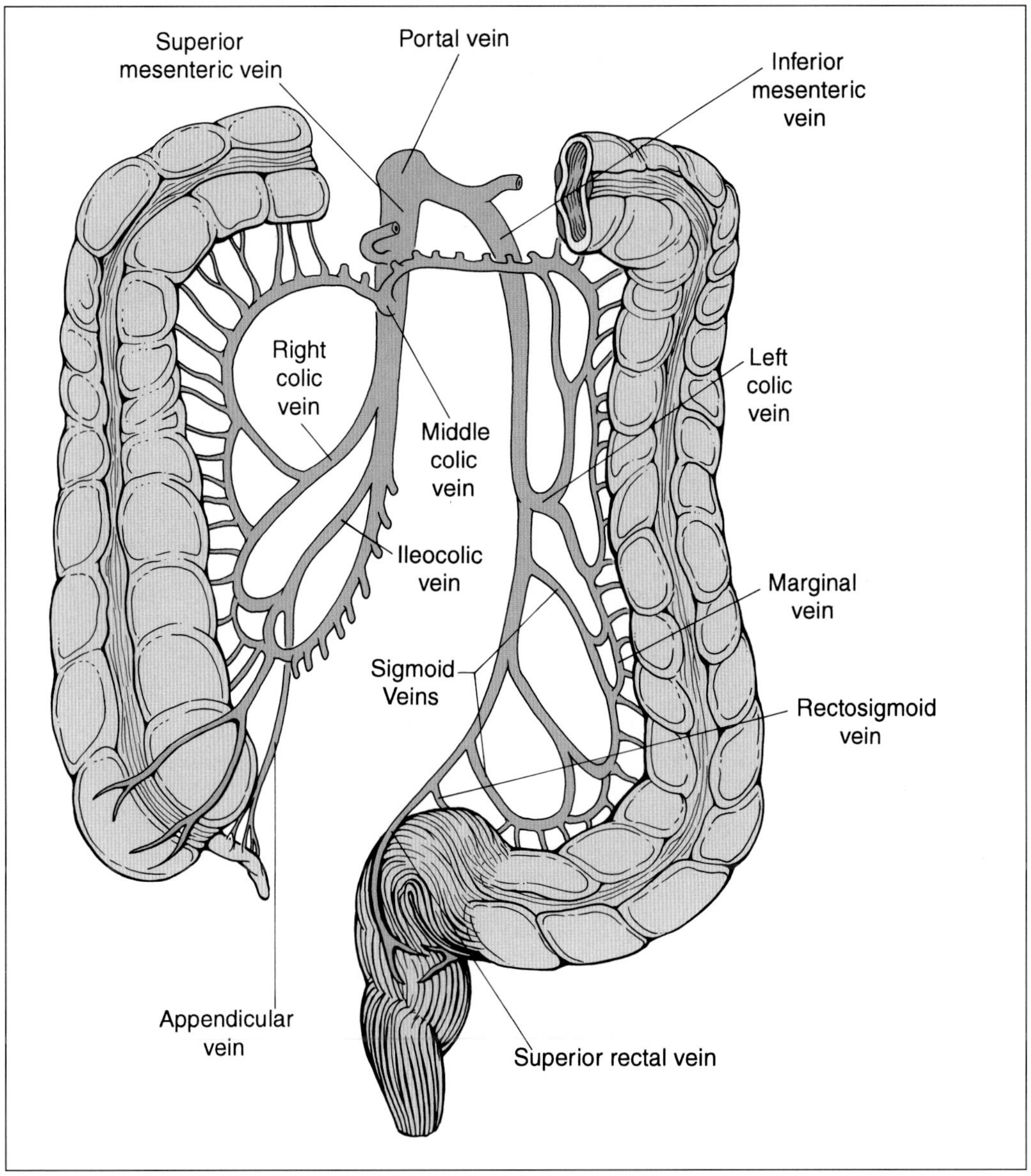

FIGURE 1-10.

The venous system that drains the colon is shown. The venous drainage of the colon empties into the portal venous system of the liver. The cecum, ascending colon, and transverse colon drain into the superior mesenteric vein via the ileocolic, right colic, and middle colic veins. The descending and rectosigmoid colon drain into the inferior mesenteric vein via the left colic, sigmoid, rectosigmoid, and superior rectal veins. (*Adapted from* Melloni *et al.* [7]; with permission.)

INNERVATION

Extrinsic innervation

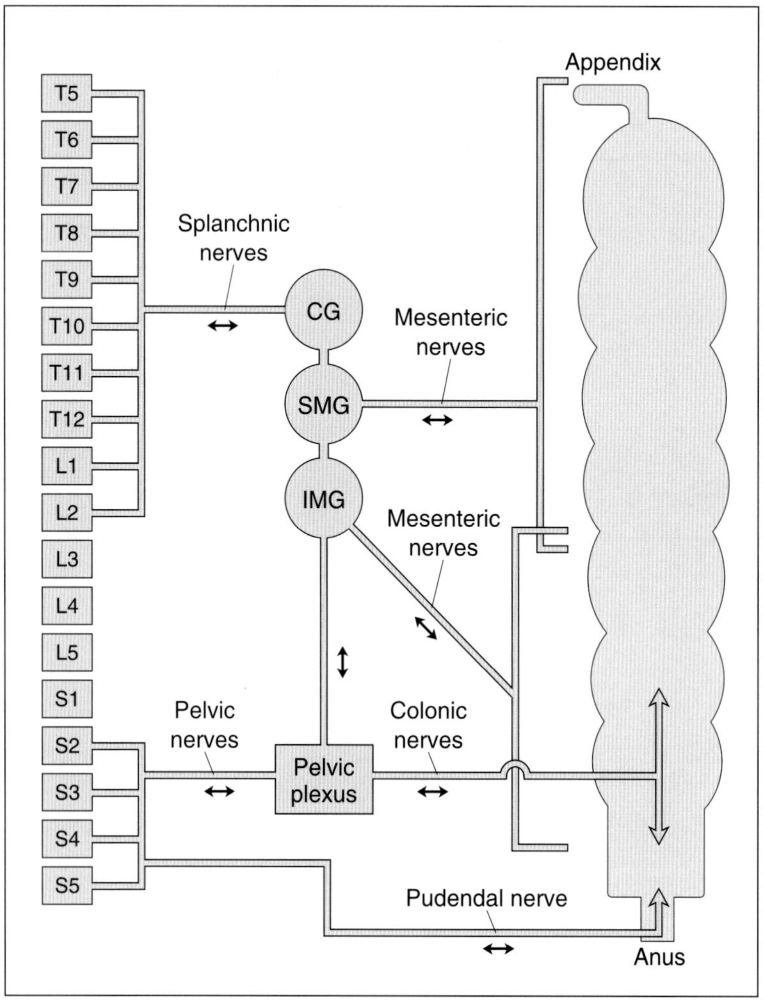

FIGURE 1-11.

The extrinsic innervation of the colon is shown. Splanchnic nerves from the thoracolumbar spinal cord serve the celiac ganglia (CG), superior mesenteric ganglia (SMG), and inferior mesenteric ganglia (IMG), which in turn project mesenteric nerves to the colonic smooth muscle and myenteric plexus. Pelvic nerves from the sacral spinal nerve supply the pelvic plexus, which in turn projects via the colonic nerve to the myenteric plexus of the distal portion of the colon and rectum. The splanchnic nerves provide predominantly a sympathetic input, whereas the pelvic nerves supply predominantly a parasympathetic input. The pudendal nerve, also from the sacral spinal nerve, provides the extrinsic neural supply to the anus. It has also been postulated from some animal studies that the most proximal regions of the colon receive extrinsic neural input from the vagus nerves (not shown). (*Adapted from* Christensen [3]; with permission.)

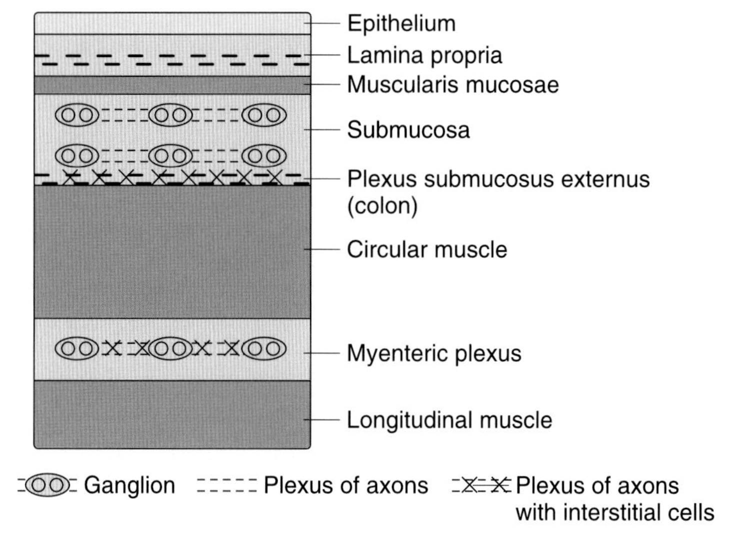

FIGURE 1-12.

The intrinsic innervation of the colonic wall is shown. Ganglia and plexuses of axons are present within the submucosal layer (submucosal plexus) and within the region between the circular and longitudinal muscle layers (myenteric plexus). These neural structures are believed to independently regulate much of the motor and secretory activity of the colon, including local reflexes. The myenteric (and to a lesser degree submucosal) plexus also receives modulatory neural input from extrinsic parasympathetic (vagal and pelvic nerves) and sympathetic (splanchnic nerves) neural pathways. (*Adapted from* Christensen [3]; with permission.)

DENSITIES OF GANGLIA

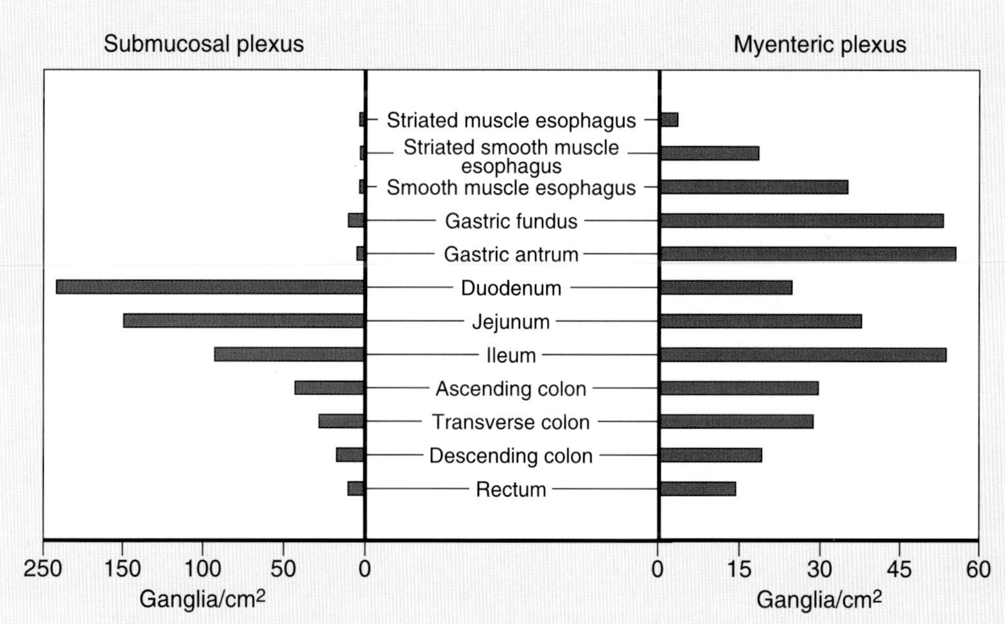

FIGURE 1-13.

The densities of ganglia in the submucosal and myenteric plexuses throughout the gastrointestinal tract are shown. The relative density of ganglia in the submucosal plexus is much less in the various colonic regions than in the small intestine. The submucosal plexus is believed to mediate secretory and absorptive activities. Thus, these functions may be more intensely controlled in the small intestine than in the colon. The discrepancies in ganglion densities in the myenteric plexuses of the small intestine and colon are less impressive. The myenteric plexus is believed to be more involved in motor function of the gut. This suggests that all regions of the gastrointestinal tract require significant neural modulation of motor activity. The relatively lower densities in the rectum suggest that this region may need less neural control. (*From* Christensen [8]; with permission.)

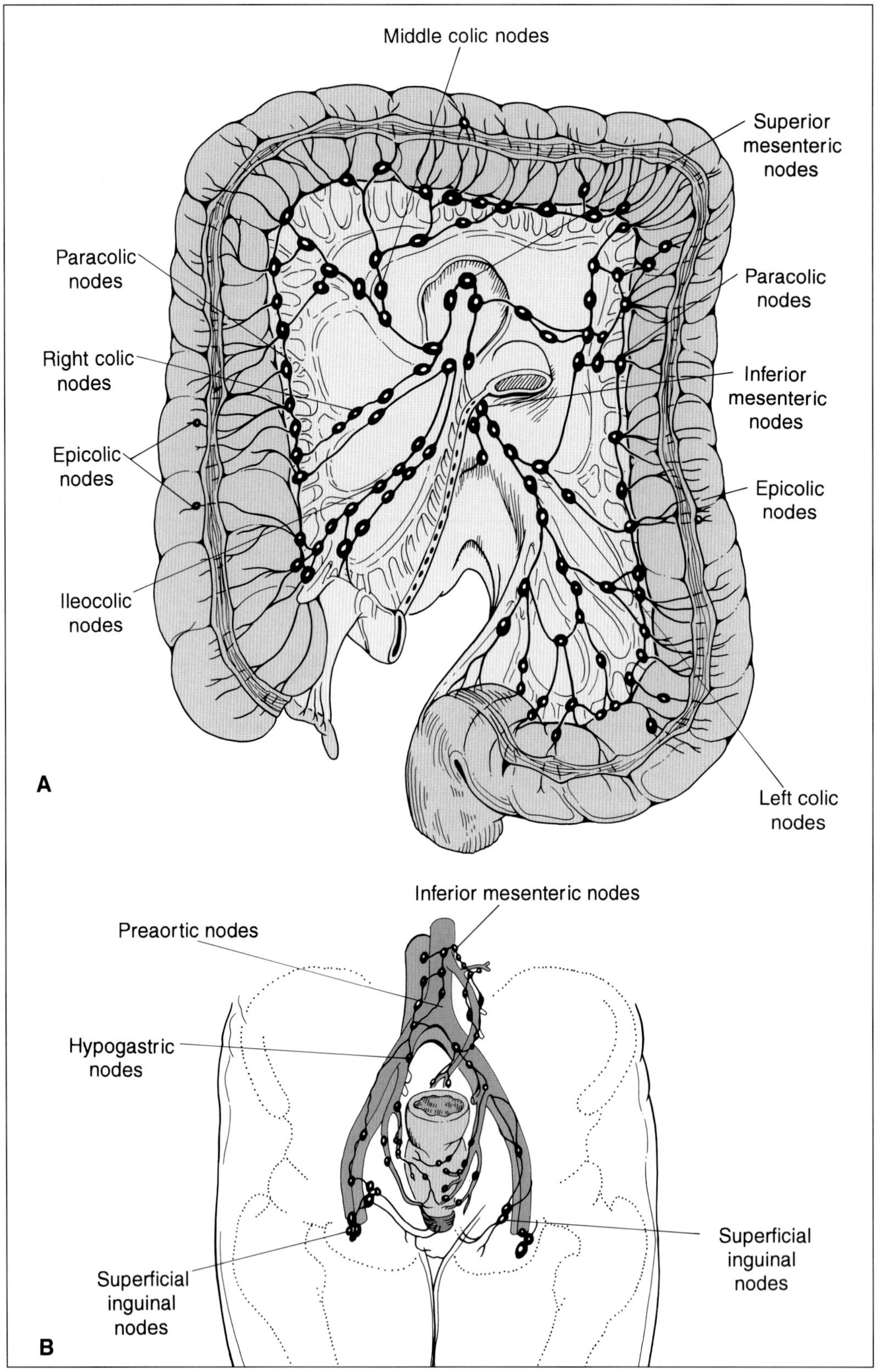

FIGURE 1-14.

The lymph nodal drainage of the colon and anus is shown. The initial chain of lymph nodes draining the colon are the epicolic nodes (**A**), which are located below the serosa. These nodes drain into the regional chains of lymph nodes (ileocolic, right colic, middle colic, and left colic). In some regions of the colon, paracolic lymph nodes are interspersed between the epicolic and the regional chains. The regional lymph nodes subsequently drain into the superior and inferior mesenteric lymph nodes. The lymph drainage of the rectum and anus proceeds via two pathways (**B**). From the lower portion of the anus the lymphatics drain into the superficial inguinal lymph nodes. The upper portion of the anus and the rectum drain into various intermediate chains, including the hypogastric lymph nodes, which then drain into the preaortic lumbar nodes, a system that merges with the inferior mesenteric nodal system.

COLONIC TRANSIT

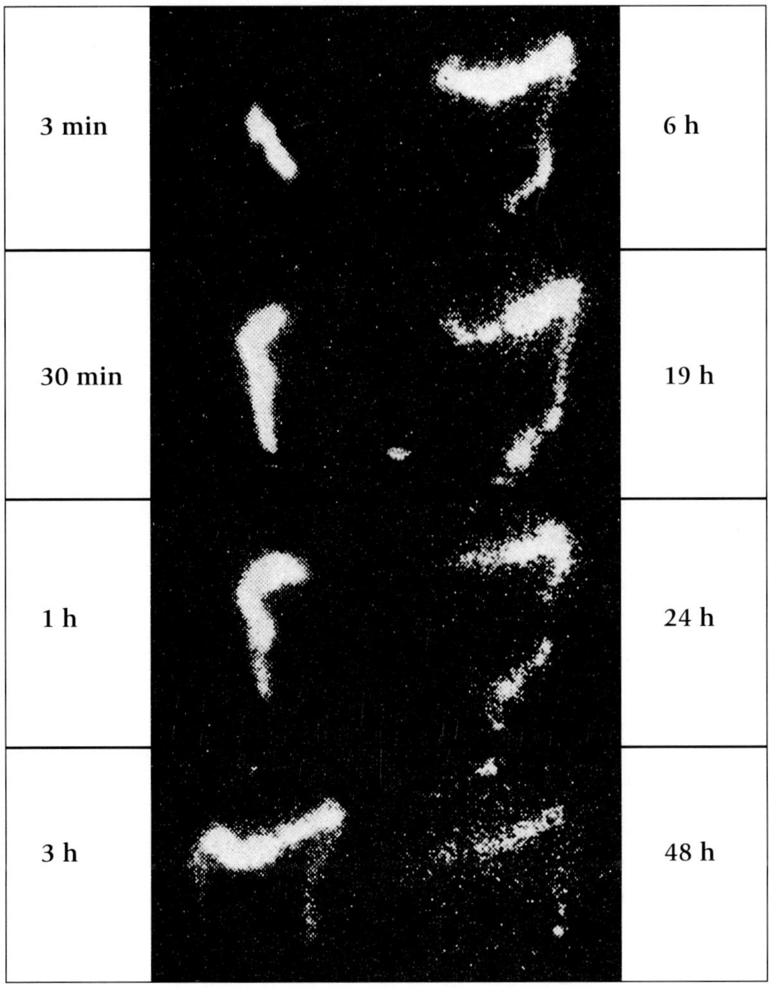

FIGURE 1-15.

The scintigraphic pattern of colonic transit in a normal individual is shown after cecal perfusion of a radiolabelled marker. In the earliest images, tracer activity concentrates in the right colon, but by 6 hours the radioligand has migrated to the transverse colon. Over the course of 1 to 2 days, the tracer is propelled into the ascending colon and rectosigmoid colon to be expelled in the feces. (*From* Krevsky *et al.* [9]; with permission.)

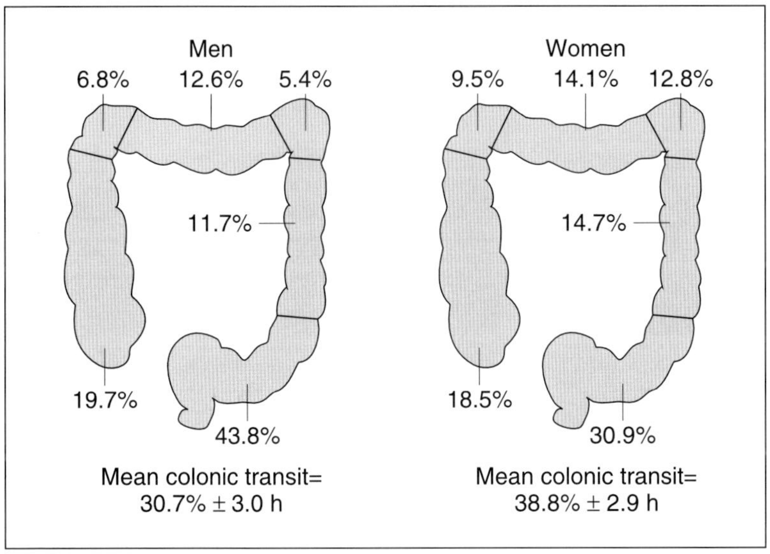

FIGURE 1-16.

From studies in which the colonic transit of orally ingested radioopaque markers is measured, it is possible to determine the percent of time that a substance spends in each region of the colon. In both men and women, the markers reside in the rectosigmoid region for the longest period of time, indicative of a storage function for this region. There is also prolonged residence of the markers in the ascending colon. This portion of the colon has been hypothesized to possess storage capabilities as well, based on the directionality of contractile patterns in this region. The mean colonic transit is slightly longer in women than in men. (*From* Metcalf *et al.* [10]; with permission.)

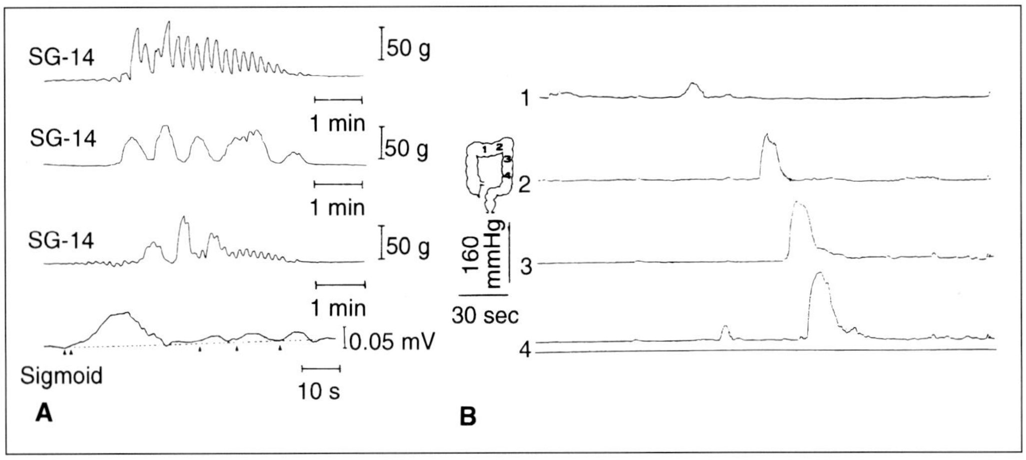

FIGURE 1-17.

Distinct motor patterns as measured by manometry are shown. **A**, The top three tracings display motor activity from a canine measured from a strain gauge (SG) transducer at a single site at different time points. These tracings show the presence of short-duration contractions in the top tracing, long-duration contractions in the second tracing, and a mix of short- and long-duration contractions in the third tracing. In the bottom tracing from a human colon, a long-duration contraction (*double arrows*) is followed by three short-duration contractions (*single arrows*). In general, short-duration contractions are present only over short sections of colon, are nonmigratory, and are believed to be responsible for the mixing of fecal material. Long-duration contractions may be stationary or migrate for short distances in either an orad or aboral direction and assist in transit of the fecal material. **B**, A high-amplitude propagated contraction is shown sequentially migrating over four consecutive recording sites in the human transverse and descending colons. High-amplitude propagated contractions are believed to be the manometric correlates to mass movements of feces in the colon. (**A**, *Adapted from* Sarna [11]; with permission.) (**B**, *Adapted from* Narducci *et al.* [12]; with permission.)

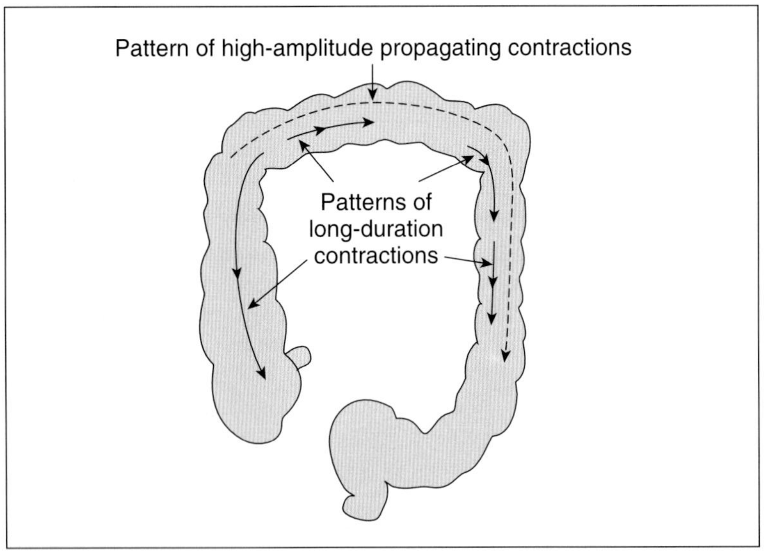

FIGURE 1-18.

The patterns of migration of long-duration contractions and high-amplitude propagated contractions are shown. Long-duration contractions may be stationary or migrate over short distances (*solid lines*). In the right and proximal transverse colons, many long-duration contractions migrate in an orad direction, whereas in the more distal regions of the colon, they migrate in an aboral fashion. In contrast, high-amplitude contractions (*dashed line*) propagate over extended distances in the colon in an aboral direction, corresponding to mass movements of feces. (*Adapted from* Christensen [3]; with permission.)

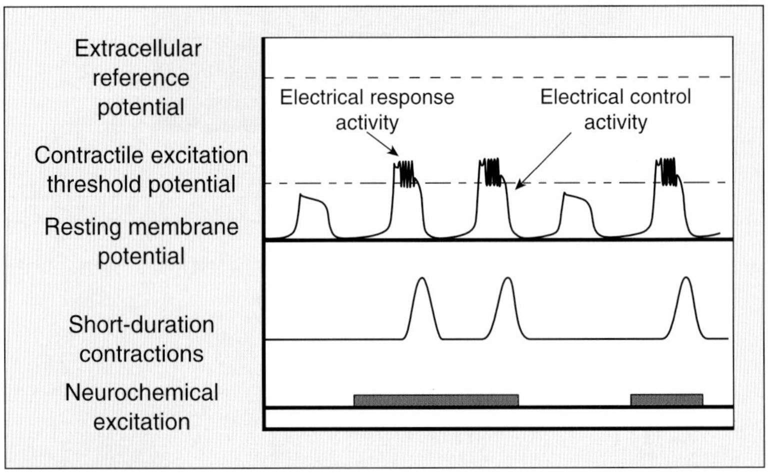

FIGURE 1-19.

The presence and intensity of short-duration contractions in the colon are regulated by characteristic electrical patterns as shown. The top tracing demonstrates the myoelectric activity of colonic smooth muscle recorded by intracellular electrodes. Under conditions of no neurochemical excitation, there is a rhythmic oscillation of the resting membrane potential, known as the *electrical control activity* or *colonic slow wave*, which does not reach a contractile excitation threshold potential. Under these conditions, contraction does not occur and the colon is quiescent. With neurochemical excitation, there is an increase in the amplitude of the electrical control activity with generation of electrical response activity or spike potentials that exceed the contractile excitation threshold potential. Thus with neurochemical excitation, there is induction of short-duration contractions in the colon. (*Adapted from* Sarna [13]; with permission.)

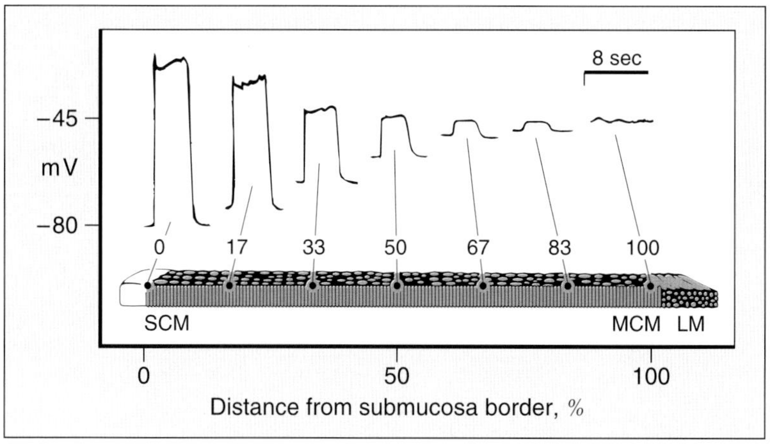

FIGURE 1-20.

Studies have been performed in canine colon muscle tissue to determine the source of colonic electrical control or slow-wave activity. These investigations reveal the spontaneous oscillatory electrical control activity to exhibit a maximal amplitude at the submucosal border of the circular muscle layer (SCM), with a continual decrease toward the myenteric border of the circular (MCM) and longitudinal (LM) muscle layers. Associated with this decrease in rhythmic electrical activity is a corresponding less negative resting membrane potential. Anatomic studies of the SCM reveal the presence of specialized cells, the interstitial cells of Cajal, which are believed to possess pacemaker capabilities for the colon. (*From* Smith *et al.* [14]; with permission.)

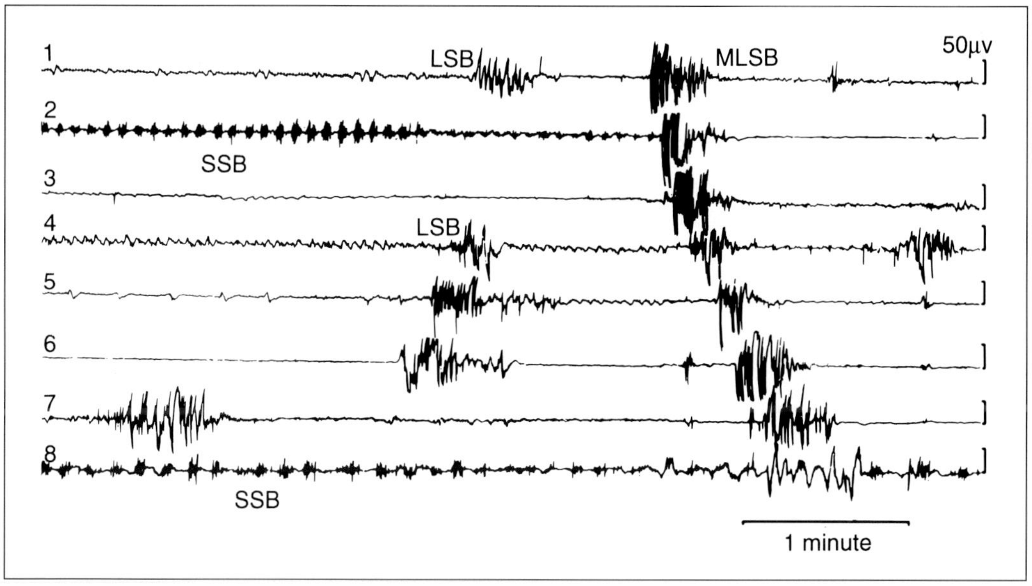

FIGURE 1-21.

Electrical activity from the human colon recorded extracellularly from eight sites is shown. Short spike bursts (SSBs) are shown in a single lead, which occur at the same frequency as the electrical control activity and represent the electrical response activity reacting to neurochemical excitation. SSBs are the electrical phenomena responsible for generation of short-duration contractions in the colon, which are generally stationary in character. Long spike bursts (LSBs) are shown in several leads and may be stationary (lead 1) or propagate in an orad or aboral direction over short distances (leads 4–6). LSBs are the electrical phenomena responsible for long-duration contractions in the colon and are not constrained by the electrical control activity of the colon. Migrating long spike bursts (MLSBs) are intense electrical complexes that propagate in an aboral direction over long distances (leads 1–8) and are the electrical phenomena responsible for the high-amplitude propagating contractions that produce mass movements of feces. (*From* Frexinos *et al.* [15]; with permission.)

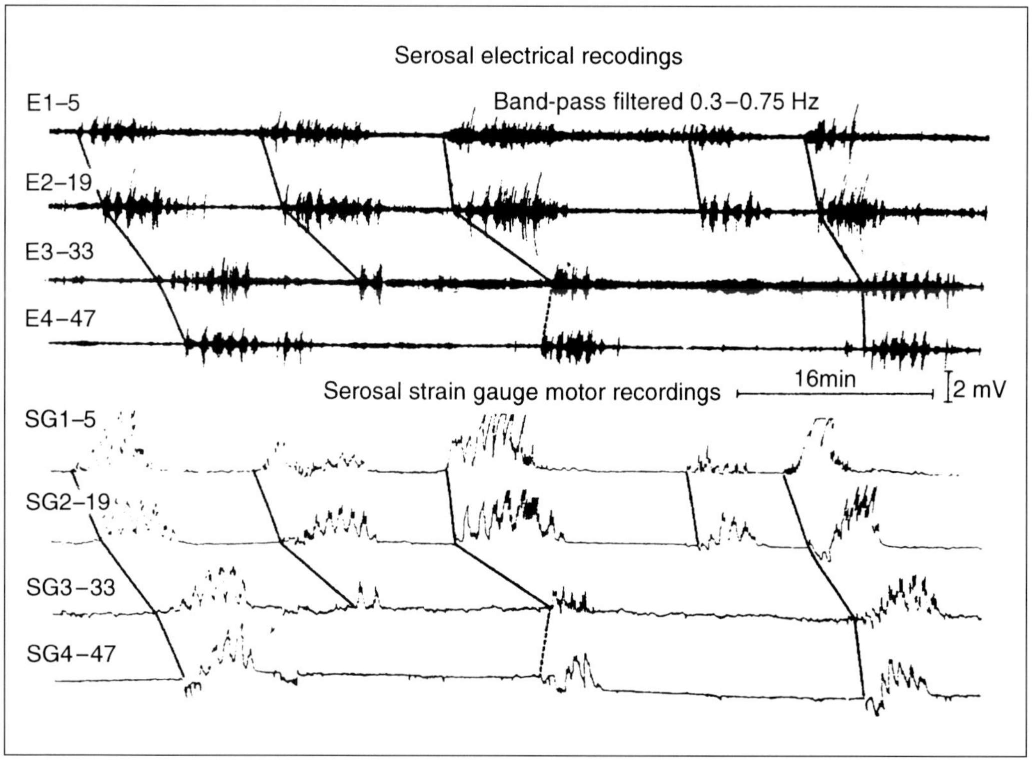

FIGURE 1-22.

Recordings from dogs demonstrate characteristic patterns of motor and myoelectric activity in addition to short- and long-duration contractions and high-amplitude propagated contractions and their electrical correlates. In electrical (E) recordings from several sites along the canine colon (upper tracings), migrating myoelectrical complexes propagate over several sites in aboral (*solid lines*) and orad (*dashed lines*) directions. These electrical complexes correlate with contractile patterns known as colonic migrating motor complexes, as measured by strain gauges (SGs) placed on the serosal layer of the canine colon (lower tracings). These E and SG recording phenomena are reproducibly demonstrated in dogs who have not undergone colonic preparation. They have not been reported in humans undergoing colonic manometry after colonic lavage. It is unknown if similar phenomena are present in the unprepared human colon. (*Adapted from* Sarna [16]; with permission.)

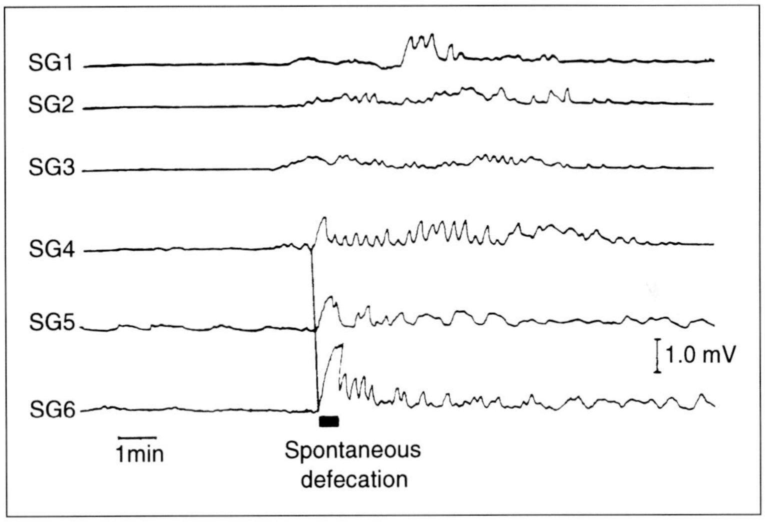

Figure 1-23.

The need to defecate is often preceded by the development of high-amplitude propagating contractions, suggesting an important role for this motor pattern in the expulsion of feces. This series of motor tracings from strain gauges (SGs) affixed to the serosa of canine colon demonstrate high-amplitude propagating contractions that develop in the proximal colon and migrate through to the distal leads and are associated with spontaneous defecation. (*Adapted from* Karaus and Sarna [17]; with permission.)

The relationship of pressure waves to fecal movements

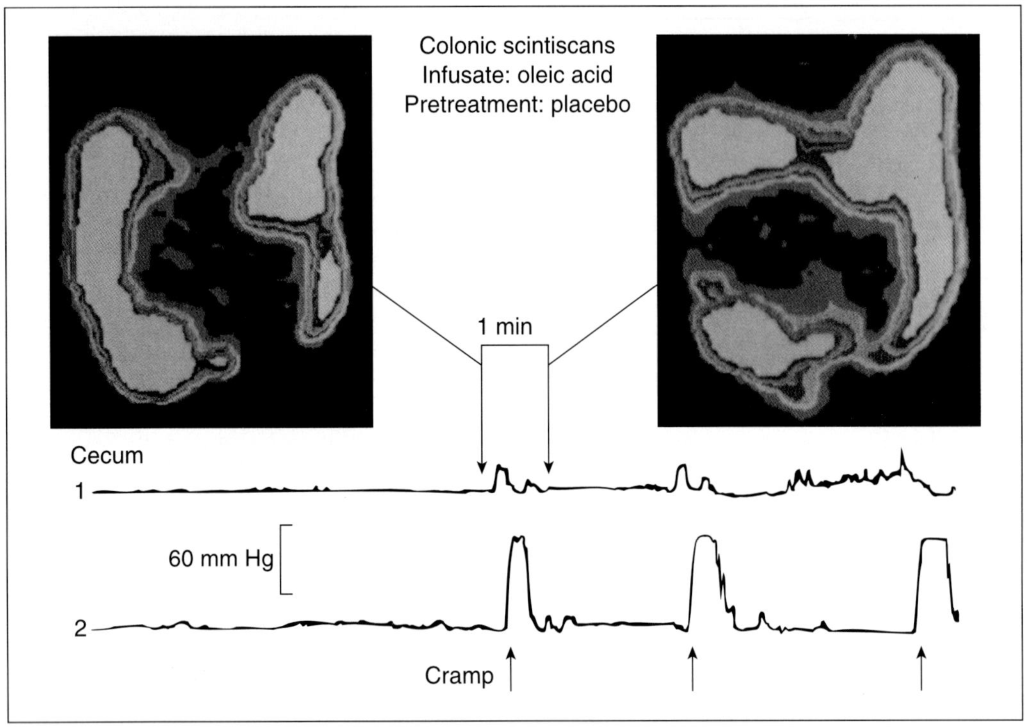

Figure 1-24.

The relationship between mass movements of colonic contents and motor activity in the colon is shown to illustrate the relationship of pressure waves to fecal movements. This figure shows movements of a radiolabelled scintigraphic tracer before and 1 minute after infusion of oleic acid into the cecum. Oleic acid infusion causes a significant shift of the tracer from the ascending colon to the splenic flexure and descending colon. The motor tracing below shows the corresponding motor response to oleic acid infusion, which demonstrates induction of multiple high-amplitude propagating contractions in temporal association with mass movements of the tracer. (*From* Kamath *et al.* [18]; with permission.)

Motility

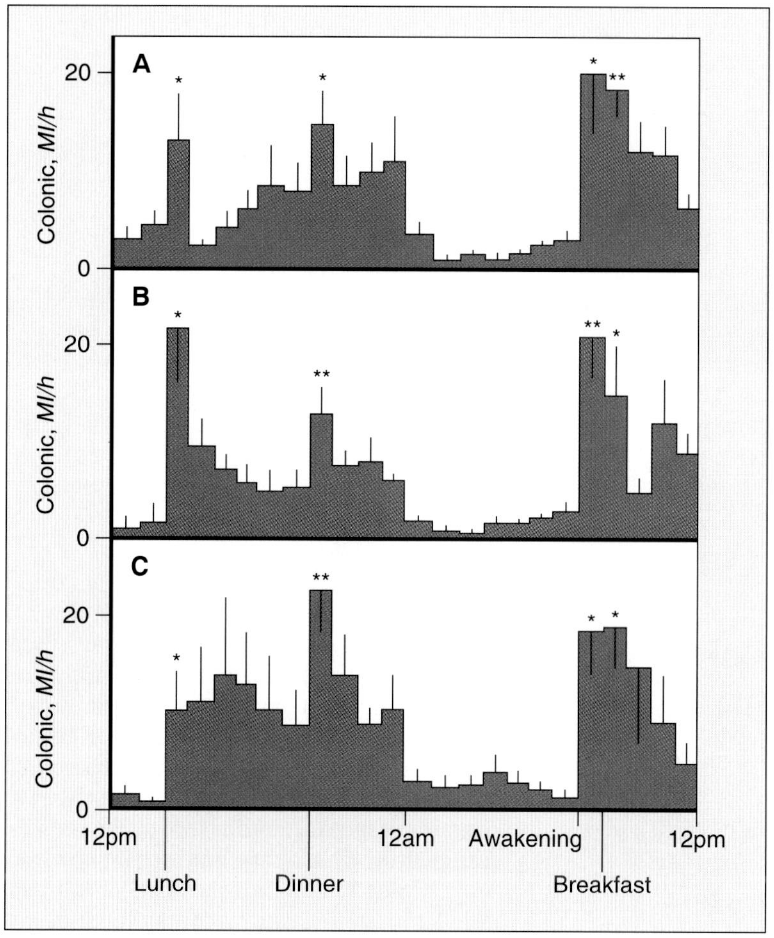

FIGURE 1-25.

The motility of the colon from the transverse, descending, and rectosigmoid colons over a 24-hour period from healthy individuals is shown. Data are expressed as a motility index (MI) calculated by measuring the area under pressure waves for each hour of recording. *Asterisks* indicate significant differences (*$P<0.05$, **$P<0.01$) compared with fasting and preawakening values. During sleep (12 AM to 6 AM), colonic motor activity is very low but increases soon after awakening. Further increases in colonic motor activity occur after meal ingestion (lunch at 2 PM, dinner at 8 PM), indicative of the gastrocolonic response. Motor activity shows similar diurnal and nocturnal changes in all three regions of the colon. (*From* Narducci *et al.* [12]; with permission.)

Motor response

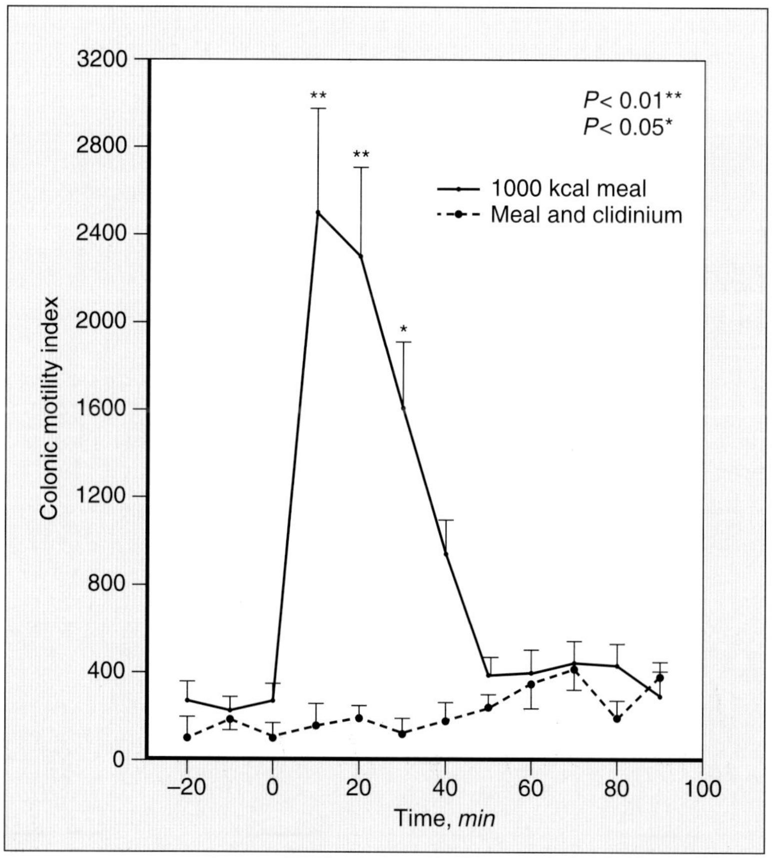

FIGURE 1-26.

The profile of the gastrocolonic motor response to meal ingestion from healthy humans is shown. Almost immediately after ingestion of a 1000 kcal meal, there is a marked increase in colonic motor activity (*solid line*) (expressed as a motility index calculated from the area under the colonic pressure waves) that persists for nearly 1 hour. When the subjects are pretreated with the anticholinergic agent clidinium (*dashed line*), there is abolition of the increase in motor activity, indicating that the gastrocolonic response to a meal is mediated by cholinergic neural pathways. (*Adapted from* Snape *et al.* [19]; with permission.)

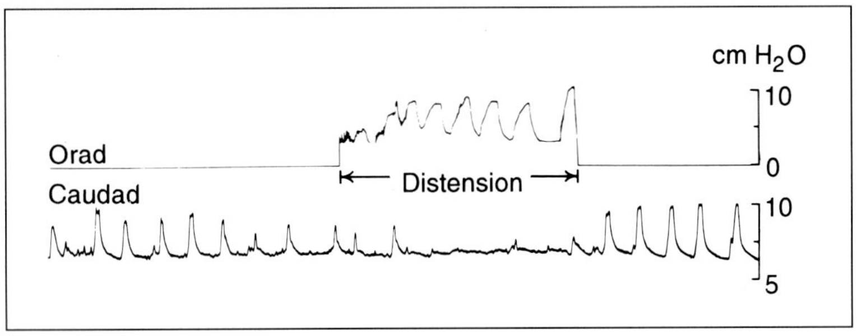

FIGURE 1-27.

The presence of a fecal bolus in the colon has been postulated to induce a physiologic motor response known as the *peristaltic reflex*, which serves to propel the bolus aborally. An experimental model of the peristaltic reflex is shown. Inflation of a colonic balloon induces an increase in phasic and tonic motor activity in the segment orad to the stimulus, known as the *ascending contraction*, and a reduction in phasic motor activity caudad to the distending stimulus, known as the *descending relaxation*. This activity results in an increase in pressure proximally and a decrease in pressure distally, providing the force necessary to propel the bolus in an antegrade direction. (*Adapted from* Kreulen and Szurszewski [20]; with permission.)

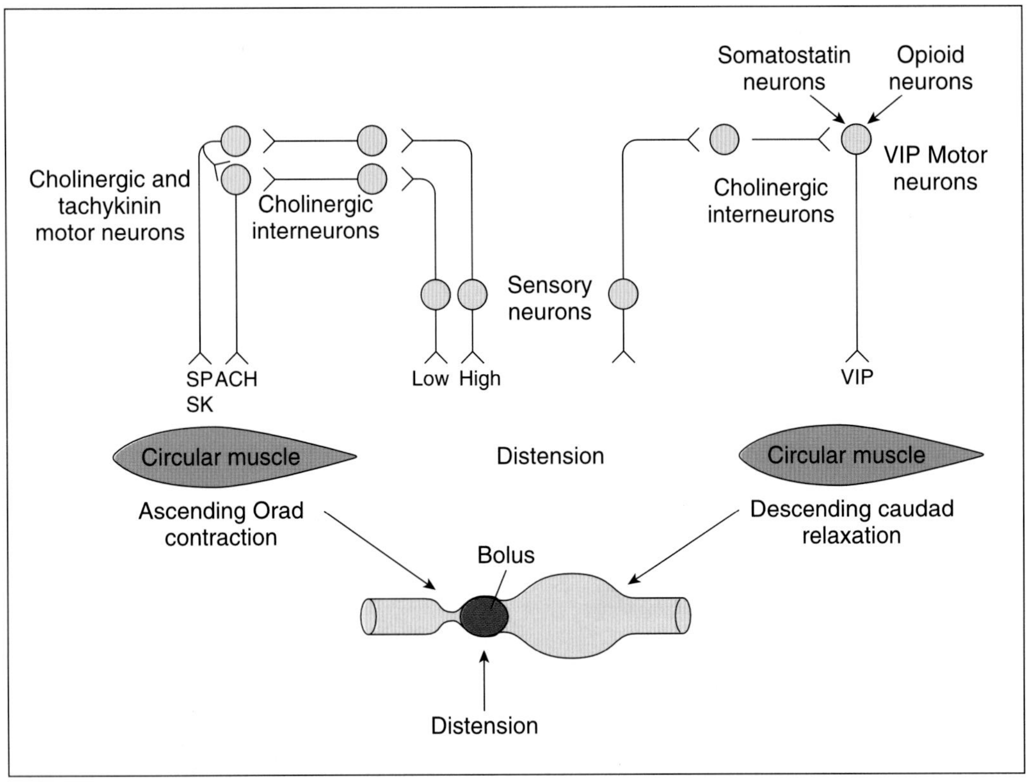

FIGURE 1-28.

Numerous animal studies have been performed to provide a model of the neural pathways involved in mediation of both limbs of the colonic peristaltic reflex. For the ascending contraction, balloon distention of a colonic segment activates sensory neural pathways. A low-threshold pathway activates cholinergic interneurons that subsequently stimulate acetylcholine (ACH)-containing motor neurons that evoke muscle contraction. A high-threshold sensory pathway also activates interneurons which then stimulate tachykinin motor neurons containing substance P (SP) and substance K (SK), neurotransmitters that also cause contraction of the circular muscle. For the descending relaxation, colonic balloon distention activates sensory neurons that stimulate cholinergic interneurons. These interneuronal pathways then activate vasoactive intestinal polypeptide (VIP)-containing neurons that induce circular muscle relaxation caudad to the distending stimulus. Activities of the VIP neurons are modulated by input from somatostatin and opioid neurons. (*From* Grider and Makhlouf [21]; with permission.)

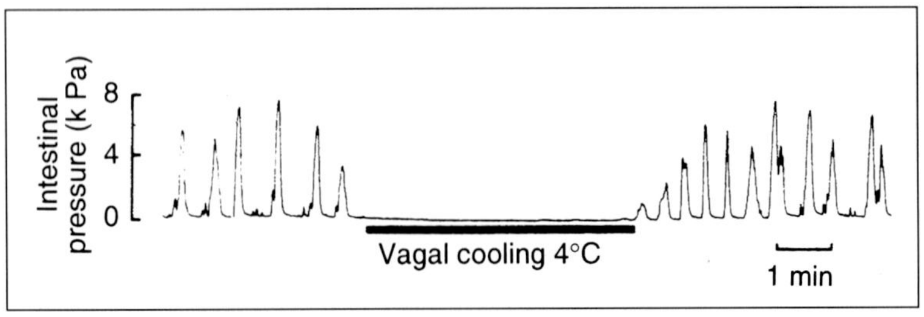

FIGURE 1-29.

The motor activity of the colon is modulated by activity from neural pathways extrinsic to the colonic wall. The effects of vagal function on colonic motor activity are shown in a ferret model. Cooling the vagus nerves to below 4 °C, which induces a temporary vagotomy, abolishes spontaneous phasic motor activity in the proximal colon, indicating that there is vagal nerve input to the colon. (*Adapted from* Collman *et al.* [22]; with permission.)

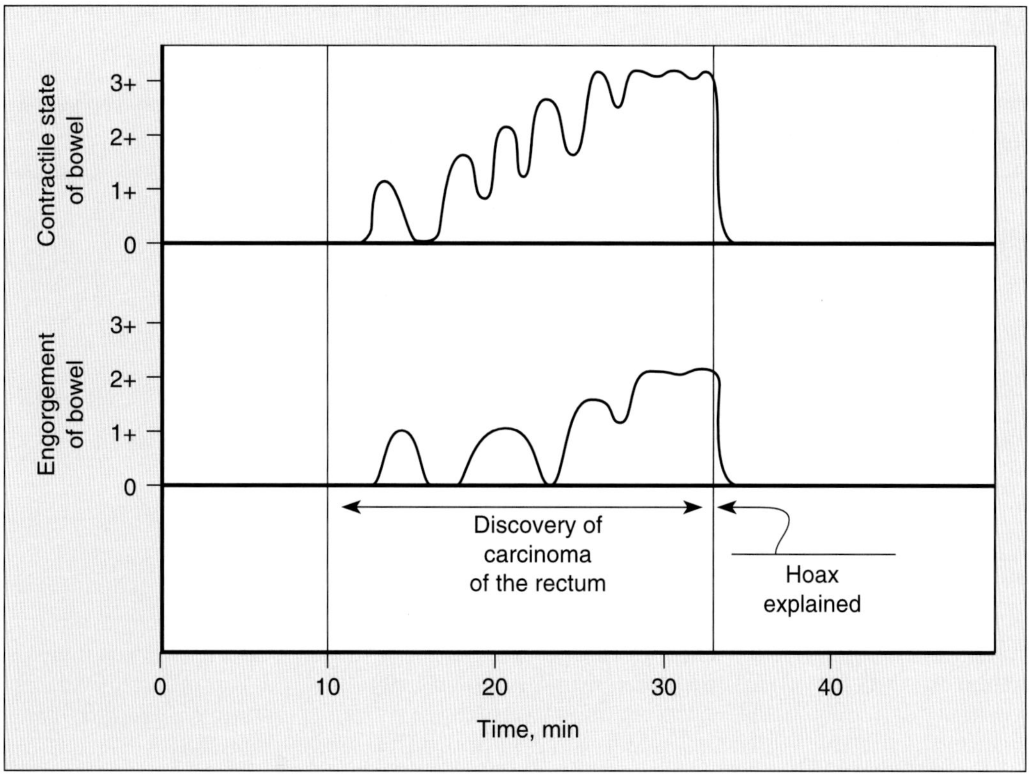

FIGURE 1-30.

In addition to modulation by extrinsic nerves, colonic motor function can be significantly altered by input from the central nervous system. This figure shows the motor and vascular responses to verbal suggestion in a medical student undergoing proctoscopic examination. During the examination, the examiner informs the student that he has discovered a malignancy in his rectum. During this hoax, the motor activity and redness of the rectum increase markedly. After the examiner reveals the true nature of the hoax, these parameters return quickly to normal. Thus stress can increase motor and vascular responses of the colon. (*From* Almy [23]; with permission.)

SMALL INTESTINAL AND COLONIC FLUID BALANCE

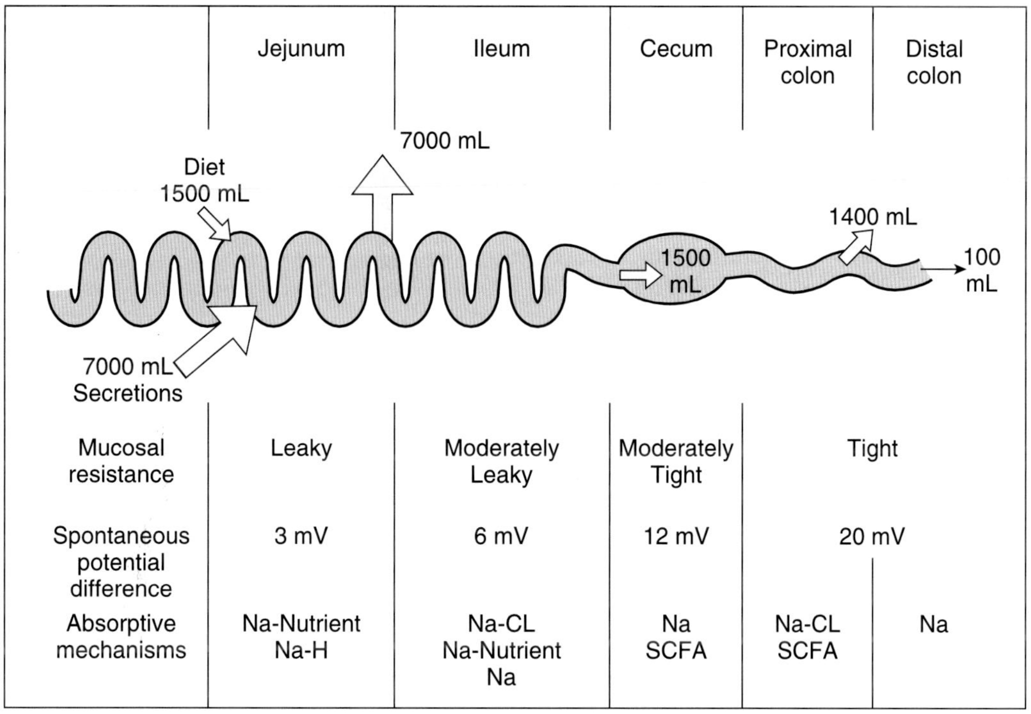

FIGURE 1-31.

A summary of small intestinal and colonic fluid balance is shown. Approximately 8500 mL of fluid are added to the gastrointestinal tract daily, 1500 mL coming from the diet and 7000 mL coming from endogenous secretions from the stomach, small intestine, pancreas, and biliary tree. Of this amount, roughly 7000 mL is absorbed in the small intestine, leaving 1500 mL of fluid for the cecum to handle. In the cecum, proximal colon, and distal colon, a further 1400 mL is absorbed, leaving approximately 100 mL of fluid to be expelled with the solid fecal material in the stool. In contrast to the relatively leaky mucosal resistance of the jejunum and ileum, resistance in the colon becomes much tighter, thus preventing back diffusion of electrolytes and water. Associated with this prevention is an increase in the spontaneous membrane potential difference, which further restricts ionic movement into the lumen. The absorptive processes are different in the distinct regions of the gastrointestinal tract, with absorption of sodium, chloride, and short chain fatty acids (SCFA) predominantly in the colon. (*Adapted from* Sellin [24]; with permission.)

ELECTROLYTE TRANSPORT MECHANISMS

TABLE 1-1. MAJOR ELECTROLYTE TRANSPORT MECHANISMS

	Pumps	Carriers	Channels
Electrogenic Na^+ absorption	Na^+, K^+-ATPase		Na^+
Electroneural Na^+ absorption	Na^+, K^+-ATPase	Na^+/H^+ Exchange Cl^-/HCO_3^- Exchange	
K^+ Secretion	Na^+, K^+-ATPase	Na^+, K^+, Cl^- Cotransport	K^+
Cl^- Secretion	Na^+, K^+-ATPase	Na^+, K^+, Cl^- Cotransport	Cl^-
HCO_3^- Secretion	Na^+, K^+-ATPase	Cl^-/HCO_3^- Exchange	

TABLE 1-1.

The major electrolyte transport mechanisms and the transcellular pathways involved are shown in this table. Sodium is absorbed, against an electrochemical gradient, in both electrogenic and electroneutral fashions. Net water transport is directly dependent on net sodium transport. Thus these pathways are responsible for the majority of fecal dehydration that occurs in the colon. Electrogenic sodium transport involves a Na^+, K^+-ATPase, whereas electroneutral sodium transport involves Na^+/H^+ and Cl-/HCO_3 exchange. Chloride secretion is handled by Na^+, K^+, Cl^- cotransport, whereas HCO_3 secretion is handled by Cl-/HCO_3 exchange. (*Adapted from* Barrett and Dharmsathaphorn [25]; with permission.)

ABSORPTION AND SECRETION

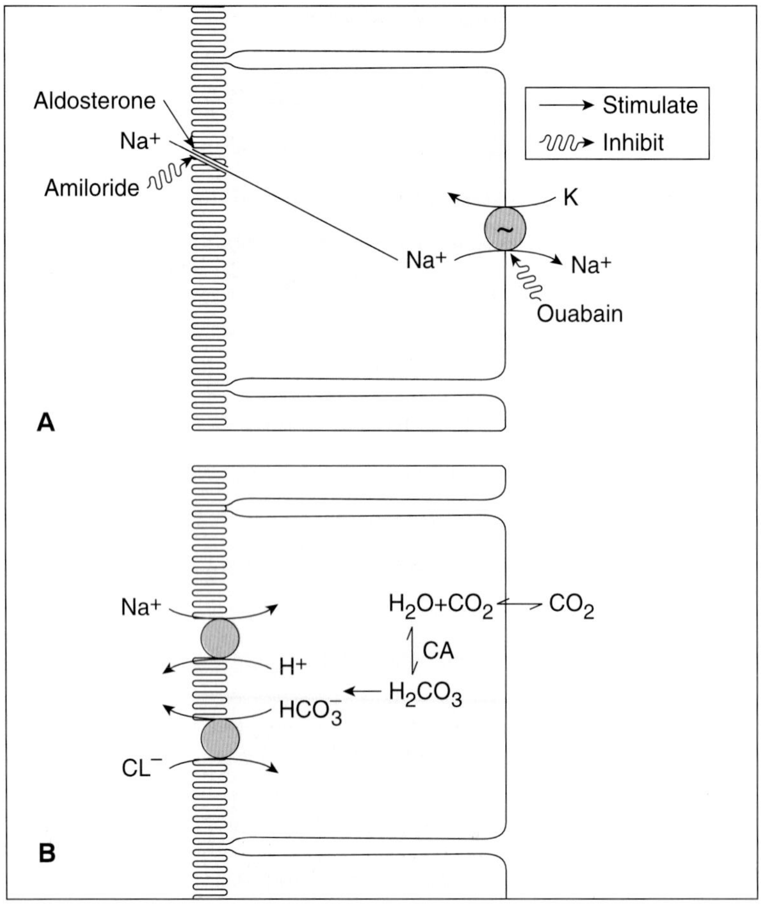

FIGURE 1-32.

The two proposed pathways of active sodium transport in the colon, which also regulate the bulk of water absorption, are shown. In the top diagram (**A**), electrogenic sodium transport is accomplished via action of a ouabain-sensitive Na^+, K^+-ATPase on the basolateral membrane. This allows the absorption of sodium ions through an aldosterone-stimulatable and an amiloride-inhibitable Na^+ channel on the mucosal surface. In the bottom diagram (**B**), electroneutral sodium transport is accomplished via the action of two ion exchangers, the Na^+/H^+ and Cl^-/HCO_3^- carriers, on the mucosal side. This pathway also provides absorption of Cl^- ions from the colonic lumen. The relative importance of these two sodium pathways in the human colon is uncertain, although amiloride-sensitive Na^+ channels have been described in the human distal colon. (*From* Binder and Sandle [26]; with permission.)

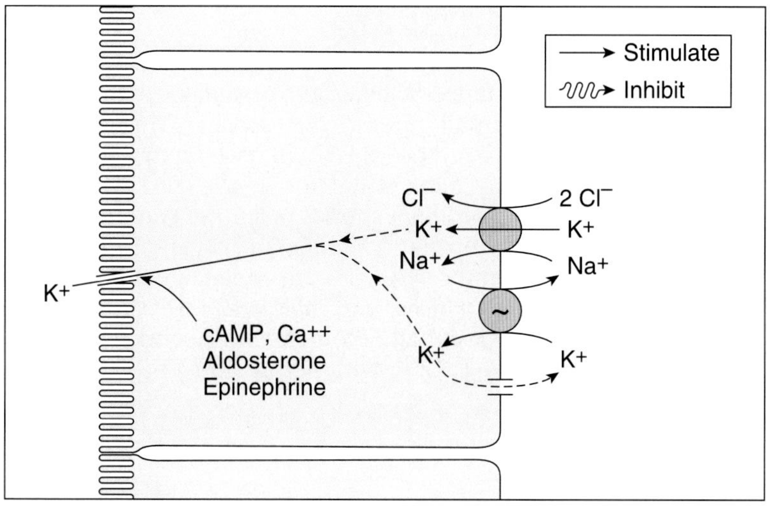

FIGURE 1-33.

The colon exhibits a net secretion of potassium when perfused with an electrolyte solution, which explains the relatively high levels of potassium in normal feces. The pathways of K^+ secretion are shown. Potassium enters the colonic epithelial cell from the basolateral surface via a Na^+, K^+-ATPase and via a Na^+, K^+, Cl^- exchanger. Potassium is then transported out into the colonic lumen via a specific K^+ channel that is sensitive to the stimulatory effects of cyclic AMP (cAMP), calcium (Ca^{++}), aldosterone, and epinephrine. (*From* Binder and Sandle [26]; with permission.)

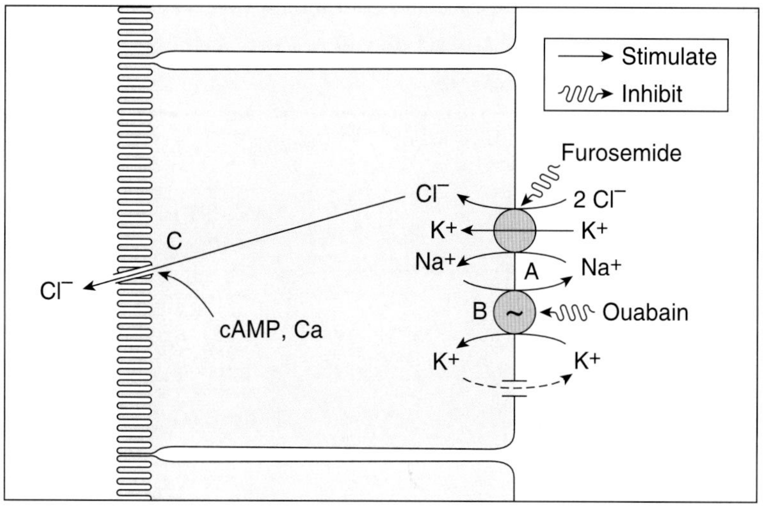

FIGURE 1-34.

The experimental models of sodium absorption and potassium secretion predict a net absorption of chloride as well. An active secretory pathway for the disposition of chloride is shown. With this transport pathway, chloride is transported into the cell via the concerted actions of the Na^+, K^+, Cl^- exchanger (**A**) and the Na^+, K^+-ATPase (**B**). Active chloride secretion is stimulated by cyclic AMP (cAMP) or increases in intracellular calcium, which then serve to normalize intracellular Cl^- (**C**). (*From* Binder and Sandle [26]; with permission.)

COLONIC FLORA

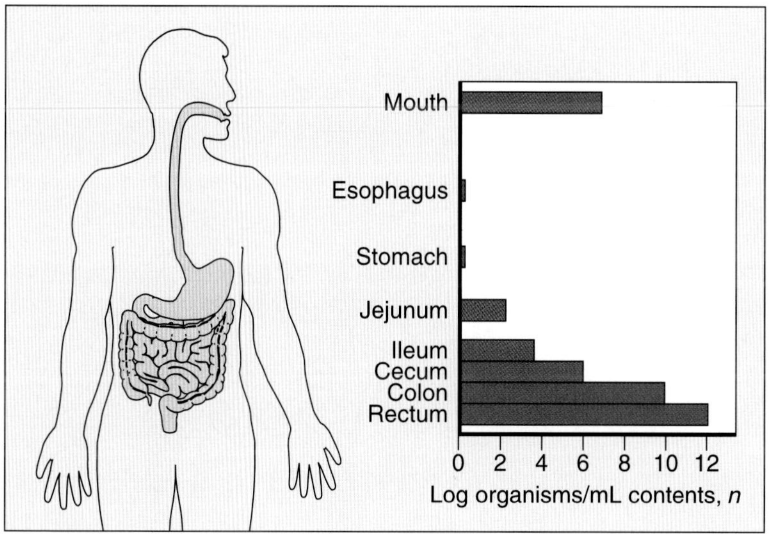

FIGURE 1-35.

The colonic lumen possesses a luxuriant flora that assists in fermentation of the fecal material, suppresses overgrowth of pathogens, affects hydration status and weight of the individual, alters stool pH for certain chemical reactions, and degrades intestinal mucins. The mouth contains a large number of flora, but the esophagus, stomach, jejunum, and ileum normally contain trivial numbers of colonies. In the colon there is a gradient in numbers of organisms ranging from 10^6/mL in the cecum to 10^{12}/mL in the rectum. (*From* Laissue and Gebbers [27]; with permission.)

TABLE 1-2. THE FECAL FLORA ORGANISMS FOUND IN HEALTHY HUMANS

Genus	Flora, %: Moore and Holdeman [27]	Flora, %: Finegold et al. [28]
Bacteroides	30	56
Eubacterium	26	14
Bifidobacterium	11	4
Peptostreptococcus	9	4
Fusobacterium	8	0.1
Ruminococcus	4	9
Clostridium	2	2
Lactobacillus	2	1
Unclassifiable	2	–
Streptococcus	2	6
Facultative gram-negatives	0.5	0.1
Propionibacterium and *Actinomyces*	0.3	0.6
Staphylococcus	0.1	0.01
Coprococcus	0.1	0.1
Acidaminococcus	–	0.2

**Organisms found to make up 0.1% or more of the flora*

Table 1-2.

The colonic flora consists of a predominance of anaerobic organisms with far smaller numbers of aerobes. This table lists those species of bacteria that make up most of the flora in the colon. The predominant species in studies conducted by Moore and Holdeman [27] and by Finegold and coworkers [28] are anaerobes such as *bacteriodes* and *eubacterium*. (*Data from* Moore and Holdeman [28] and Finegold *et al.* [29]; with permission.)

ANATOMY OF THE RECTUM AND ANUS

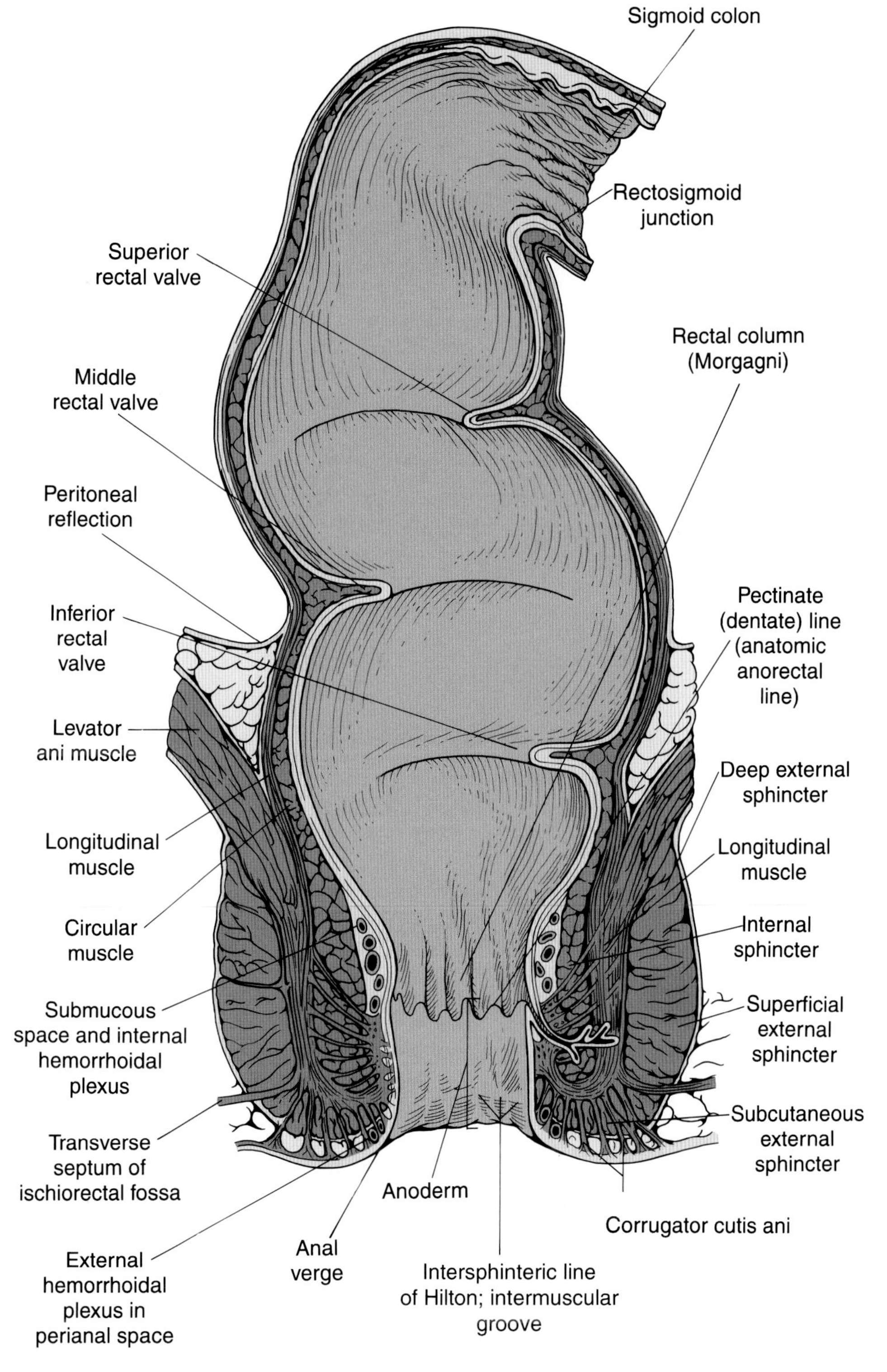

FIGURE 1-36.

The anatomy of the rectum and anus is shown. The most distal 7 to 8 cm of rectum is infraperitoneal and is thereby fixed by surrounding supporting tissues. More orad regions of the rectum and sigmoid colons are intraperitoneal and more mobile. The rectal mucosa is smoother and less corrugated than the more proximal colon, and the rectum is capacious owing to its physiologic function as a storage receptacle for feces before defecation. The rectal mucosa forms three eccentric rectal valves, also known as the *valves of Houston*. The most distal rectum is marked by the rectal columns of Morgagni, which terminate at the pectinate or dentate line delineating the junction of the rectal and anal mucosae. The transition from columnar to squamous mucosa occurs gradually in the distal rectum, usually above the pectinate line. The hemorrhoidal plexuses reside under the mucosa of both the rectum and anus and are believed to serve a cushioning role. The anal musculature is specialized with the circular muscle layer forming a prominent internal anal sphincter. The longitudinal muscle of the rectum projects to the region of the internal anal sphincter but is not as prominent. The external anal sphincter, a skeletal muscle structure, is composed of three muscle groups, the deep external sphincter, the superficial external sphincter, and the subcutaneous external sphincter. The internal sphincter is responsible for much of the resting anal tone. The external sphincter responds to voluntary squeeze commands to maintain continence when feces have moved into the rectum. Finally, the levator ani muscles, three skeletal muscles (puborectalis, pubococcygeus, and iliococcygeus), form the sling musculature surrounding the distal rectum that maintain continence when contracted. When the puborectalis component of the levator ani apparatus relaxes, defecation is permitted.

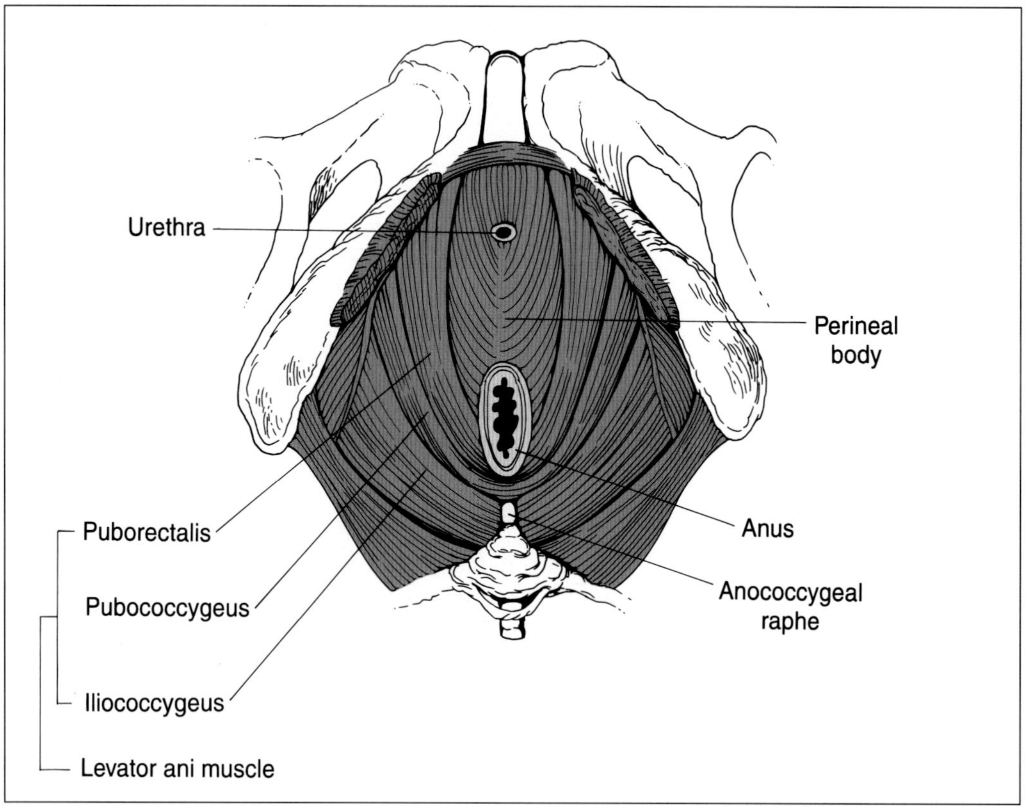

FIGURE 1-37.

The muscular arrangement of the levator ani muscles is shown in relation to the anorectum and pelvis. Some of the levator ani muscles merge with fibers of the external anal sphincter. Each of the levator muscles has a bony attachment on the anterior of the pelvis. Only the iliococcygeus is fixed posteriorly to the coccyx via the anococcygeal raphe. The puborectalis is tonically contracted under resting conditions, pinching closed the distal rectum and aiding the anal sphincter in maintenance of continence. With defecation, the puborectalis component of the levator ani muscles relaxes and permits expulsion of the fecal bolus. (*Adapted from* Mulholland [2]; with permission.)

Histology of rectal and anal mucosae

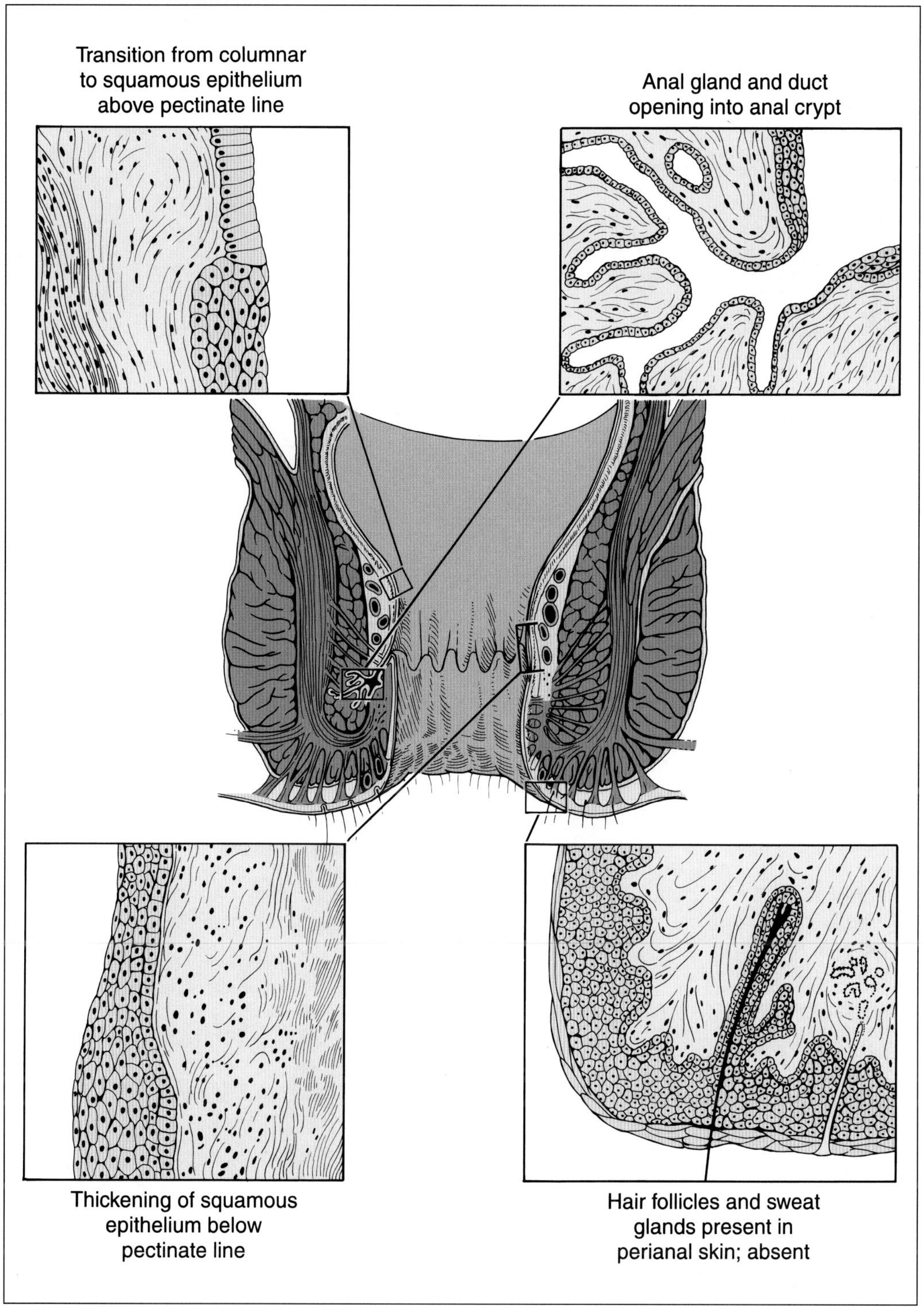

FIGURE 1-38.

The histology of the rectal and anal mucosae is shown. There is a transitional region above the pectinate line from the columnar epithelium present throughout most of the colon to the squamous epithelium of the anus. Above the pectinate line, the squamous epithelium is relatively thin, but in the anal canal, the epithelium thickens. At the pectinate line, tubular anal glands drain into ducts that feed the anal crypts. No hair or sweat glands are present in the anal canal itself, but the perianal skin is richly served with these structures.

ARTERIAL BLOOD SUPPLY FOR THE ANUS

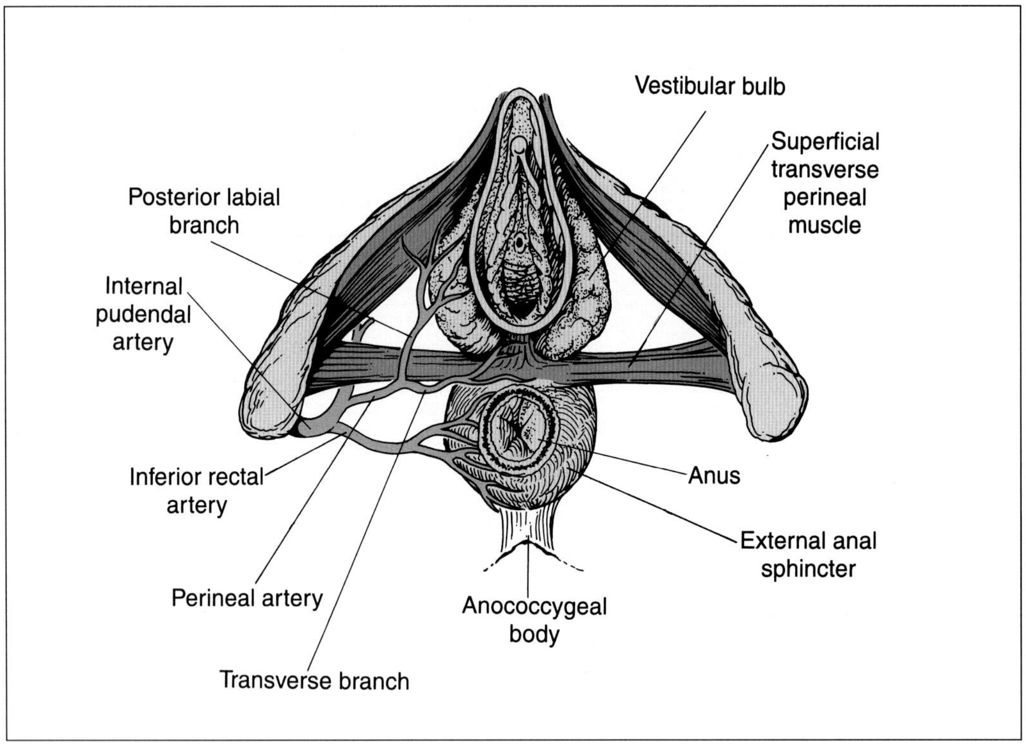

FIGURE 1-39.

The arterial blood supply specific for the anus is shown. The external anal sphincter receives blood from several branches of the inferior rectal artery, which is itself a branch of the internal pudendal artery. (*From* Melloni *et al.* [7]; with permission.)

FECAL CONTINENCE

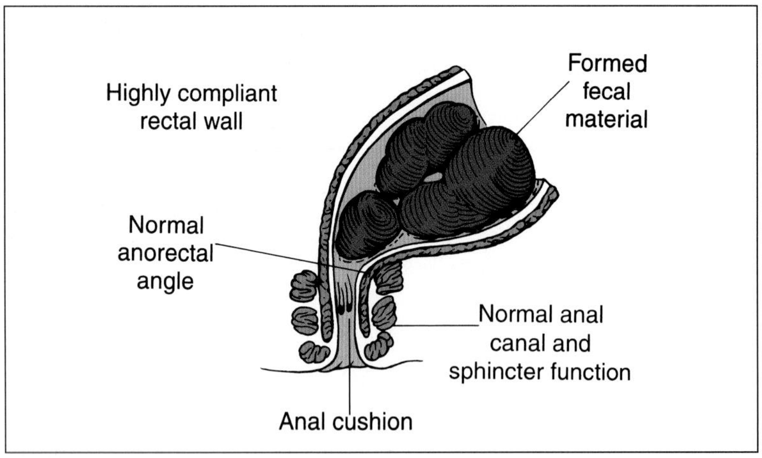

FIGURE 1-40.

The factors necessary for maintenance of fecal continence are shown. During its passage through the colon, fecal material becomes dehydrated and formed such that the stool that reaches the rectum is semisolid to solid. The rectum itself exhibits a highly compliant wall that allows it to serve as a reservoir for the fecal material until it can be conveniently expelled. The internal anal sphincter provides sufficient tone to prevent accidental loss of fecal material, whereas the external sphincter muscles voluntarily contract if unwanted loss of feces is impending. The anal cushions, made up of mucosa, hemorrhoidal plexuses, and the subepithelial-supporting tissue provide a seal that does not permit passage of liquid material under resting conditions. Finally, the anorectal angle created by the puborectalis muscle provides a functional obstruction to accidental loss of stool at rest. (*Adapted from* Irving and Catchpole [30]; with permission.)

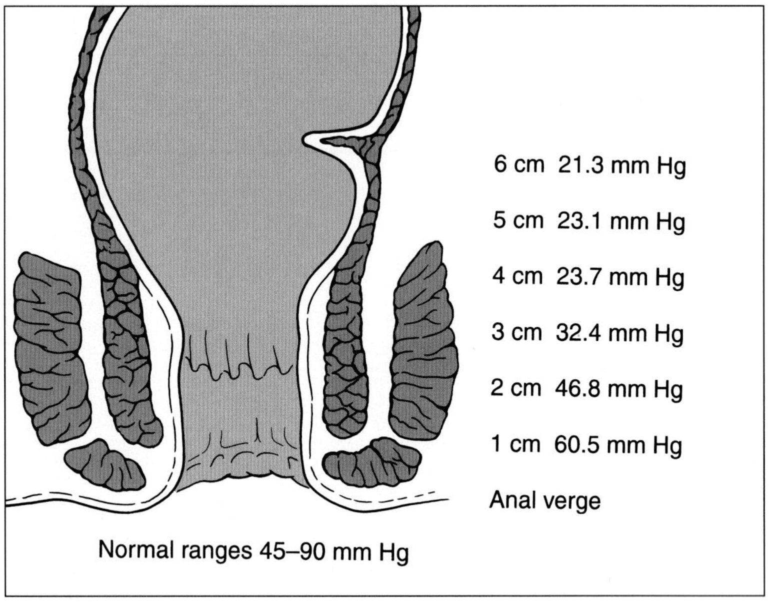

FIGURE 1-41.

The pressure profile of the anal canal is shown. The mean length of the anatomic anal canal is 3.7 cm, being slightly shorter in women than in men. However, there is a functional region of elevated pressure that extends above this level, which helps to maintain fecal continence. The maximal anal pressure occurs in the first 1 to 2 cm of the anus, but pressures elevated above intrarectal levels are measured for 6 cm from the most external aspect of the anus. (*Adapted from* Irving and Catchpole [30]; with permission.)

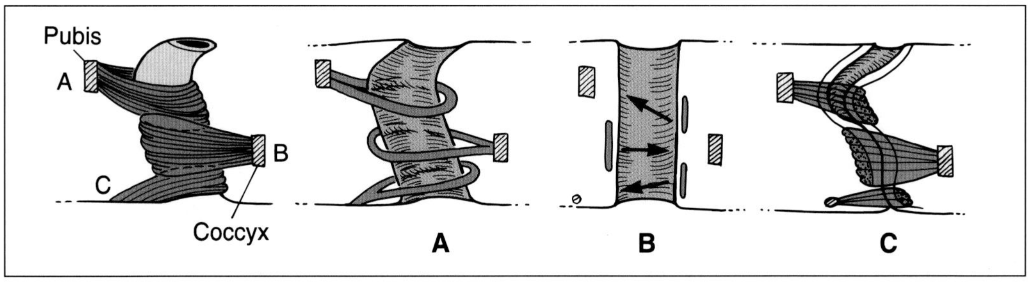

FIGURE 1-42.

The external anal sphincter assists in the maintenance of fecal continence by way of the triple loop mechanism shown in this figure. On the left, the three loops are formed by the three distinct muscles of the external anal sphincter. The uppermost loop, formed from the deep external sphincter muscle, attaches anteriorly on the pubis. The intermediate loop, formed from the superficial external sphincter, attaches posteriorly to the coccyx. The base loop, formed from the subcutaneous external sphincter, attaches to the perianal skin. On the right, a diagrammatic representation of the mechanism of anal occlusion by the triple loop system of the external anal sphincter is shown. **A**, The external sphincter at rest. With external sphincter contraction (**B**), the direction of contraction of each of the loops is shown (anterior to the left, posterior to the right). Tight contraction of these three loops results in tight anal occlusion as shown in **C**. (*Adapted from* Shafik [31] and Shafik [32]; with permission.)

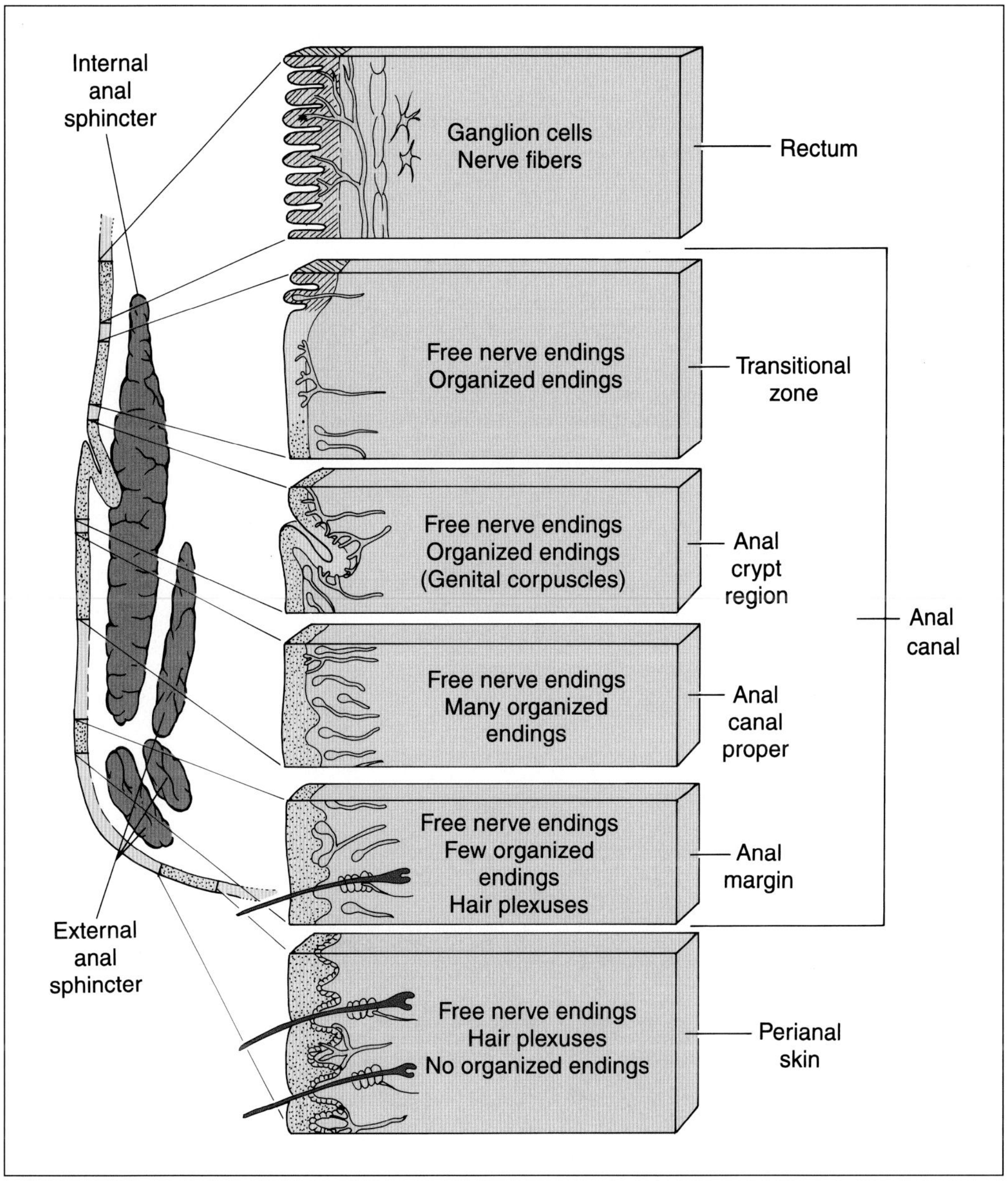

FIGURE 1-43.

The epithelial nerve endings of the rectum and anus provide a specialized system for the differentiation of solid, liquid, and gaseous material to be expelled from the rectum. The rectum is innervated with ganglion cells and nerve fibers that mediate the reflex activities of the rectoanal region, including the reflex relaxation of the internal anal sphincter upon rectal distension. The rectum has few free or organized nerve endings and is insensitive to most mucosal stimuli. The transitional zone above the pectinate line, the anal crypt region, and the anal canal itself possess numerous free nerve endings as well as organized nerve endings, which serve to sense anal contents before their controlled passage. These nerve endings allow the individual to discriminate between solid, liquid, and gaseous material so that a conscious decision may be made for its evacuation from the rectum. In the perianal cutaneous region, there is a loss of the organized nerve endings that are so prominent in the anal canal. In this region, numerous hair plexuses are present. (*Adapted from* Duthie and Gairns [33]; with permission.)

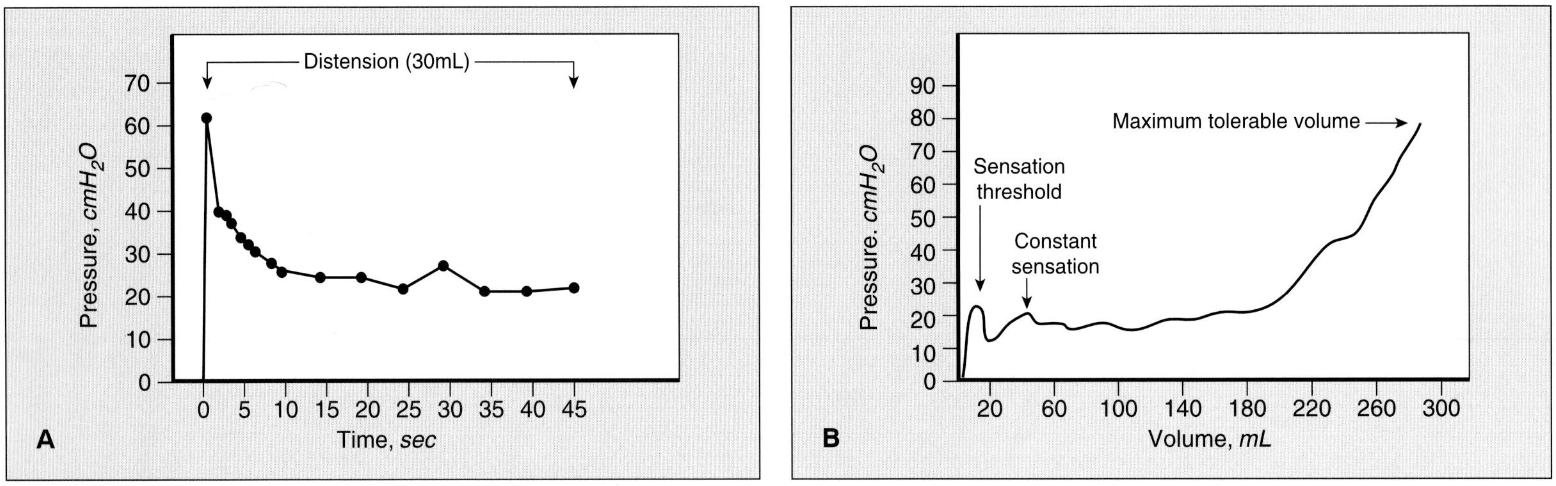

FIGURE 1-44.

Fecal continence is aided by the presence of a highly compliant rectum that allows the rectum to accommodate large amounts of formed stool before its evacuation. **A**, Abrupt inflation of an intrarectal balloon produces a sudden increase in rectal pressure that abates as the rectum accommodates to the presence of a distending stimulus. **B**, The elastic properties of the rectum are shown. As an intrarectal balloon is gradually inflated, there is a minimal increase in intrarectal pressure until large volumes (> 200 mL) are infused. This process demonstrates the highly compliant nature of the rectal vault. (*From* Schiller [34]; with permission.)

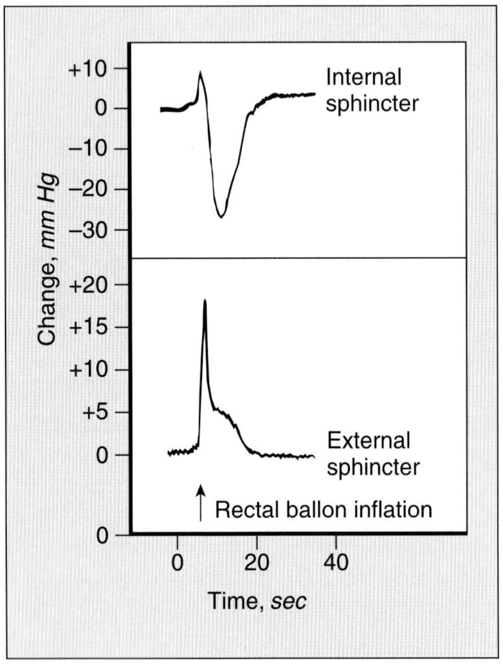

FIGURE 1-45.

The reflex responsiveness of the anal region to a distending stimulus in the rectum is shown. Rectal balloon inflation results in an abrupt decrease in pressure in the internal anal sphincter, known as the *rectoanal inhibitory reflex* (*top*). In contrast, there is a normal increase in pressure in the external anal sphincter upon rectal distention (*bottom*). These physiologic responses are important for two reasons. The presence of a rectoanal inhibitory reflex allows the anus to relax upon filling of the rectal vault to permit efficient defecation. The reflex contraction of the external sphincter prevents accidental leakage of rectal contents until they may be evacuated in a socially convenient setting. (*Adapted from* Alva *et al.* [35]; with permission.)

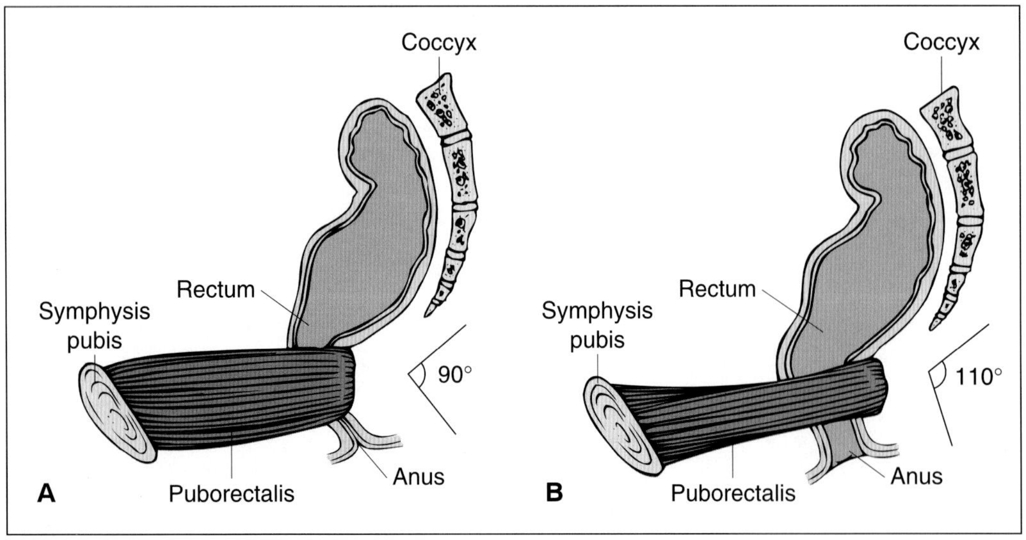

FIGURE 1-46.

Defecation involves the coordinated interaction of several different muscular structures in and surrounding the rectum and anus. For maintenance of fecal continence, an anorectal angle of approximately 90° is maintained by the tonic contraction of the puborectalis muscle of the levator ani apparatus (**A**). With defecation, there is relaxation of the puborectalis with development of a more obtuse rectoanal angle (110°), associated with relaxation of the internal anal sphincter (**B**). This relaxation allows the effortless evacuation of the contents of the rectal vault. (*Adapted from* Schiller [34] and Goei [36]; with permission.)

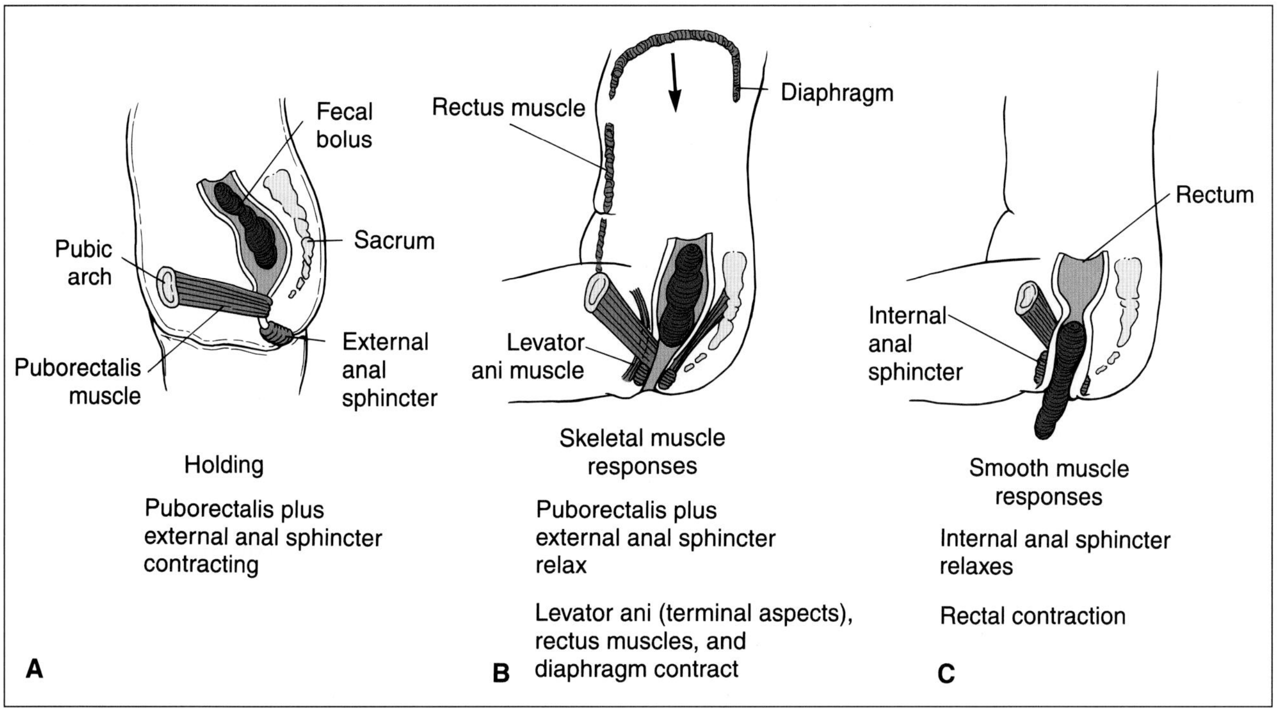

FIGURE 1-47.

A summary of the muscular actions required for defecation is shown. **A**, Passage of the fecal bolus into the rectum evokes contraction of the puborectalis component of the levator ani muscles and the external anal sphincter until defecation may voluntarily proceed in a more desirable environment. **B**, The skeletal muscle responses involved in voluntary defecation are shown. There is voluntary relaxation of the puborectalis and external anal sphincter which straightens the recto-anal angle to afford unimpeded passage of the fecal bolus. The relaxation is associated with contraction of the rectus abdominis muscles, diaphragm, and terminal aspects of the other levator ani muscles that increase intra-abdominal pressure to provide additional force for effective defecation. **C**, The smooth muscle responses are shown. Contraction of the rectal smooth muscle increases intrarectal pressure to provide a propulsive force for defecation. Concomitant relaxation of the internal anal sphincter permits easy passage of the stool. (*Adapted from* Schiller [34]; with permission.)

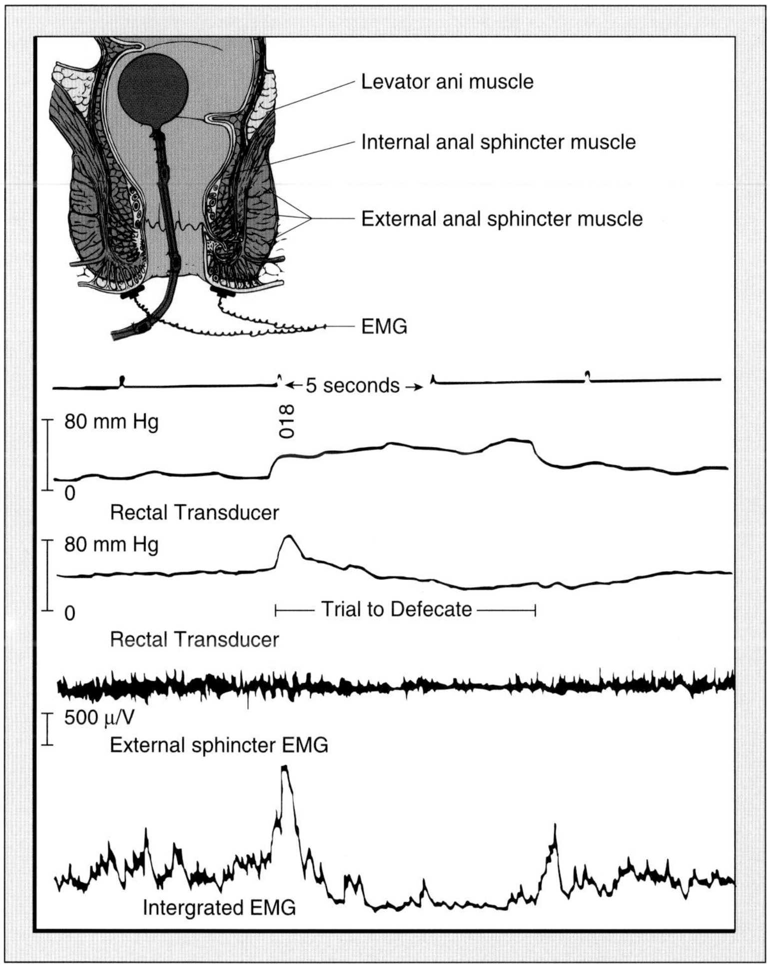

FIGURE 1-48.

The manometric and electromyographic responses to defecation are shown. Upon attempted defecation, there is an increase in pressure as measured by an intrarectal pressure transducer. In contrast, after a brief increase there is a prolonged decrease in anal pressure as determined by a transducer in the anal canal. Electromyographic (EMG) activities measured by cutaneous electrodes at the external anal sphincter in an integrated fashion show a decrease in firing coincident with the attempted defecation maneuver. (*Adapted from* Wald [37]; with permission.)

REFERENCES AND RECOMMENDED READING

1. Carlson BM: *Human Embryology and Developmental Biology*. St. Louis: Mosby; 1994:307–339.
2. Mulholland MW: Colon: Anatomy and structural anomalies. In *Textbook of Gastroenterology*. Edited by Yamada T. Philadelphia: JB Lippincott; 1991:1582–1587.
3. Christensen J: Motility of the intestine. In *Gastrointestinal Disease: Pathophysiology, Diagnosis, Management*, edn 5. Edited by Sleisenger MH, Fordtran JS. Philadelphia: WB Saunders; 1994:822–837.
4. Staubesand J: *Sobotta Atlas of Human Anatomy*, vol 2. Baltimore-Munich: Urban and Schwarzenberg; 1990:86–245.
5. Williamson RC: Intestinal adaptation: Structural, functional, and cytokinetic changes. *N Engl J Med* 1978, 298:1393–1401.
6. Trier JS, Winter HS: Anatomy, embryology, and developmental abnormalities of the small intestine and colon. In *Gastrointestinal Disease: Pathophysiology, Diagnosis, Management*, edn 5. Philadelphia: WB Saunders; 1994:793–822.
7. Melloni JL, Fox I, Melloni HP, Melloni BJ: *Melloni's Illustrated Review of Human Anatomy*. Philadelphia: JB Lippincott; 1988:1–51.
8. Christensen J: Gastrointestinal motility. In *Best and Taylor's Physiologic Basis for Medical Practice*. Edited by West JB. Baltimore: Williams and Wilkins; 1991:614–644.
9. Krevsky B, Melmud LS, D'Ercole F, *et al.*: Colonic transit scintigraphy: A physiologic approach to the quantitative measurement of colonic transit in humans. *Gastroenterology* 1986, 91:1102–1112.
10. Metcalf AM, Phillips SF, Zinsmeister AF, *et al.*: Simplified assessment of segmental colonic transit. *Gastroenterology* 1987, 92:40–47.
11. Sarna SK: Physiology and pathophysiology of colonic motor activity [Part 1]. *Dig Dis Sci* 1991, 36:827–862.
12. Narducci F, Bassotti G, Gaburri M, *et al.*: Twenty four hour manometric recording of colonic motor activity in healthy man. *Gut* 1987, 28:17–25.
13. Sarna SK: In vivo myoelectric activity: Methods, analysis, and interpretation. In *Handbook of Physiology: A Critical, Comprehensive Presentation of Physiological Knowledge and Concepts*. Edited by Wood JD. Bethesda: American Physiological Society; 1989:817–863.
14. Smith TK, Reed JB, Sanders KM: Origin and propagation of electrical slow waves in circular muscle of canine proximal colon. *Am J Physiol* 1987, 252:C215–C224.
15. Frexinos J, Bueno L, Fioramonti J: Diurnal changes in myoelectrical spiking activity of the human colon. *Gastroenterology* 1985, 88:1104–1110.
16. Sarna SK: Myoelectric correlates of colonic motor complexes and contractile activity. *Am J Physiol* 1986, 250:G213–G222.
17. Karaus M, Sarna SK: Giant migrating contractions during defecation in the dog colon. *Gastroenterology* 1987, 92:925–933.
18. Kamath PS, Phillips SF, O'Connor MK, *et al.*: Colonic capacitance and transit in man: Modulation by luminal contents and drugs. *Gut* 1990, 31:443–449.
19. Snape WJ, Wright SH, Battle WM, *et al.*: The gastrocolonic response: Evidence for a neural mechanism. *Gastroenterology* 1979, 77:1235–1240.
20. Kreulen DL, Szurszewski JH: Reflex pathways in the abdominal prevertebral ganglia: Evidence for a colocolonic inhibitory reflex. *J Physiol* 1979, 295:21–32.
21. Grider JR, Makhlouf GM: Regulation of the peristaltic reflex by peptides of the myenteric plexus. *Arch Int Pharmacodyn Ther* 1990, 303:232–251.
22. Collman PI, Grundy D, Scratcherd T: Vagal control of colonic motility in the anaesthetized ferret: Evidence for a non-cholinergic excitatory innervation. *J Physiol* 1984, 348:35–42.
23. Almy TS: Experimental studies on the irritable colon. *Am J Med* 1951, 10:60–67.
24. Sellin JH: Intestinal electrolyte absorption and secretion. In *Gastrointestinal Disease: Pathophysiology, Diagnosis, Management*, edn 5. Edited by Sleisenger MH, Fordtran JS. Philadelphia: WB Saunders; 1994:954–976.
25. Barrett KE, Dharmsathaphorn K: Secretion and absorption: Small intestine and colon. In *Textbook of Gastroenterology*. Edited by Yamada T. Philadelphia: JB Lippincott; 1991:265–294.
26. Binder HJ, Sandle GI: Electrolyte absorption and secretion in the mammalian colon. In *Physiology of the Gastrointestinal Tract*, edn 2. Edited by Johnson LR. New York: Raven Press; 1987:1389–1418.
27. Laissue JA, Gebbers JO: The intestinal barrier and the gut-associated lymphoid tissue. *Curr Stud Hematol Blood Transfus* 1992, 59:19–43.
28. Moore WEC, Holdeman LV: Human fecal flora: The normal flora of 21 Japanese-Hawaiians. *Appl Microbiol* 1974, 27:961–979.
29. Finegold SM, Sutter VL, Mathisen BE: Normal indigenous flora. In *Human Intestinal Microflora in Health and Disease*. Edited by Hentges DJ. New York: Academic Press; 1983:3–31.
30. Irving MH, Catchpole B: ABC of colorectal diseases. Anatomy and physiology of the colon, rectum, and anus. *BMJ* 1992, 304:1106–1108.
31. Shafik A: A new concept of the anatomy of the anal sphincter mechanism and the physiology of defecation. The external anal sphincter: A triple-loop system. *Invest Urol* 1975, 12:412–49.
32. Shafik A: A new concept of the anatomy of the anal sphincter mechanism and the physiology of defecation. III. The longitudinal anal muscle and role in anal sphincter mechanism. *Invest Urol* 1976, 13:271–277.
33. Duthie HL, Gairns FW: Sensory nerve endings and sensation in the anal region of man. *Br J Surg* 1960, 47:585–595.
34. Schiller LR: Fecal incontinence. In *Gastrointestinal Disease: Pathophysiology, Diagnosis, Management*, edn 5. Edited by Sleisenger MH, Fordtran JS. Philadelphia: WB Saunders; 1994:934–953.
35. Alva J, Mendeloff AI, Shuster MM: Reflex and electromyographic abnormalities associated with fecal incontinence. *Gastroenterology* 1967, 53:101–106.
36. Goei R: Defecography: Principles of technique and interpretation. *Radiologe* 1993, 33:356–360.
37. Wald A: Anorectum. In *Atlas of Gastrointestinal Motility in Health and Disease*. Edited by Schuster MH. Baltimore: Williams & Wilkins; 1993:229–249.

Chapter 2

Colonoscopy of the Anus, Rectum, and Normal Colon

TIMOTHY T. NOSTRANT

The colonoscope has become the tool of choice for diagnosing many colonic disorders, including those abnormalities appearing on radiographs, lower gastrointestinal bleeding, and acute and chronic inflammatory bowel disease. The colonoscope is also useful in screening for and monitoring colonic cancer. Colonoscopy offers therapeutic options in patients with gastrointestinal bleeding and colonic polyps as well as dilation treatment for inflammatory and postsurgical strictures.

This chapter introduces the reader to the many variations normally encountered in routine colonoscopy and shows what can happen during treatment of colonic polyps. A thorough knowledge of normal variations allows the endoscopist to appropriately direct biopsy specimens and to interpret histologic changes in light of what is seen during endoscopy. Equipment used in both diagnostic and therapeutic colonoscopy is presented.

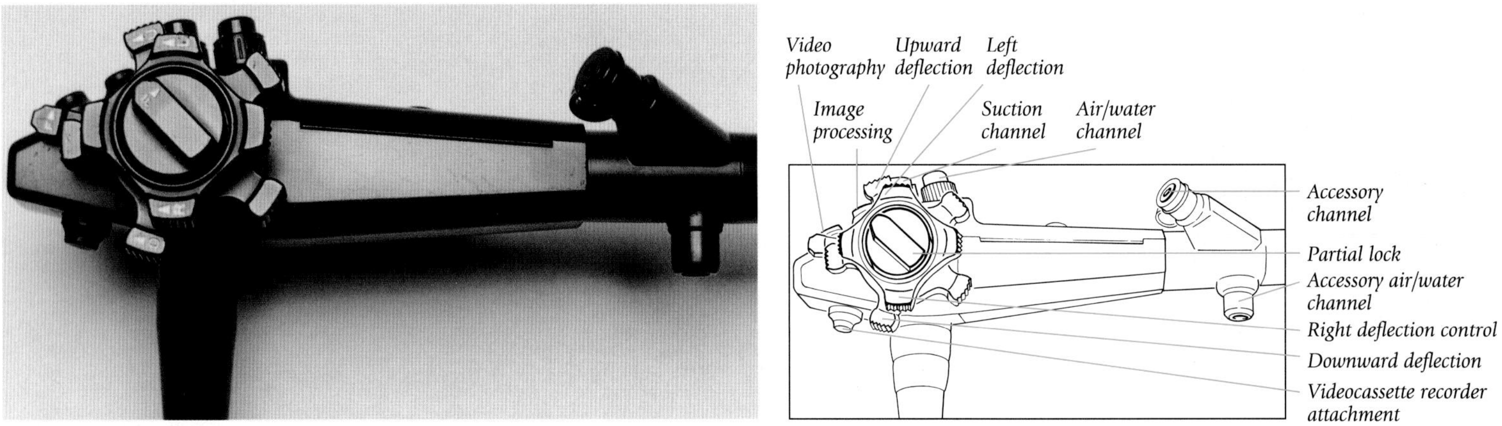

FIGURE 2-1.

The control chassis of the Pentax EC 3801 video colonoscope (Pentax Precision Instrument Corp., Orangeburg, NY). The control chassis has three basic elements. The first element is the deflection controls (dual rotary knobs). The inner control is for upward and downward deflection (180°). The outer control is for right and left deflection (160°). Both controls have partial locks to make the distal insertion tube more rigid for easier passage. The second element is the function buttons on the top of the chassis. The larger buttons are for air or water and for suction. The two smaller buttons are for video photography and image processing. The button on the under carriage of the scope is for a videocassette recorder attachment. The third element is the accessory channel, which is used for insertion of all accessories. The final channel is an accessory air or water channel to clean the lens and potentially to clean soiled or bloody areas during colonoscopy.

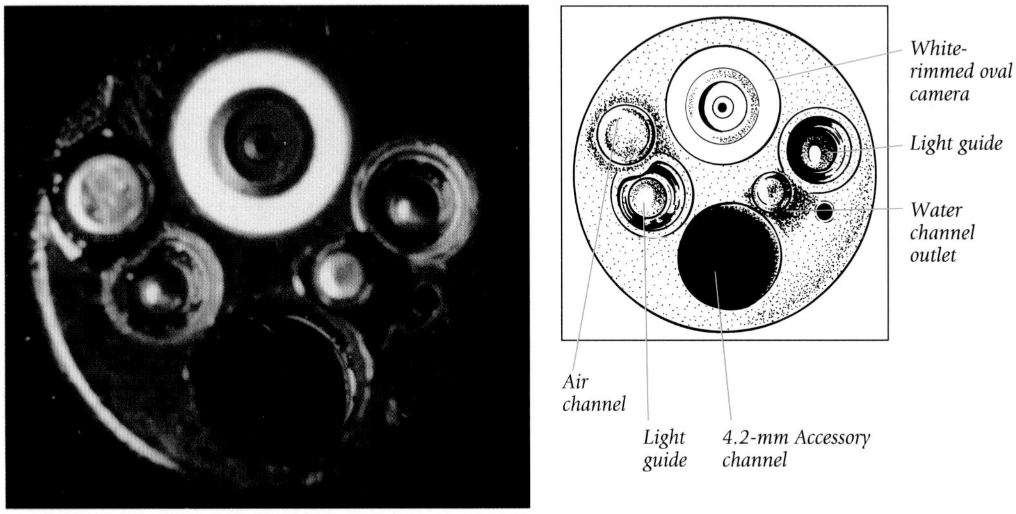

FIGURE 2-2.

The working end of the colonoscope. The two metal attachments represent the separate air or water channels that primarily insufflate the bowel and clean the lens, respectively. A tiny hole just below the water channel is the outlet for the accessory air or water channel on the chassis that facilitates cleaning. The 4.2-mm accessory channel facilitates passage of therapeutic accessories. The white-rimmed oval camera is for video imaging of the colon. The input is passed back into the video processor and displayed on a video monitor. Two light guides for illumination are also shown. Low-level illumination is used for video work, and xenon (high intensity light) is used for transillumination to help localize scope position.

Colonoscopy accessories

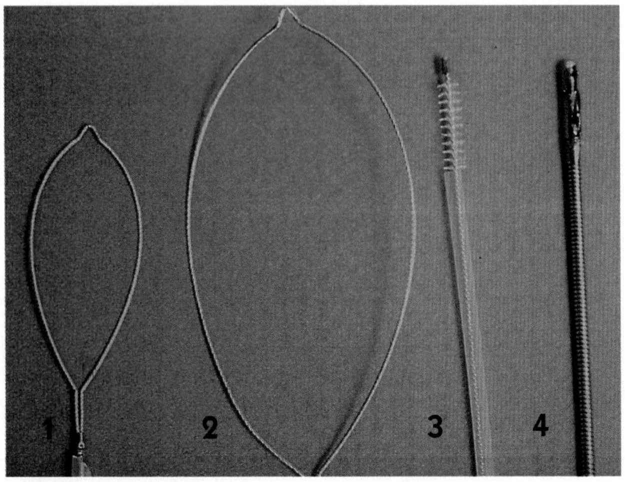

FIGURE 2-3.

The two wire loop snares (*1* and *2*) are used to remove both pedunculated (stalked) and nonpedunculated (sessile) polyps. Size of snare can vary with size of polyp as shown here. Hexagon, sickle-shaped, and crescent-shaped wires can be used in special circumstances. Rotatable snares to cover the colonic wall and facilitate removal of polyps are also available. Cytology brushes (*3*) and standard biopsy forceps (*4*) are used to obtain specimens for diagnosis. Cytology brushes are useful predominantly when there is concern about bleeding after biopsy and are less commonly used in the colon compared with the upper gastrointestinal tract. Needle probes in the middle of the standard cup biopsy forceps allow retrieval of two specimens with one passage.

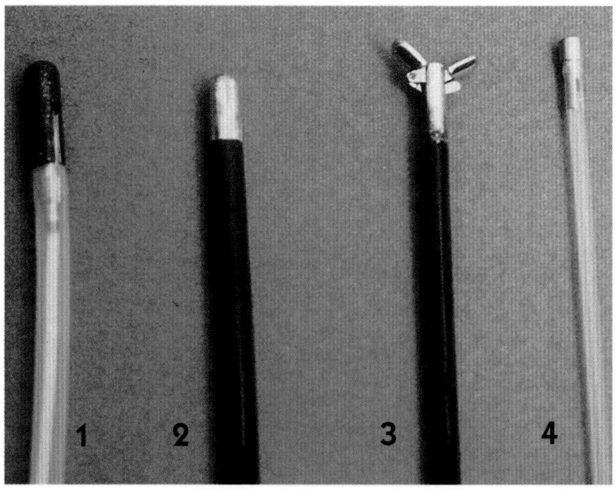

FIGURE 2-4.

The four types of devices used for bleeding control or electrocoagulation. The heater probe (*1*) and bicap probe (*2*) are most commonly used to stop bleeding after polypectomy or to obliterate vascular lesions such as arteriovenous malformations. Both rely on the same principle of sealing the vessel with pressure and heat. Heat is generated directly by the heater probe and indirectly in tissue by electrical resistance using the bicap probe. Both probes and their accessories are reasonably priced. The hot biopsy forceps (*3*) is a monopolar device used to grasp polyps and to coagulate the stalk or pseudostalk created by retraction of a polyp off the colonic wall. Because current passes through the wall, there is a greater concern for deep tissue injury. The laser probe (*4*) is used predominantly for lesions not amenable to the above therapies, such as extensive telangiectases or arteriovenous malformations. Tumor destruction is another possible use but is used less commonly for colonic tumors when compared with esophageal tumors. Cost for laser equipment is high.

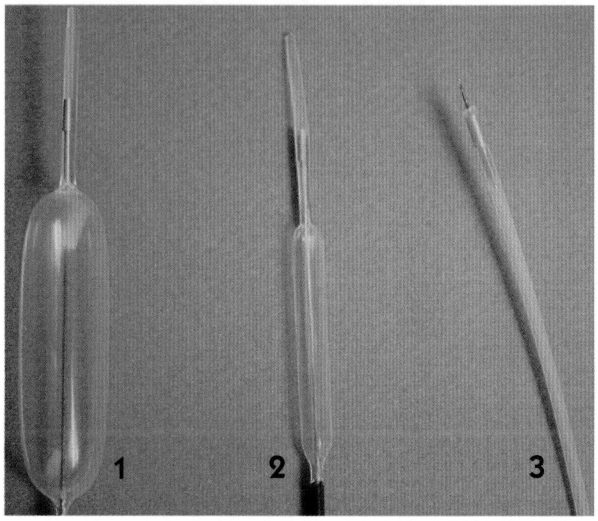

FIGURE 2-5.

Colonic dilators and needle injectors. Through the scope balloon dilators range from 18 to 60F in diameter. Dilation of postoperative strictures or strictures secondary to inflammatory bowel disease are the major indications. The balloons depicted here are 45F (*1*) and 18F (*2*). The injecting needle (*3*) can be used to inject saline to facilitate polypectomy, to infiltrate a bleeding source with epinephrine or other sclerosant, or to mark an area with methylene blue to help the surgeon locate a lesion for surgical treatment (colon polyp removal, vascular lesion removal).

EXAMINATION OF THE PERINEUM

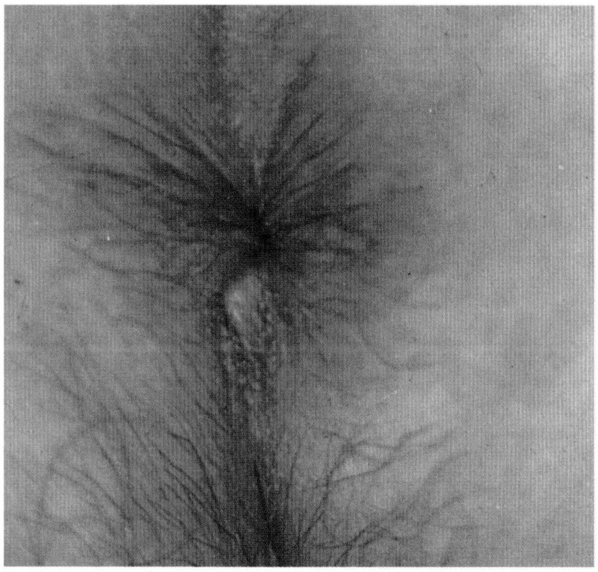

FIGURE 2-6.

A normal perineal examination. An examination of the perineum is the first part of the colonoscopy. Separation of both buttocks with the hands allows full evaluation of the anal and perianal skin. Perianal skin and anal mucosa are normally more granular. No breakdown should be seen. Excoriations may point to pruritus ani, and an evaluation for pin worms would be appropriate. Anal fissures can be seen and are usually observed on the posterior and anterior anal walls. Fistulas can be seen anywhere in the perineal area but are usually concentrated within 3 to 5 cm of the anal verge. Examination of the perineum from the posterior aspect of the anus all the way to the coccyx should be done to exclude pilonidal tracts and cysts.

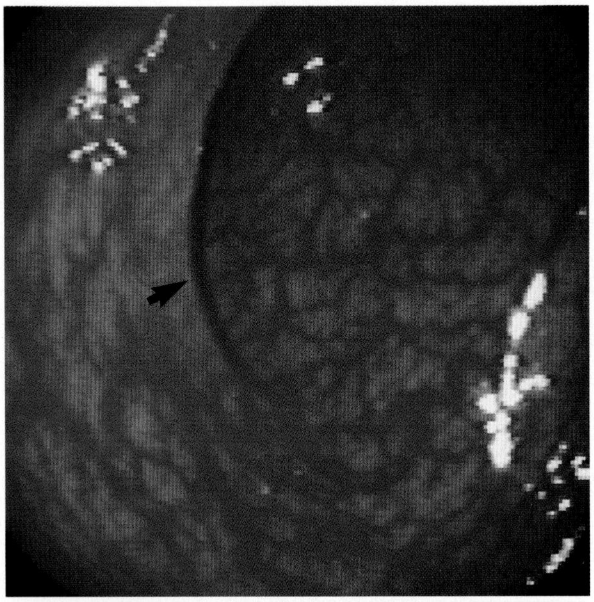

FIGURE 2-7.

Colonoscopic evaluation of the rectum. Light reflection off the clear colonic mucosa should be glistening and not granular as shown. Venous channels as well as capillaries with many side branches are easily visible. This figure presents prominent subepithelial vascular detail with major subbranching. The first valve of Houston's valves (rectal valves) is shown on the left (*arrow*).

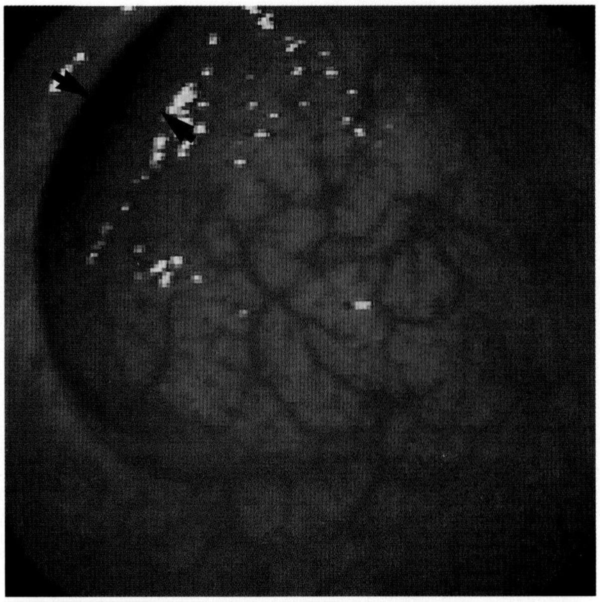

FIGURE 2-8.

A mucosa with less prominent vascular detail and longer capillary channels. Venous vessels are easily seen and clearly demarcated. The first two rectal valves are visible on the left (*arrows*). The lumen of the rectum is much wider than the sigmoid, descending, and transverse colons. Examination behind each of the rectal valves is mandatory to exclude lesions.

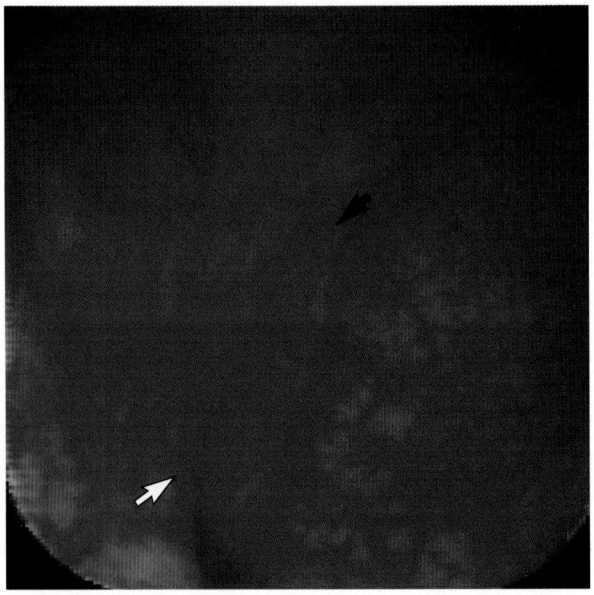

FIGURE 2-9.

Examination of the rectal wall. This figure enables the endoscopist to compare the rectal wall 3 cm from the anus (*open arrow*) with the rectal mucosa (*closed arrow*). As the mucosa goes from the distal rectum to the proximal rectum, vessels become more distinct, thinner, and occupy less surface area. Vessels in the distal rectum appear less prominent, larger, less distinct, and more venous in character as the anal plexus is approached.

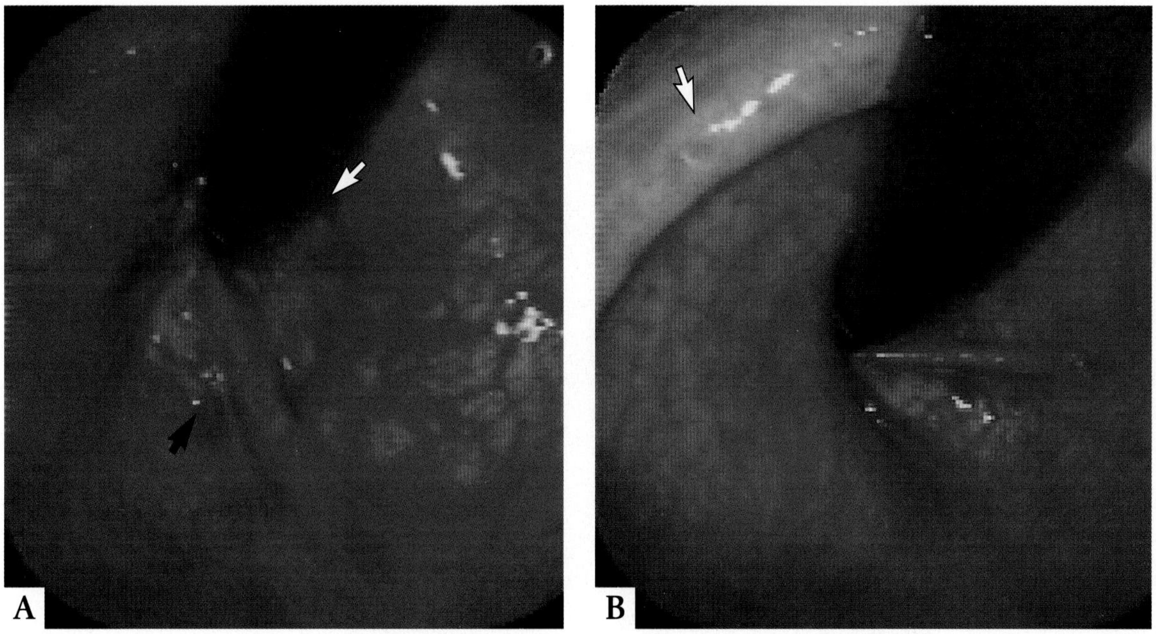

FIGURE 2-10.

Retroflexion of the colonoscope in the rectum. This maneuver can be accomplished easily by raising the tip of the colonoscope upward and backward. As the maneuver is accomplished, the colonoscope can be advanced and torqued such that the distal rectal and anal mucosa are directly visualized. **A**, Pushing the colonoscope further in will bring the anal canal closer. The anal canal and scope (*open arrow*) are easily visible. The anal venous plexus and anal folds (*closed arrow*) are seen with puckering of the anal mucosa. No internal hemorrhoids are observed. The heavy density of vessels as the colonoscope approaches the anus is again appreciated. **B**, Pulling out the colonoscope gives a more panoramic view, with the first rectal valve easily seen at the top (*arrow*).

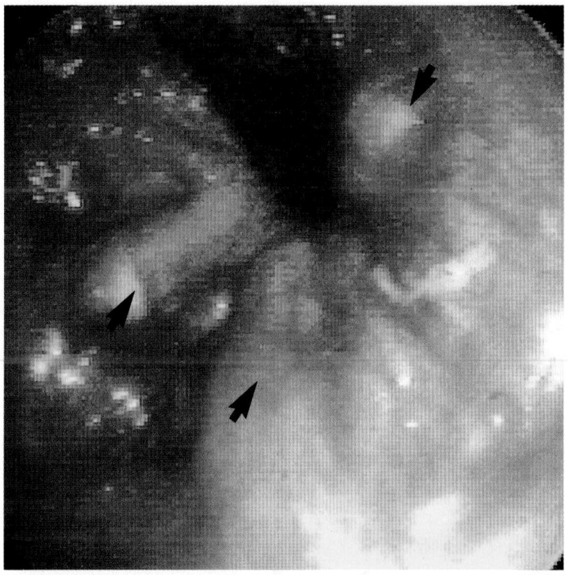

FIGURE 2-11.

Skin tags can be seen at the beginning of the hemorrhoidal plexus. Skin tags (*arrows*) are particularly common in patients with internal hemorrhoids that prolapse. These skin tags usually represent squamous hyperplasia secondary to continuous movement irritation. If they enlarge, they can become polypoid and be mistaken for colon polyps. If biopsied or cauterized, skin tags can be painful because they maintain normal anal or skin innervation.

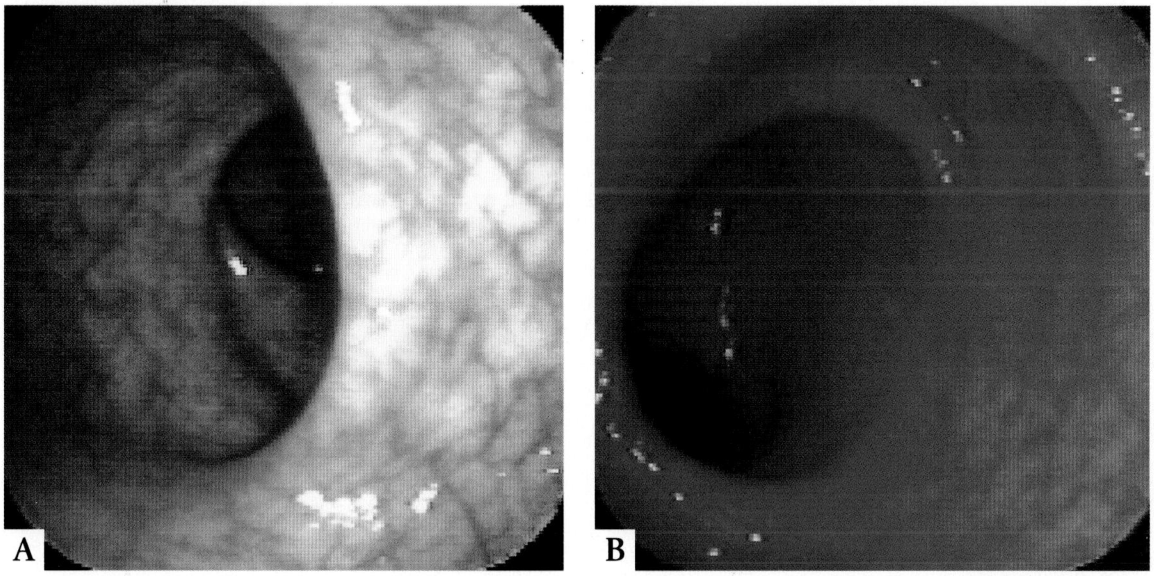

FIGURE 2-12.

Approaching the rectosigmoid junction. As the colonoscope proceeds up the rectum, mucosal vessels become less prominent, and all three rectal valves can be seen (**A**). Just beyond these three rectal valves is the rectosigmoid junction (**B**).

EXAMINATION OF THE COLON

Sigmoid colon

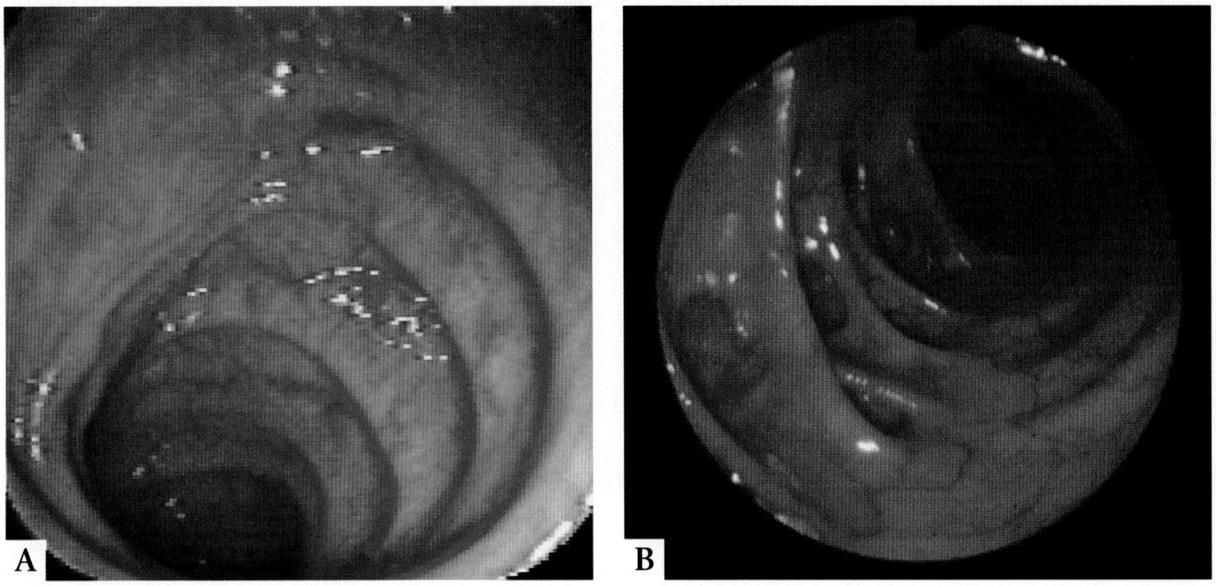

Figure 2-13.

The sigmoid colon. **A**, Passing into the sigmoid colon, the caliber of the lumen narrows and becomes more tubular. Folds are usually thin and easily seen continuing deeper in the colon. **B**, Diverticula with fold thickening should be closely evaluated in the sigmoid colon. Knowledge of the existence of diverticula is important in evaluating patients with left lower quadrant pain.

Descending colon

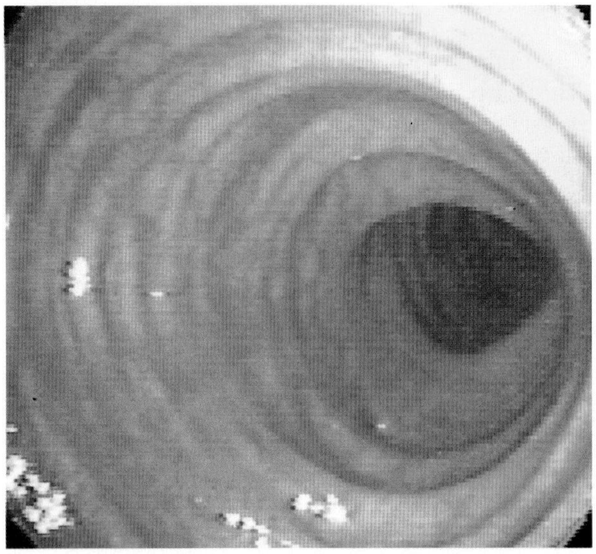

Figure 2-14.

The descending colon is frequently more tubular than the sigmoid colon. The splenic flexure, one of the major turns in the colon, is seen in the distance as a faint bluish hue.

Splenic flexure

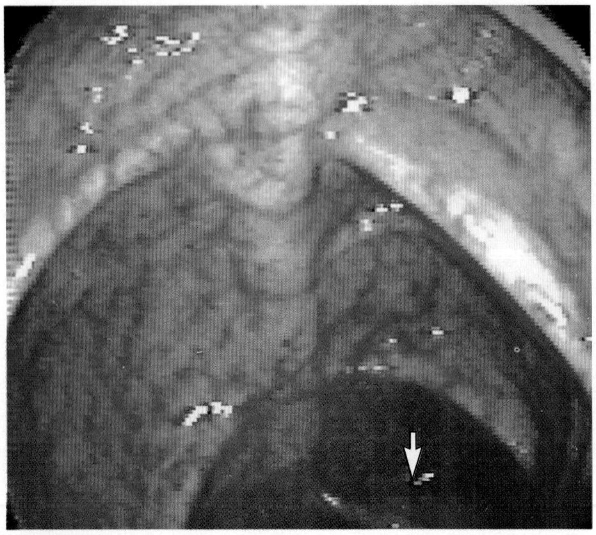

Figure 2-15.

Approaching the splenic flexure, a focal discrete area of bluish hue is seen through the colonic mucosa. The hue is produced by the impression of the spleen on the colon. A large turn is visible at the bottom right of the mucosa (*arrow*).

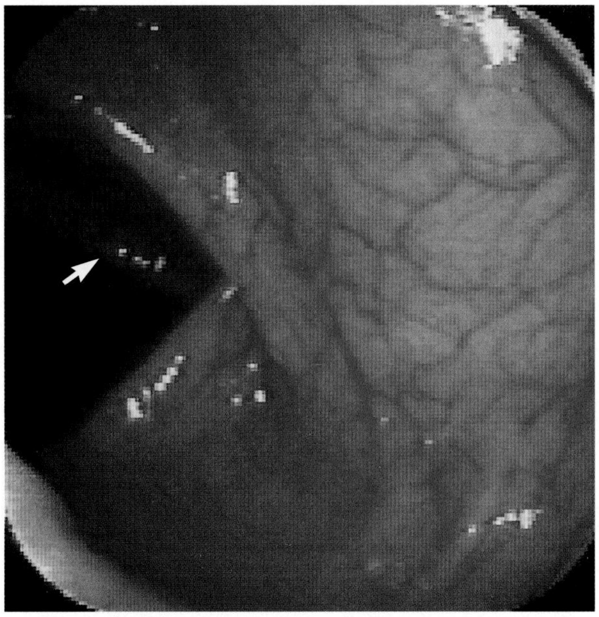

FIGURE 2-16.

The splenic flexure may be redundant and offer both true and false passages. Endoscopists should pay close attention to detail and appreciate the fact that the true passage is almost always found by following the direction of the folds. The transverse colon is seen in the left upper quadrant (*arrow*).

Transverse colon

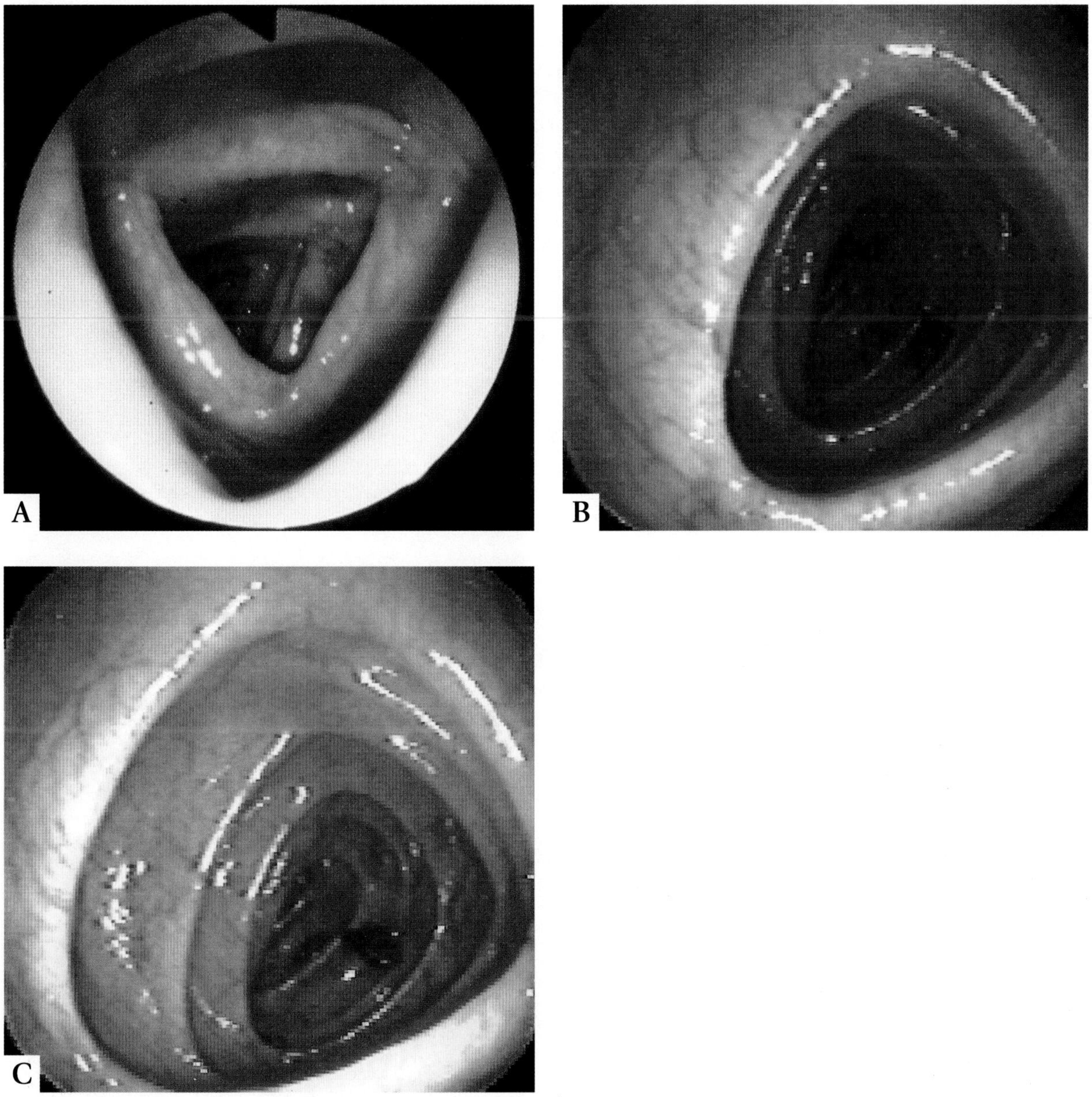

FIGURE 2-17.

The transverse colon is the most varied in contour of all of the colon sections. **A**, Bound by the splenic flexure on the left and the hepatic flexure on the right, the transverse colon can have the characteristic triangular folds. **B** and **C**, Variants of this configuration include a more tubular transverse colon presented here.

Hepatic flexure

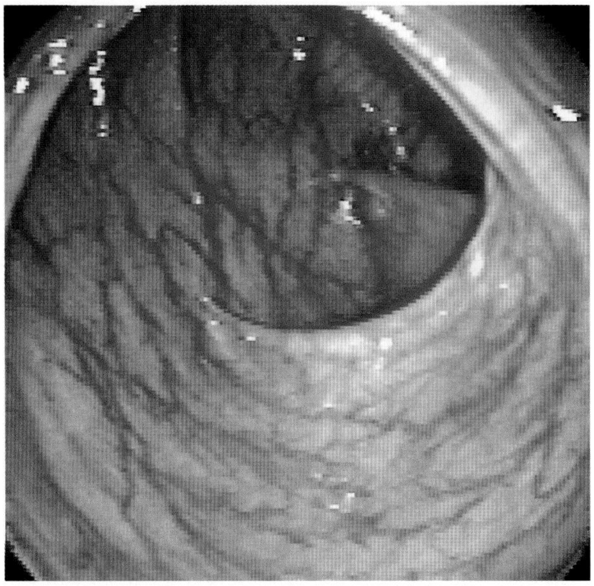

FIGURE 2-18.

Hepatic flexure is similar in configuration to the splenic flexure but is usually less redundant. Once again a bluish hue is seen secondary to hepatic impression.

Ascending colon

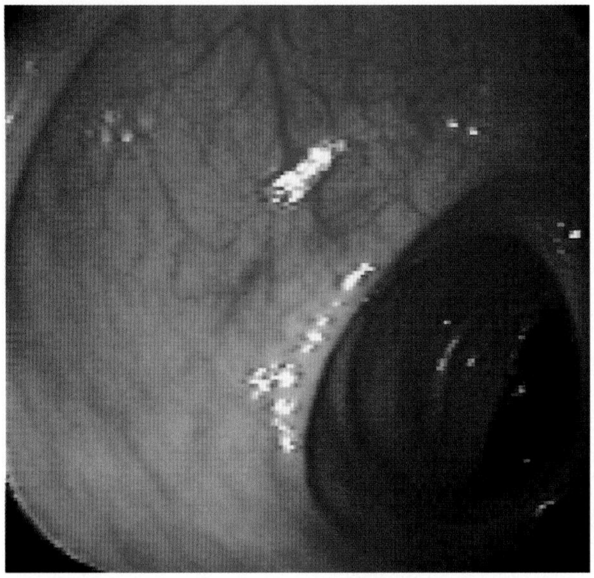

FIGURE 2-19.

The ascending colon is more capacious than the transverse and left colons. Mucosal vessels are harder to see. Compared with the left and transverse colons, folds in the right colon are usually semilunar or incomplete. Similar to the transverse colon, triangular folds can be visible in the right colon.

Cecum

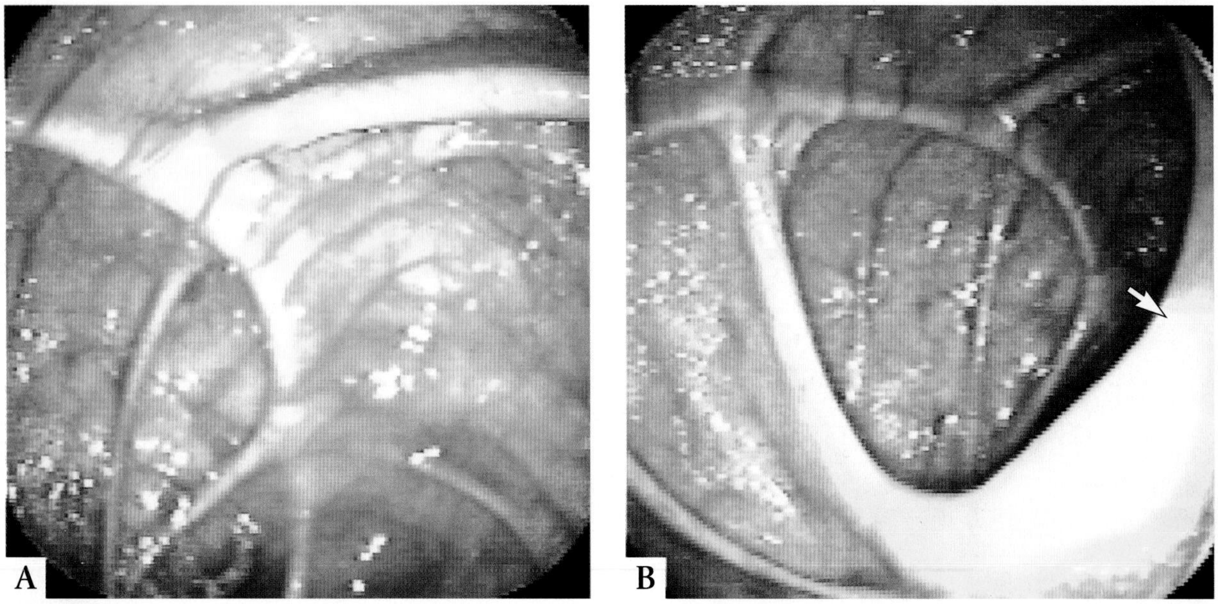

FIGURE 2-20.

The cecum is identified by three different characteristics: fusing of the taeniae coli, the ileocecal valve, and the appendiceal orifice. **A**, The fusing of the taeniae coli is depicted. The taeniae coli represent the three longitudinal muscular strands that begin in the base of the appendix, run to the anus, and fuse into the longitudinal muscle of the external anal sphincter. **B**, The ileocecal valve (distal lip) and the fusion of the taeniae coli. The appearance (*Continued on next page*)

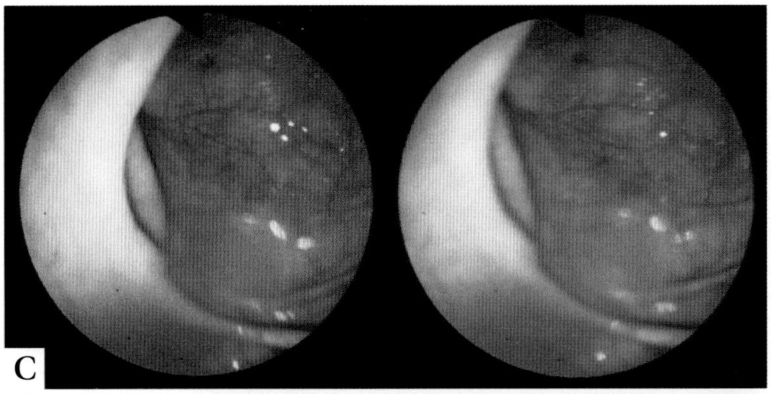

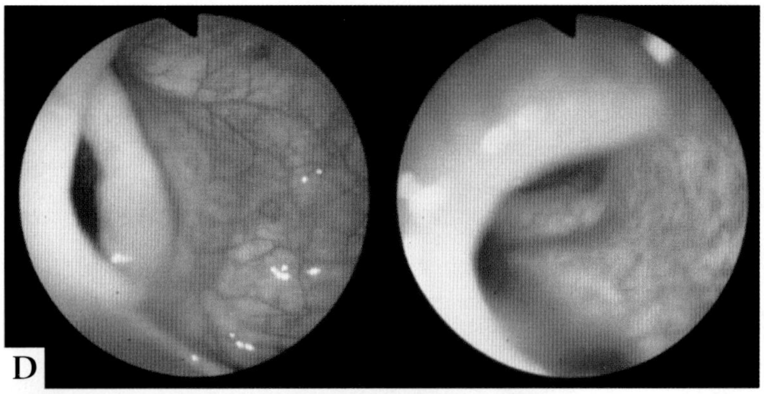

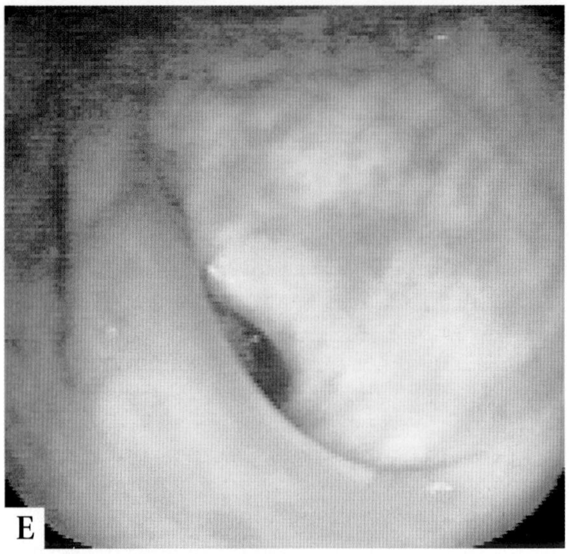

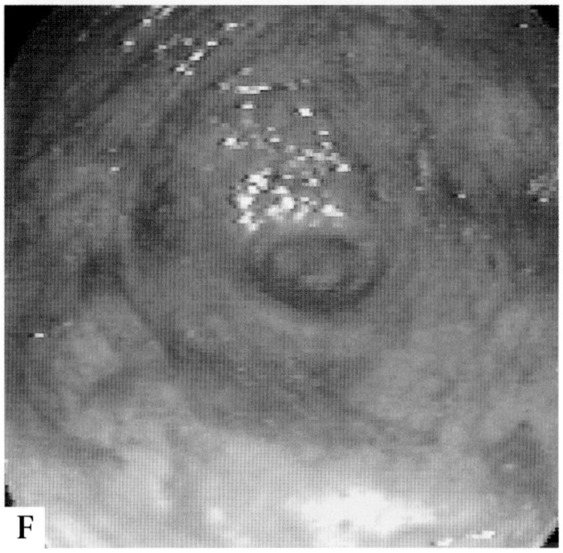

FIGURE 2-20. ***(CONTINUED)***

of the proximal cecum may appear cuplike or dome-shaped if the taeniae coli fuse with the lips of the ileocecal valve. A small notch (*arrow*) signifies the superior aspect of the ileocecal valve. **C** and **D**, The distal and proximal lips of the ileocecal valve. The valve is usually approached in this position, and the scope tip is turned into the valve and will usually pop into the terminal ileum. With modern instrumentation, the terminal ileum can be intubated if necessary in 80% or more of cases. Biopsy forceps placed into the terminal ileum may allow the endoscopist to pull the scope into the small bowel in difficult cases. **E** and **F**, The appendix is varied in its appearance. It most commonly presents as a slitlike opening (*E*) at the base of the taeniae fusion or as a circular orifice (*F*). Fecal particles are seen frequently obliterating the orifice and do not point to possible appendicitis.

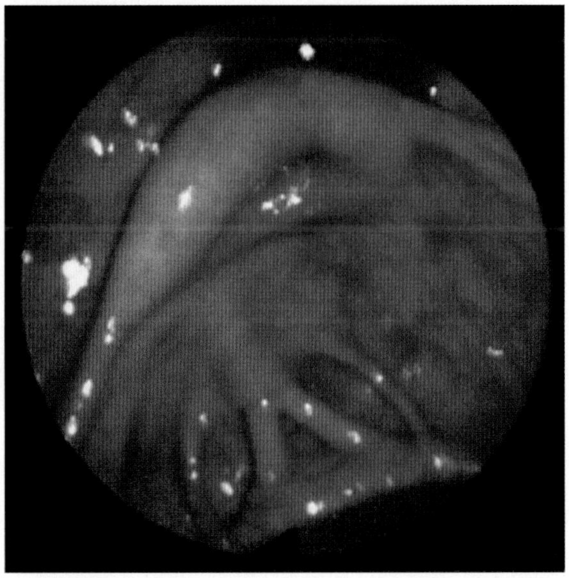

FIGURE 2-21.

The appendix, taeniae coli fusion, and ileocecal valve. This view is produced by rectroflexing the colonoscope tip in the cecum. Although this position allows good visualization, colonoscopic biopsy and entrance into the terminal ileum may not be possible because of instrument angulation.

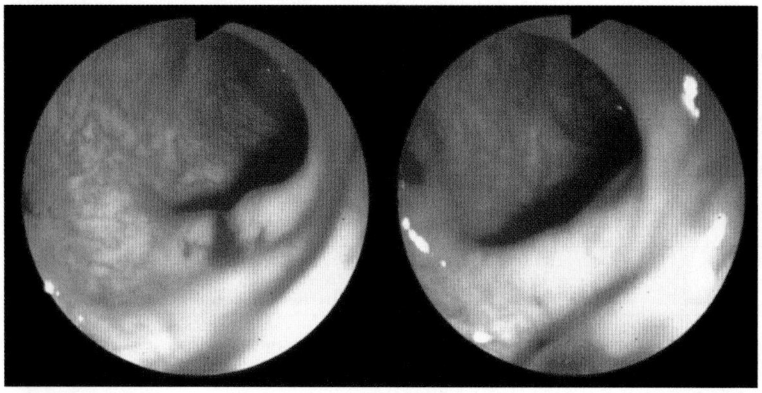

FIGURE 2-22.

The terminal ileum is usually easily differentiated from the colon. Kercking rings are usually seen but are not as prominent as in the duodenum. The mucosa is less glistening and more villous and dull than the colon, similar to the duodenum. Active peristalsis and contractions moving toward the colonoscope tip point to the small bowel over colon. Kercking rings and a dull mucosa are depicted in this figure of the terminal ileum. The red spots are secondary to biopsy artifact.

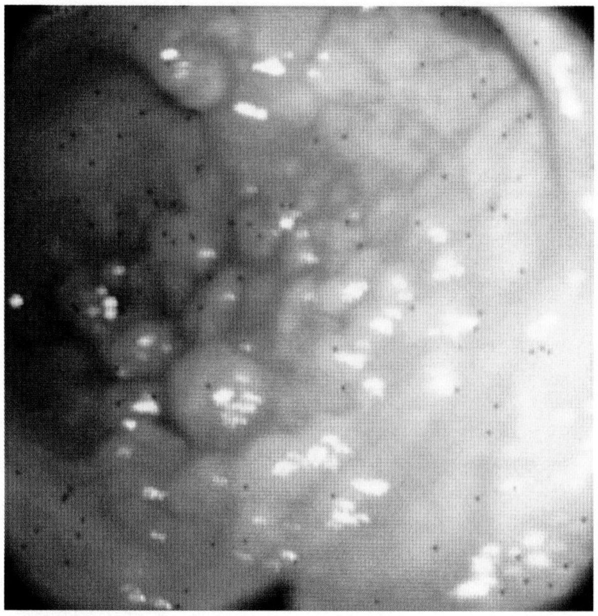

FIGURE 2-23.

Lymphoid modules can be seen in a normal terminal ileum. These modules vary from 1 to several millimeters in size and can be matted. Mucosal changes may point to Crohn's disease or infections like yersinosis or tuberculosis. Diffuse lymphoid nodules throughout the small intestine may be seen in patients with immunoglobulin-A antibody deficiency.

MISCELLANEOUS FINDINGS IN THE COLON

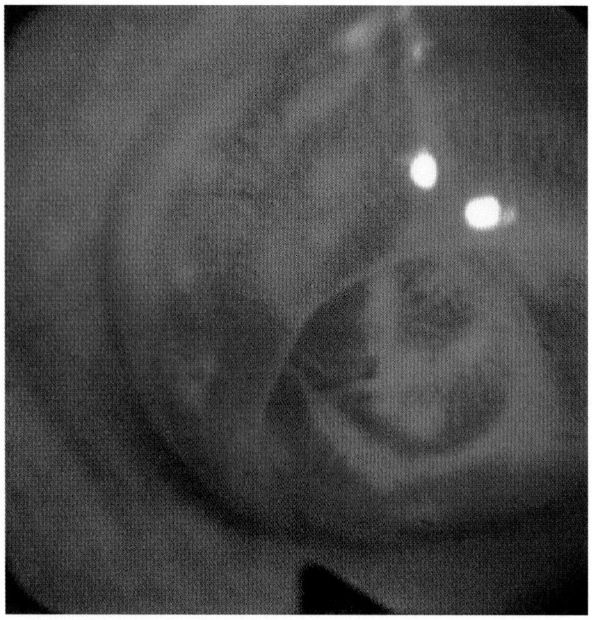

FIGURE 2-24.

Acute inflammation around a slitlike opening in the cecum. This inflammation occurred in a 60-year-old man presenting with a fever of unknown origin lasting 4 months and a mass in the cecum visible with barium enema. Surgery revealed appendicitis.

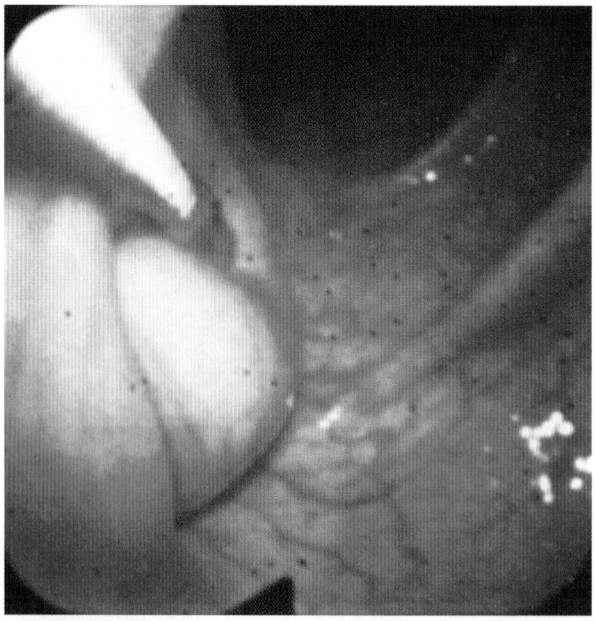

FIGURE 2-25.

Large masses in the right colon can mimic carcinoma or colon polyps. A 5-cm mass was discovered in the right colon. A biopsy forceps easily compresses the mass. Grabbing the mucosa allowed the endoscopist to pull the mucosa off the mass (tenting), suggesting a submucosal mass. Numerous biopsy samples revealed lipid globules consistent with a colonic lipoma.

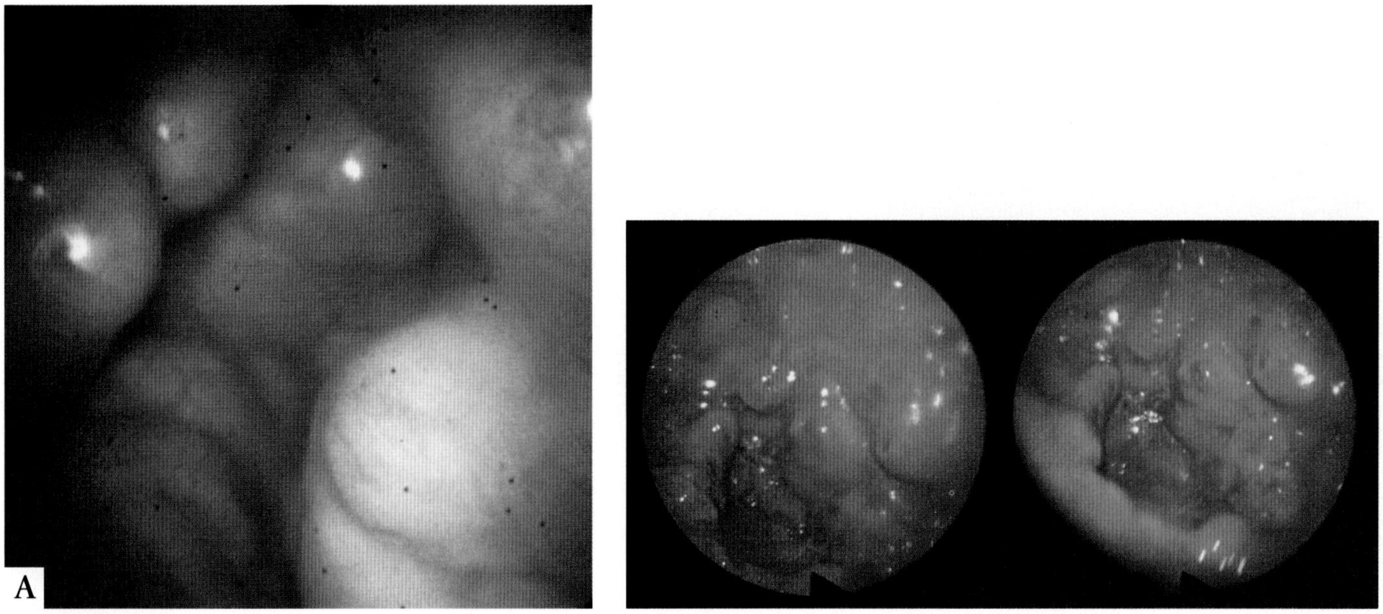

Figure 2-26.

Pneumotosis cystoides intestinalis is an uncommon condition characterized by multiple gas-filled endothelial-lined cysts occurring either in the subserosa or submucosa of the intestinal tract. Proposed mechanisms include forced passage of air from the colon lumen or pulmonary alveoli into the colon walls. The second mechanism is anaerobic fermentation and trapping of diffused gas. **A**, Submucosal gas is presented. Biopsy will usually cause the bleb to disappear. **B**, Submucosal or subserosal gas accumulation is shown. Biopsy specimens may show overlying inflammation. Biopsy specimens demonstrate firm tissue; their appearance may mimic neoplastic disease. Radiographs or computed tomography may confirm the diagnosis.

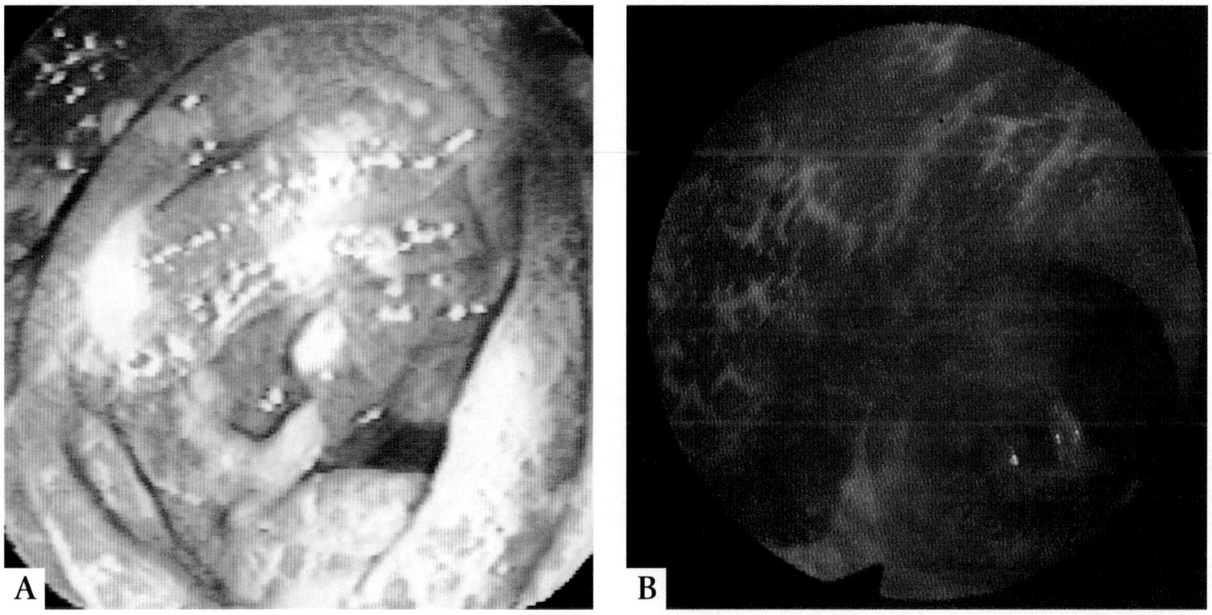

Figure 2-27.

Melanosis coli is an accumulation of lipofuscin-like pigment in macrophages in the lamina propria below the colonic crypt epithelium. Pigment can also be seen in the deeper bowel layers and lymph nodes. Degenerated lipid membranes damaged by the anthraquinone laxatives (senna, cascara, danthron, aloe) are the source for the pigmentation. Distribution is variable, but most often predominates in the cecum and rectum. Polyps and cancers do not pigment and therefore are easily seen against the dark background. The condition is benign and usually takes a year to both accumulate or disappear with taking or abstaining from laxatives. **Panel A** demonstrates mild "tigroid" pigmentation predominantly on the folds, whereas **panel B** demonstrates heavy accumulation of pigment and "black bowel".

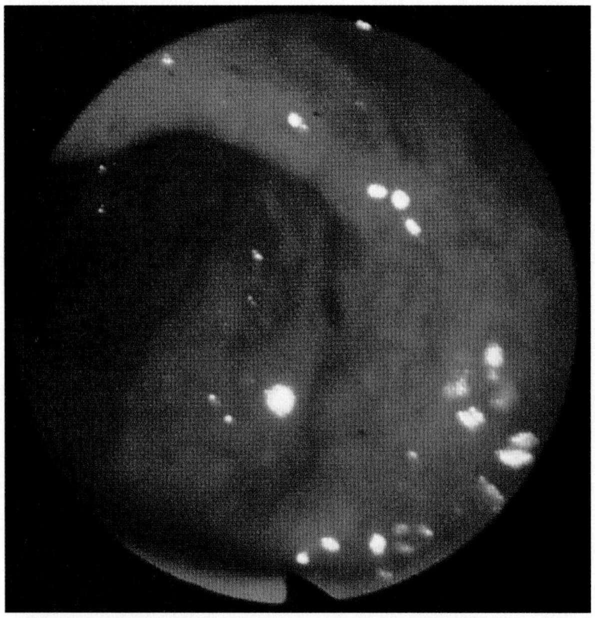

FIGURE 2-28.

Abnormalities of rectal vasculature are uncommon. Prominent rectal veins are normal variants. Dilated rectal veins (rectal varices) in a patient with portal hypertension are shown. These veins represent true communications between the portal–splanchnic circulation. The veins extend from the squamous epithelium across the dentate line and into the rectal mucosa; they are serpentine and can cause severe bleeding. Optimal treatment is unknown, but treatments used for esophageal varices have also been used for rectal varices.

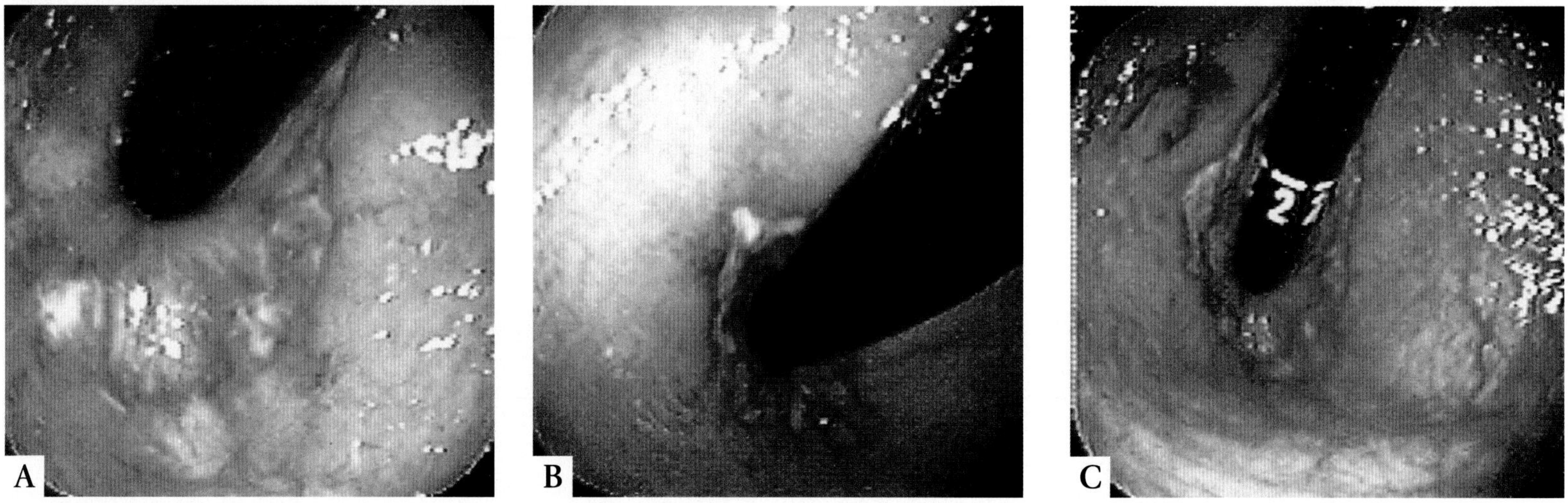

FIGURE 2-29.

A–C, Solitary rectal ulcer is a condition produced by difficult defecation and straining. Rectal prolapse is common (90%). Ulcers are usually seen on the anterior rectal wall 7 to 10 cm from the anal verge. This location serves as a lead point for rectal prolapse.

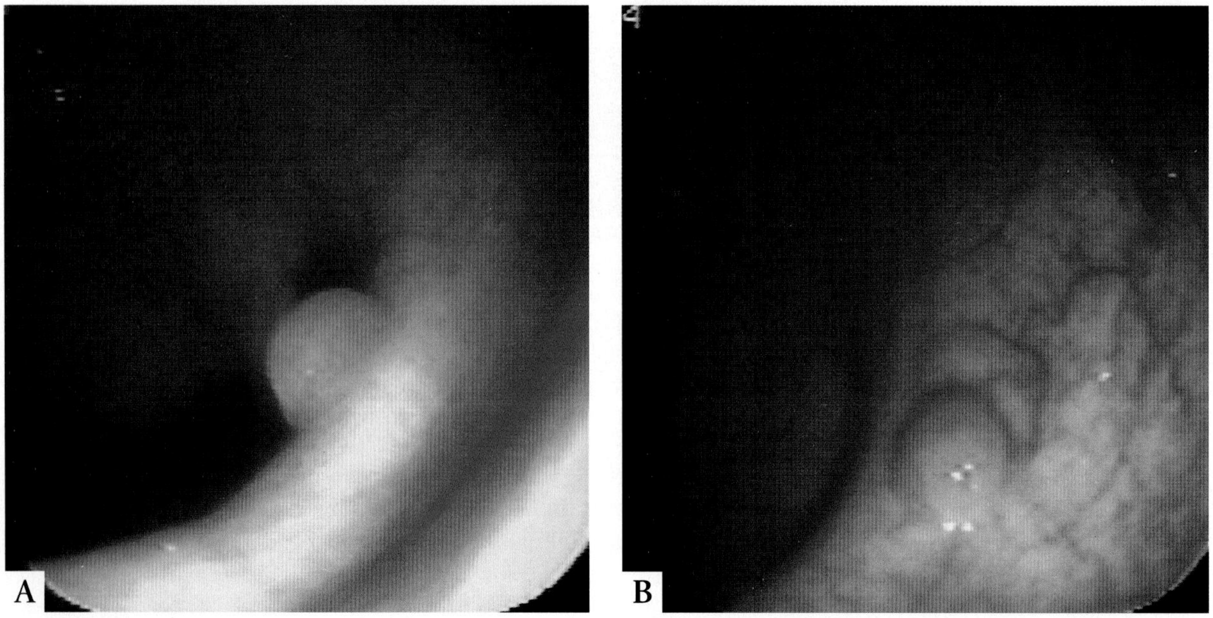

FIGURE 2-30.

Two 3-mm polyps in the rectum before and after hot biopsy are shown. The base of both polyps is cauterized, and the head sloughs with time. **A**, A polyp on the upper side of a sigmoid fold. **B**, A polyp just distal to the polyp on the upper side of a sigmoid fold.

(Continued on next page)

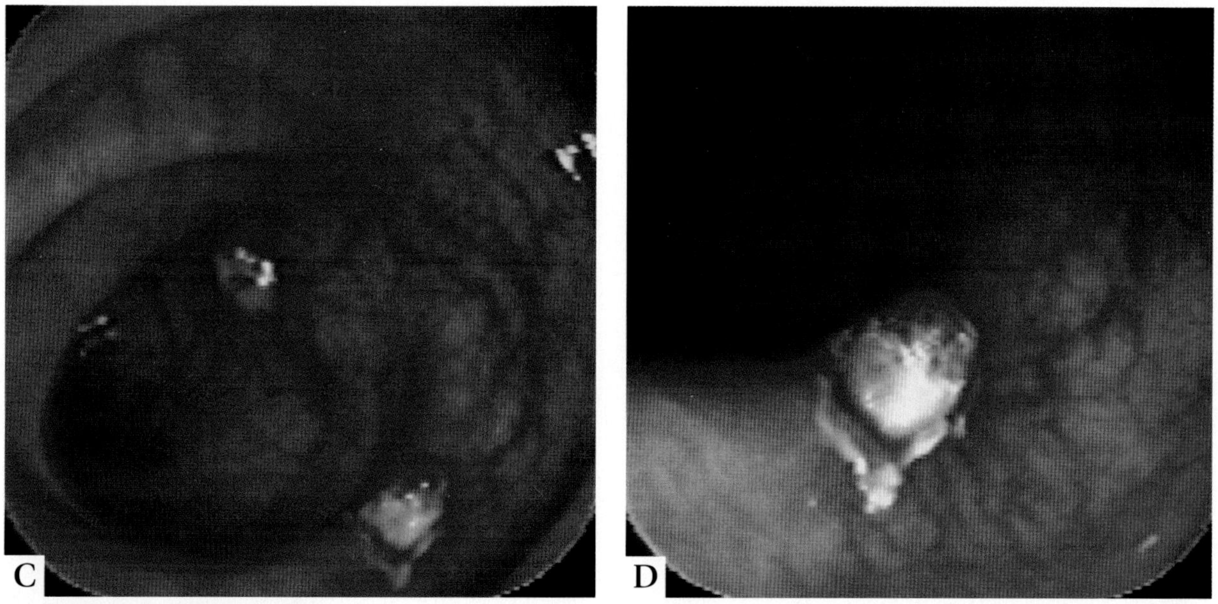

FIGURE 2-30. *(CONTINUED)*

C, Both polyps after cauterization. **D**, A detailed view of the distal polyp with its cauterized base.

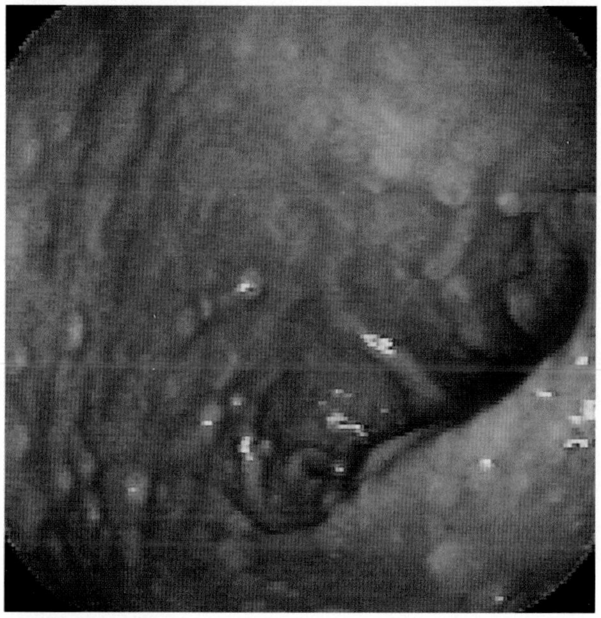

FIGURE 2-31.

Lymphoid nodules in the rectum are commonly seen but are usually few in number. Lymphogranuloma venereum is presented in a patient with AIDS.

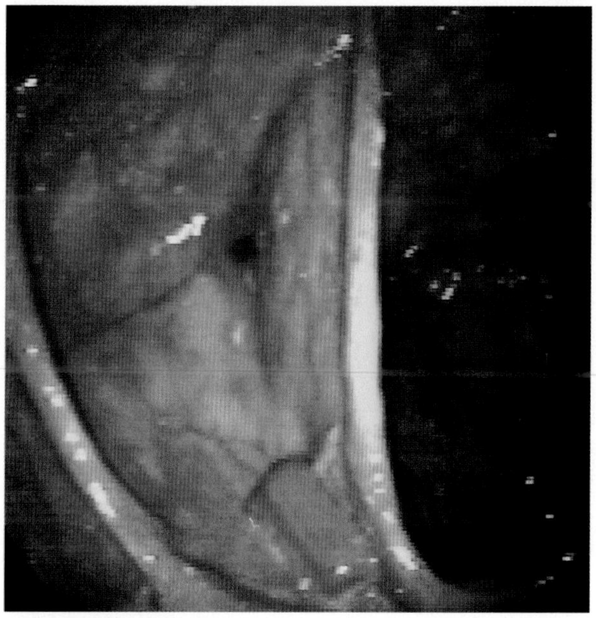

FIGURE 2-32.

Undissolved pills are commonly seen in the colon. Rapid transit, low pH, and older tablets are possible causes. An undissolved Asacol tablet (Procter and Gamble, Norwich, NY) in the proximal colon is shown.

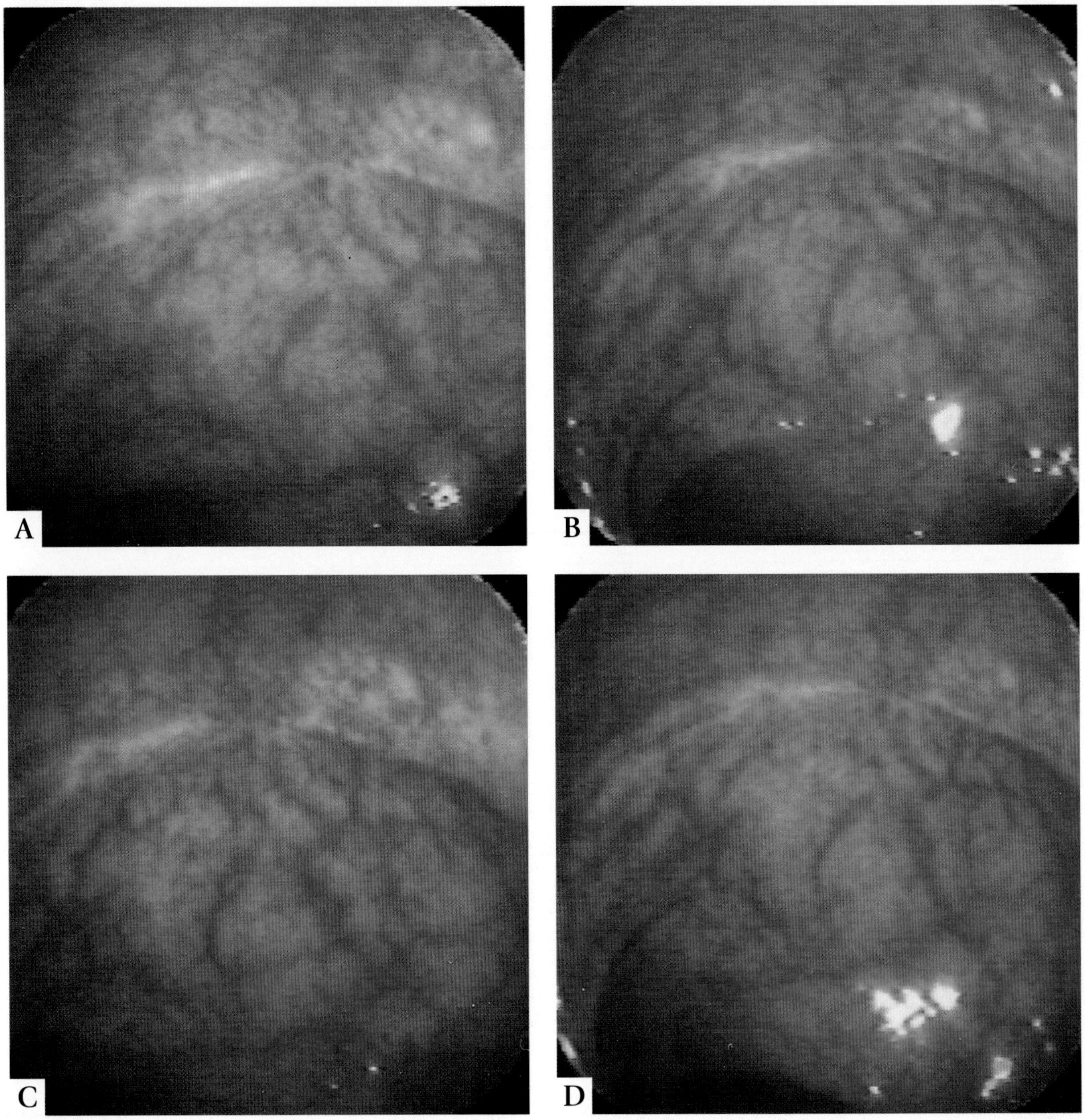

FIGURE 2-33.

A–D, Postpolypectomy artifacts are common and can be confused with carcinoma if previous colon treatments are unknown. A white scar along the surface of a rectal fold secondary to a surgical transanal polypectomy is shown.

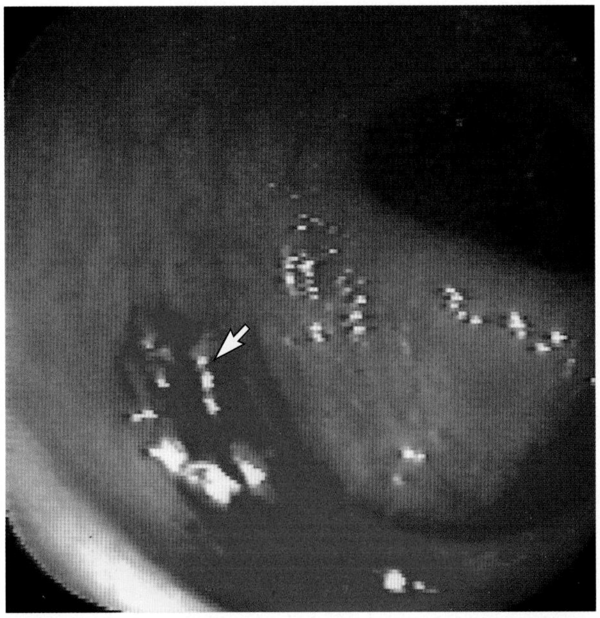

FIGURE 2-34.

Bleeding after a hot biopsy polypectomy. The polyp tissue is represented by the yellowish mount (*arrow*) at the beginning of the heme trail. Bleeding was stopped with repeated cautery using the bicap probe.

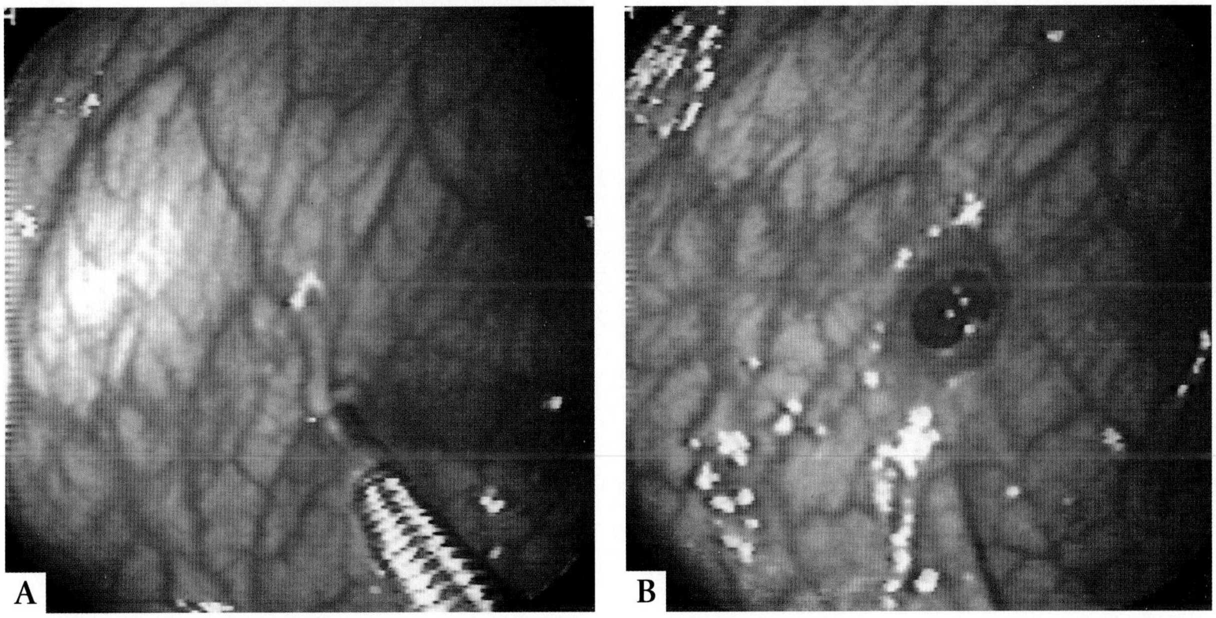

FIGURE 2-35.

A and **B**, Biopsy forceps can sometimes produce submucosal edema with mild epithelial bleeding. These edemas will almost always resolve unless there is an underlying vascular disorder. If possible, samples should be taken from areas devoid of large subepithelial vessels.

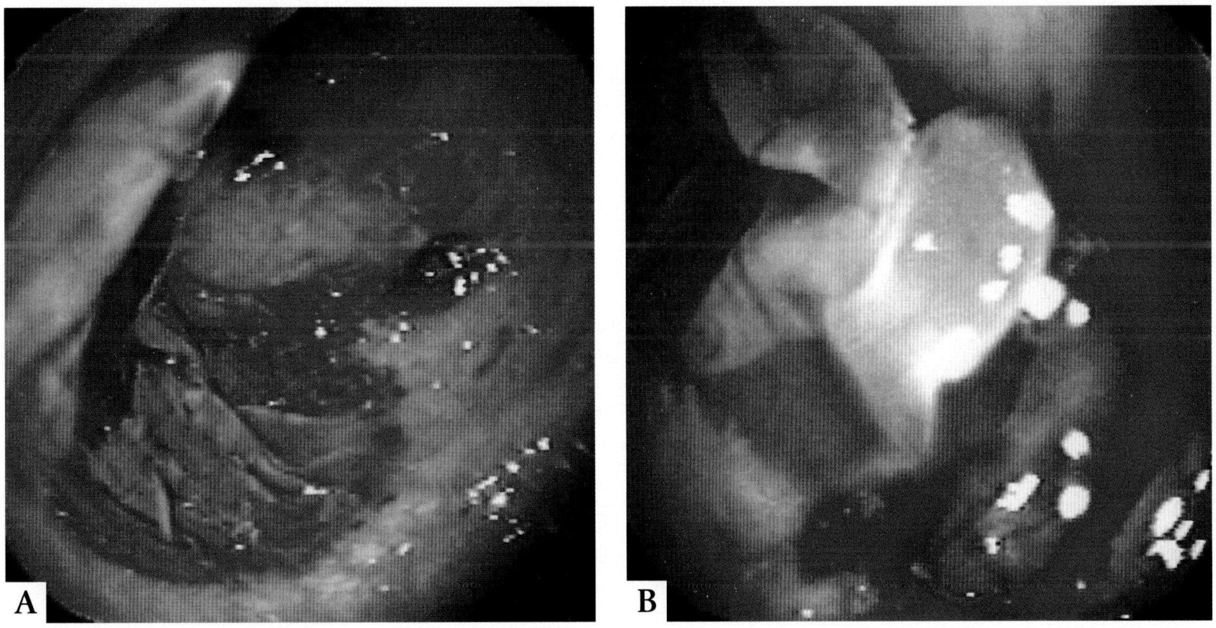

FIGURE 2-36.

Rupture of a large submucosal hematoma. This rupture occurred in a patient with unsuspected Ehler-Danlos syndrome after a simple mucosal biopsy. Mucosal biopsies can be associated with submucosal hematomas, but they are rarely of clinical importance, even in patients with mild coagulopathy. Biopsy specimens should be taken from areas void of visible vessels. **Panel A** represents the ruptured hematoma. **Panel B** represents the denuded membrane seen 5-cm distal to the hematoma.

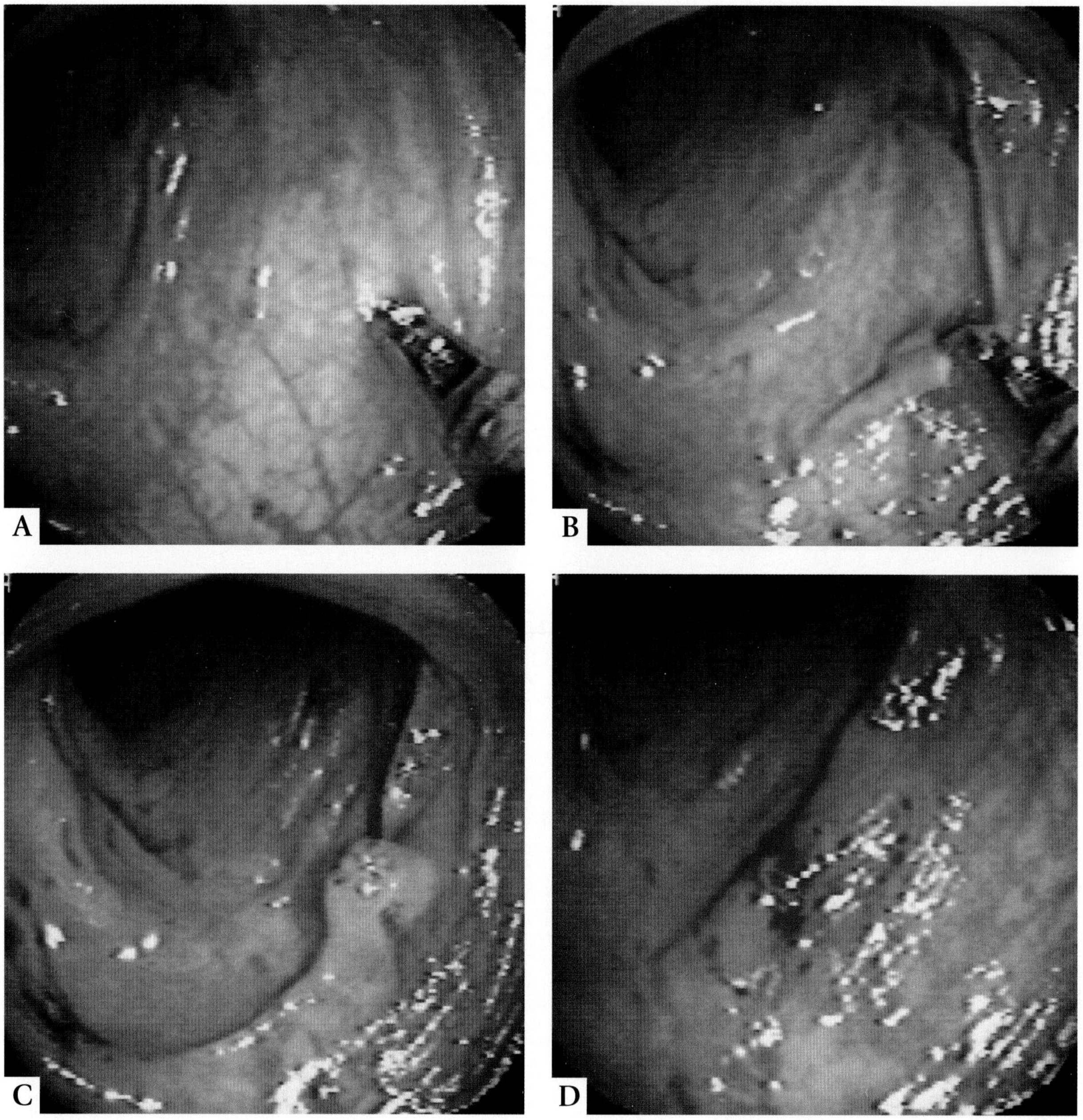

FIGURE 2-37.

The biopsy sequence with a standard forceps. **A**, The unopened forceps is passed into the colon through the biopsy channel. **B**, The biopsy forceps is opened and the mucosa is grasped. **C**, The biopsy forceps is retrieved and leaves a biopsy artifact simulating a suction artifact. **D**, With time, small amounts of heme are seen and the pulled-up mucosa flattens. This sequence is similar when using the "hot biopsy" forceps but a whitish cautery will be seen.

Chapter 3

Neoplasia of the Colon and Rectum

ROBERT S. BRESALIER

Cancers of the colon and rectum (colorectal cancers) represent a major cause of morbidity and mortality in the United States and other Westernized countries. It is estimated that in 1995 there will be 149,000 new cases of colorectal cancer and 56,000 related deaths in the United States. Overall colorectal cancer represents the second most common cause of cancer-related deaths in this country (second only to lung cancer).

This chapter covers a wide variety of topics related to neoplasia of the colon and rectum. Epidemiology of colorectal cancer and the roles of environmental and genetic factors that play a role in causation are examined. Preneoplastic adenomatous polyps and the hereditary adenomatous and harmartomatous syndrome are covered as is the topic of carcinoma arising in ulcerative colitis. Gross and histologic characteristics of preneoplastic and neoplastic lesions are viewed through endoscopic photographs, radiographs, and photomicrographs of histologic specimens. Tables and charts review the clinical and pathologic features of colorectal neoplasia, including staging of diseases. Screening for adenomatous polyps and colorectal cancers is examined, including the use of fecal occult blood testing and sigmoidoscopy. The vast majority of colorectal cancers are adenocarcinomas. Lymphomas and carcinoid tumors of the large bowel are briefly covered as well.

Rates, incidences, and causes

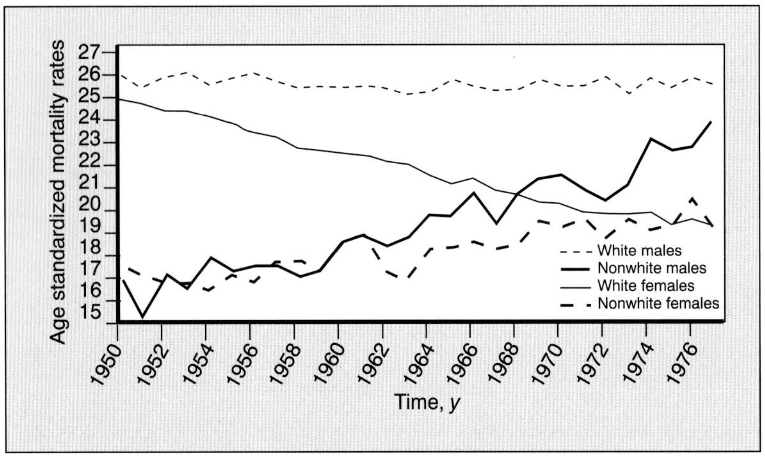

FIGURE 3-1.

Colorectal cancer mortality rates among white and nonwhite populations by gender in the United States. Mortality rates have remained relatively stable during the past several decades in white males, have decreased in white females, and have increased substantially in the nonwhite population. (*From* Boyle *et al.* [1]; with permission.)

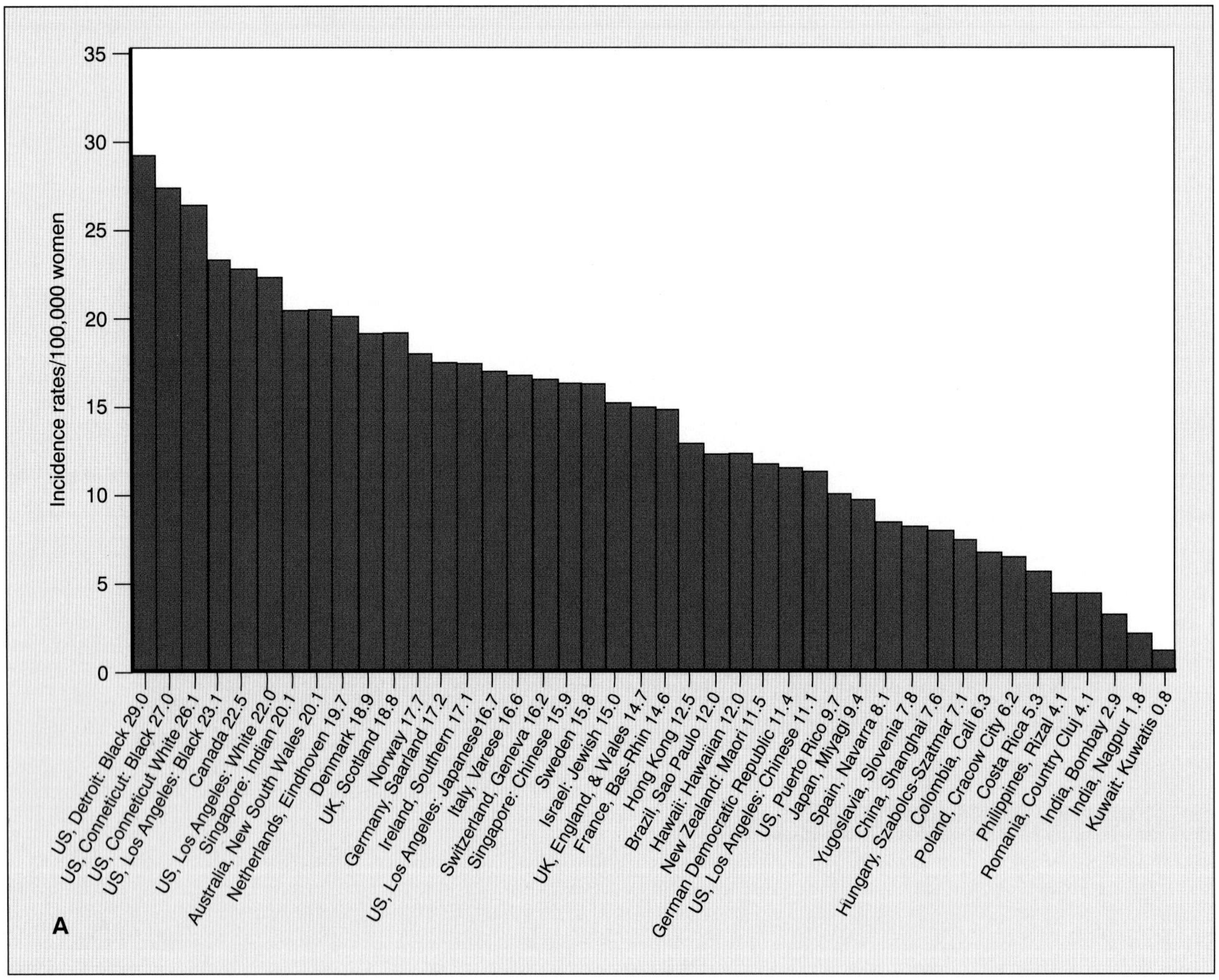

FIGURE 3-2.

Age-standardized rates of colon cancer in populations having the highest and lowest rates worldwide. Incidence is per 100,000 population in men (**A**) and women (**B**).
(Continued on next page)

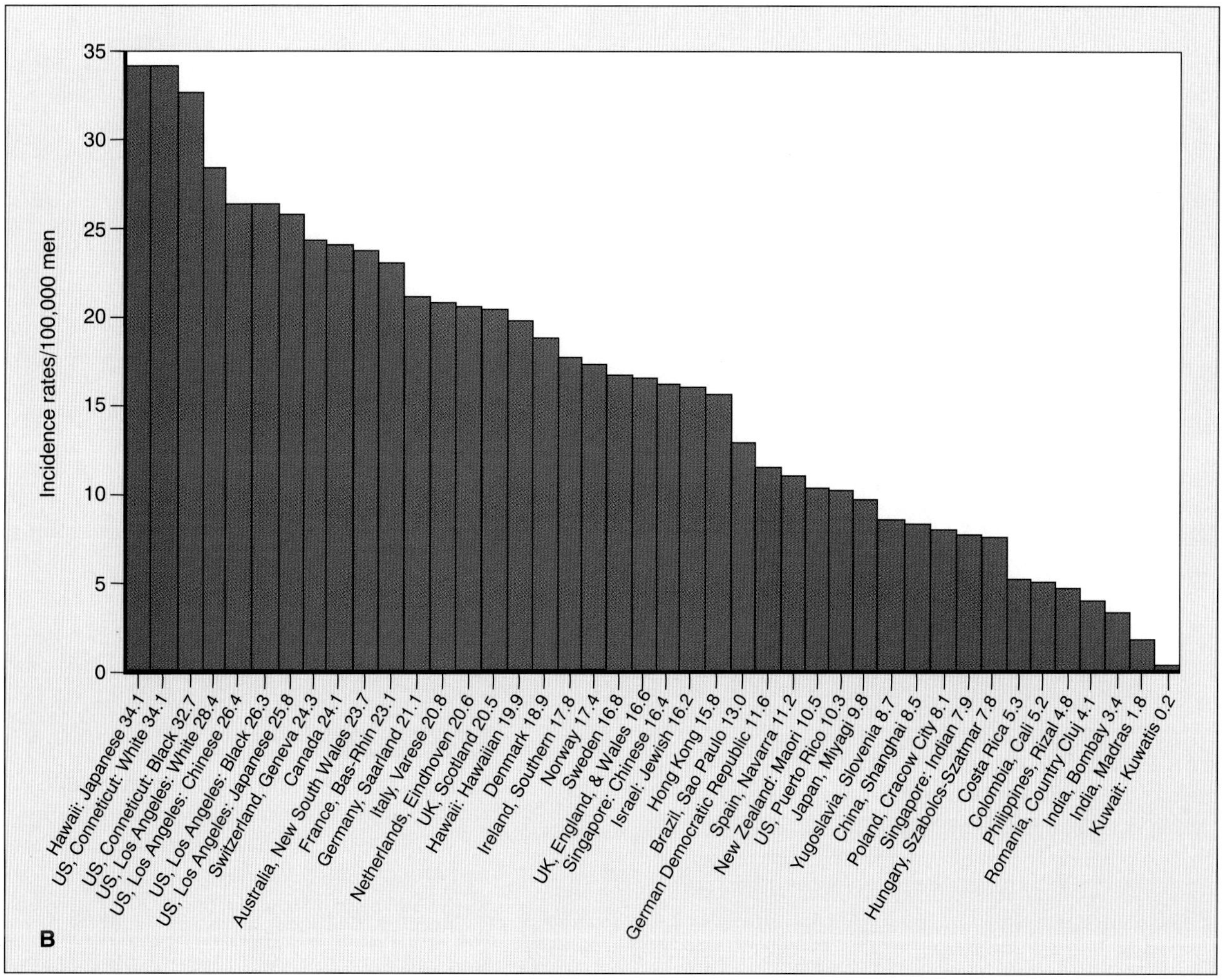

FIGURE 3-2. *(CONTINUED)*

The incidence of colon and rectal cancer varies substantially worldwide, with high incidence rates in the westernized countries of North America, Australia, and New Zealand, intermediate rates in Europe, and low rates in regions of Asia, South America, and sub-Saharan Africa. (*Data from* Whalen *et al.* [2].)

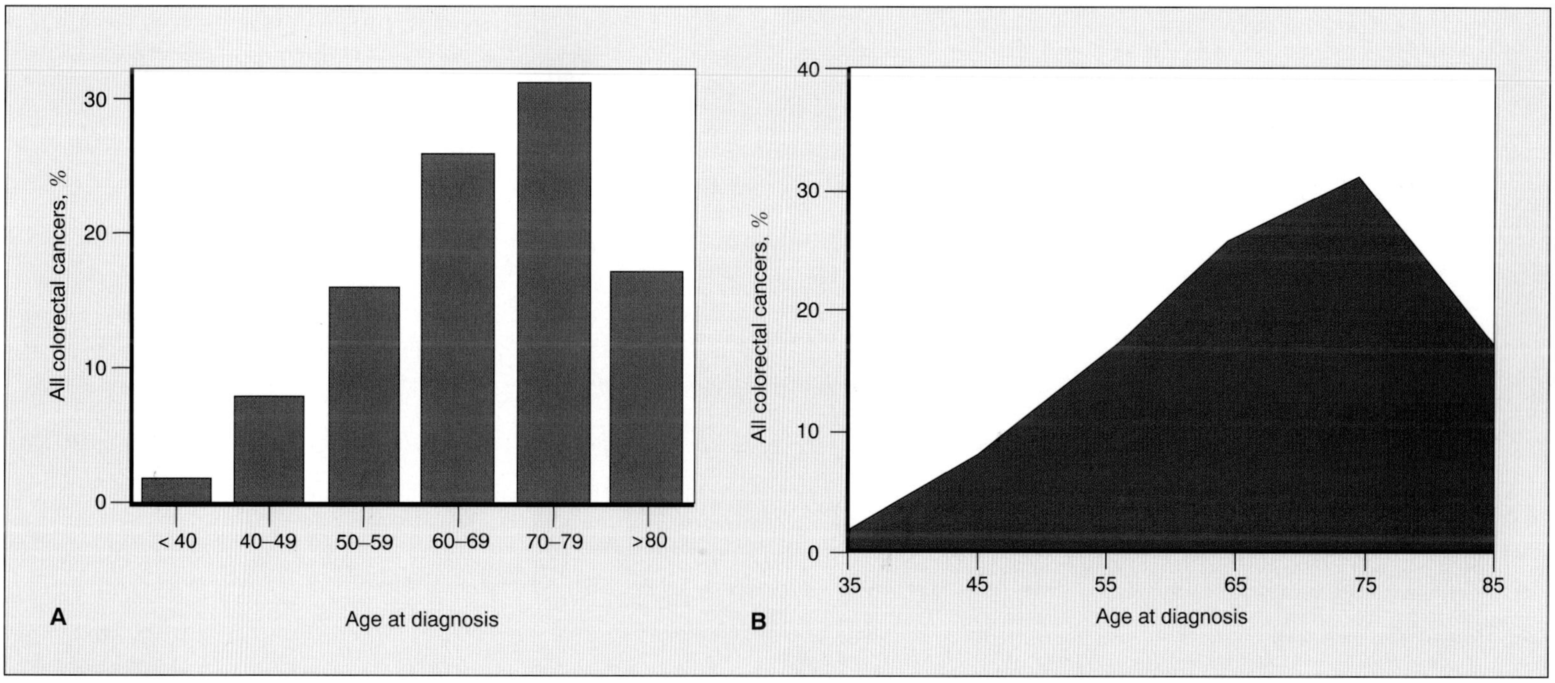

FIGURE 3-3.

A and **B**, Colorectal cancer incidence by age in the United States. The percent of colorectal cancers by age at diagnosis is shown. The majority of colon cancer in the general population occurs after the age of 50. (*Data from* The Surveillance, Epidemiology and End Results (SEER) Program.)

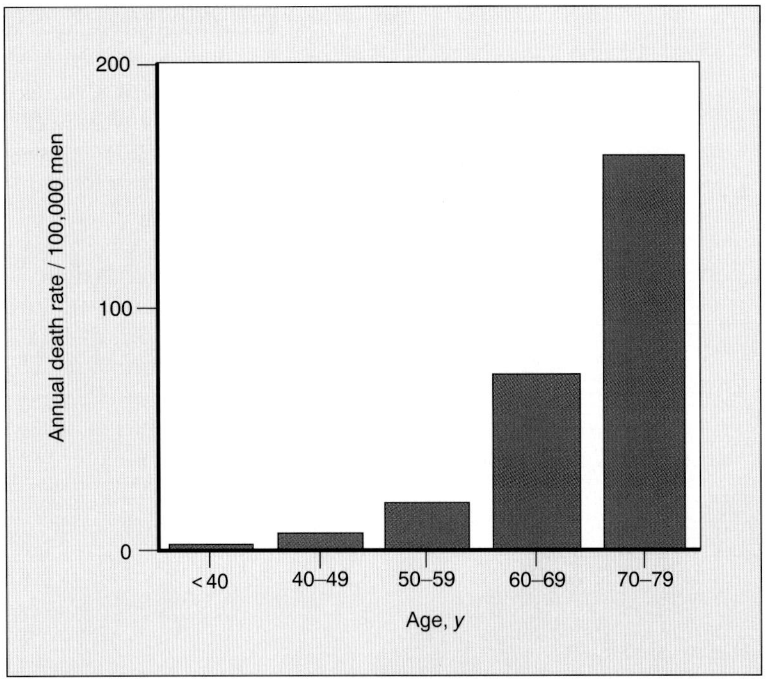

FIGURE 3-4.

Colorectal cancer death rates in men in the United States according to age. Death rate reflects the age-related incidence of colorectal cancer in the general population.

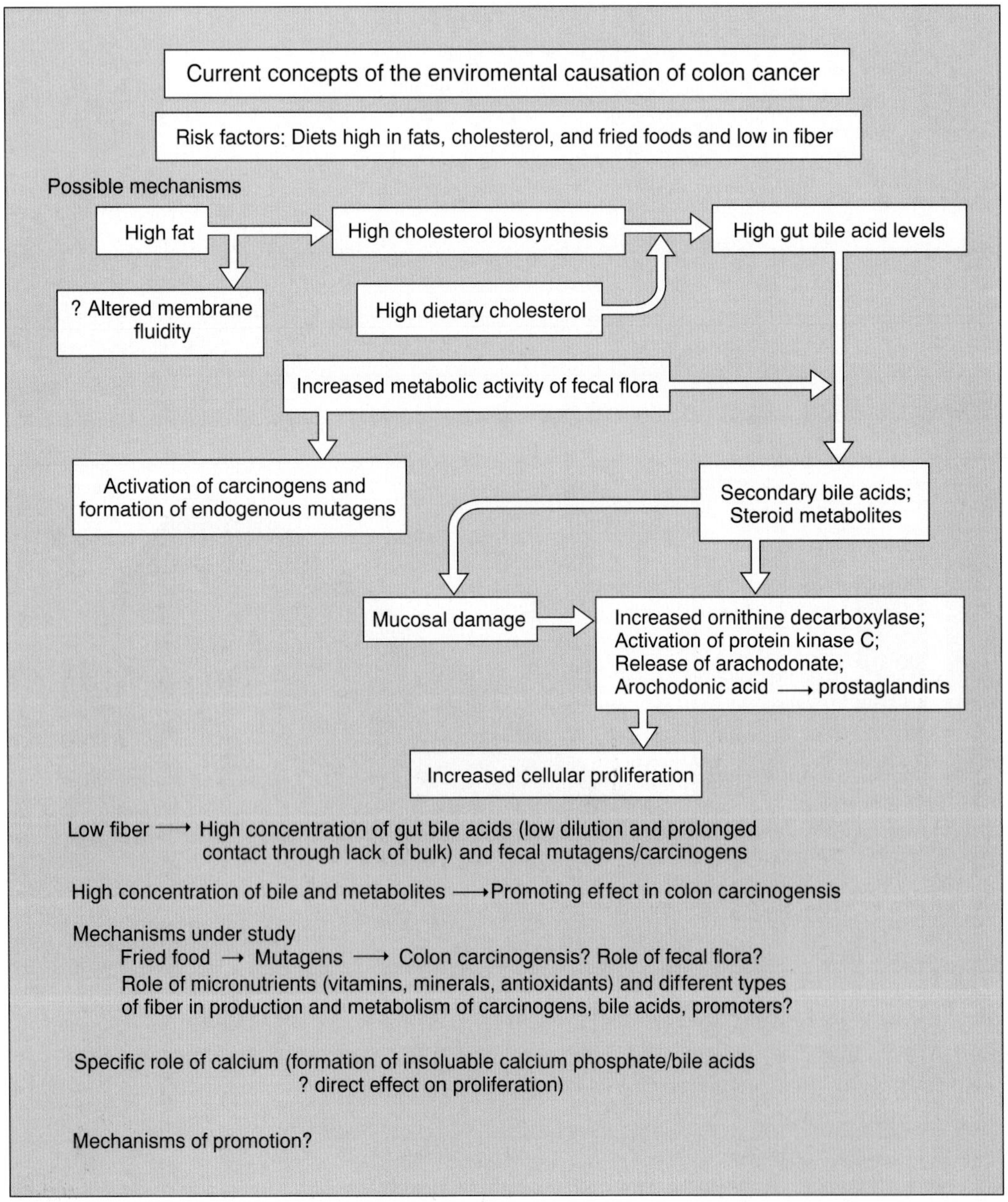

FIGURE 3-5.

Current concepts of the environmental causation of colon cancer. Mechanisms by which high-fat, low-fiber diets influence carcinogenesis in the colon are based on epidemiologic associations, animal models, and laboratory investigations. The exact mechanisms, however, remain speculative. The role of macronutrients and micronutrients in the diet in promoting carcinogenesis or in protecting the mucosa remain to be fully determined. (*From* Bresalier and Kim [3]; with permission.)

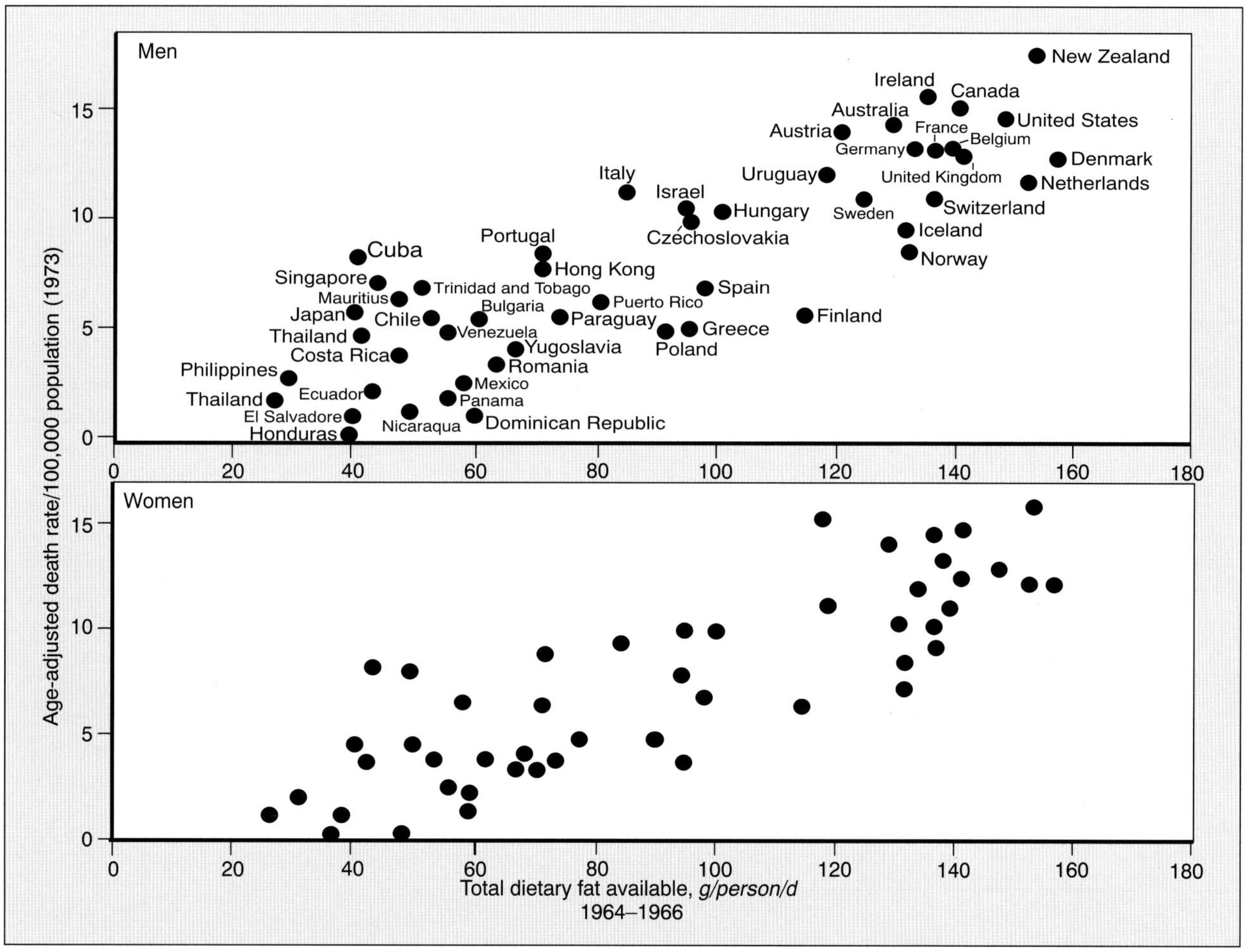

FIGURE 3-6.

Correlation between age-adjusted mortality from colon cancer and consumption of fat. Total dietary fat intake parallels the colon cancer-associated death rate. Potential mechanisms by which high fat intake may promote carcinogenesis in the colon are outlined in Figure 3-5. (*From* Reddy *et al.* [4]; with permission.)

Abnormal proliferation of neoplasia

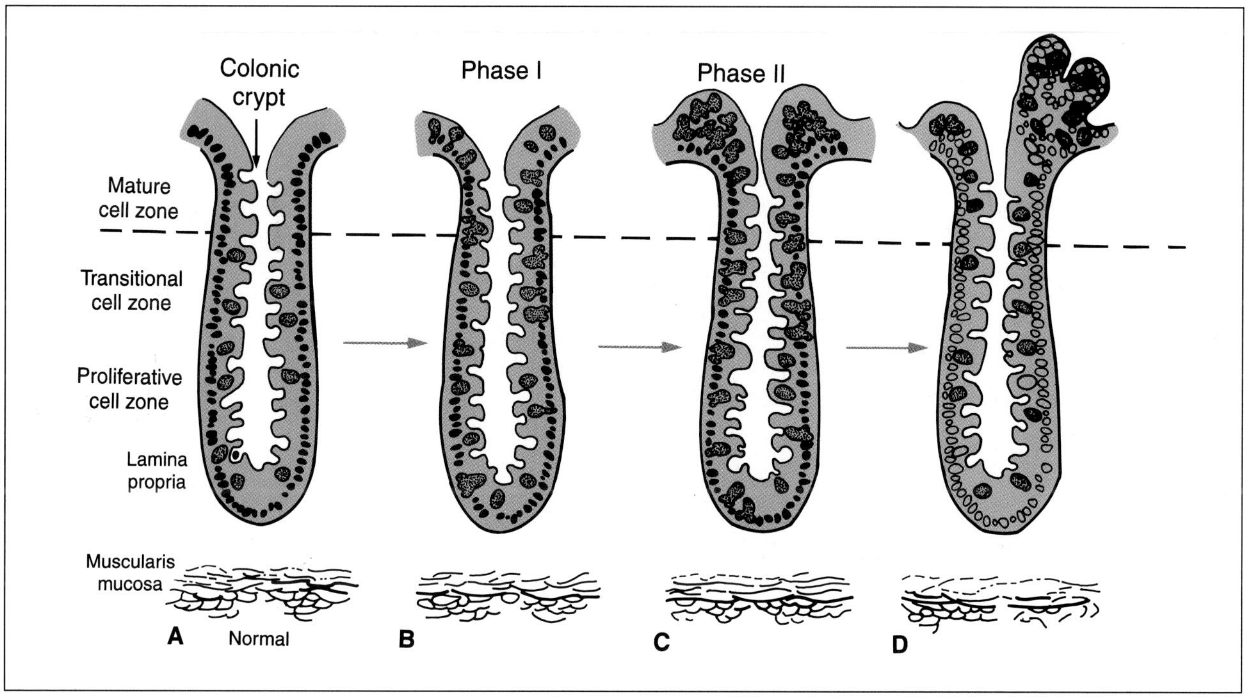

FIGURE 3-7.

Abnormal proliferation is a hallmark of neoplasia. This figure depicts a sequence of events to account for the location of abnormally proliferating colonic epithelial cells before and during the formation of polypoid neoplasms in humans. **A**, Location of proliferating and differentiating epithelial cells in normal colonic crypt. Dark cells illustrate thymidine labeling in cells that are synthesizing DNA and preparing to undergo cell division. As cells pass from the proliferative zone through the transitional zone, DNA synthesis and mitosis are repressed, and migrating epithelial cells leave the proliferative cell cycle to undergo normal maturation before they reach the surface of the mucosa. **B**, Development of a phase I proliferative lesion in the colonic epithelial cells as they fail to repress the incorporation of thymidine^{3}H into DNA and begin to develop an enhanced ability to proliferate. The mucosa is flat and the number of new cells born equals the number extruded without excess cell accumulation in the mucosa. **C**, Development of a phase II proliferative lesion in colonic epithelial cells. The cells incorporate thymidine ^{3}H into DNA and also have developed additional properties that enable them to accumulate in the mucosa as neoplasms begin to form. **D**, Further differentiation of abnormally retained proliferating epithelial cells into pathologically defined neoplastic lesions, including adenomatous polyps and villous adenomas. (*Adapted from* Lipkin [5]; with permission.)

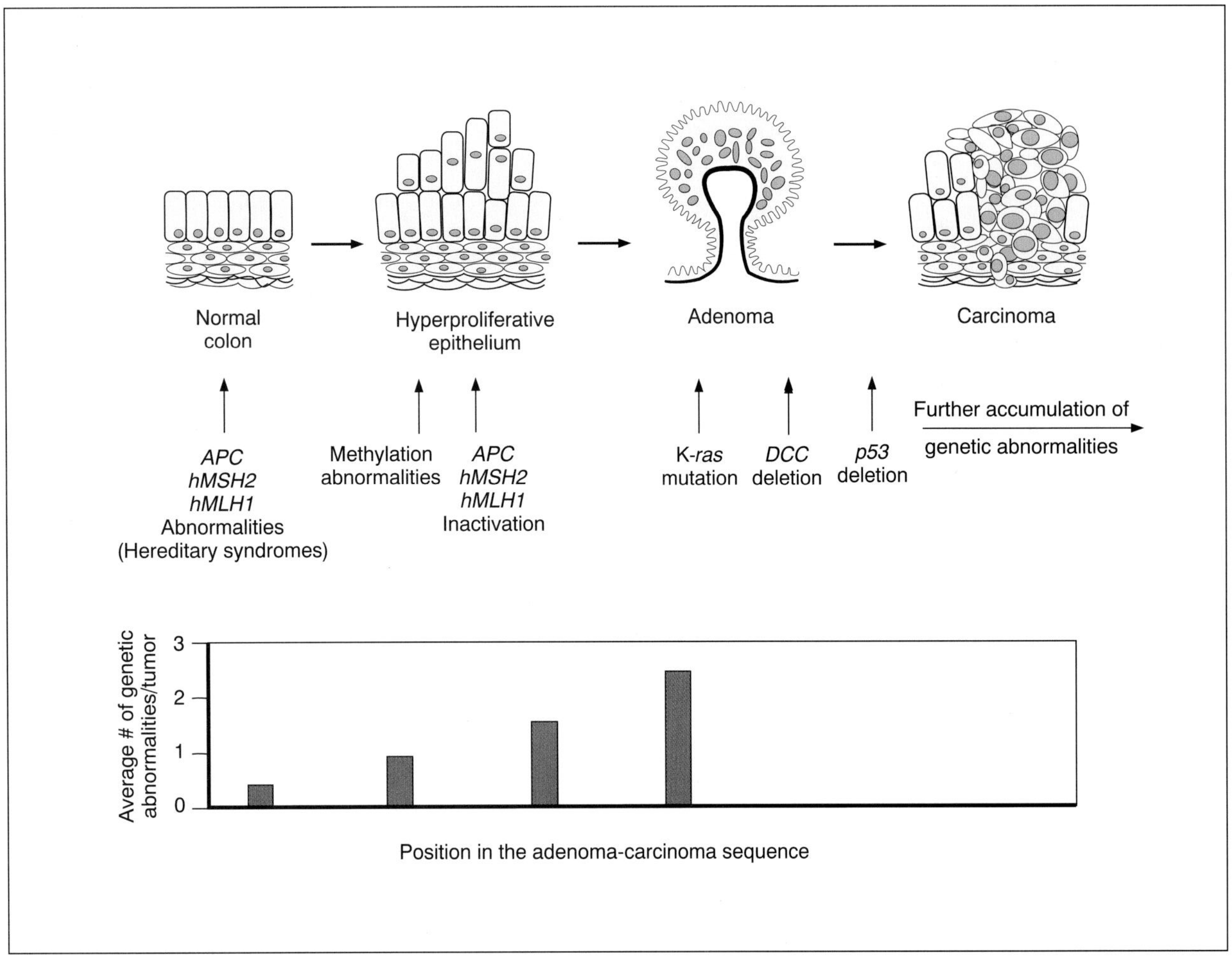

FIGURE 3-8.

Molecular genetic events in the evolution of colon cancer. The progression to colorectal cancer is associated with an accumulation of genetic alterations, including alterations in oncogenes (K-*ras*), tumor suppressor genes (*APC, DCC, p53*), and DNA repair genes (*hMSH2, hMLH1*). The exact sequence of events is approximate and may vary in sporadic cancers compared with those arising in hereditary syndromes or inflammatory bowel disease. (*Adapted from* Bresalier *et al.* [6]; with permission.)

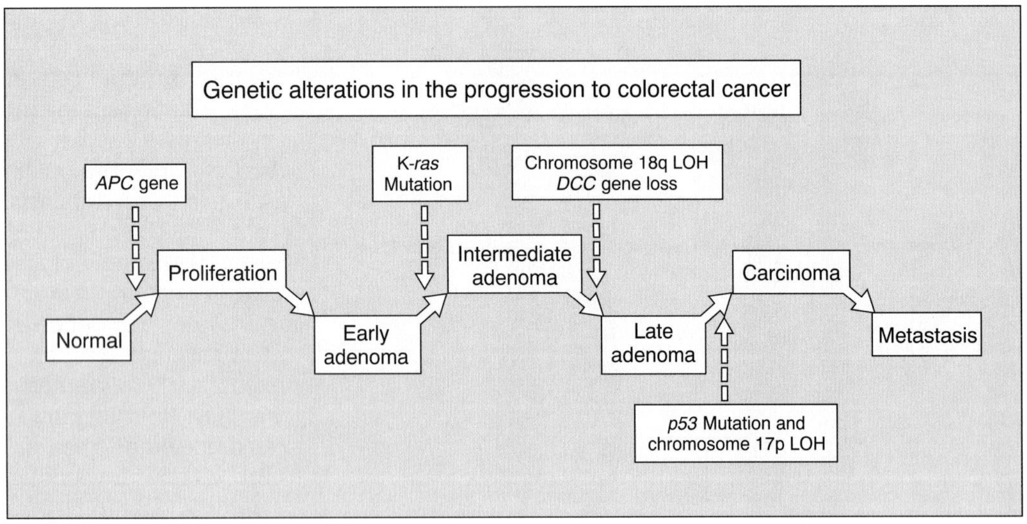

FIGURE 3-9.

Genetic alterations in the progression to colorectal cancer. Colorectal cancers arise through an accumulation of genetic events, which include alterations in oncogenes, tumor suppressor genes, and DNA repair genes. These alterations may be inherited (germ line mutations) or acquired (*see* Fig. 3-8) [7]. LOH—loss of heterozygosity.

TABLE 3-1. GENES ALTERED IN COLON CANCER

GENE	CHROMOSOME	SPORADIC TUMORS WITH ALTERATIONS, %	CLASS	FUNCTION
K-ras	12	50	Protooncogene	Signal transduction
APC	5	60	Tumor supressor	?Cell adhesion
DCC	18	70	Tumor supressor	?Cell adhesion
p53	17	75	Tumor supressor	Cell cycle control (G1/S arrest)
hMSH2	2		DNA Mismatch repair	Maintains fidelity of DNA replication
hMLH1	3		DNA Mismatch repair	Maintains fidelity of DNA replication

TABLE 3-1.

Genes altered in sporadic colon cancer. Percentages of tumors with altered genes are approximate. The genes *hMSH2* and *hMLH1* are commonly altered in nonpolyposis hereditary colon cancer, but the incidence of gene abnormalities in sporadic cancers is unknown. Replication errors are present in about 15% of sporadic cancers.

Hereditary nonpolyposis colorectal cancer

TABLE 3-2. HEREDITARY NONPOLYPOSIS COLORECTAL CANCER

Three or more relatives with colorectal cancer (one must be first-degree relative of other two)

Colorectal cancer involving at least two generations

One or more colorectal cancer cases before age 50

TABLE 3-2.

Criteria for diagnosis of hereditary nonpolyposis colorectal cancer established by the International Collaborative Group on Hereditary Nonpolyposis Colorectal Cancer [8]. This familial syndrome is inherited in an autosomal dominant manner. Defects in DNA mismatch repair genes on chromosomes 2 and 3 that maintain the fidelity of DNA replication have been linked to a high percentage of nonpolyposis hereditary colon cancer kindreds.

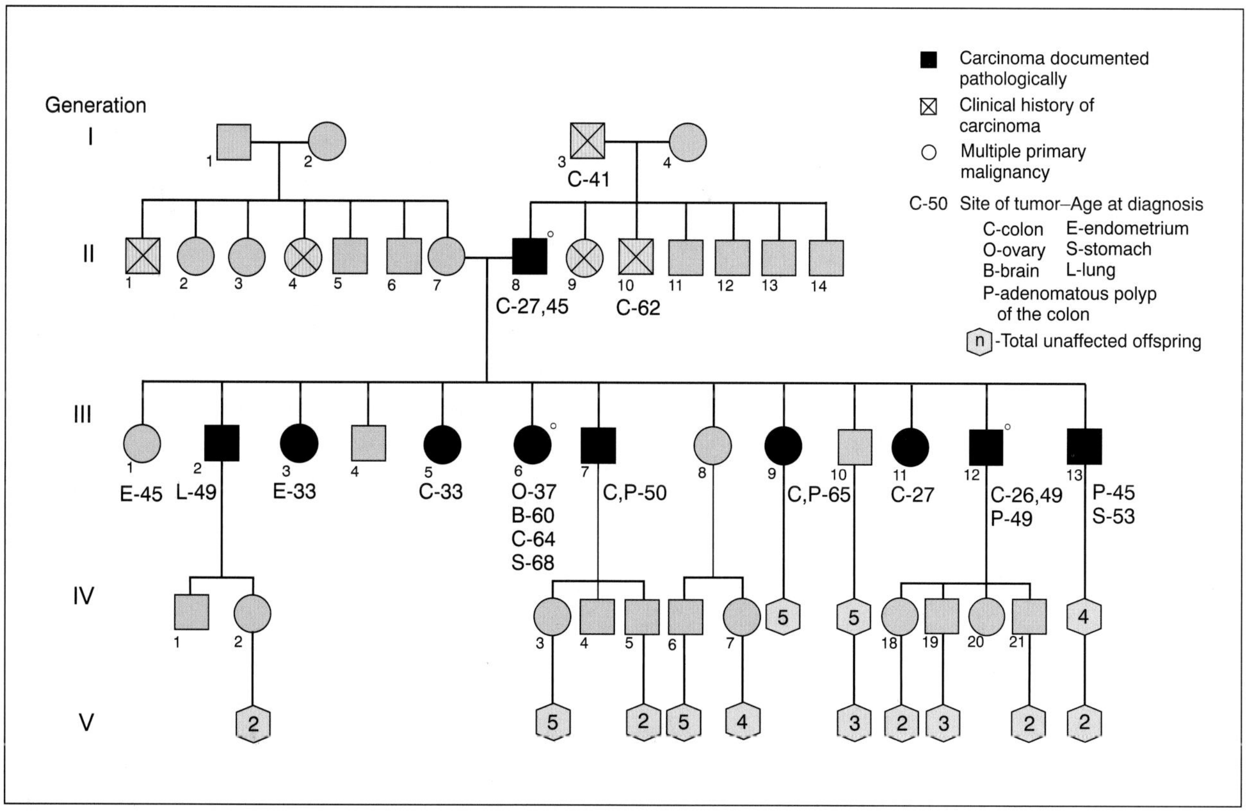

FIGURE 3-10.

Pattern of inheritance of cancer in a family with cancer family syndrome (hereditary nonpolyposis colorectal cancer type b, Lynch syndrome II). Affected members are found in generations I, II, and III; members of generations IV and V are young and still at risk for developing cancer. Family members are prone to cancers of the female genital tract and other sites in addition to colorectal cancer. (*From* Boland [9]; with permission.)

TABLE 3-3. HNPCC CLINICAL CHARACTERISTICS

Characteristics	HNPCC	Sporadic
Mean age at diagnosis, y	44.6	67
Multiple colon cancers, %	34.5	4–11
Synchronous	18.1	3–6
Metachronous	24.3	1–5
Proximal location, %	72.3	35
Excess malignancies at other sites	Yes	No
Mucinous and poorly differentiated cancers	Common	Infrequent
RER + %	79	17

Table 3-3.

Comparison of clinical characteristics of cancers arising in hereditary nonpolyposis colorectal cancer (HNPCC) with those of sporadic colon cancer. Cancers arising in this setting occur at a younger age and are often multiple and proximally located. RER—replication errors. (*Data from* Lynch *et al.* [10].)

Polyps and adenomas

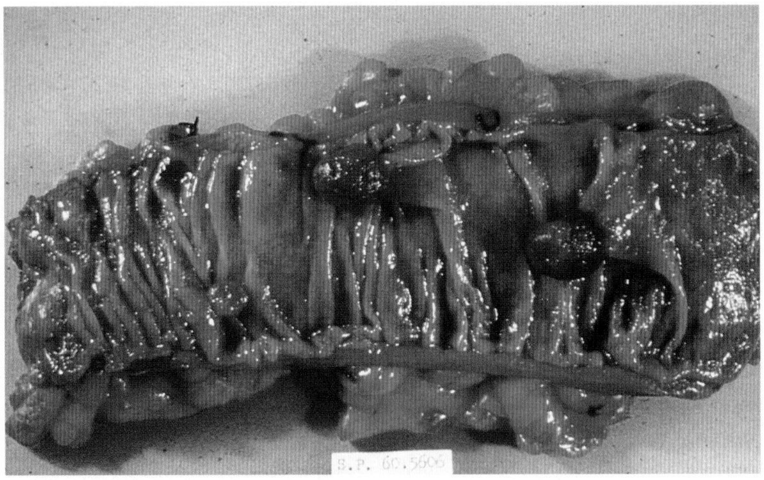

Figure 3-11.

Segmental colectomy specimen containing multiple pedunculated polyps. The vast majority of colorectal cancers arise in adenomatous polyps. These cancers may be pedunculated (on a stalk) or sessile.

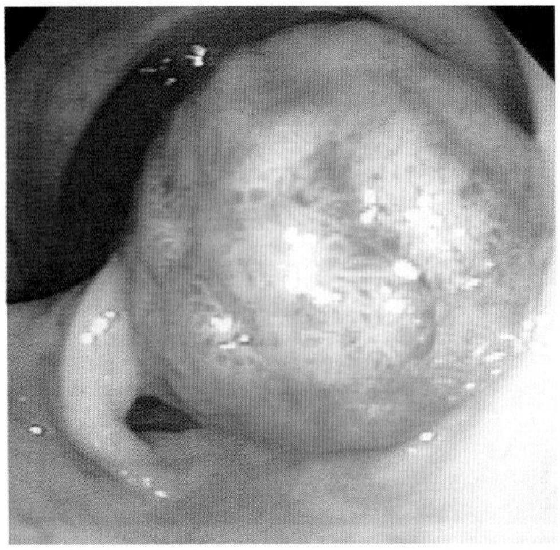

Figure 3-12.

Large pedunculated polyp seen at colonoscopy. The polyp extends from the colonic mucosa by way of a fibrovascular stalk (*see* Fig. 3-14).

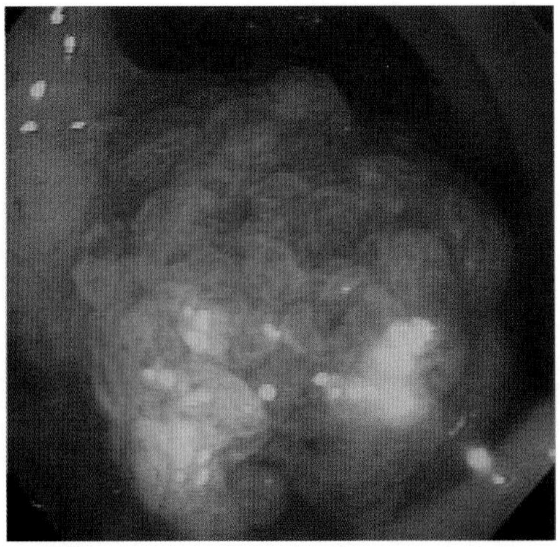

Figure 3-13.

Large sessile polyp seen at colonoscopy (villous adenoma). The polyp extends directly from the colonic wall. This large polyp was found to be a villous adenoma (*see* Fig. 3-15B).

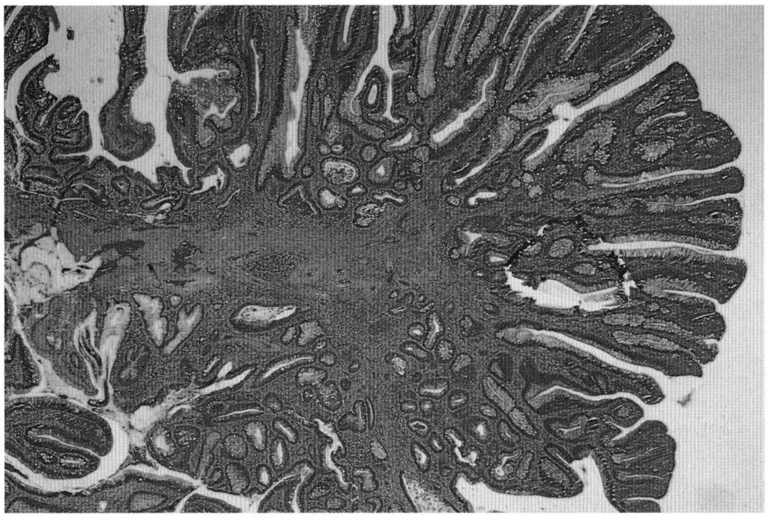

FIGURE 3-14.

Photomicrograph of tubular adenoma of the colon cut in cross section to demonstrate stalk. Tubular adenomas are characterized by a complex network of branching adenomatous glands.

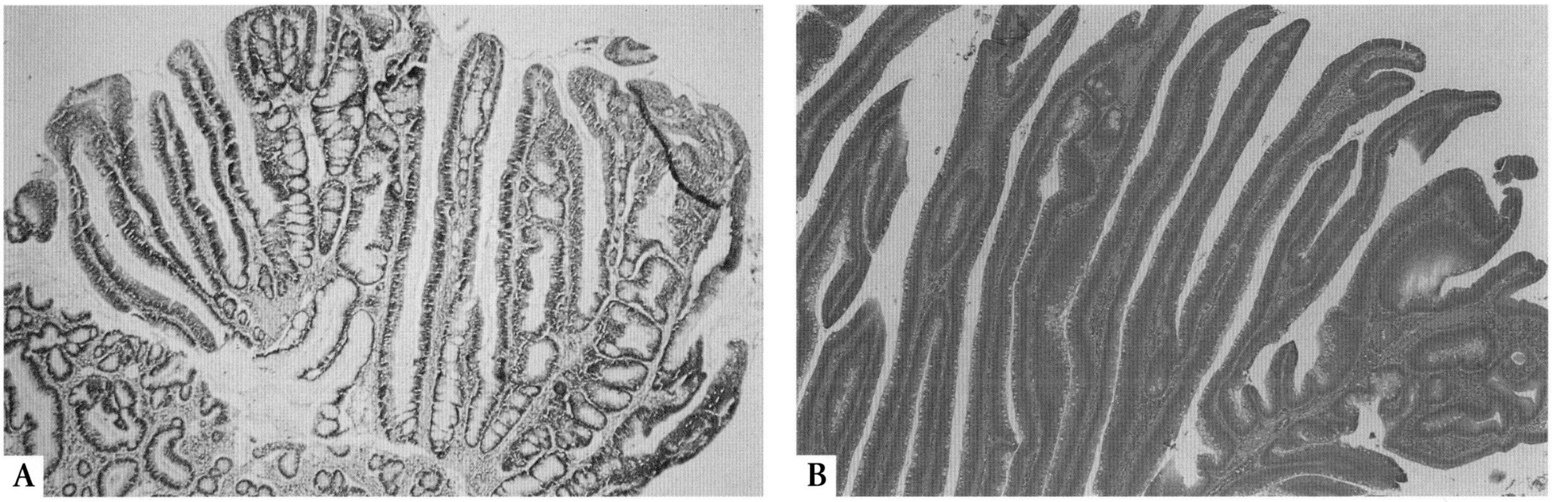

FIGURE 3-15.

Photomicrograph of a tubulovillous adenoma (**A**). This polyp has the characteristics of a tubular adenoma as well as adenomatous glands that extend straight down from the surface to the center of the polyp, which are characteristic of villous adenomas (**B**).

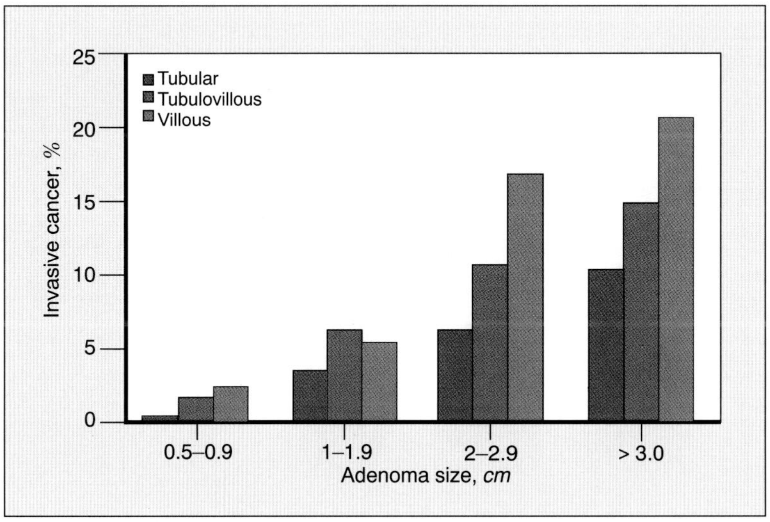

FIGURE 3-16.

The percent of adenomas containing invasive cancer by size and histology. An analysis of 7000 endoscopically removed polyps was performed. Potential for malignant degeneration is associated with increased size and villous histology. (*Adapted from* Bresalier [11]; with permission.)

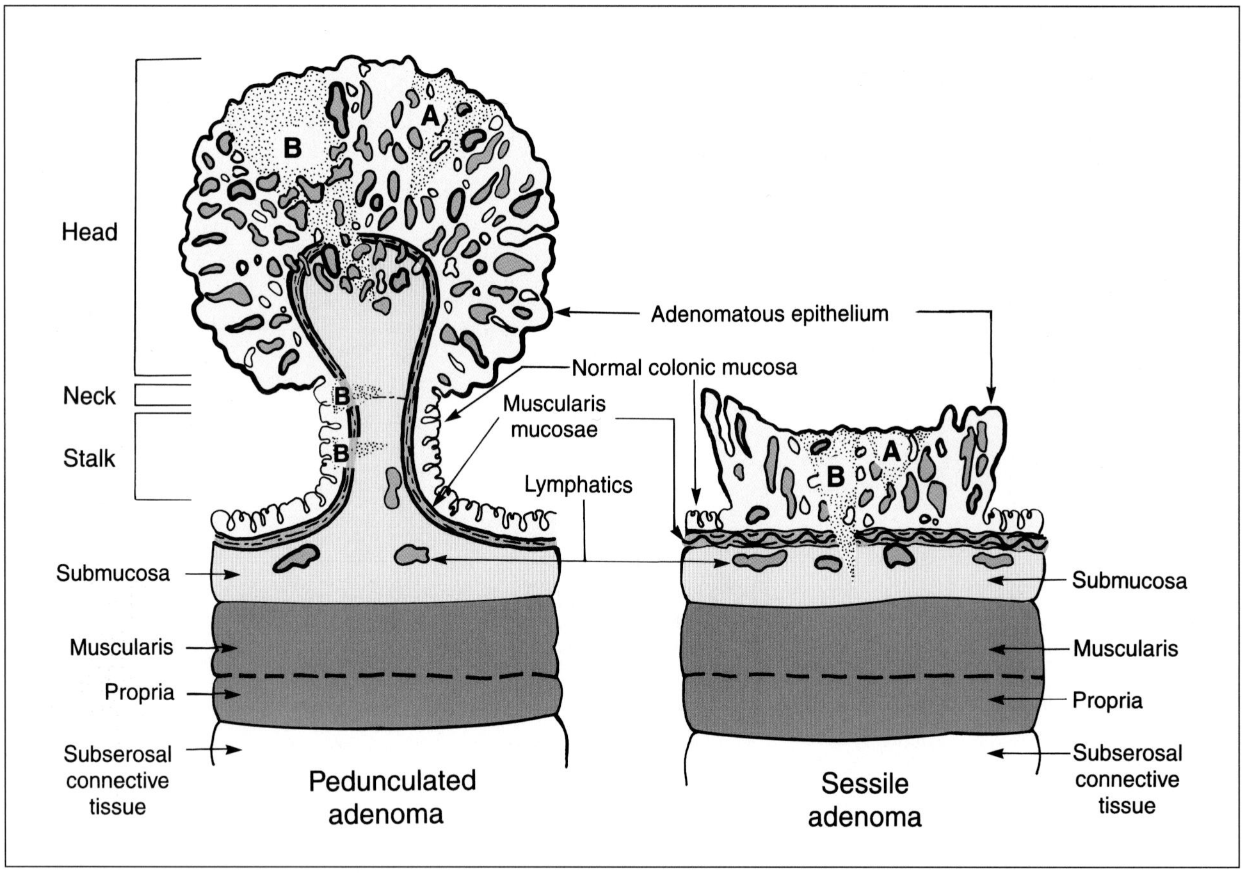

FIGURE 3-17.

Diagrammatic representation of carcinoma within a polyp. *Black wedges* represent foci of carcinoma. *A wedges* indicate carcinoma *in situ;* malignant cells do not traverse the muscularis mucosae. *B wedges* indicate invasive carcinoma; malignant cells have breached the muscularis mucosae. (*Adapted from* Haggitt *et al.* [12]; with permission.)

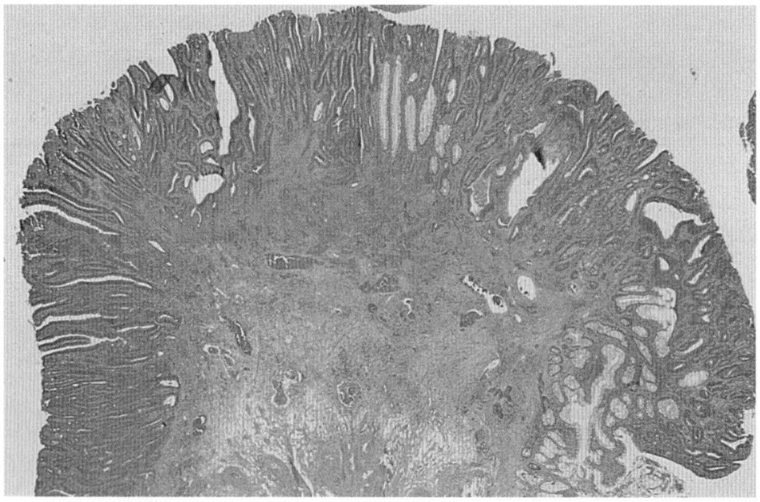

FIGURE 3-18.

Low-power photomicrograph of pedunculated adenoma containing focus of adenocarcinoma. Malignant glands can be seen invading stalk. This figure is analogous to the *B wedges* in Figure 3-17.

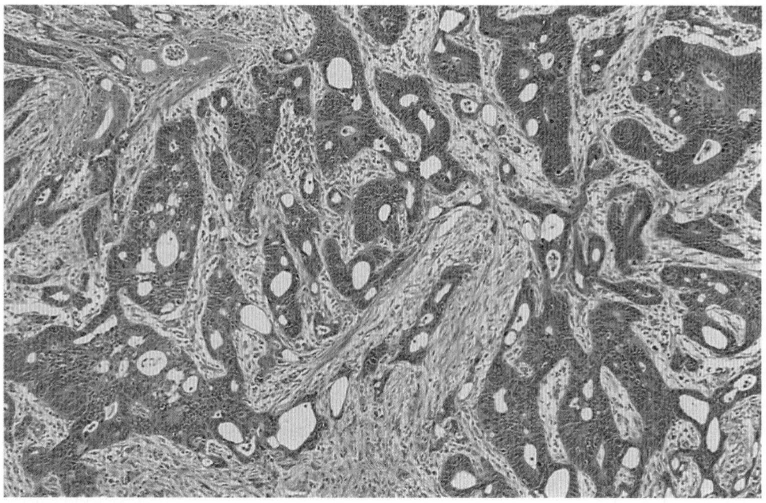

FIGURE 3-19.

High-power view of the stalk of polyp seen in Figure 3-18. Well-differentiated carcinomatous glands are seen invading the polyp stalk.

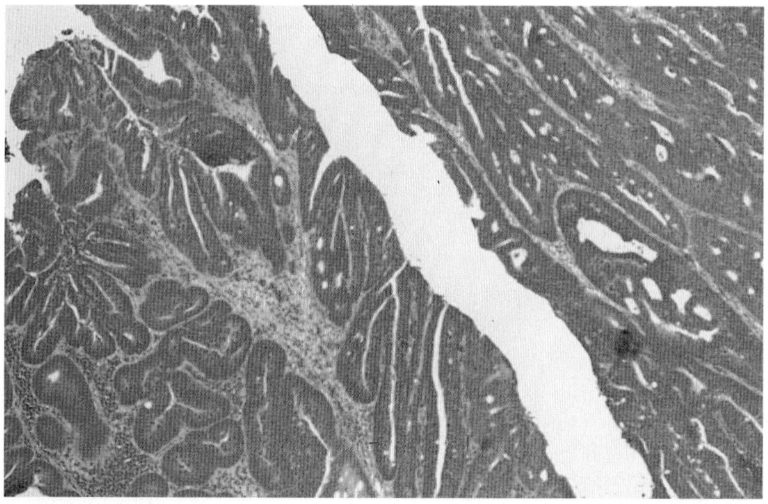

FIGURE 3-20.

Severe atypia (carcinoma *in situ*) in the head of an adenomatous polyp. Glands are irregular and crowded. The cells have a high nuclear to cytoplasmic ratio.

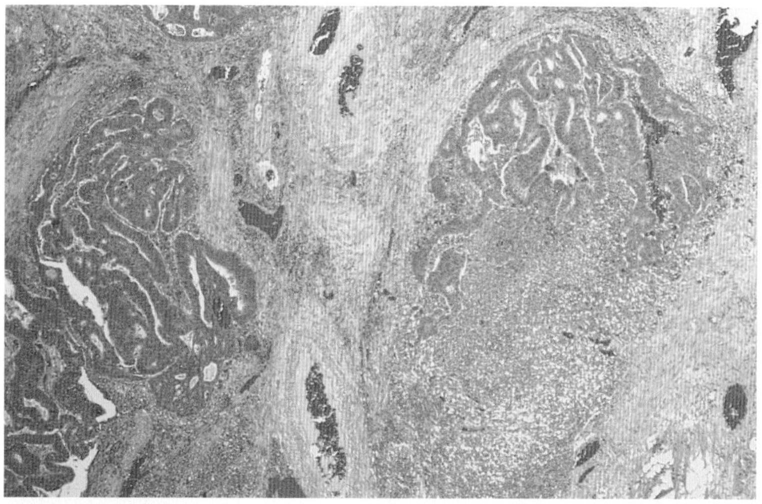

FIGURE 3-21.

Well-differentiated adenocarcinoma invading the neck of an adenomatous polyp (*ie*, submucosal invasion). Malignant glands are seen in close proximity to vascular structures and are at the resection margin, indicating high likelihood of extension beyond the confines of the polyp.

Familial adenomatous polyposis

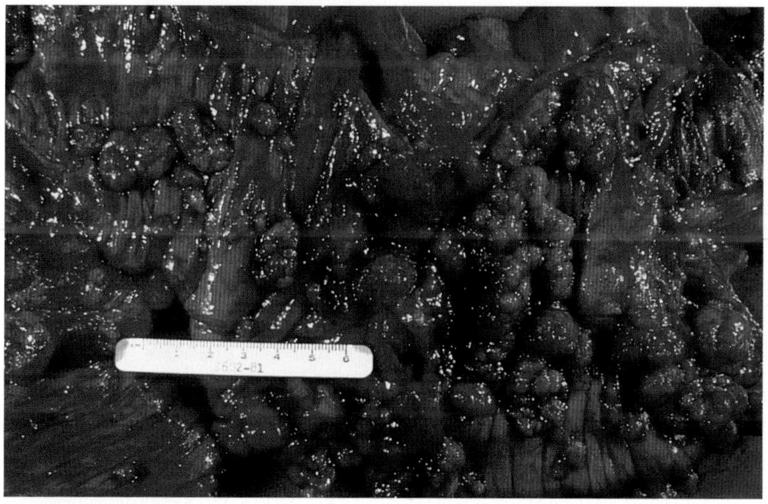

FIGURE 3-22.

Colectomy specimen from a patient with familial adenomatous polyposis coli. In this syndrome, hundreds to thousands of adenomatous polyps arise in the colon. This disease is inherited as an autosomal dominant gene located on chromosome 5q (*APC*). If the colon is not removed in these individuals, the development of colon cancer is inevitable.

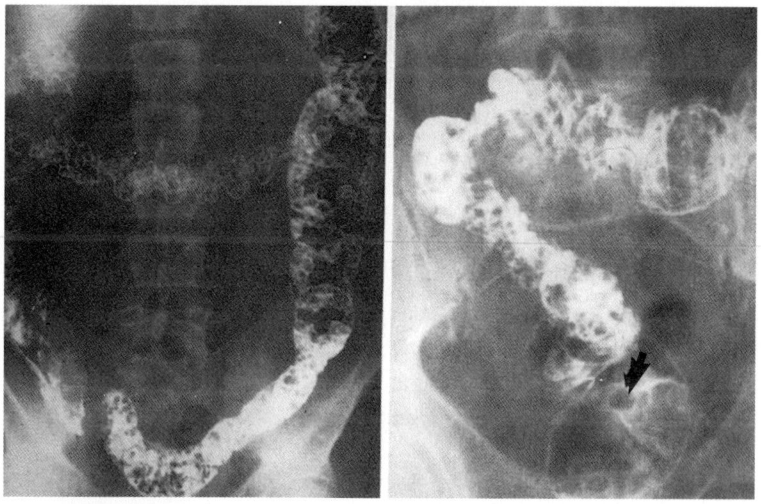

FIGURE 3-23.

Radiograph of a barium enema from a patient with familial adenomatous polyposis. Thousands of polyps are seen as filling defects in the barium column. The *arrow* points to a carcinoma arising in this setting.

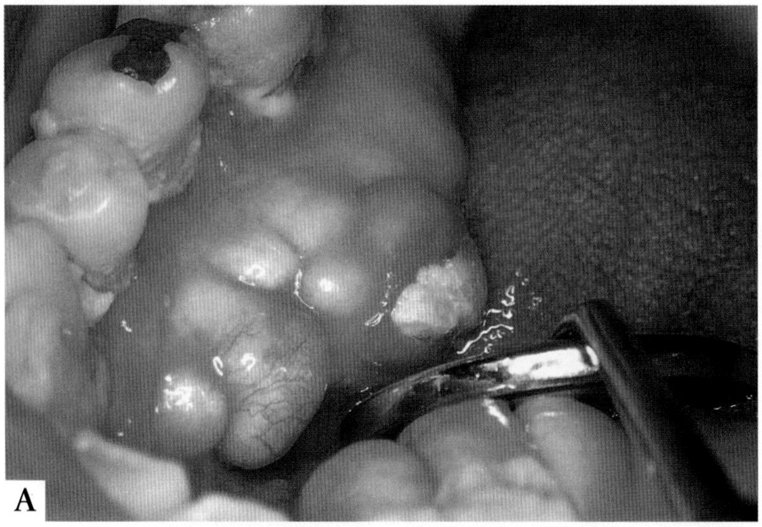

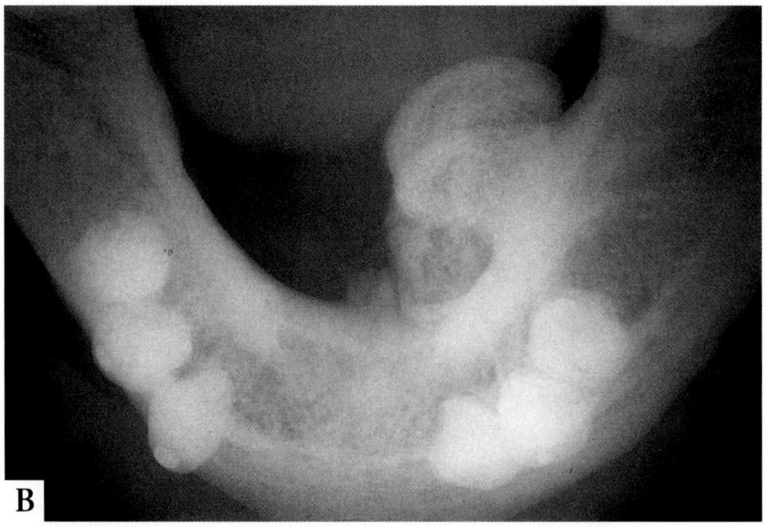

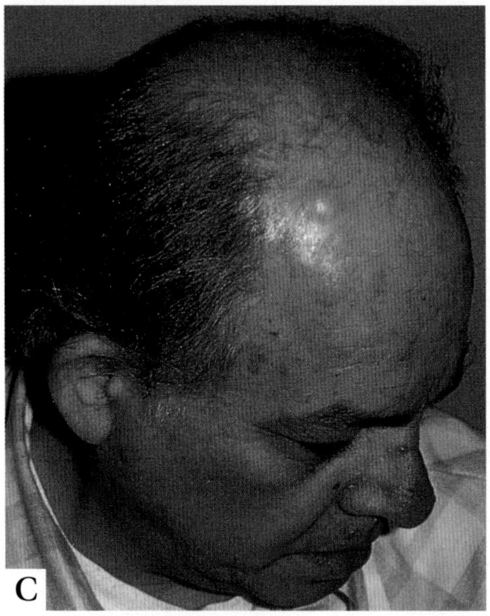

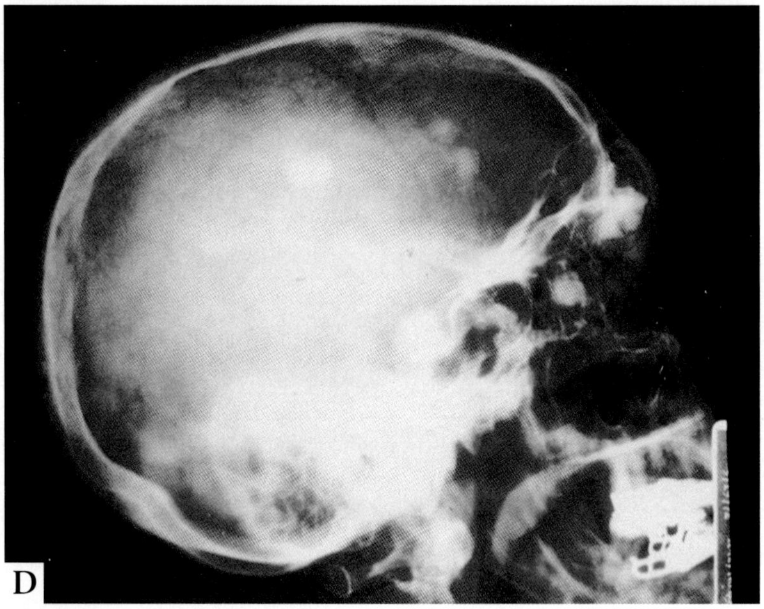

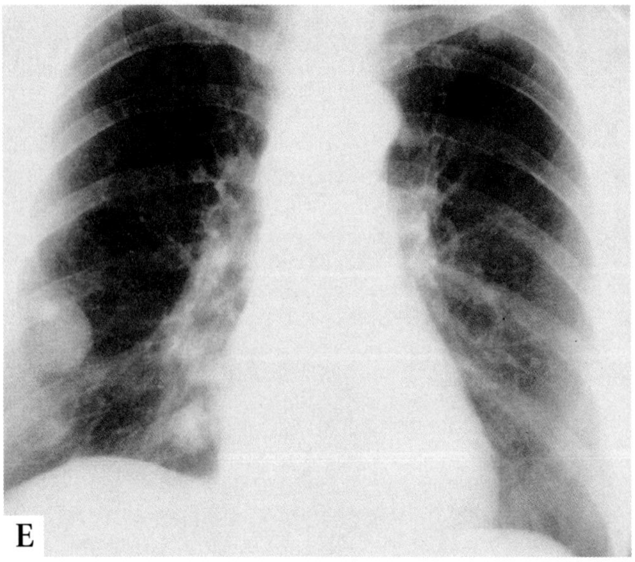

FIGURE 3-24.

Gardner's syndrome is a subset of familial adenomatous polyposis. Familial adenomatous polyposis and Gardner's syndrome are variable manifestations of a disease that may be traced to a single gene locus. The primary features of this syndrome are colonic polyposis, osteomas (particularly in the skull and mandible), and soft-tissue tumors. Periampullary tumors of the duodenum including carcinomas are also common. Soft-tissue tumors include epidermoid cysts, fibromas, lipomas, and desmoid tumors. **A**, Mandibular osteoma in a patient with Gardner's syndrome. **B**, Radiograph of a mandible demonstrating mandibular osteoma. **C**, Osteoma of the skull in a patient with gross Gardner's syndrome. **D**, Skull radiograph showing multiple osteomas. **E**, Fibroma seen as soft-tissue density on chest radiograph in a patient with Gardner's syndrome.

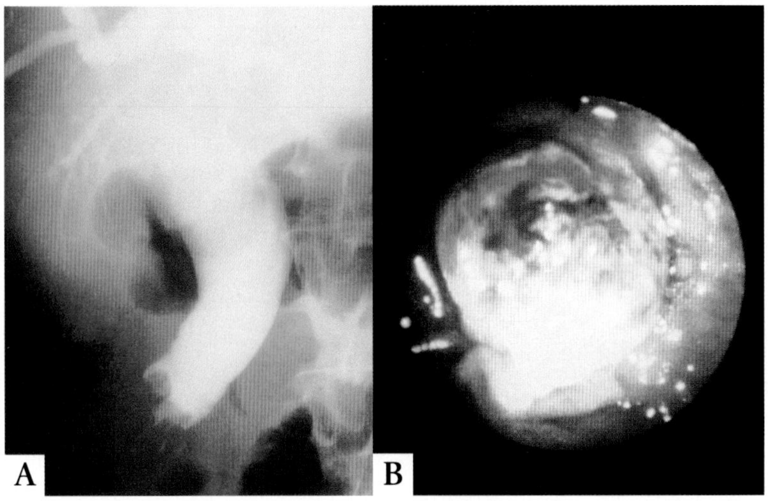

FIGURE 3-25.

Ampullary carcinoma arising in a patient with Gardner's syndrome. Cholangiogram demonstrates the dilated common bile duct (**A**). An endoscopic view of ampullary tumor (**B**) is also depicted.

Hamartomatous polyposis syndromes

Hamartomatous polyposis syndromes are characterized by multiple hamartomatous polyps of the gastrointestinal tract, including the colon. Although the hamartomas themselves carry no malignant potential, carcinomas of the colon do arise in adenomatous tissue associated with juvenile polyposis, the Peutz-Jeghers syndrome, and the Cronkhite-Canada syndrome.

Peutz-Jeghers syndrome

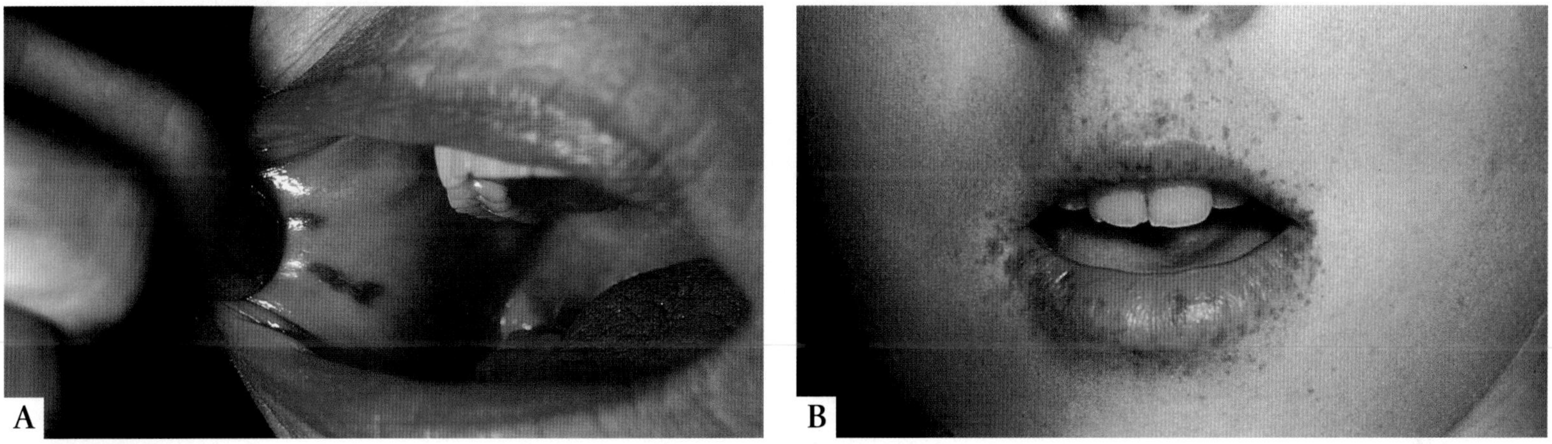

FIGURE 3-26.

A and **B**, Mucocutaneous pigmentation is depicted in a patient with Peutz-Jeghers syndrome. Hamartomas of gastrointestinal tract and mucocutaneous pigmentation define this familial syndrome (autosomal dominant with variable penetrance). Carcinomas of the colon and small intestine may arise in associated adenomatous epithelium.

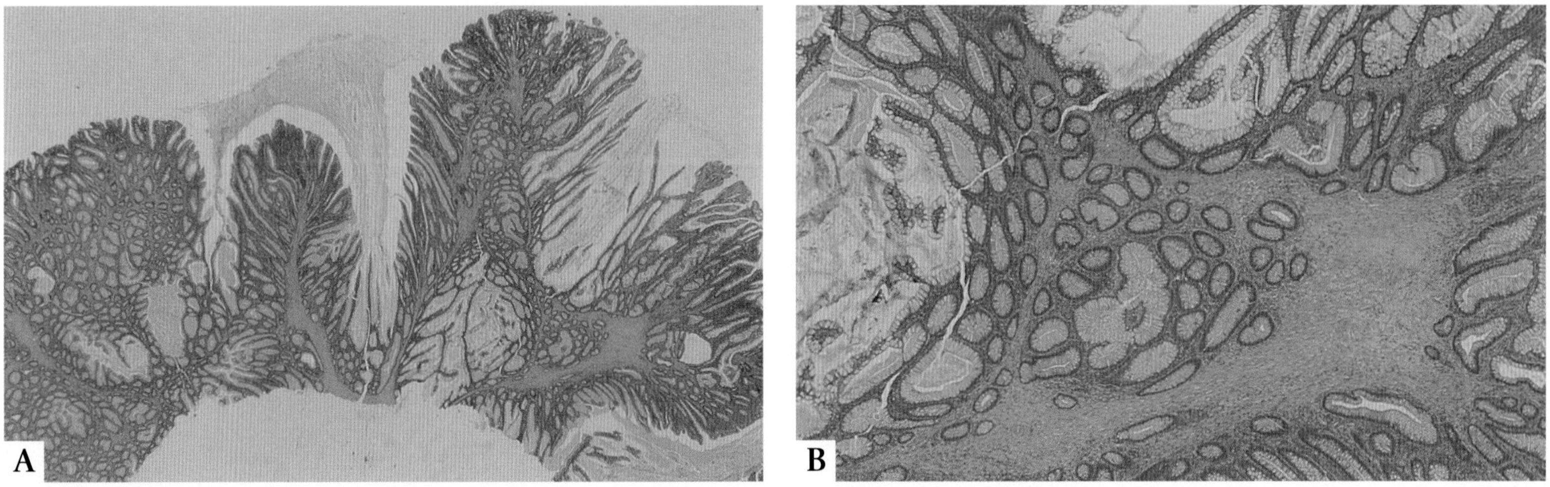

FIGURE 3-27.

Low-power (**A**) and high-power (**B**) photomicrograph of a Peutz-Jeghers polyp. In this type of polyp, the glandular epithelium is supported by an arborizing framework of well-developed smooth muscle that is contiguous with the muscularis mucosae.

Hamartomatous polyp

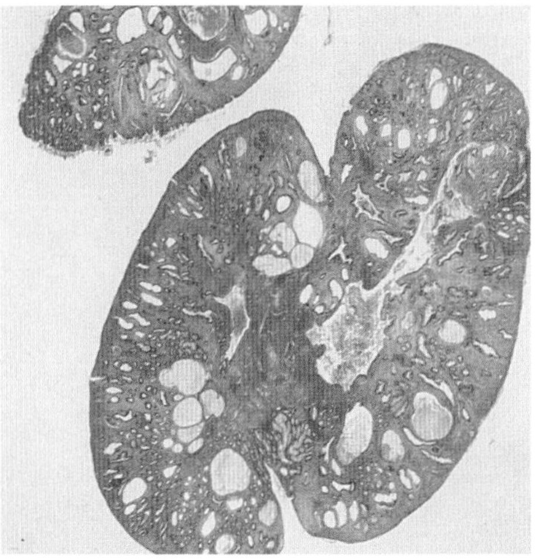

FIGURE 3-28.

Juvenile polyp. This low-power photomicrograph demonstrates a hamartomatous polyp with dilated mucus-filled glands and extensive edema and inflammation in the lamina propria. Hamartomas of the colon, small intestine, and stomach characterize familial juvenile polyposis. The risk of colon cancer is increased in this syndrome because of the presence of synchronous adenomatous polyps.

Cronkhite-Canada syndrome

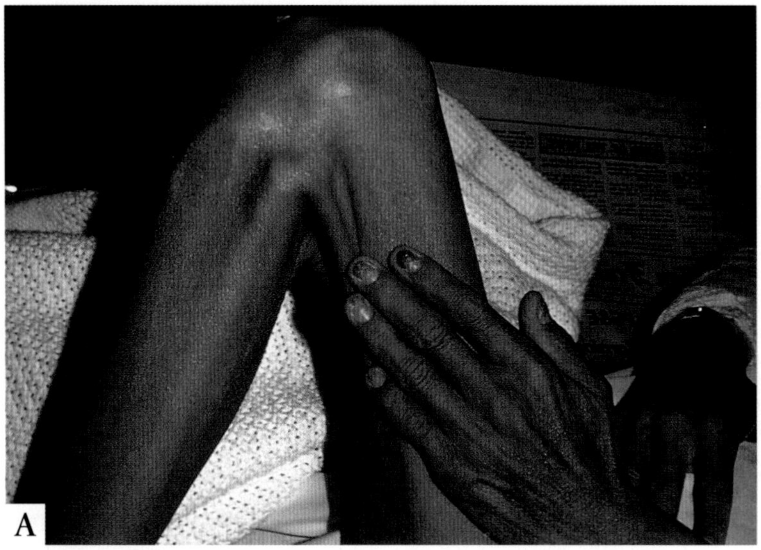

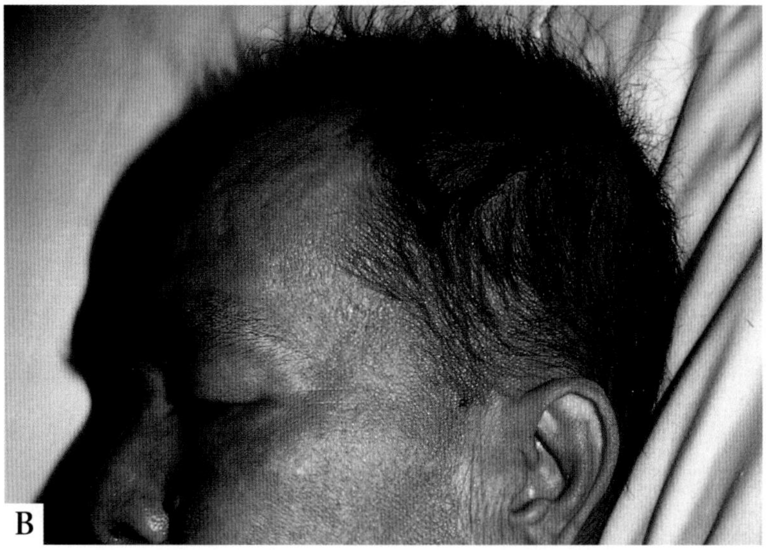

FIGURE 3-29.

The Cronkhite-Canada syndrome. This spontaneously arising syndrome is characterized by diffuse gastrointestinal polyposis (inflammatory polyps similar to juvenile polyps), cutaneous hyperpigmentation and dystrophic changes in the fingernails (**A**), alopecia (**B**), and intestinal malabsorption. Similar to juvenile polyposis, adenomatous epithelium may occur in conjunction with hamartomas, conferring a risk of carcinoma.

Torre's or Muir's syndrome

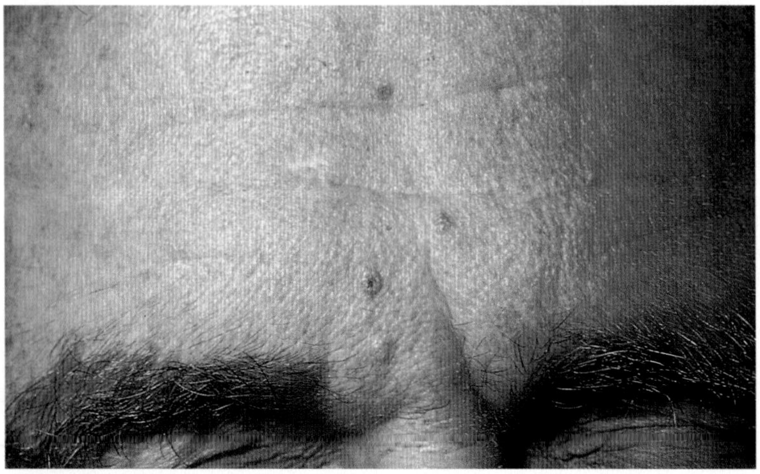

FIGURE 3-30.

Sebaceous skin adenomas in a patient with Torre's or Muir's syndrome. This syndrome consists of multiple skin lesions (sebaceous adenomas and carcinomas, basal and squamous carcinoma, keratoacanthomas) in conjunction with adenomas and adenocarcinomas of the colon. This syndrome has recently been shown to represent a subset of nonpolyposis hereditary colon cancer.

Ulcerative colitis and colorectal carcinoma

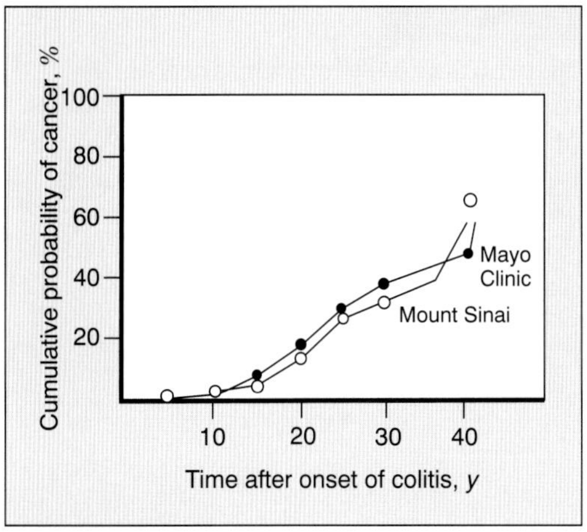

FIGURE 3-31.

Cumulative probability of developing colorectal carcinoma in patients with ulcerative colitis. Data from tertiary referral centers such as the Mayo Clinic and Mount Sinai Medical Center indicate a 1% per year cumulative incidence after 10 years duration of disease. Data from primary care settings suggest an approximately 0.5% per year cumulative incidence. (*From* Bresalier and Kim [3]; with permission.)

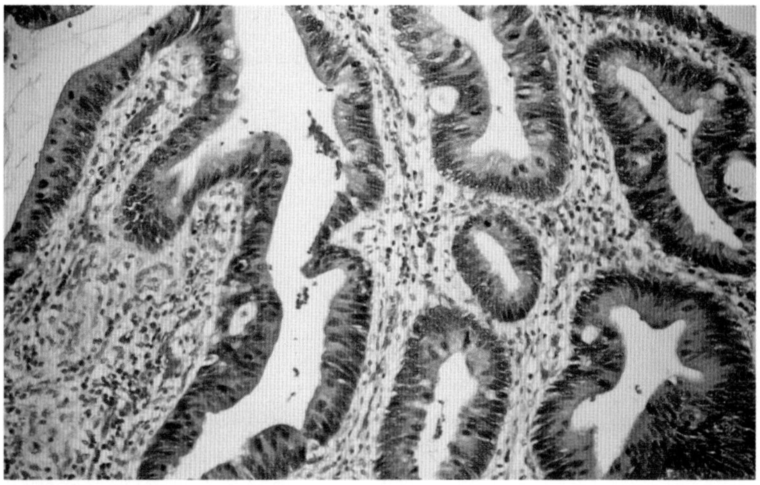

FIGURE 3-32.

Photomicrograph of colonic dysplasia in a patient with ulcerative colitis. Crowded back-to-back glands and pseudostratification of nuclei are seen. Adenocarcinomas of the colon arise in dysplastic epithelium in patients with long-standing colitis. Such dysplasia may occur in flat epithelium or in dysplasia-associated mass lesions (*see* Figs. 3-33 and 3-34).

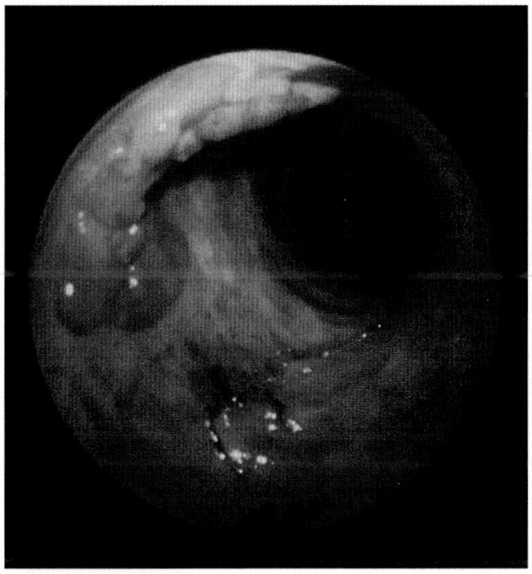

FIGURE 3-33.

Dysplasia-associated mass lesions seen at colonoscopy in a patient with ulcerative colitis. Such lesions may be plaquelike as shown in Figure 3-32 or polypoid and contain dysplastic epithelium. These lesions are highly associated with synchronous carcinoma of the colon.

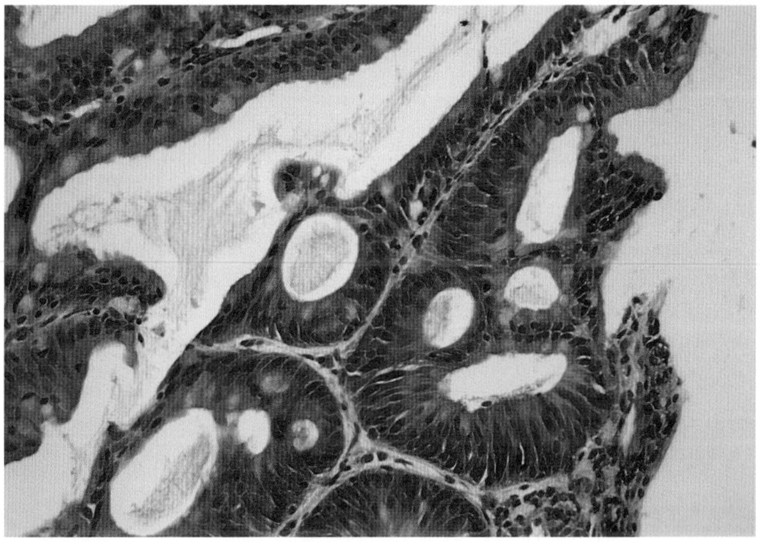

FIGURE 3-34.

High-grade dysplasia in a dysplasia-associated mass lesion. The appearance of high-grade dysplasia in such a lesion is highly suggestive of coincident carcinoma and is an indication for total colectomy.

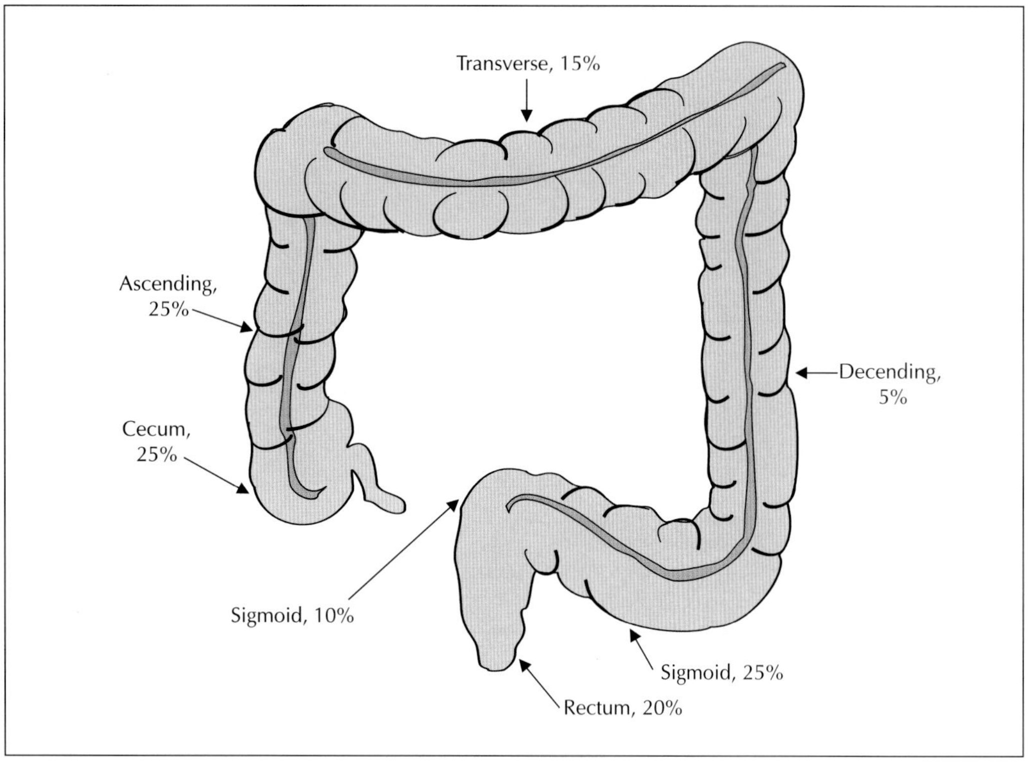

FIGURE 3-35.

Distribution of colorectal cancer in the colon. Although approximately two-thirds of cancers still arise distal to the splenic flexure, an increasing number of cancers are being found in the right colon.

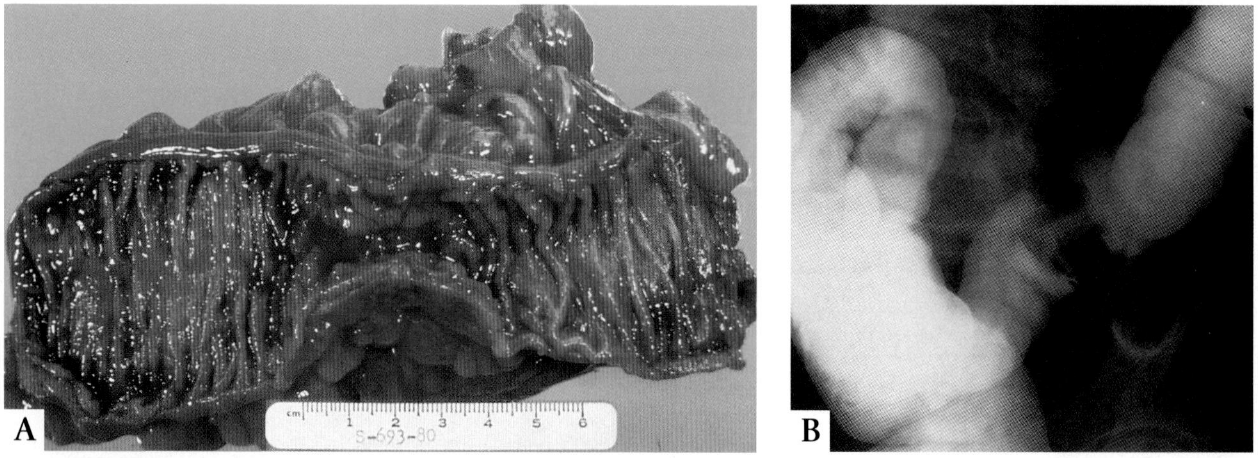

FIGURE 3-36.

A, A gross surgical specimen of annular constricting or napkin-ring carcinoma of the colon. **B**, Full-column barium enema demonstrating the annular constricting lesions.

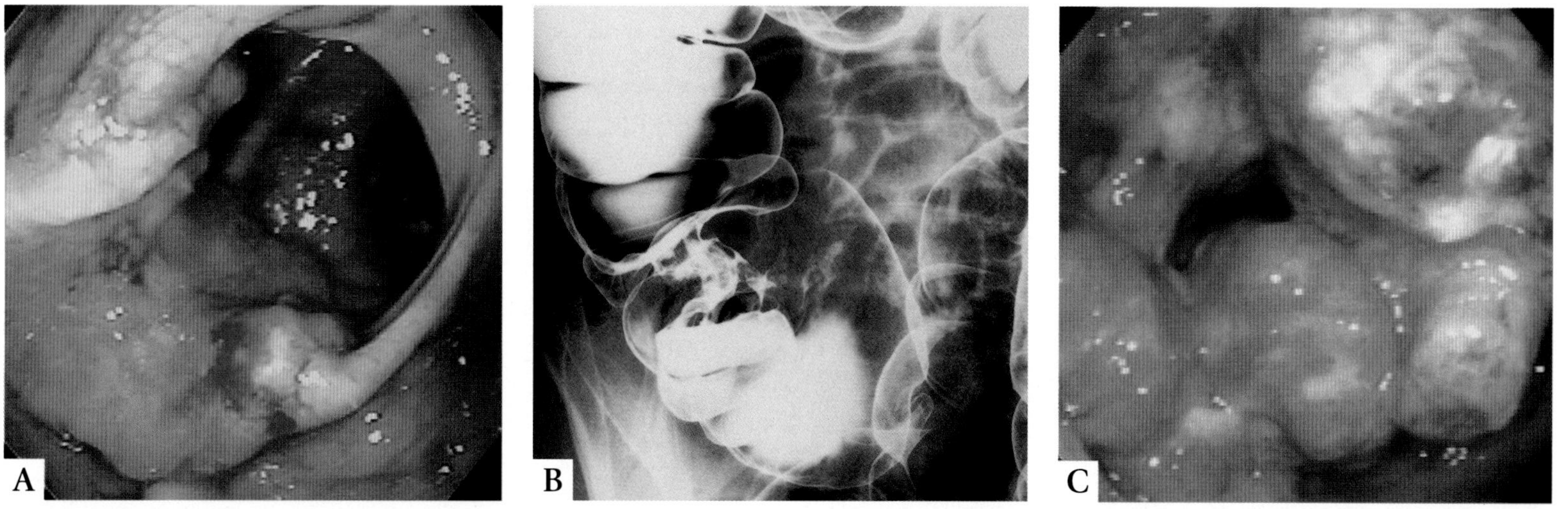

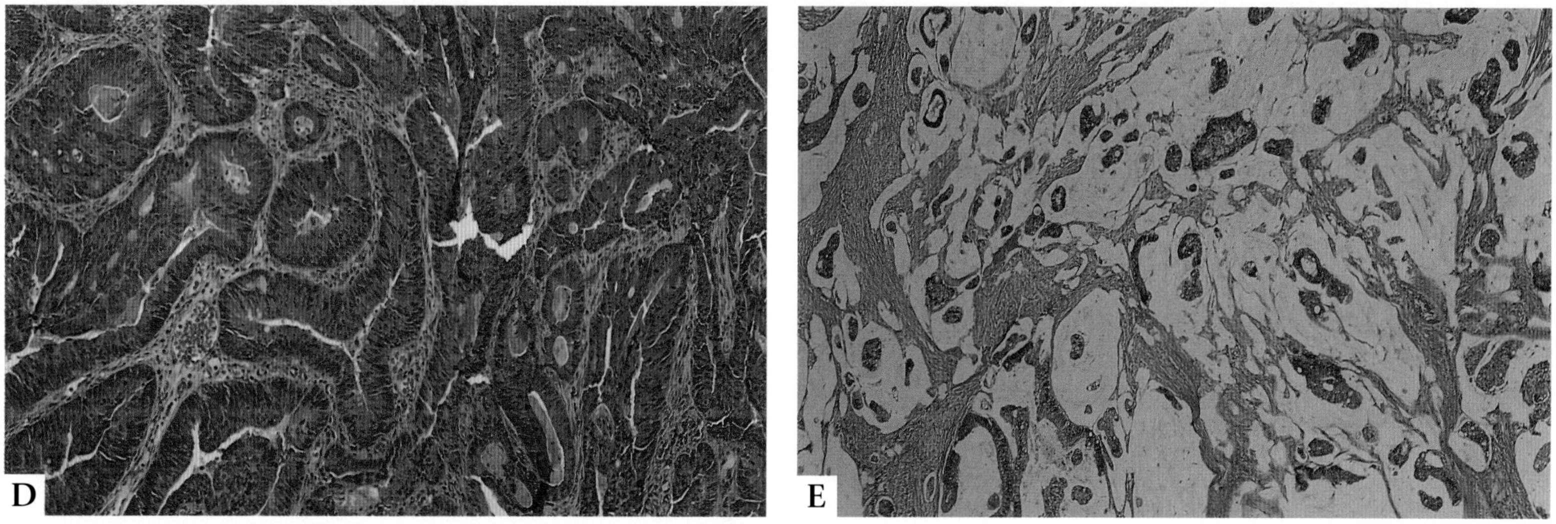

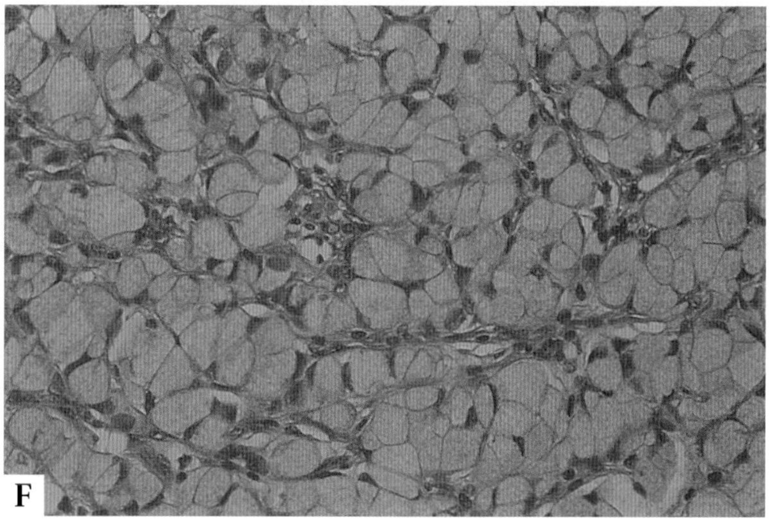

FIGURE 3-37.

Miscellaneous adenocarcinomas and carcinomas affecting the colon. **A**, Adenocarcinoma of the colon infiltrating a gross colonic fold seen at colonoscopy. **B**, Air-contrast barium enema demonstrating mucosal involvement by cecal carcinoma. **C**, An obstructing polypoid carcinoma of the colon seen at colonoscopy. **D**, Well-differentiated adenocarcinoma of the colon. This histologic section demonstrates crowded neoplastic glands. **E**, Colloid carcinoma of the colon with scattered nests of tumor cells floating in "lakes of mucin." **F**, Signet cell carcinoma of the colon. Large vacuoles of mucin displace the nuclei of individual cells.

TABLE 3-4. DUKES' CLASSIFICATION FOR CARCINOMA OF THE RECTUM AND ITS MODIFICATIONS FOR COLORECTAL CARCINOMA

Stage	Dukes, 1932 (*Rectum*)	Gabriel, Dukes, Bussey, 1935 (*Rectum*)	Kirklin *et al.*, 1949 (*Rectum & sigmoid*)	Astler-Coller, 1954 (*Rectum & colon*)
A	Limited to bowel wall	Limited to bowel wall	Limited to mucosa	Limited to mucosa
B	Through bowel wall	Through bowel wall	—	—
B1	—	—	Into muscularis propria	Into muscularis propria
B2	—	—	Through muscularis propria	Through muscularis propria (and serosa)
B3	—	—	—	—
C	Regional nodal metastases	—	Regional nodal metastases	—
C1	—	Regional nodal metastases near primary lesion	—	Same as B1 plus regional nodal metastases
C2	—	Proximal node involved at point of ligation	—	Same as B2 plus regional nodal metastases
C3	—	—	—	—
D	—	—	—	—

Stage	Turnbull *et al.*, 1967 (*Colon*)	Modified Astler-Coller (Gunderson & Sosin, 1974) (*Rectum & colon*)	GITSG, 1975 (*Rectum & colon*)
A	Limited to mucosa	Limited to mucosa	Limited to mucosa
B	Tumor extension into periodic fat	—	—
B1	—	Into muscularis propria	Into muscularis propria
B2	—	Through serosa m = microscopic m + g = gross	Through serosa
B3	—	Adherent to or invading adjacent structures	—
C	Regional nodal metastases	—	—
C1	—	Same as B1 plus regional nodal metastases	1–4 regional nodes positive
C2	—	Same as B2 plus regional nodal metastases	>4 regional nodes positive
C3	—	Same as B3 plus regional nodal metastases	—
D	Distant metastases (liver, lung, bone) or caused by parietal or adjacent organ invasion	—	—

TABLE 3-4.

Dukes' classification for colorectal carcinoma and its modifications. (*From* Bresalier and Kim [3]; with permission.)

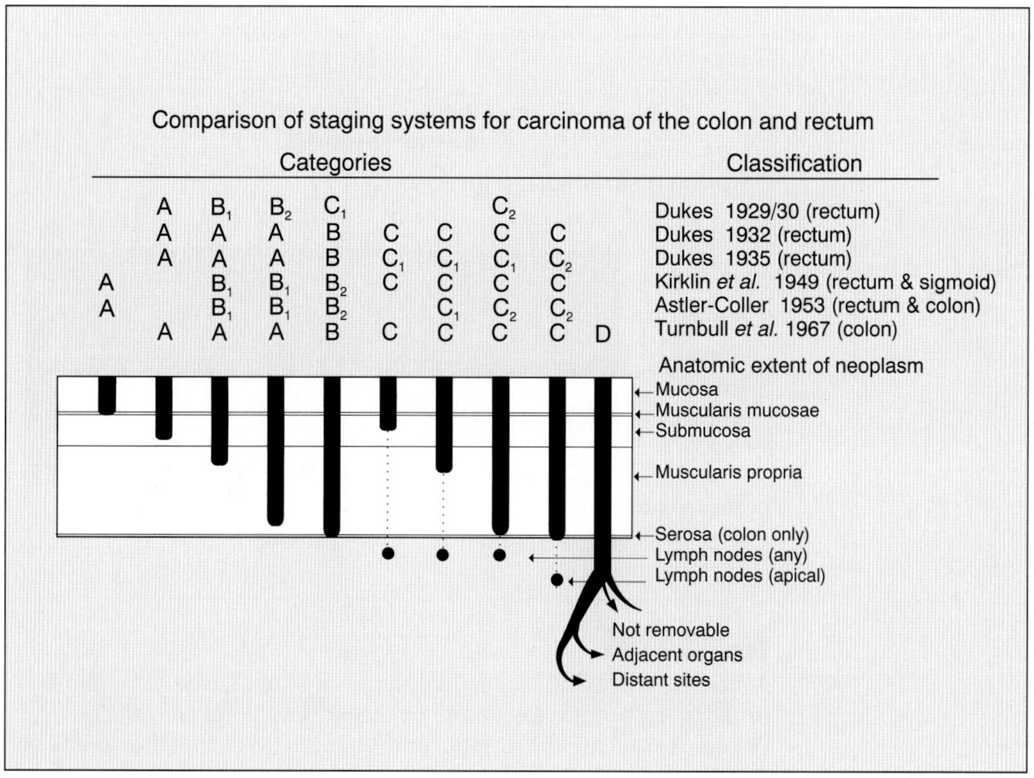

FIGURE 3-38.

Comparison of modifications of the Dukes' staging system for carcinoma of the colon and rectum. The Astler-Coller and Turnbull modifications are commonly used, but existence of multiple classifications is confusing. This confusion has led to more standardized classifications of colorectal cancer, such as the Tumor, Node, and Metastases (TNM) classification of the American Joint Committee for Cancer (*see* Table 3-5). (*From* Donnegan and DeCosse [13]; with permission.)

TABLE 3-5. STAGING OF COLORECTAL CANCER—AMERICAN JOINT COMMITTEE ON CANCER USING THE TNM CLASSIFICATION

Stage 0
Carcinoma in situ Tis N0 M0

Stage I
Tumor invades submucosa T1 N0 M0
Tumor invades muscularis propria T2 N0 M0

Stage II
Tumor invades through muscularis propria into subserosa or into nonperitonealized pericolic or perirectal tissues T3 N0 M0
Tumor perforates the visceral peritoneum or directly invades other organs or structures T4 N0 M0

Stage III
Any degree of bowel wall perforation with regional lymph node metastasis
N1 1 to 3 pericolic or perirectal lymph nodes involved
N2 4 or more pericolic or perirectal lymph nodes involved
N3 Metastasis in any lymph node along a named vascular trunk
Any T N1, M0
Any T N2,N3 M0

Stage IV
Any invasion of bowel wall with or without lymph node metastasis but with evidence of distant metastasis
Any T Any N M1

Dukes' B (corresponds to Stage II) is a composite of better (T3, N0, M0) and worse (T4, N0, M0) prognostic groups as is Dukes' C (corresponds to Stage III) (any T, N1, M0) and (any T, N2, N3, M0)

TABLE 3-5.

Staging of colorectal cancer according to the American Joint Committee for Cancer using the Tumor, Node, and Metastasis (TNM) classification. This system was developed to provide more uniform staging of colorectal cancer. Tis–tumor in situ. (*From* American Joint Committee for Cancer Staging and End Result Reporting [14]; with permission.)

Survival probabilities

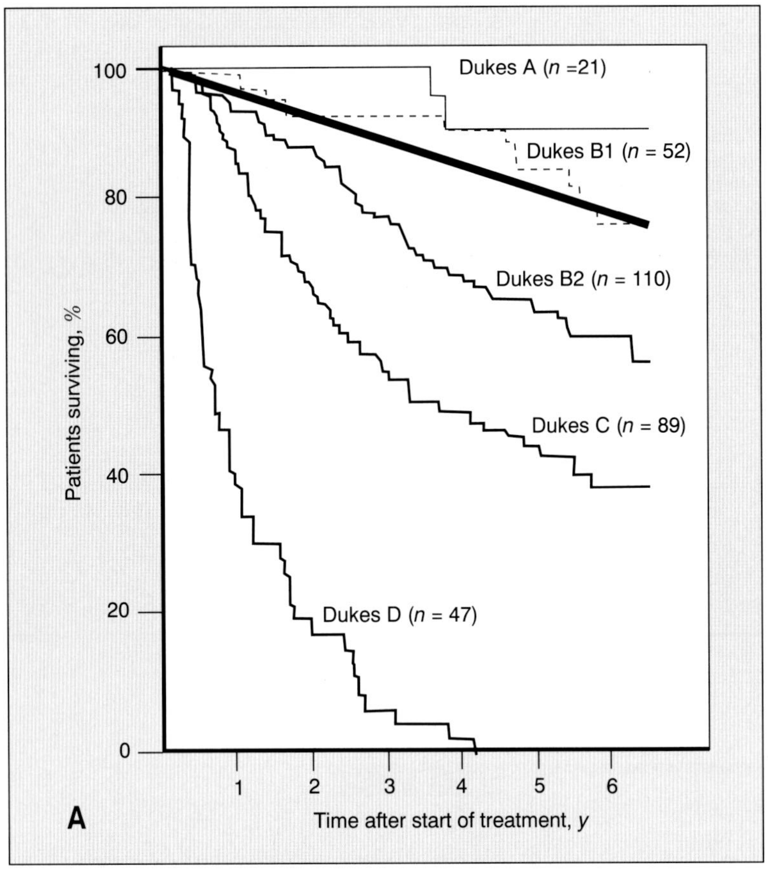

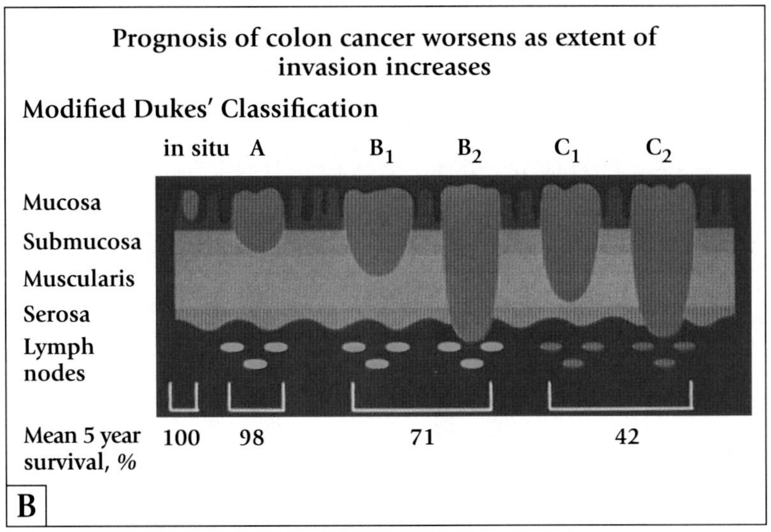

FIGURE 3-39.

A, Survival probabilities according to stage of disease in patients undergoing potentially curative surgery for colorectal cancer. Expected survival among age- and sex-matched general population is indicated by heavy line. **B**, Prognosis worsens as the extent of invasion increases. (**A**, *From* Moertel *et al.* [15]; with permission.) (**B**, *From* Podolsky [16]; with permission.)

Factors that may affect prognosis

TABLE 3-6A. PATHOLOGIC FEATURES THAT MAY AFFECT PROGNOSIS IN PATIENTS WITH COLORECTAL CANCER

Pathologic features	Effect on prognosis
Surgical pathology stage	
Depth of bowel wall penetration	Increased penetration diminishes prognosis 1–4 nodes better than >4 nodes
Number of regional lymph nodes involved by tumor	
Tumor histology	
Degree of differentiation	Well differentiated better than poorly differentiated
Mucinous (colloid) or signet ring cell histology	Diminished prognosis
Scirrhous histology	Diminished prognosis
Venous invasion	Diminished prognosis
Lymphatic invasion	Diminished prognosis
Perineural invasion	Diminished prognosis
Local inflammation and immunologic reaction	Improved prognosis
Tumor size	No effect in most studies
Tumor morphology	Polypoid/exophytic better than ulcerating/infiltrating
Tumor DNA content	Increased DNA content (aneuploidy) diminishes prognosis

TABLE 3-6B. CLINICAL FEATURES THAT MAY AFFECT PROGNOSIS IN PATIENTS WITH COLORECTAL CANCER

Clinical features	Effect on prognosis
Diagnosis in asymptomatic patients	?Improved prognosis
Duration of symptoms	No demonstrated effect
Rectal bleeding as presenting symptom	Improved prognosis
Bowel obstruction	Diminished prognosis
Bowel perforation	Diminished prognosis
Tumor location	?Colon better than rectum ?Left colon better than right colon
Age < 30	Diminished prognosis
Preoperative serum CEA	Diminished prognosis with high CEA level
Deletions in chromosome 18 (*DCC* gene)	Diminished prognosis
Distant metastases	Markedly diminished prognosis

TABLE 3-6.

A, Pathologic features of a tumor that may affect the prognosis of a patient with colorectal cancer. **B**, Clinical features that may affect prognosis in patients with colorectal cancer. Although disease stage is the most important feature affecting prognosis, other pathologic and clinical features have modifying effects. CEA—carcinoembryonic antigen.

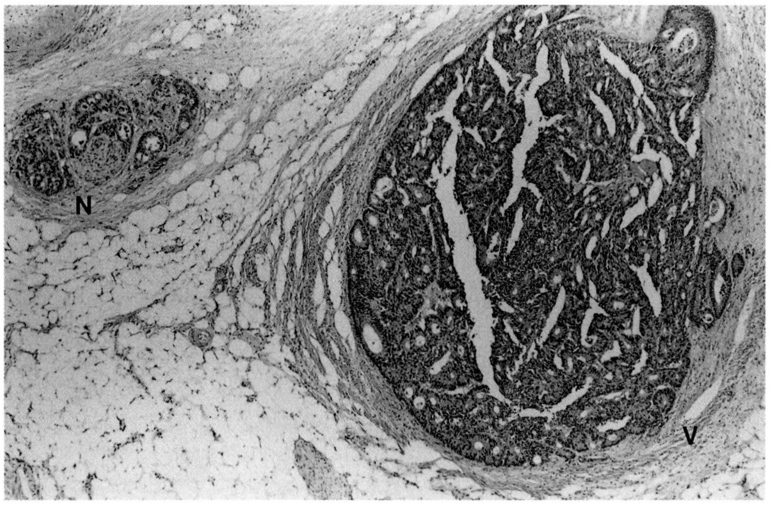

FIGURE 3-40.

Perivenous (V) and perineural (N) invasion may adversely affect prognosis in patients with colorectal cancer.

Metastasis cascade

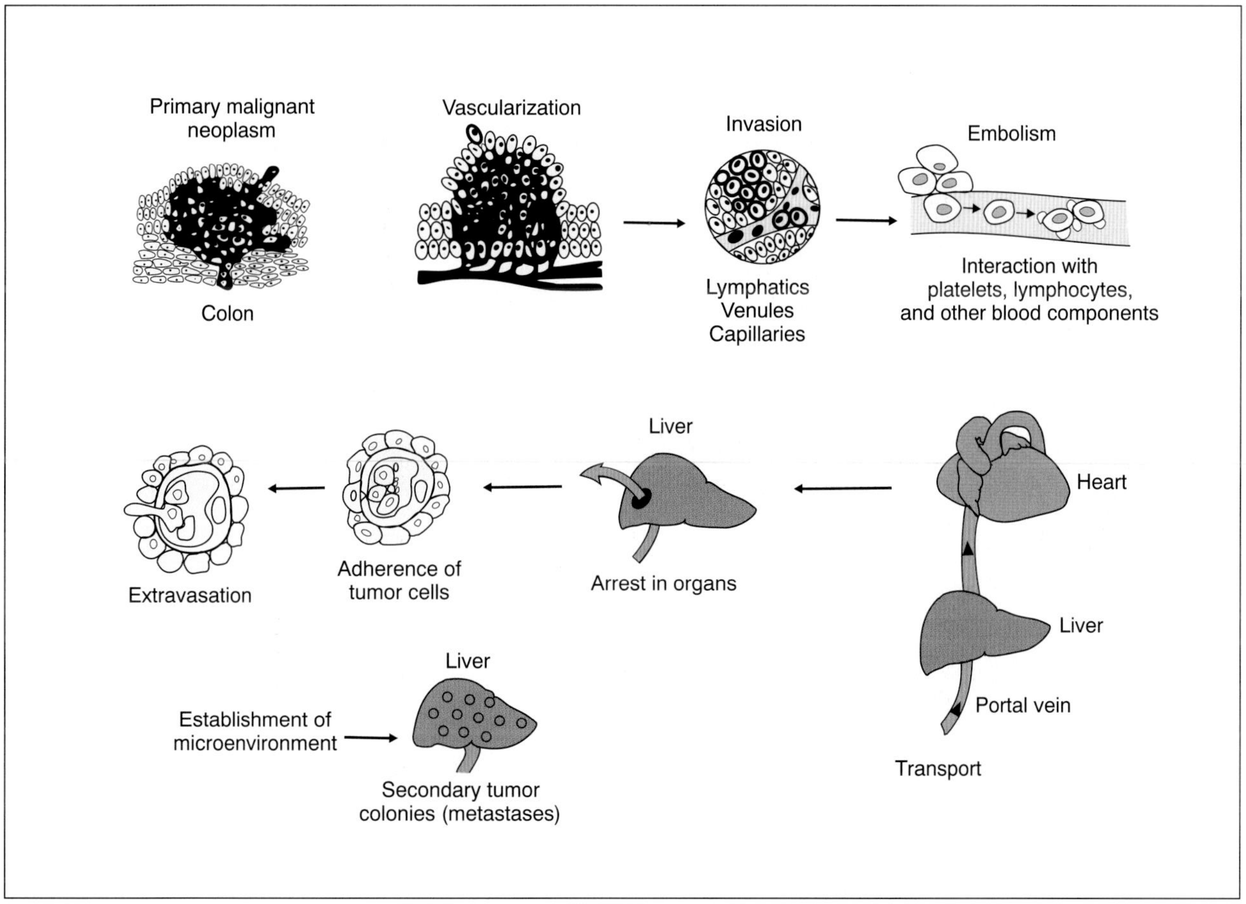

FIGURE 3-41.

Metastasis cascade. Metastasis of colorectal cancer cells from the primary site in the colon to the liver involves a complex series of events, all of which are necessary to result in distant metastatic disease. Tumors must become vascularized to grow at the primary site. Cells must then be able to invade basement membranes, avoid immune surveillance, adhere to vascular endothelia, and interact with the microenvironment to set up metastatic foci.

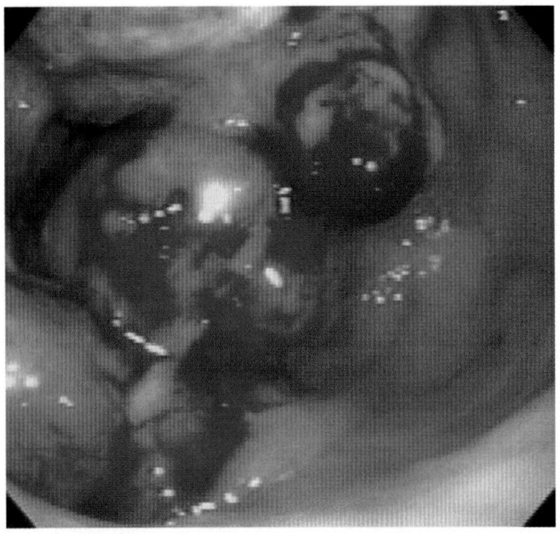

FIGURE 3-42.

Colonoscopic view of bleeding colon cancer. Colorectal cancers may present with gross bleeding (hematochezia) or result in the presence of occult blood in the stool.

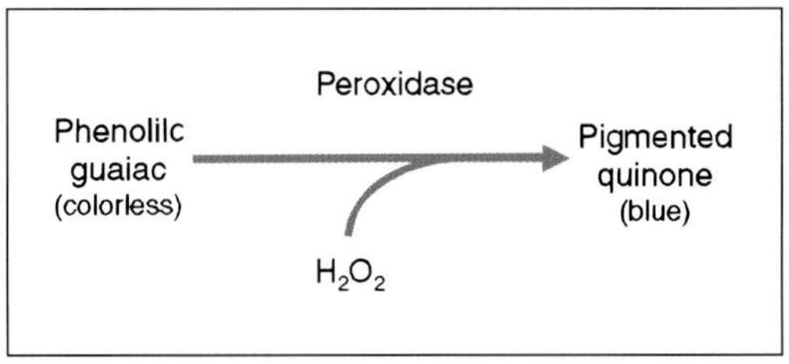

FIGURE 3-43.

Depiction of the principle behind the peroxidase-guaic–based tests for fecal occult blood such as Hemoccult (SmithKline Diagnostics, San Jose, CA). The colorless guaiac indicator, which is impregnated in the card, turns blue when oxidized in the presence of hydrogen peroxide and the peroxidase activity of hemoglobin. This type of test is the basis for all major screening trials of fecal occult blood testing for colorectal cancer.

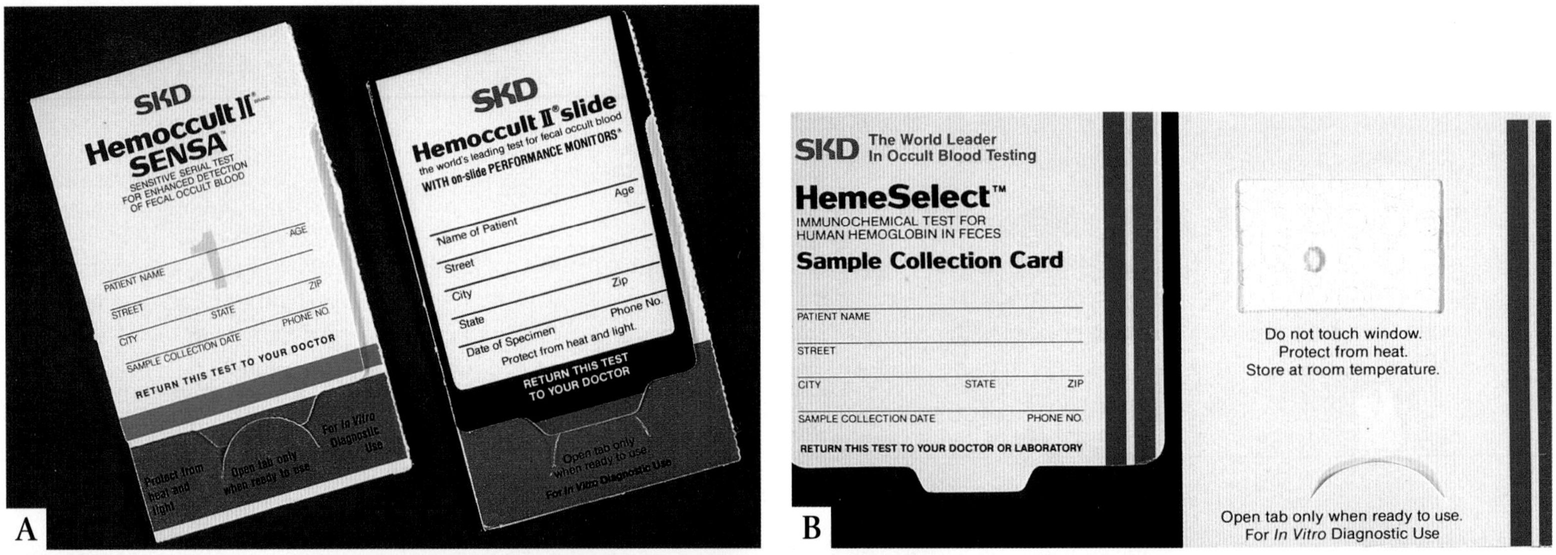

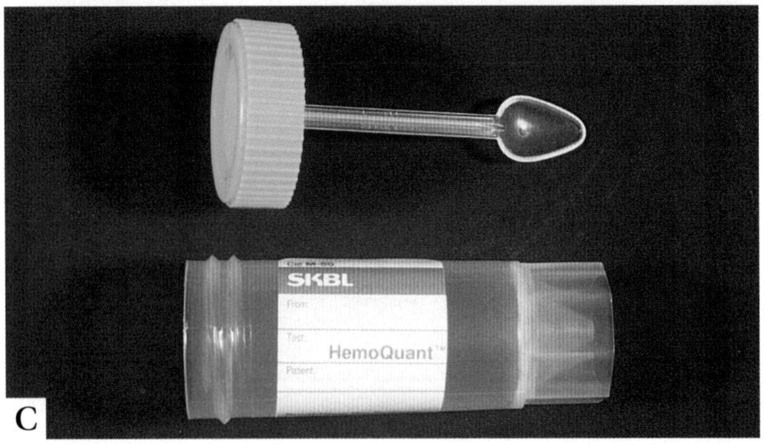

FIGURE 3-44.

Commonly used slide tests for fecal occult blood. Hemoccult SENSA (SmithKline Diagnostics, San Jose, CA) has greater sensitivity than Hemoccult (SmithKline Diagnostics) but must be used in conjunction with dietary restriction (peroxidase-containing foods) to avoid false-positive results. **B**, Immunochemical tests such as HemeSelect (SmithKline Diagnostics), are sensitive and specific for human hemoglobin in feces. **C**, The HemoQuant test (SmithKline Bioscience Laboratories, Philadelphia, PA) is a quantitative test for fecal occult blood based on fluorescence of heme-derived porphyrins. Stool is collected and sent to the laboratory for testing. Although highly sensitive for detecting occult blood in stool, this test has not been clearly proven to be superior to other tests.

TABLE 3-7. ADVANTAGES AND LIMITATIONS OF THE GUAIAC-IMPREGNATED SLIDE TEST FOR FECAL OCCULT BLOOD TESTING

- Advantages
  - Readily available
  - Convenient
  - Inexpensive
  - Good patient compliance in motivated groups
- Disadvantages
  - Depends on degree of fecal hydration
  - Affected by storage (hemoglobin degradation)
  - Affected by tumor location
- False-positive tests
  - Exogenous peroxidase activity
    - Red meat (nonhuman hemoglobin)
    - Uncooked fruits and vegetables (vegetable peroxidase)
  - Any source of gastrointestinal blood loss (epistaxis, gingival bleeding, upper gastrointestinal tract pathology, hemorrhoids, etc.)
  - Medications
    - Topical iodine
    - Aspirin, nonsteroidal anti-inflammatory agents (induce upper gastrointestinal bleeding)
- False-negative tests
  - Storage of slides
  - Ascorbic acid (vitamin C)
  - Improper sampling/developing
  - Lesion not bleeding at time of stool collection
  - Degradation of hemoglobin by colonic bacteria

TABLE 3-7.

Advantages and limitations of the guaiac-based slide tests used for fecal occult blood testing. Although readily available and widely employed clinically, care must be taken to avoid sources of false-positive and false-negative tests. (*From* Bresalier and Kim [3]; with permission.)

TABLE 3-8. CONTROLLED TRIALS OF FECAL OCCULT BLOOD TESTING IN SCREENING ASYMPTOMATIC PERSONS FOR COLORECTAL CANCER

				Dukes stage A or B, %	
Site	Cohort	Screening interval, *mo*	Rehydrated	Screened	Control
New York	21,961	—	No	66	33
Minnesota	46,551	12 and 24	Yes	61*	58
England	142,690	24	No	76	46
Sweden	51,325	14–22	Yes	64	35
Denmark	61,938	24	No	81	46

**A significant decrease in stage D cancers in the screened group and a significant decrease in mortality of colorectal cancer*

TABLE 3-8.

Controlled screening trials of fecal occult blood testing for colorectal cancer. Routine fecal occult blood testing of asymptomatic individuals has been demonstrated to significantly decrease mortality caused by colorectal cancer. (*From* Bresalier and Kim [3]; with permission.)

Flexible sigmoidoscopy

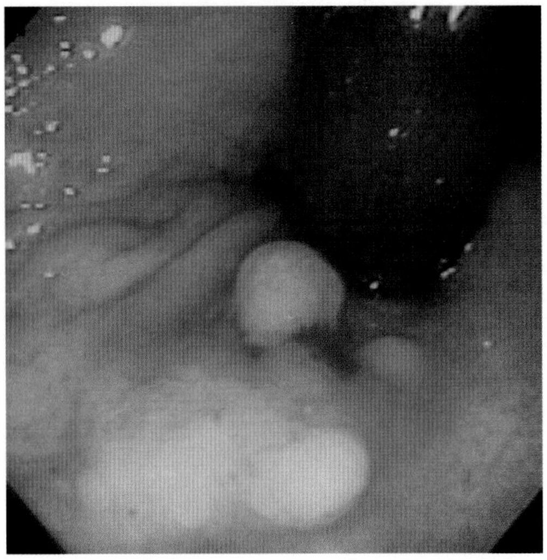

FIGURE 3-45.

Flexible sigmoidoscopic view of the distal rectum upon retroflexion of the sigmoidoscope, which demonstrates several small polyps. Flexible sigmoidoscopy has been shown to detect two- to threefold more neoplasms than rigid sigmoidoscopy. Periodic flexible sigmoidoscopy and polypectomy may reduce cancer incidence and mortality caused by cancer within the reach of the endoscope by approximately 70%.

Endoscopic polypectomy

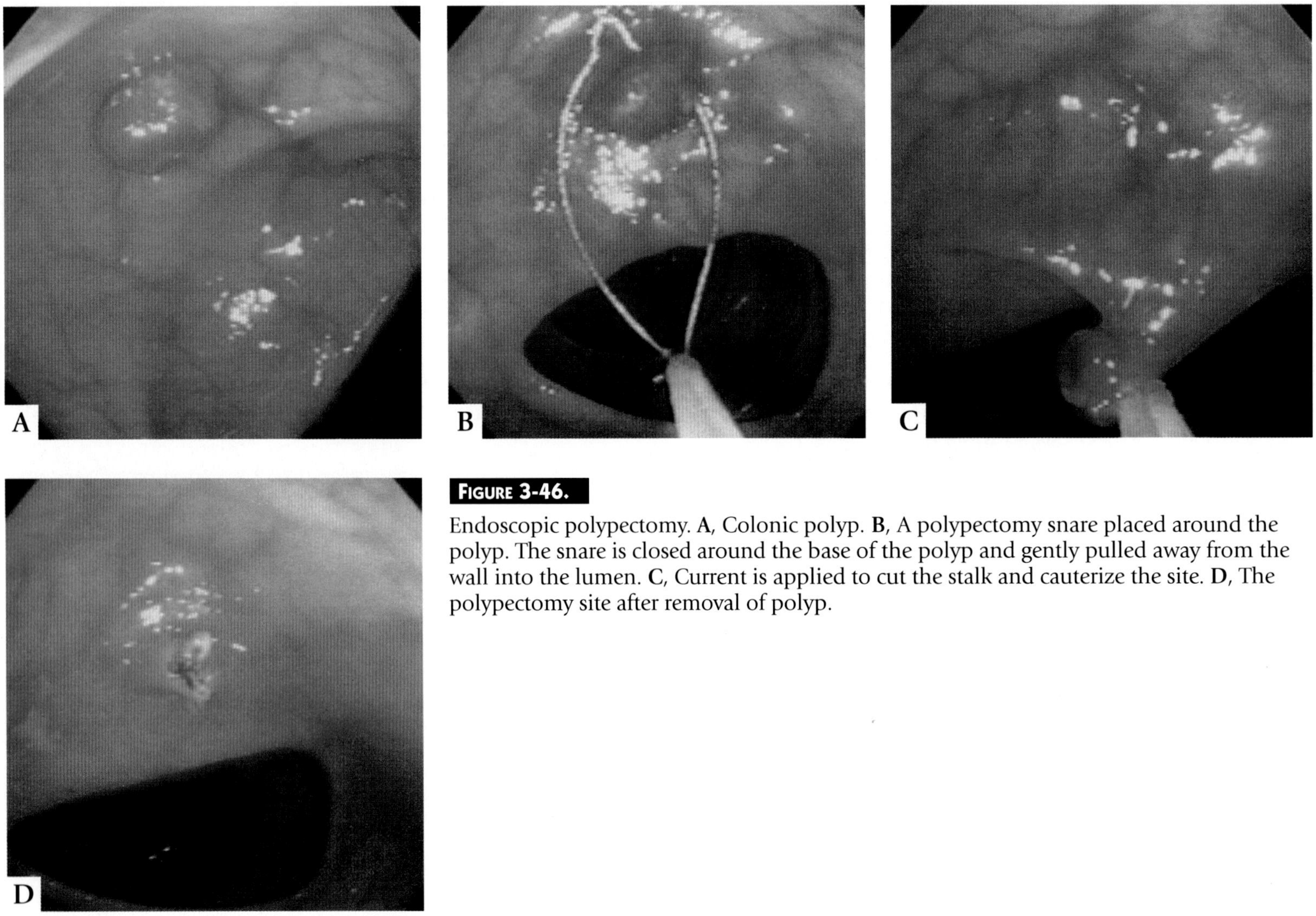

FIGURE 3-46.

Endoscopic polypectomy. **A**, Colonic polyp. **B**, A polypectomy snare placed around the polyp. The snare is closed around the base of the polyp and gently pulled away from the wall into the lumen. **C**, Current is applied to cut the stalk and cauterize the site. **D**, The polypectomy site after removal of polyp.

TABLE 3-9. NATIONAL POLYP STUDY

Surveillance intervals after colonoscopic removal of newly diagnosed adenomas
Follow-up interval
3 years
1 and 3 years

FINDING	PATIENTS		RELATIVE RISK (95%CI)	P VALUE
Adenoma	Two examinations, *n*(%)	One examination, *n*(%)		
Any	141 (41.7)	137 (32.0)	1.3 (1.1–1.6)	0.006
Advanced*	11 (3.3)	14 (3.3)	1.0 (0.5–2.2)	0.99

TABLE 3-9.

Data from the national polyp study indicate that a 3-year surveillance interval is adequate after colonoscopic removal of an uncomplicated adenoma in average-risk individuals. The study consisted of two groups that differed in the interval between colonoscopies; the first group included 428 patients rescreened 3 years after index polypectomy, and the second group included 338 patients rescreened 1 and 3 years after polypectomy. Although more adenomas were detected when patients had surveillance colonoscopy more frequently, there was no difference in detection of important advanced lesions.

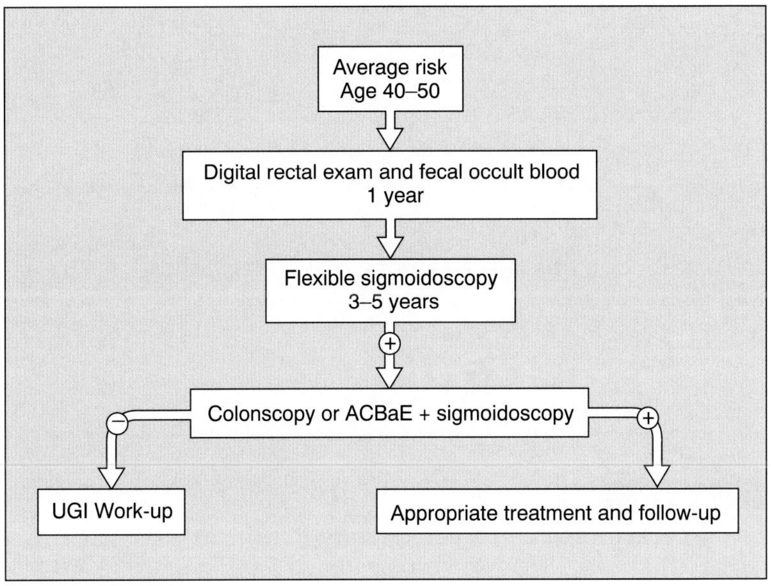

FIGURE 3-47.

Algorithm for colon cancer surveillance of average-risk individuals in the general population. Current data indicate that screening with fecal occult blood testing and sigmoidoscopy can significantly reduce mortality from colorectal cancer. (*From* Bresalier and Kim [3]; with permission.)

Surgical resection

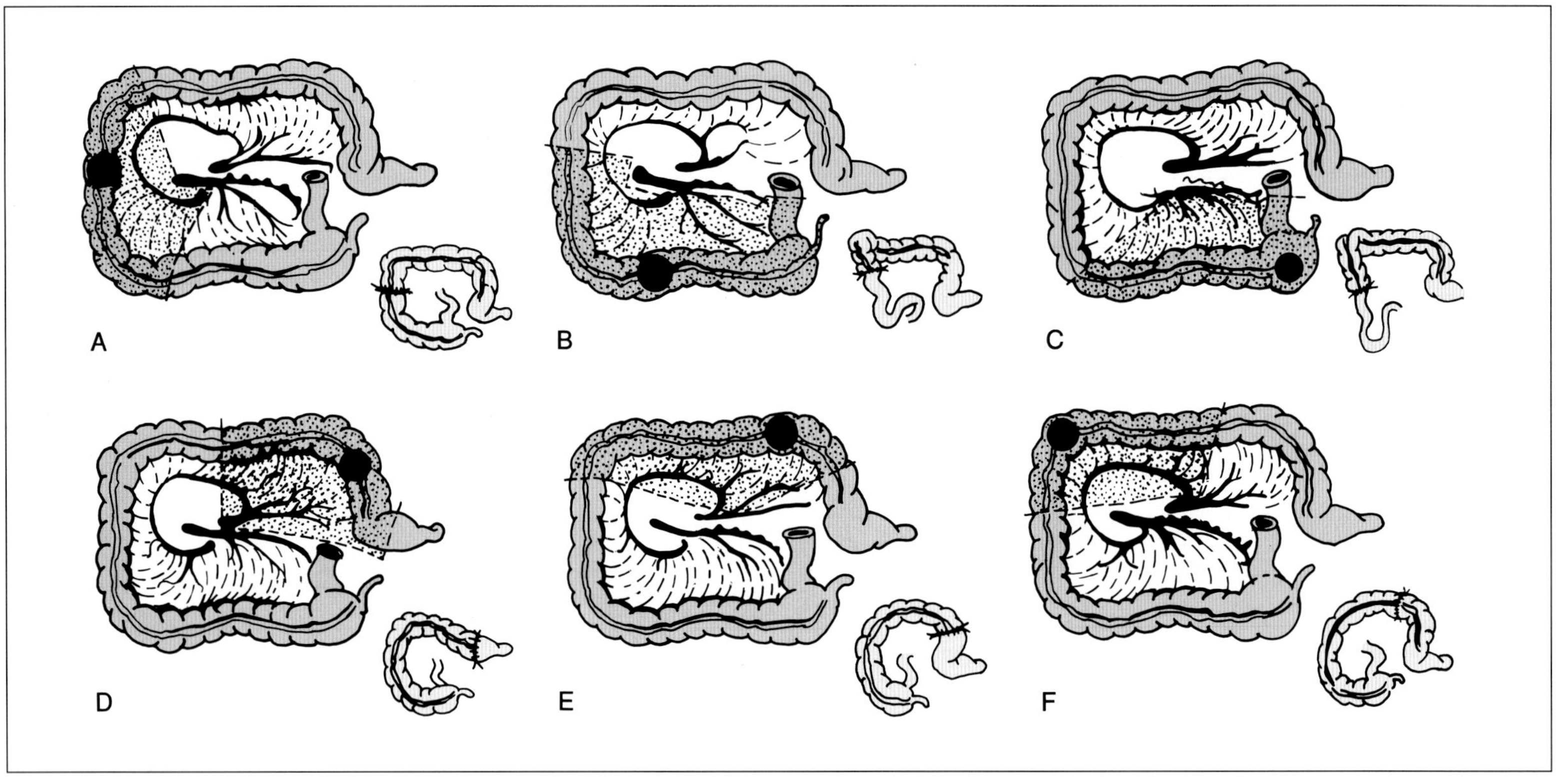

FIGURE 3-48.

A–F, Extent of surgical resection for cancer of the colon at various sites. The extent of colonic resection is determined by blood supply and distribution of regional lymph nodes. (*From* Schrock [17]; with permission.)

Adjuvant therapy

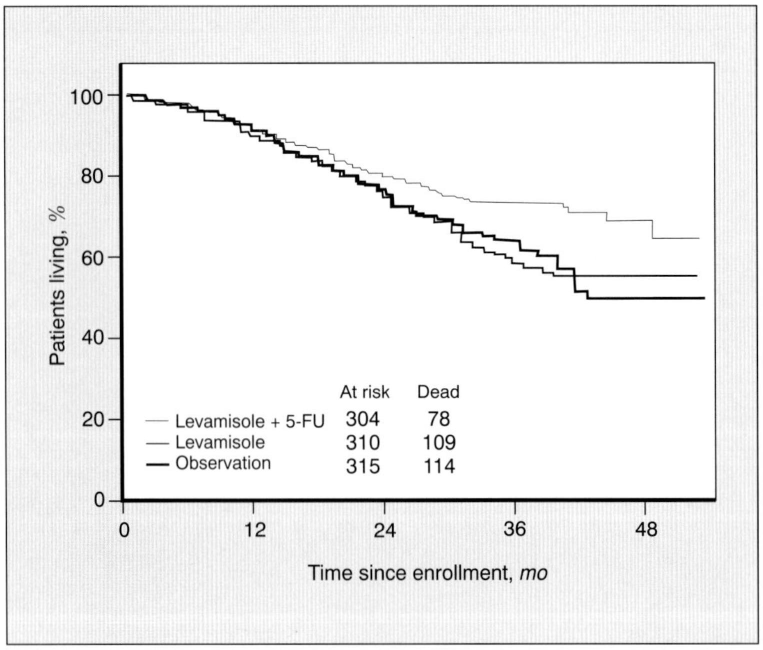

FIGURE 3-49.

Adjuvant chemotherapy of colon cancer in patients with Dukes' C (stage III) disease. Therapy with combined 5-fluorouracil (5-FU; a chemotherapeutic agent) and levamisole (a reported immune system stimulant) results in significantly improved patient survival compared with observation or levamisole alone. (*From* Moertel *et al.* [18]; with permission.)

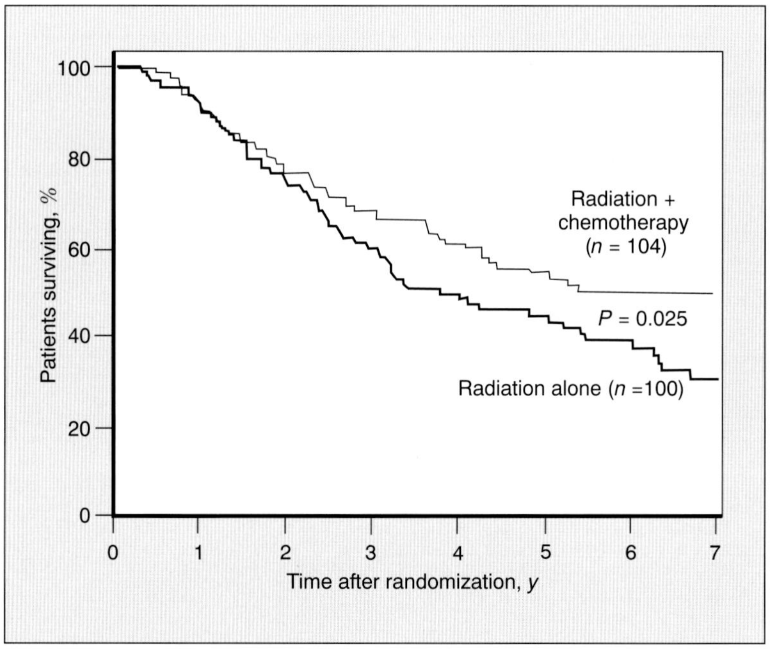

FIGURE 3-50.

Combined modality adjuvant therapy with postoperative radiation (for local disease) and chemotherapy (for microscopic metastatic disease) significantly improves survival in patients with stages II and III rectal cancer. (*From* Krook *et al.* [19]; with permission.)

Lymphomas

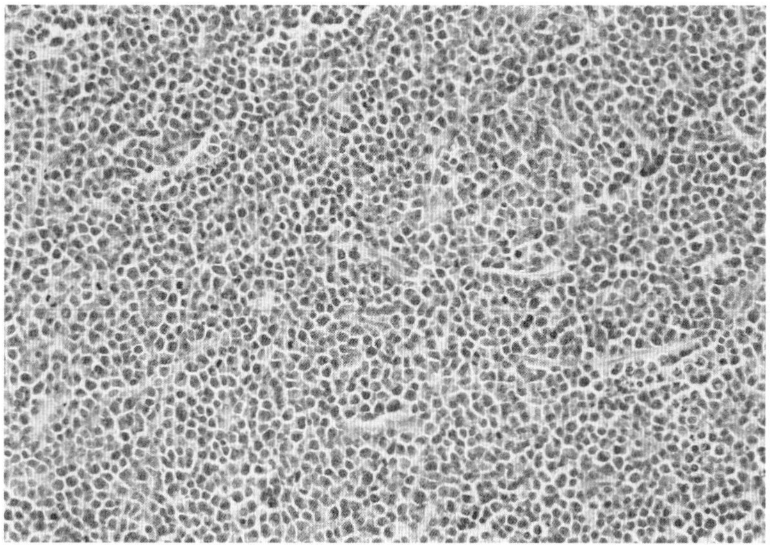

FIGURE 3-51.

Photomicrograph of a primary lymphoma of the large bowel. These tumors are rare, representing approximately 0.5% and 0.2%, respectively, of all malignant colonic and rectal tumors. The cecum is the most common site of primary large bowel lymphoma, followed by the rectum. Immunohistochemical studies indicate that most are B-cell lymphomas.

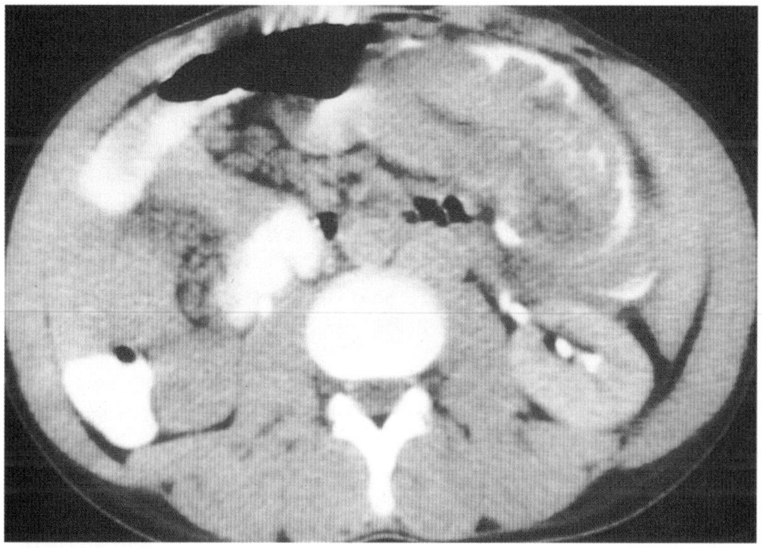

FIGURE 3-52.

Computed tomographic scan of the abdomen demonstrating intussusception of the bowel caused by lymphoma in a patient with AIDS. Non-Hodgkins lymphomas have been reported in up to 6% of patients with AIDS overall and occur in both the small and large intestine.

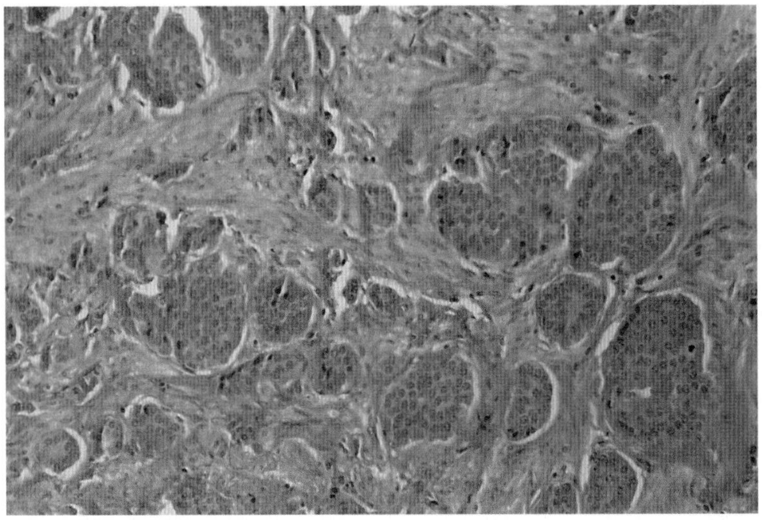

FIGURE 3-53.

Photomicrograph of a rectal carcinoid. Carcinoids of the rectum are rare. These tumors are usually small (80% are less than 1 cm) and rarely, if ever, metastasize. They do not cause the carcinoid syndrome. Carcinoid tumors of the appendix are relatively common but are often an incidental finding at appendectomy and rarely metastasize.

REFERENCES

1. Boyle P, Zaridze DG, Smans M: Descriptive epidemiology of colorectal cancer. *Int J Cancer* 1985, 36:9–18.
2. Whalen SL, Parkin DM, Masayer E: Patterns of cancer incidence in five continents. Lyon International Agency for Research on Cancer, 1990. [IARC Scientific Publication 102.]
3. Bresalier RS, Kim YS: Malignant neoplasms of the large intestine. In *Gastrointestinal Disease: Pathophysiology/Diagnosis/Management*, edn 5. Edited by Sleisenger, Fordtran. Philadelphia: WB Saunders; 1993: 1449–1493.
4. Reddy BS, Cohen LA: Nutrition and its relationship to cancer. *Adv Cancer Res* 1980, 32:237–245.
5. Lipkin M: Phase I and phase 2 proliferative lesions of colonic epithelial cells in diseases leading to colonic cancer. *Cancer* 1974, 34:878–888 .
6. Bresalier RS, *et al.*: Familial colon cancer. In *Premalignant Conditions of the Gastrointestinal Tract.* Edited by Eastwood GL. New York: Elsevier Publishing Co., 1991:227–243.
7. Vogelstein B, Fearon ER, Hamilton SR, *et al.*: Genetic alterations during colorectal-tumor development. *N Engl J Med* 1988, 319:525–532.
8. Lynch HT, Smyrk TC, Watson P, *et al.*: Genetics, natural history, tumor spectrum, and pathology of the hereditary and nonpolyposis colorectal cancer: An updated review. *Gastroenterology* 1993, 104:1535–1549.
9. Boland CR: Familial colonic cancer syndromes. *West J Med* 1983, 139:351–359.
10. Lynch HT, Watson P, Lanspa S, *et al.*: Natural history of colorectal cancer in hereditary colorectal cancer (Lynch Syndromes I and II). *Dis Colon Rectum* 1988, 31:439–444.
11. Bresalier R: Colorectal cancer. In *Principles and Practices of Gastroenterology and Hepatology*. Edited by Gitrick G, Hollander D, Sanloff JM, *et al.* Appleton & Lange; 1994:343–367.
12. Haggitt RC, Glutzbach RE, Soffer EE, Wruble LD: Prognostic factors in colorectal carcinomas arising in the adenomas: Implications for lesions removed by endoscopic polypectomy. *Gastroenterology* 1985, 89:328–336.
13. Donnegan WL, DeCosse JJ: Pitfalls and controversies in staging of colorectal cancer. In *Carcinoma of the Colon and Rectum*. Edited by Enker WF. Chicago: Year Book, 1978:49–70.
14. American Joint Committee for Cancer Staging and End Result Reporting: *Manual for Staging Cancer*, edn 3. Philadelphia: JB Lippincott, 1988.
15. Moertel CG, O'Fallon JR, Go VLW, *et al.*: The preoperative carcinogenic antigen test in the diagnosis, staging and prognosis of colorectal cancer. *Cancer* 1986, 58: 603–610.
16. Podolsky DK: Gastrointestinal Oncology, Unit 22. American Gastroenterological Association; 1989.
17. Schrock TR: Large intestine. In *Current Surgical Disease and Treatment*. Edited by Way LW. Norwalk: Lange Medical Publishers, 1985:594–601.
18. Moertel CG, Fleming TR, MacDonald JS, *et al.*: Levamisole and fluorouracil for adjuvant therapy of resected colorectal carcinoma. *N Engl J Med* 1990, 322:352–358.
19. Krook JE, Moertal CG, Gunderson LL, *et al.*: Effective adjuvant therapy for high risk carcinoma. *N Engl J Med* 1991, 324:705–715.

Chapter 4

Inflammatory Colitides

LAWRENCE S. FRIEDMAN
FIONA GRAEME-COOK
ROBERT H. SCHAPIRO

The idiopathic inflammatory diseases include ulcerative colitis and Crohn's disease. Most evidence suggests that these two forms of inflammatory bowel disease are distinct entities but share pathophysiologic processes; however, their precise causes remain unknown. Genetic factors are thought to play a role as suggested by an increased prevalence of inflammatory bowel disease (5% to 10%) among first-degree relatives of affected patients and an increased incidence in certain populations. Recently, an increased frequency of HLA-DR2 has been observed in patients with ulcerative colitis. Moreover, about 70% of patients with ulcerative colitis, as well as those with primary sclerosing cholangitis, have been found to have circulating antineutrophil cytoplasmic antibodies. Specific alterations in the composition of mucin glycoproteins have been observed in patients with ulcerative colitis. In patients with Crohn's disease, granulomatous angiitis, possibly related to an earlier measles infection, has been suggested to be an underlying pathophysiologic process. In both diseases, altered immune regulation is observed and characterized by increased mucosal antibody production, complement deposition in intestinal mucosa, and increased numbers of cytotoxic T cells. Mucosal immune activation is also suggested by increased expression of various cytokines and inflammatory mediators, but the precise stimulus or stimuli remain uncertain.

Patients with ulcerative colitis typically present with bloody diarrhea, although those with proctitis may actually complain of constipation. The inflammatory process is confined to the mucosa of the colon. The clinical presentation of Crohn's disease is more varied, reflecting the patchy and transmural nature of the inflammatory process. The colon alone is involved in 30% of cases, the small intestine in 40%, and both the large and small intestine in 30% of cases. Diagnosis depends on demonstration of characteristic endoscopic, radiologic, and histologic features in the appropriate clinical setting. The differential diagnosis often includes acute colitis, most typically caused by an infectious agent. The idiopathic inflammatory bowel diseases may be associated with a variety of extraintestinal manifestations, including peripheral and axial arthritis, a variety of skin lesions, primary sclerosing cholangitis, and an increased risk of thromboembolic disease. Increased risks of colonic cancer in patients with longstanding ulcerative colitis and small intestinal cancer in patients with small intestinal Crohn's disease are well established, and an association between Crohn's disease and an increased risk of colonic cancer has been suggested.

Medical therapy of inflammatory bowel disease is based on nonspecific suppression of the inflammatory process. The mainstays of therapy include corticosteroids and aminosalicylates. In disease unresponsive to corticosteroids or in the setting of a high corticosteroid requirement, the immunosuppressive agents azathioprine or 6-mercaptopurine may be added. Cyclosporine has shown promise in the treatment of acute, severe ulcerative colitis. Oral antibiotics, including metronidazole, are useful in the treatment of colonic and perineal Crohn's disease. Colectomy is curative in ulcerative colitis and may be required in up to 30% of cases. When feasible, ileoanal anastomosis is the surgical treatment of choice. In Crohn's disease, surgery is ultimately required in most cases. In patients with small intestinal strictures, strictureplasty, rather than resection, is preferable when the stricture is fibrotic and uninflamed.

ULCERATIVE COLITIS

Endoscopic features

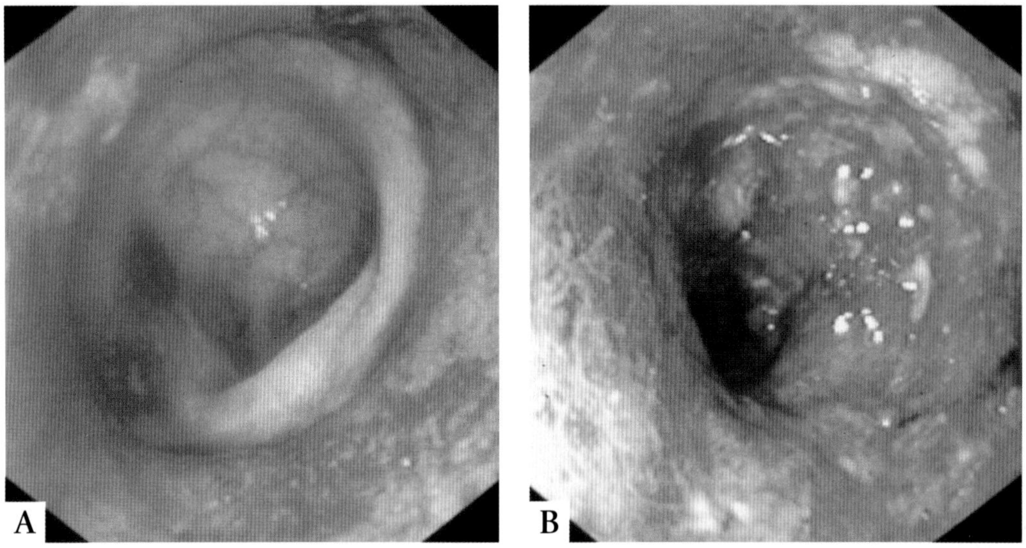

FIGURE 4-1.
Endoscopic features of active ulcerative colitis. Findings include diffusely erythematous, edematous, and granular mucosa with areas of submucosal hemorrhage and, when severe, frank mucopurulent exudate. Inflammation invariably begins in the rectum and extends proximally for varying extents. The chronicity of the process is suggested by the loss of colonic haustrations; otherwise, the endoscopic picture is nonspecific and could be consistent with acute infectious colitis, chronic ulcerative or Crohn's colitis, or any number of other specific causes of colitis. **A**, Mild distal ulcerative colitis with diffuse erythema and friability well demarcated from the normal mucosa more proximally is depicted. **B**, This example shows moderately severe ulcerative colitis with irregular, inflamed, ulcerated mucosa and a patchy exudate.

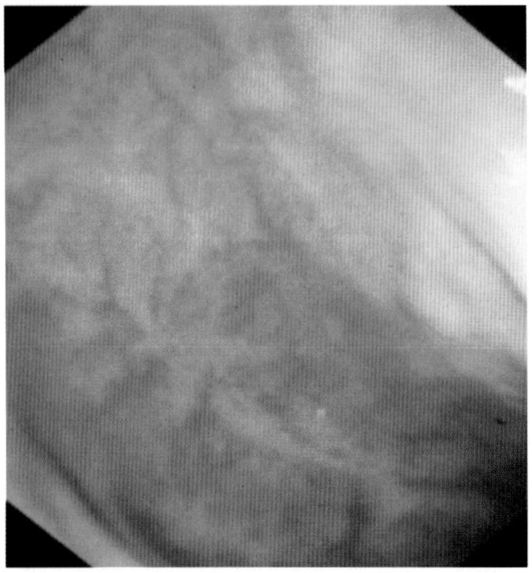

FIGURE 4-2.
Ulcerative colitis in remission. The normal vascular pattern is absent and a white scar indicates the site of a previous ulcer.

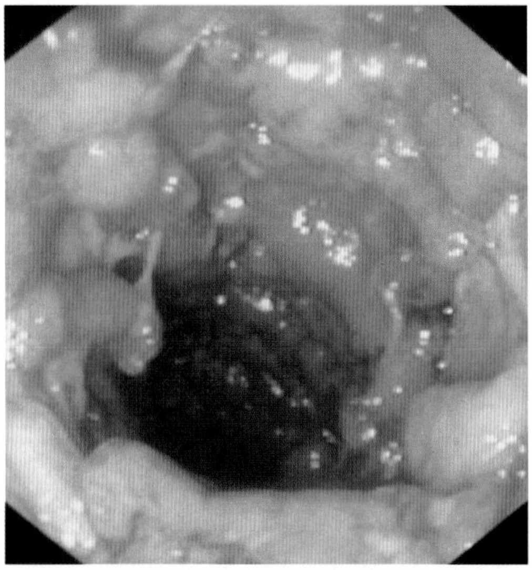

FIGURE 4-3.
Severe ulcerative colitis. The mucosa shows extensive ulceration and diffuse thickening with an inflammatory infiltrate. In contrast to Crohn's colitis, the ulceration lacks depth.

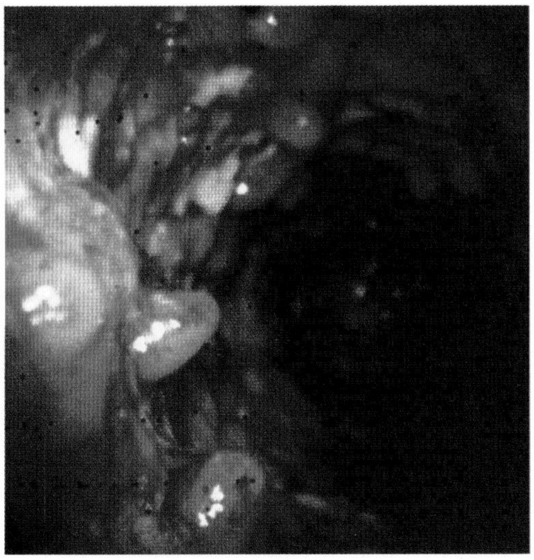

FIGURE 4-4.

Severe ulcerative colitis with pseudopolyps. In addition to severe mucosal ulceration and inflammation, chronic ulcerative colitis is often associated with the formation of pseudopolyps, which represent islands of regenerating mucosa and exuberant inflammation amidst diffuse mucosal destruction. Pseudopolyps have no malignant potential.

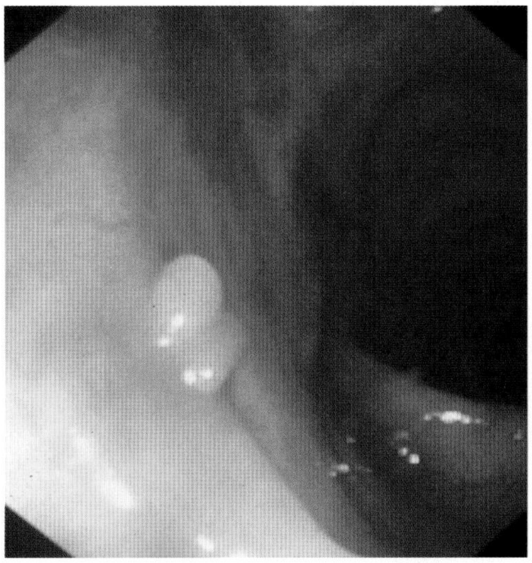

FIGURE 4-5.

Chronic ulcerative colitis. In longstanding ulcerative colitis, the mucosa has an atrophic and scarred appearance with a blunted vascular pattern. Pseudopolyps are often present.

Radiographic appearance

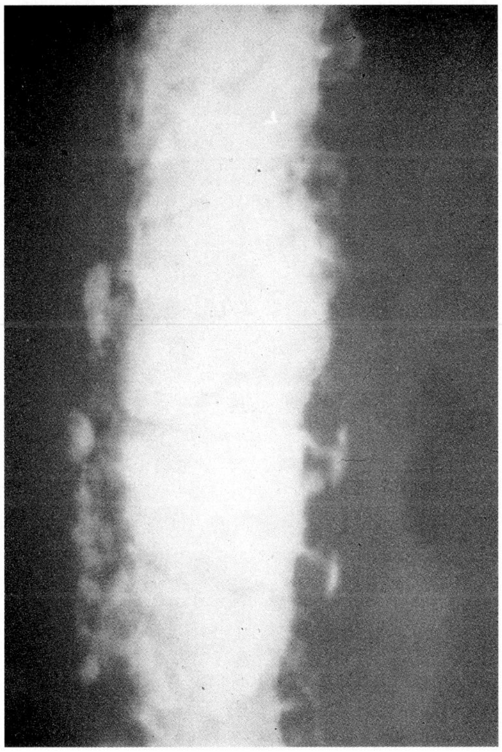

FIGURE 4-6.

Radiographic appearance of severe ulcerative colitis. This single-contrast barium enema demonstrates the typical ragged and ulcerative appearance of the mucosa in active ulcerative colitis. Characteristic collar-button or undermining ulcers are seen. In general, barium enema and colonoscopy should be avoided in fulminant ulcerative colitis because of the possibility of precipitating toxic megacolon.

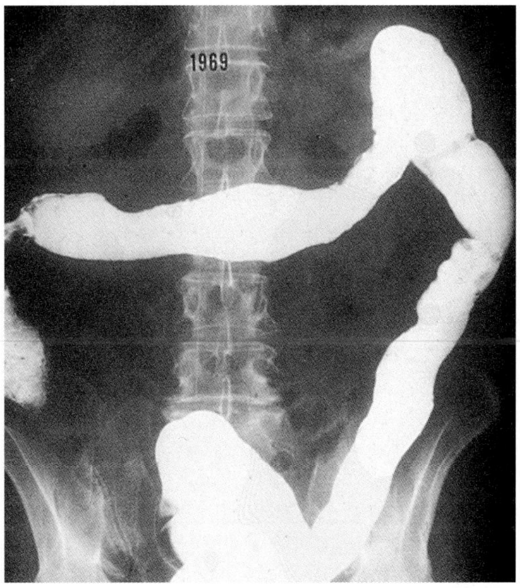

FIGURE 4-7.

Radiographic appearance of chronic ulcerative colitis. Longstanding chronic ulcerative colitis, as shown in this single-contrast barium enema, is characterized by shortening and straightening of the colon with loss of haustrations, resulting in the appearance of a featureless tube. No ulcerations are seen.

Pathologic specimen

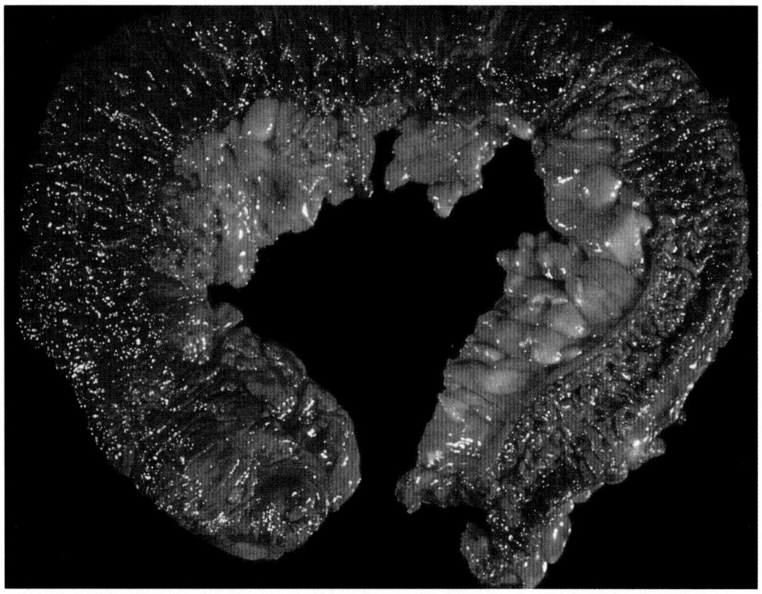

FIGURE 4-8.

Gross pathologic specimen of resected colon from a patient with severe ulcerative colitis. Inflammation is diffuse and continuous, involving the mucosa and extending from the rectum without interruption to the ascending colon.

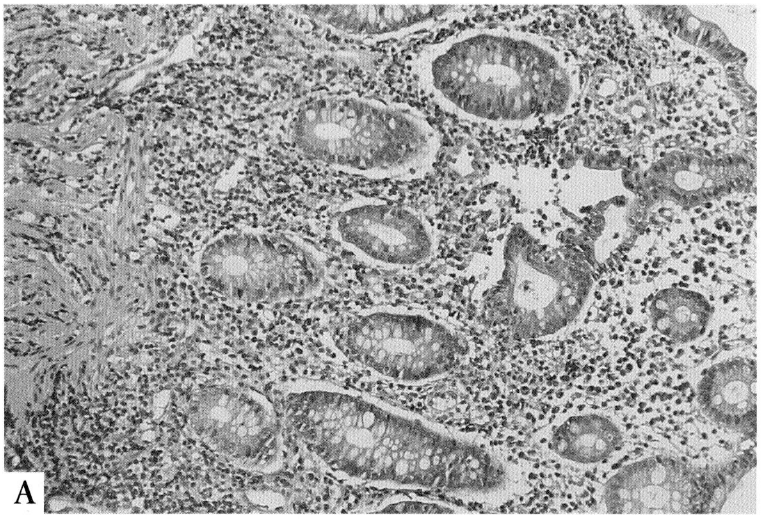

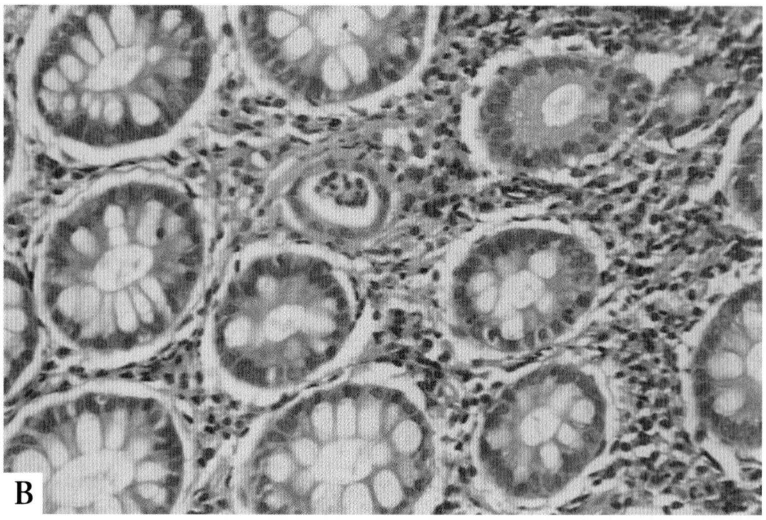

FIGURE 4-9.

Microscopic features of the specimen shown in Figure 4-8. **A**, There is diffuse acute and chronic inflammation with architectural distortion and destruction of some glands, depletion of mucin from goblet cells, and crypt abscesses. Inflammation is limited to the mucosa. **B**, A higher power microscopic feature showing diffuse inflammation and a crypt abscess.

Dysplasia

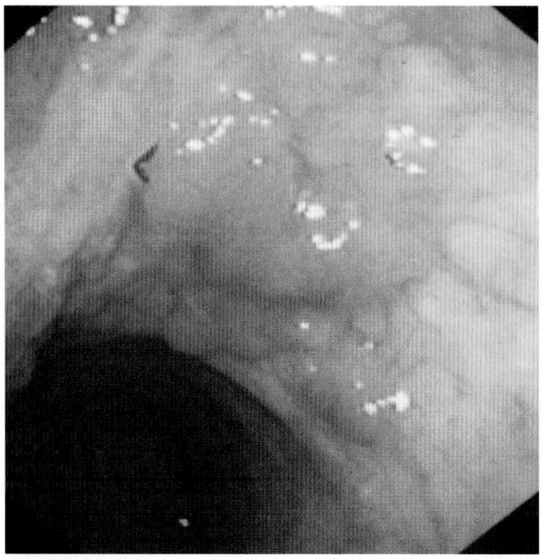

FIGURE 4-10.

Dysplasia-associated lesion or mass in chronic ulcerative colitis. Long-standing ulcerative colitis is associated with an increased risk of colonic carcinoma. The risk correlates with the duration of colitis and the extent of disease; colitis involving the entire colon (pancolitis) is associated with a much greater risk of colonic carcinoma than disease limited to the left colon, and ulcerative proctitis is not associated with an increased risk of rectal cancer in excess of that of the background (noncolitis) population. In patients with ulcerative colitis at increased risk of colonic cancer, surveillance colonoscopy is performed to screen for dysplasia or precancer, a marker of an increased likelihood of colonic cancer. Dysplasia may be found in normal-appearing mucosa but is more likely associated with raised, flat, or bumpy lesions as shown.

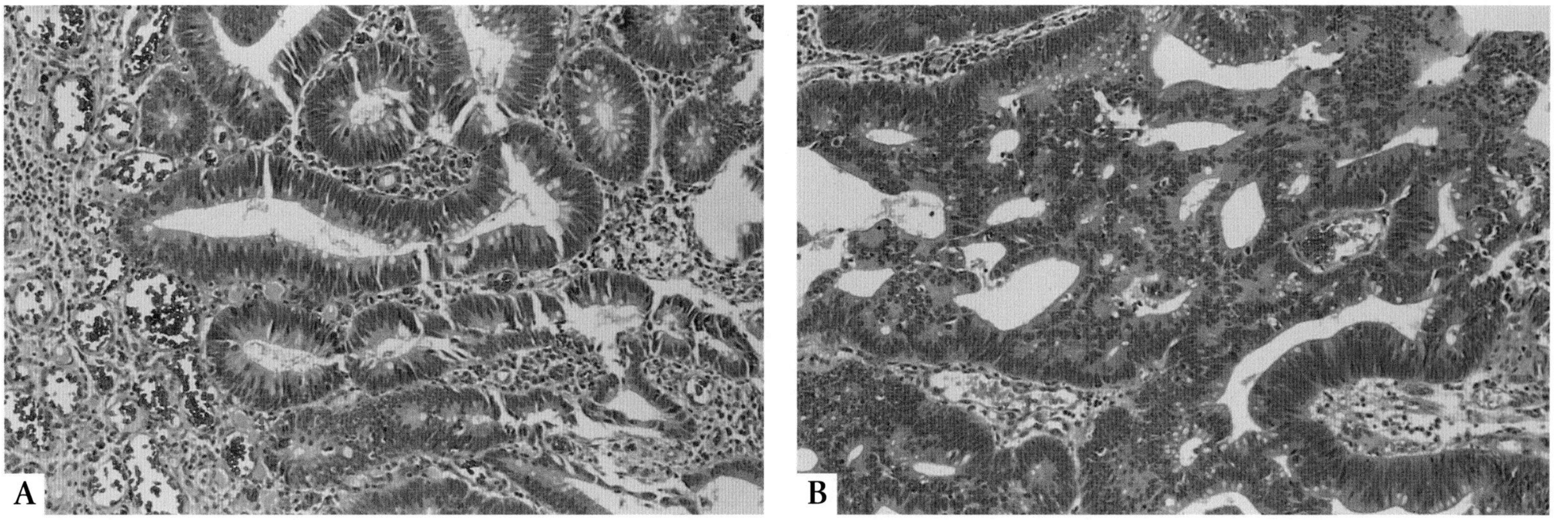

FIGURE 4-11.

Histologic features of dysplasia. **A**, Low-grade dysplasia characterized by nuclear enlargement, crowding, and hyperchromasia in the colonic epithelial cells. Nuclei are stratified but remain in the basal half of the cells. There is some depletion of mucin. **B**, In high-grade dysplasia, the changes are more pronounced. Nuclei are stratified to the surface, and there is a marked increase in nuclear pleomorphism. A branching of cribriform pattern to the glands and scattered cell necrosis is shown. No mucin goblets are evident.

Colonic carcinoma

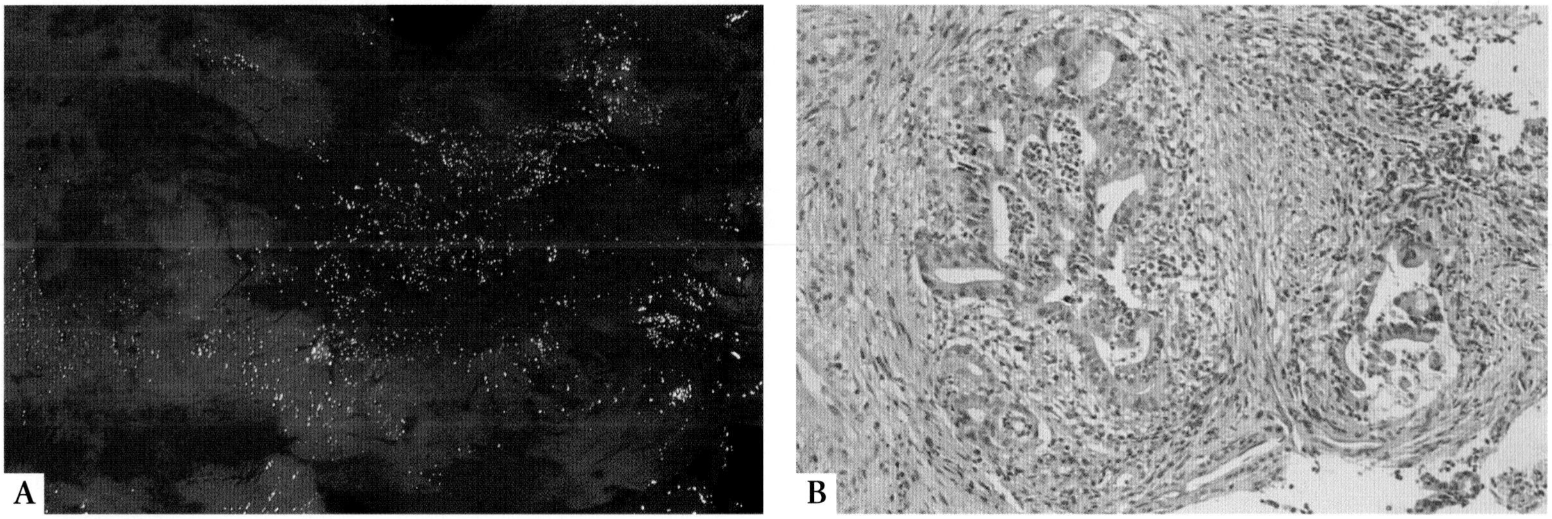

FIGURE 4-12.

Colonic carcinoma in ulcerative colitis. **A**, Gross resected specimen of the rectum showing frank rectal carcinoma in the setting of diffuse ulcerative colitis. The rectum has a loss of mucosal folds and a granular hemorrhagic surface surrounding a deeply invasive carcinoma. **B**, Microscopic section showing an infiltrating adenocarcinoma arising in a background of chronic ulcerative colitis with a surrounding desmoplastic stroma.

Endoscopic features

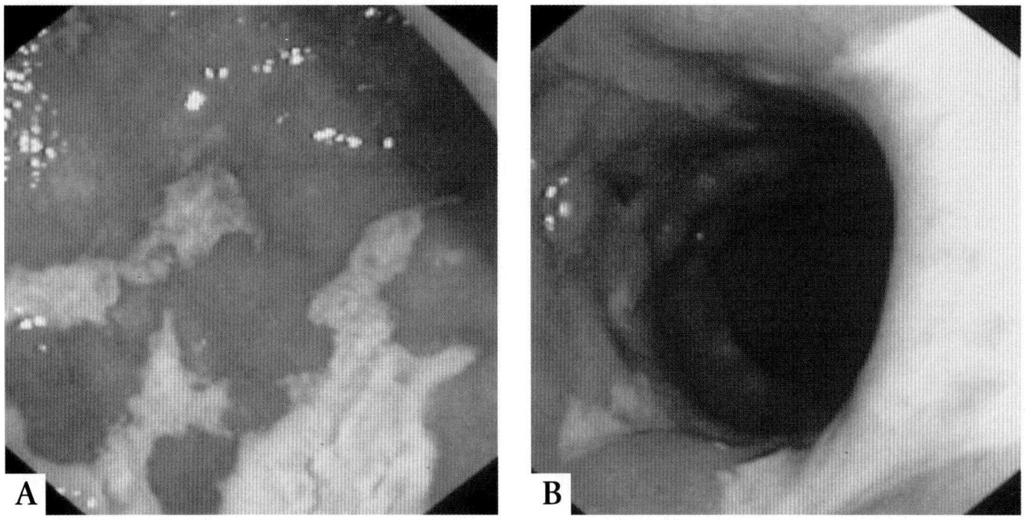

FIGURE 4-13.

A and B, Endoscopic features of Crohn's disease of the terminal ileum. A diffuse inflammation is depicted with characteristic large irregular ulcers that are often stellate or longitudinal.

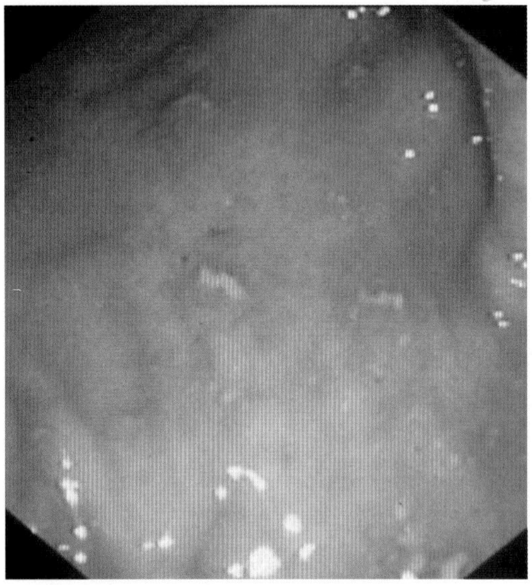

FIGURE 4-14.

Endoscopic features of early Crohn's disease. The earliest lesion of Crohn's disease, shown on colonoscopy, is aphthous ulceration, a focal mucosal defect with surrounding erythema. This finding is nonspecific and may also be seen in herpesvirus infection, cytomegalovirus infection, Yersinia infection, tuberculosis, schistosomiasis, and Behcet's disease.

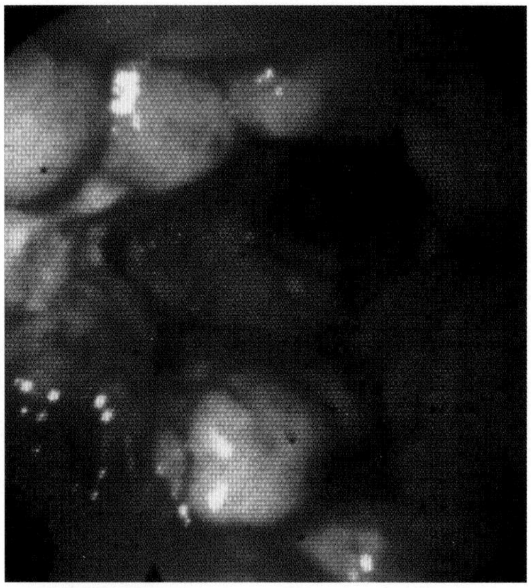

FIGURE 4-15.

Severe Crohn's colitis. A characteristic "cobblestone" appearance is the result of multiple longitudinal ulcers and exuberant inflammation with pseudopolyp formation as well as thickening of the intestinal wall because of transmural inflammation.

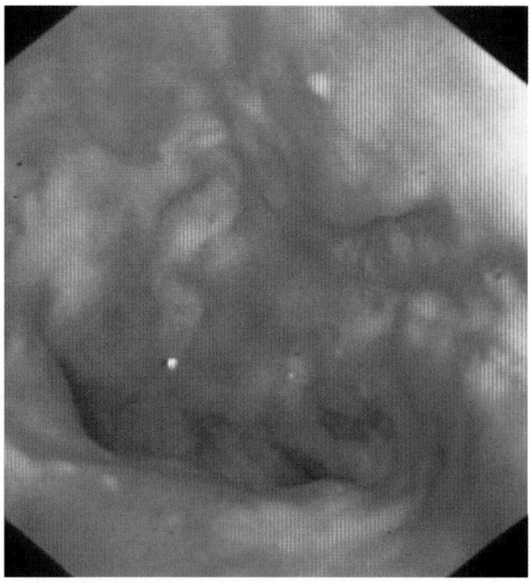

FIGURE 4-16.

Crohn's colitis in remission. Patchy erythema surrounds areas in which epithelialization of previous sites of ulceration has taken place. There is no active ulceration.

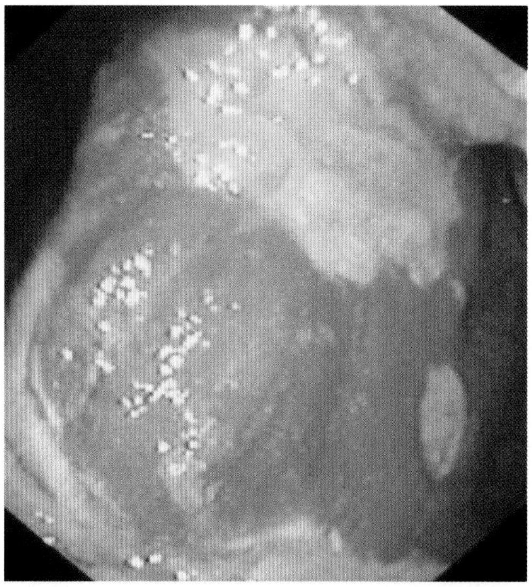

FIGURE 4-17.

Crohn's disease at an ileocolonic anastomosis. Endoscopic recurrence of disease following surgical resection is invariable and first occurs on the ileal side of an ileocolonic anastomosis, although clinical recurrence may not necessarily follow. Typical Crohn's ulcers in the neoterminal ileum at an ileorectal anastomosis are shown.

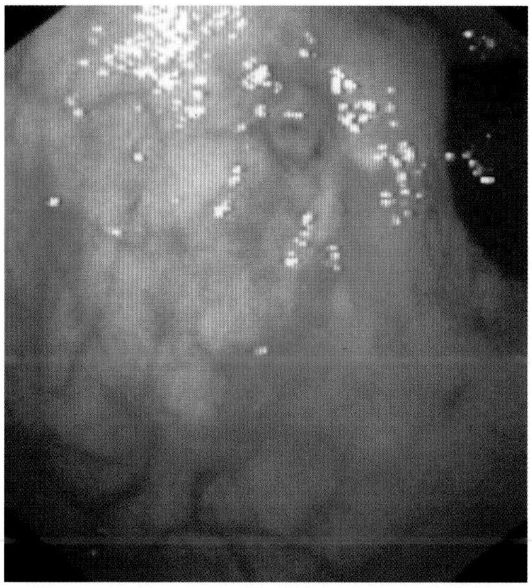

FIGURE 4-18.

Retroflexed view of the rectum showing a small fistulous opening in a patient with Crohn's disease. Because of the transmural nature of the inflammation in Crohn's disease, fistula formation is typical and may develop between segments of the bowel and between the bowel and the bladder, vagina, urethra, prostate, or skin. Abscess formation may result. Perianal fistula formation is typically, but not necessarily, associated with active proctitis.

Perianal Crohn's disease

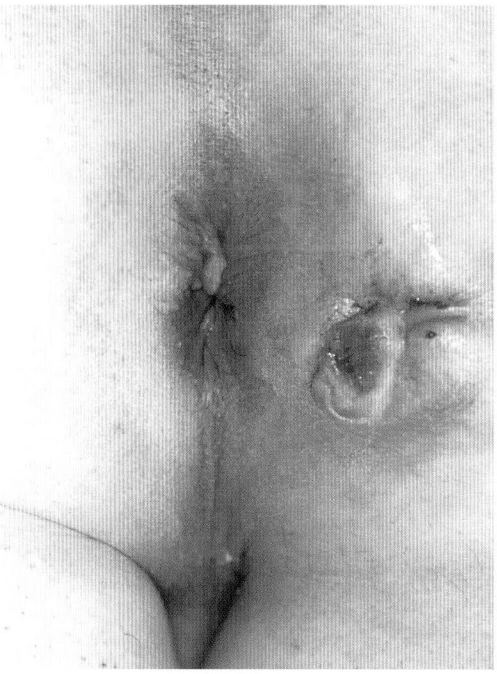

FIGURE 4-19.

The cutaneous opening of a perirectal fistula is shown. Such fistulas may arise from the crypts of Morgagni in the anus and spread through the internal anal sphincter, resulting in perineal or rectovaginal fistulas, ischiorectal abscesses, or intersphincteric abscesses.

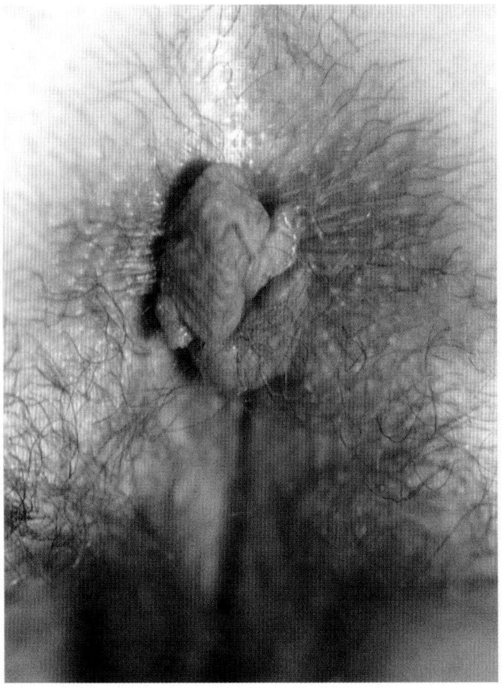

FIGURE 4-20.

Typical perianal changes of Crohn's disease. The large skin tags of granulation tissue, which are firm and thickened, give an "elephant-ear" appearance.

Small bowel

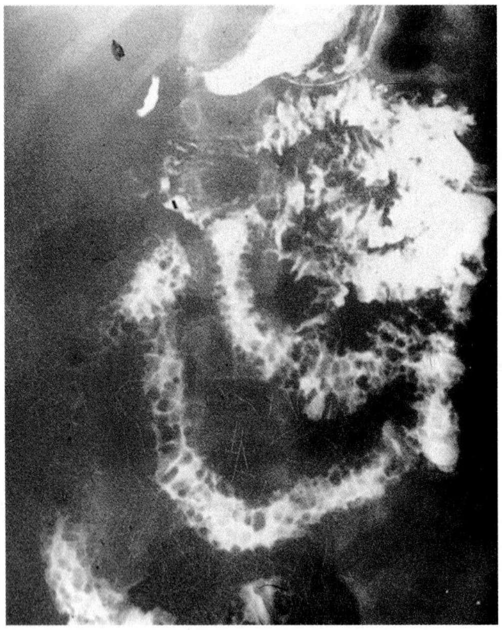

FIGURE 4-21.

Small bowel follow through in Crohn's disease. In addition to diffuse nodularity of the small intestine, lumens of involved loops of bowel appear to be widely separated as a result of a marked increase in the thickness of the bowel wall, resulting from transmural inflammation and mesenteric edema and hyperemia.

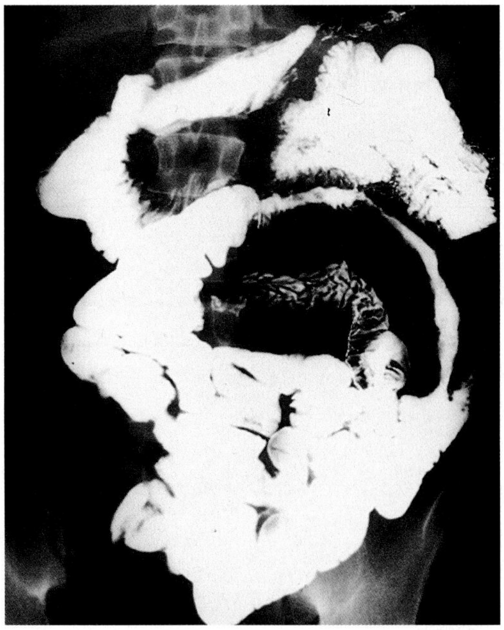

FIGURE 4-22.

Small bowel follow through showing an isolated segment of Crohn's disease of the jejunum, the so-called "string sign." Lumen of the involved segment is narrowed as a result of either diffuse inflammation of the bowel wall with spasm or a fibrotic stricture from previous inflammation.

Additional radiologic findings

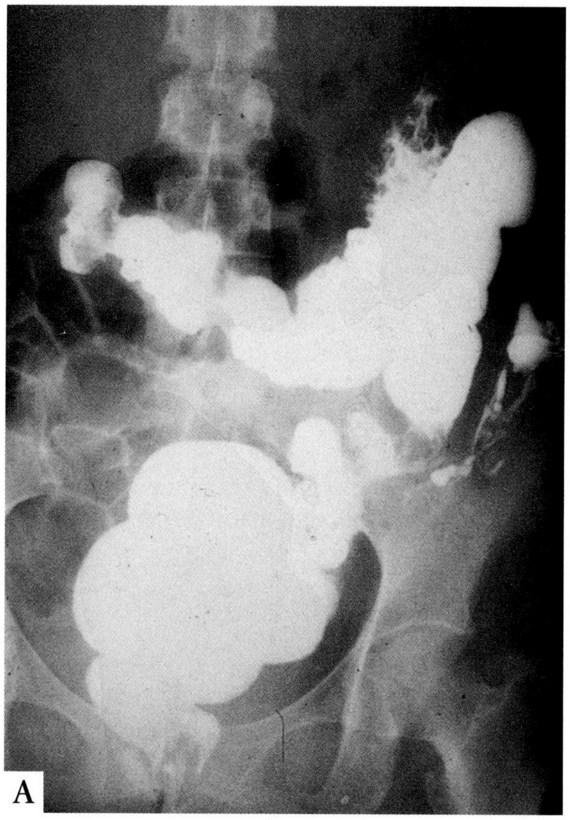

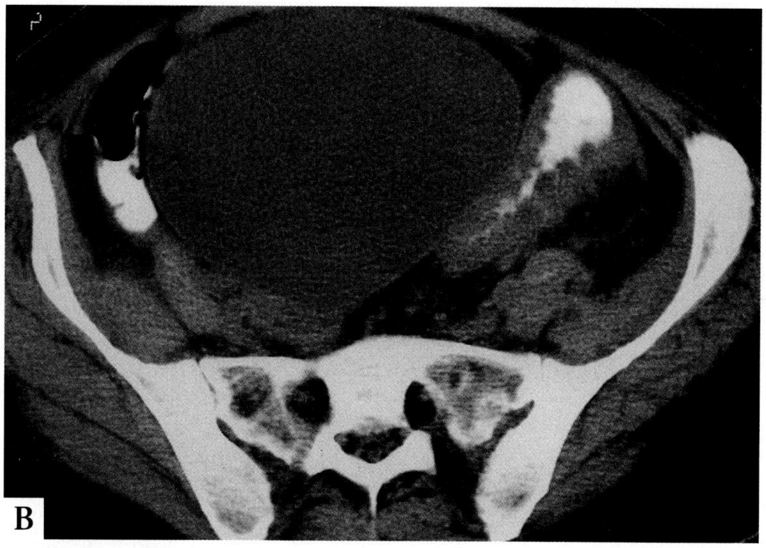

FIGURE 4-23.

Additional radiologic findings in Crohn's disease. **A**, Barium enema demonstrates a fistula from the descending colon to the left paracolonic soft tissue as a result of Crohn's disease. **B**, Computed tomographic scan showing marked thickening of the colonic wall (to the left of the bladder) typical of Crohn's disease. Computed tomographic scanning is also useful for detecting Crohn's abscesses and fistulas. (**B**, *Courtesy of* G. J. Whitman, Boston, MA)

SPECIMENS

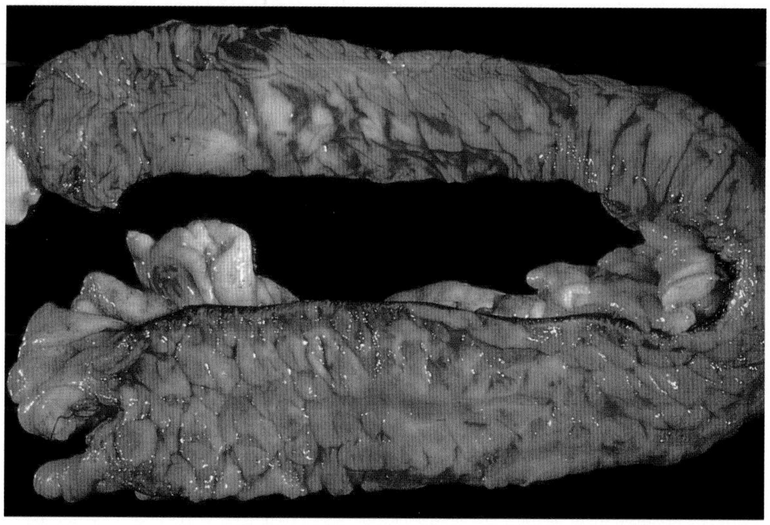

FIGURE 4-24.

Gross specimen of a colon resected from a patient with Crohn's colitis. The mucosa demonstrates a typical cobblestone appearance with linear and discrete ulcers and a narrow lumen. The inflammation is patchy with "creeping fat," reflecting extension of the transmural inflammation into the serosa.

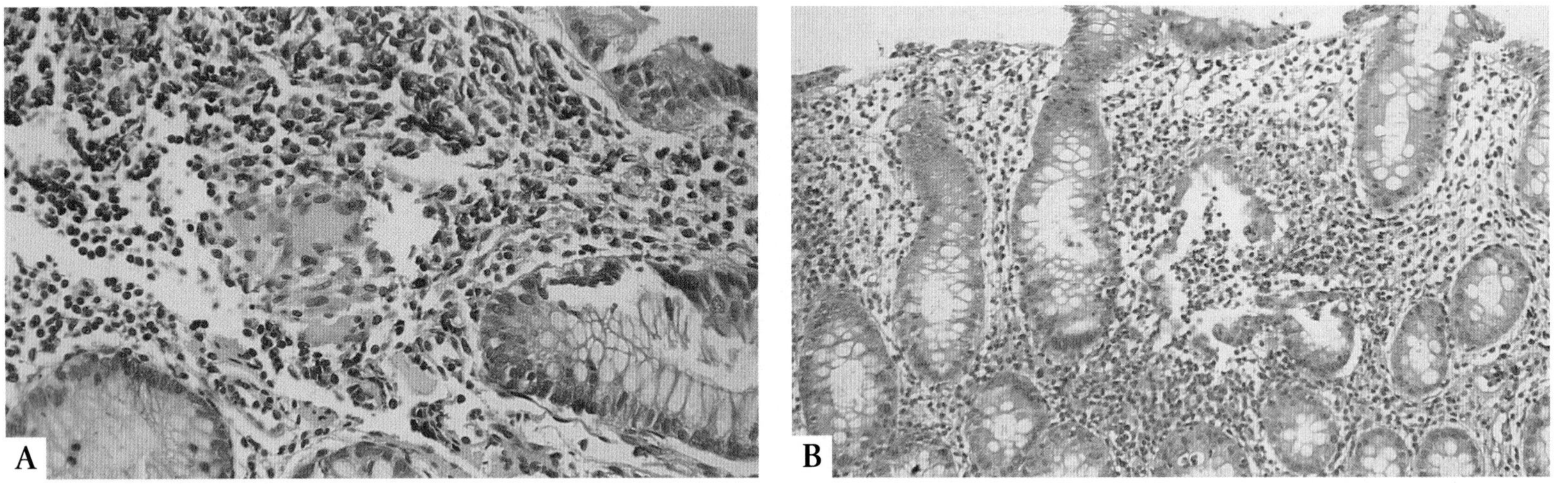

FIGURE 4-25.

Microscopic specimen from a patient with Crohn's colitis. **A**, The specimen has diffuse inflammation of the mucosa and submucosa with a small granuloma in the center. **B**, Patchy inflammation with marked enlargement of crypts and a focal abscess can be seen. In contrast to ulcerative colitis, the mucin is relatively preserved.

THEORIES OF INFLAMMATORY BOWEL DISEASE ETIOLOGY

TABLE 4-1. THEORIES OF INFLAMMATORY BOWEL DISEASE ETIOLOGY

- Toxic response to luminal contents
  - Specific microbial pathogen
  - Abnormal luminal constituents
  - Increased absorption of luminal macromolecules
- Enhanced immunologic response to normal constituents
- Autoimmune response
  - To epithelial cell or mucus glycoproteins
  - Molecular mimicry (cross-reactivity of intestinal microflora and epithelia)
  - To immune cells

TABLE 4-1.

Theories of inflammatory bowel disease etiology. The precise cause or causes of inflammatory bowel disease are unknown. The most widely held theories of pathogenesis focus on the possibility of a toxic response to a luminal antigen, enhanced immunologic responsiveness to normal luminal constituents, or an autoimmune response to an epithelial cell, mucus glycoprotein, immune cell, or cross-reacting antigen of bacterial origin. (*Adapted from* Sartor [1]; with permission.)

TISSUE DAMAGE IN INFLAMMATORY BOWEL DISEASE

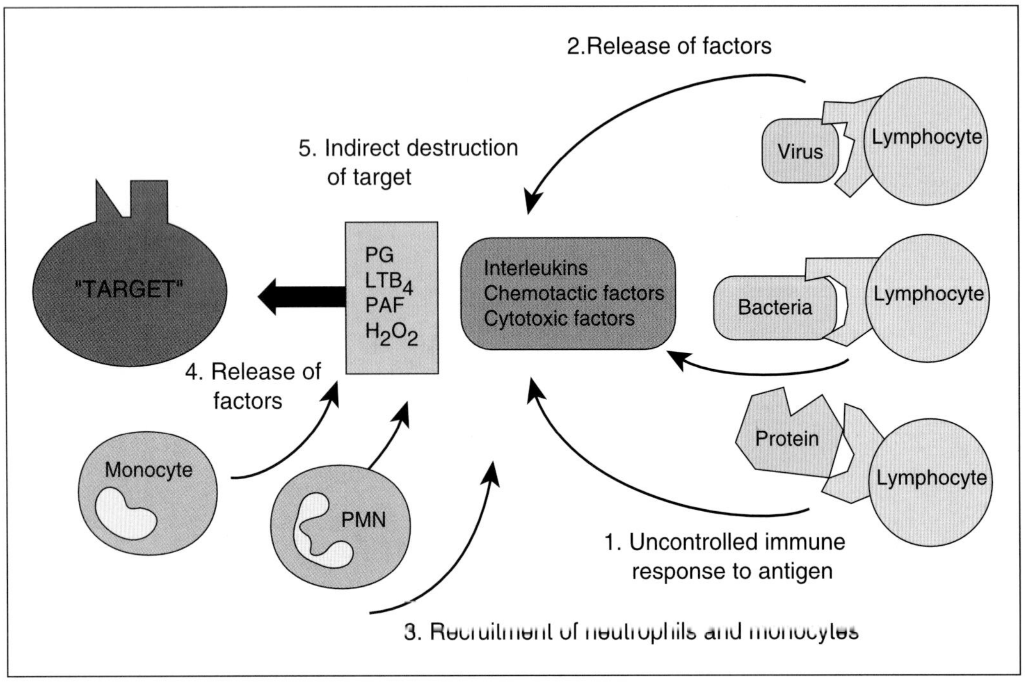

FIGURE 4-26.

Immune-mediated tissue damage in inflammatory bowel disease. A variety of immune mechanisms have been proposed to mediate attack against a specific putative target antigen in inflammatory bowel disease. In addition to a direct attack by lymphocytes or other immune cells, tissue damage may result from the release of a variety of cytokines, which in turn recruit additional inflammatory mediators and lead to further local tissue damage. LTB_4—leukotriene B_4; PAF—platelet activating factor; PG—prostaglandins; PMN—polymorphonuclear neutrophil. (*Adapted from* Targan *et al.* [2]; with permission.)

ISCHEMIC COLITIS

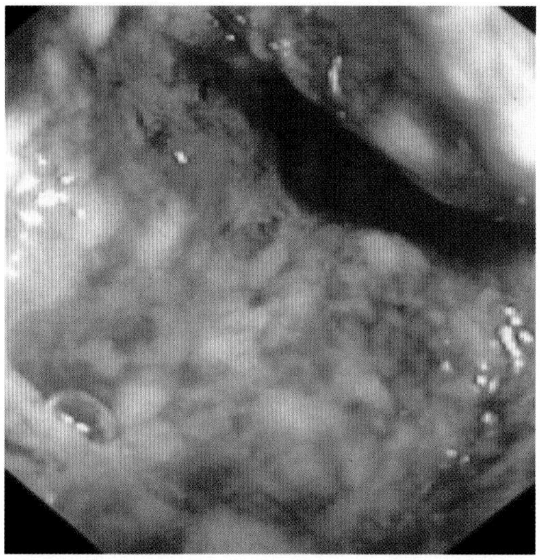

FIGURE 4-27.

Endoscopic appearance of ischemic colitis. In elderly persons, in particular, ischemic colitis enters into the differential diagnosis of inflammatory bowel disease. The etiology is usually nonocclusive ischemic damage to the colon as a result of hypotension or hypoperfusion. Iatrogenic injury to or ligation of the inferior mesenteric artery may also result in ischemic colitis. In contrast with ulcerative colitis, the rectum is typically spared, colonic involvement is segmental, and the symptoms are acute and self-limited. Typical endoscopic features include ulceration, which is patchy and in severe cases, as shown here, associated with necrosis and exudation. In some cases, resolution may be followed by stricture formation.

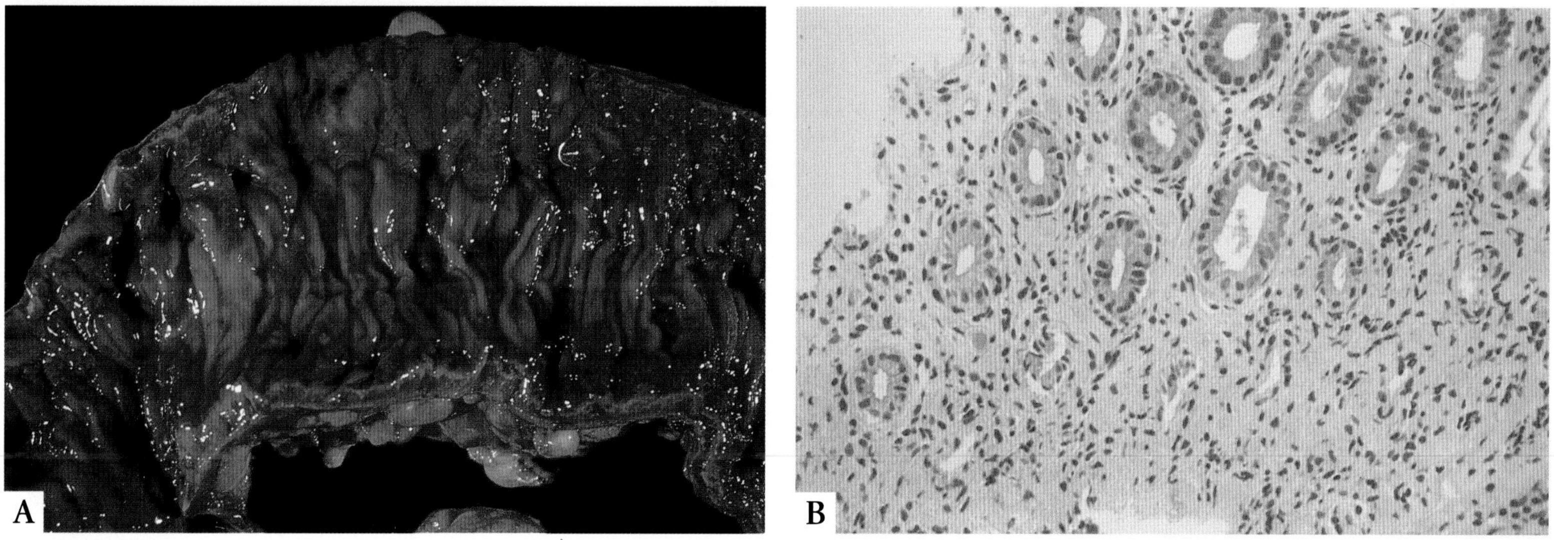

FIGURE 4-28.

Pathologic features of ischemic colitis. **A**, Grossly, the mucosa is inflamed and hemorrhagic with scattered deep ulcers and a greenish pseudomembrane representing sloughed mucosa. **B**, Microscopic examination shows little if any inflammation. There is scattered gland dropout, small fibrin thrombi in arterioles, and fibrin in the stroma. In some cases of ischemic colitis, inflammation with crypt abscesses may be present, simulating ulcerative colitis.

CHOLESTEROL EMBOLI

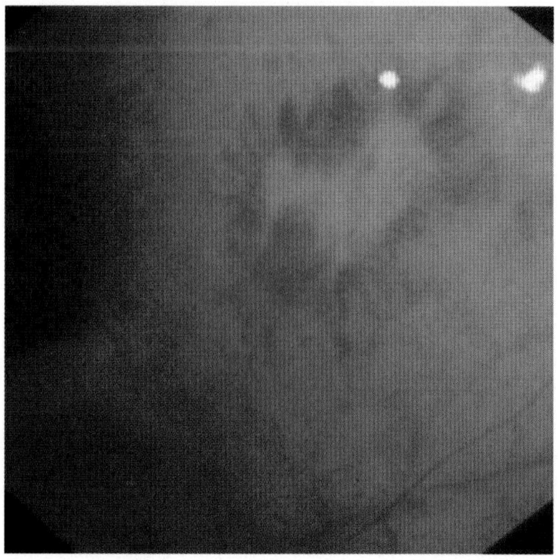

FIGURE 4-29.

Endoscopic features of cholesterol emboli. Cholesterol emboli occur in older patients with atherosclerosis often after arteriography or initiation of anticoagulation. In addition to livedo reticularis, blue toe syndrome, hypertension, and renal insufficiency, patients may develop ischemic colitis, gastrointestinal bleeding, acute pancreatitis, acute cholecystitis, or hemorrhagic gastritis. Cholesterol emboli to the colon may be detected on colonoscopy as punctate areas of ischemia with surrounding hemorrhage.

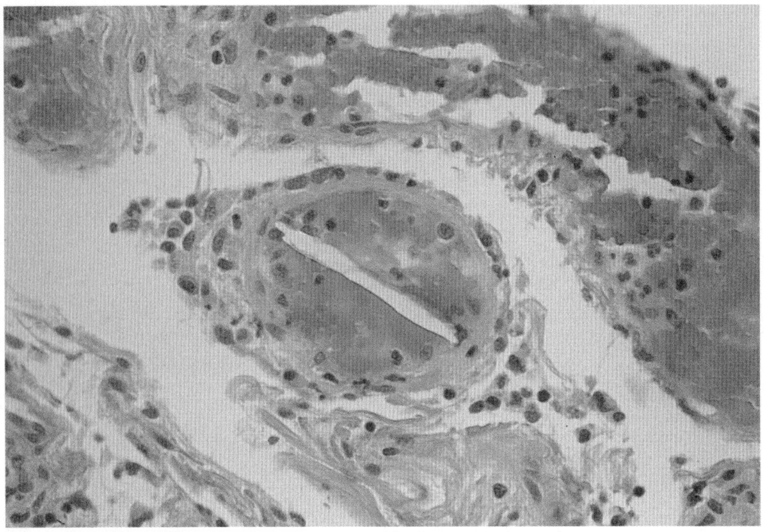

Figure 4-30.

Histologic specimen of the colon showing a cholesterol embolus with a characteristic cleft in a small submucosal arteriole.

RADIATION COLITIS

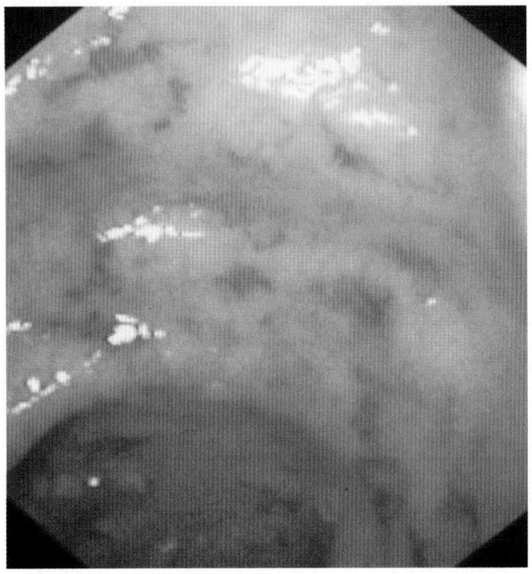

Figure 4-31.

Endoscopic features of radiation colitis. Radiation colitis is seen most commonly as a complication of pelvic irradiation for gynecologic malignancy. The endoscopic appearance may be indistinguishable from that of ulcerative colitis, but common characteristic mucosal telangiectatic lesions are seen. Luminal narrowing is frequent and solitary ulcers may occur.

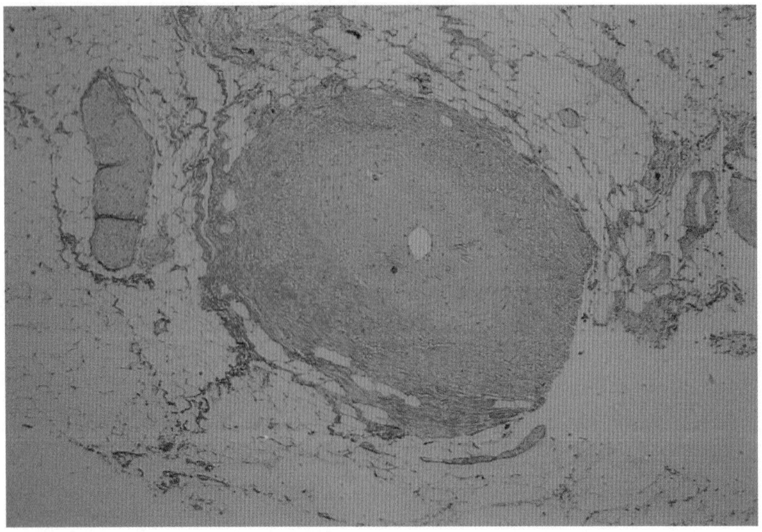

Figure 4-32.

Histologic features of radiation colitis. Radiation colitis is thought to occur in part from obliteration of the lumens of muscular arterioles in the submucosa as a result of swelling of endothelial cells and thrombosis. Large foam cells accumulate in the subintima. The process leads to ischemia with fibrosis and mucosal ulceration. Secondary calcification may also be seen.

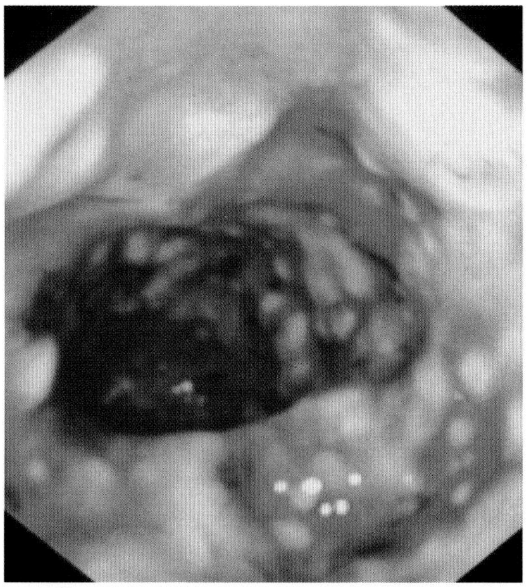

FIGURE 4-33.

Endoscopic appearance of pseudomembranous colitis. Pseudomembranous colitis characteristically results from the use of antibiotics and is caused by the toxin produced by *Clostridium difficile*. The characteristic appearance is yellow-white pseudomembranes on a background of diffuse colonic inflammation.

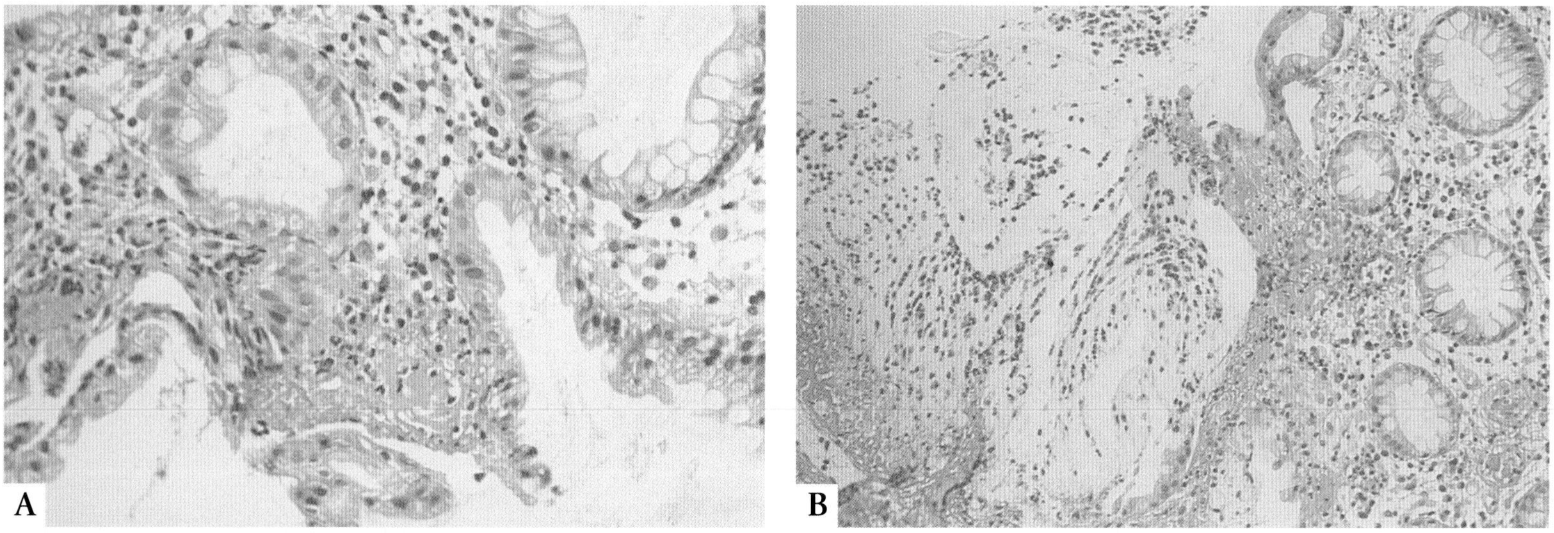

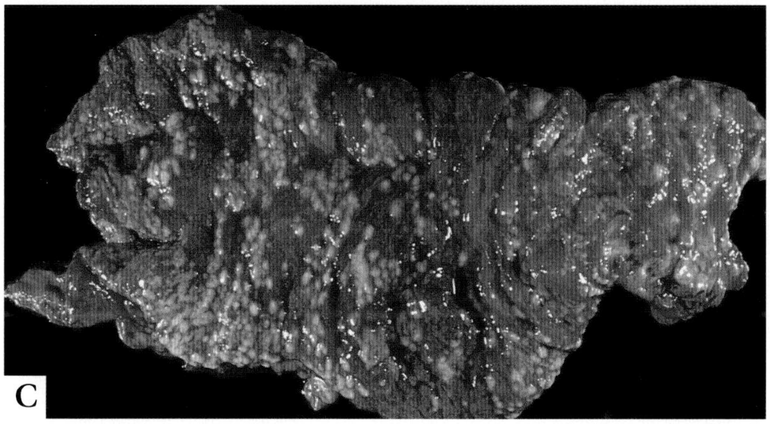

FIGURE 4-34.

Pathologic features of pseudomembranous colitis. **A**, Histologically, the early lesion is characterized by fibrin deposition and an infiltration of neutrophils under the surface epithelium. **B**, Subsequently, a characteristic volcano lesion may be seen in which crypts erupt as mucus and neutrophils stream from the destroyed gland. Surrounding crypts may appear normal. **C**, The gross appearance demonstrates the characteristic yellow-white plaquelike pseudomembranes.

ESCHERICHIA COLI INFECTION

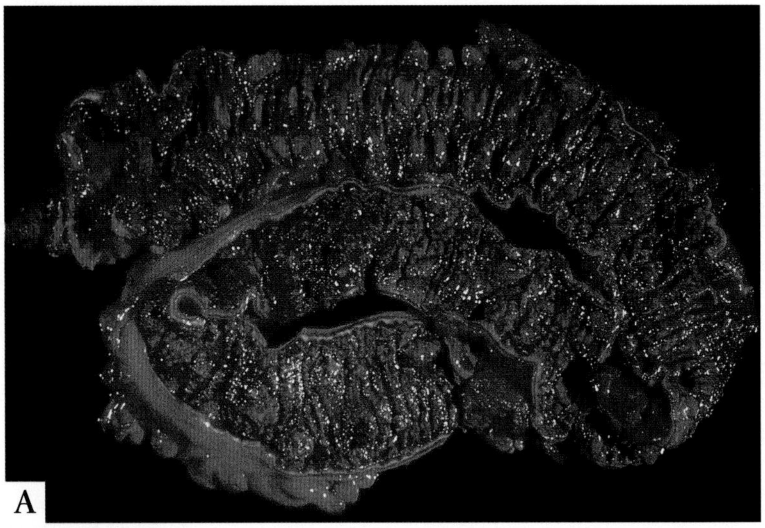

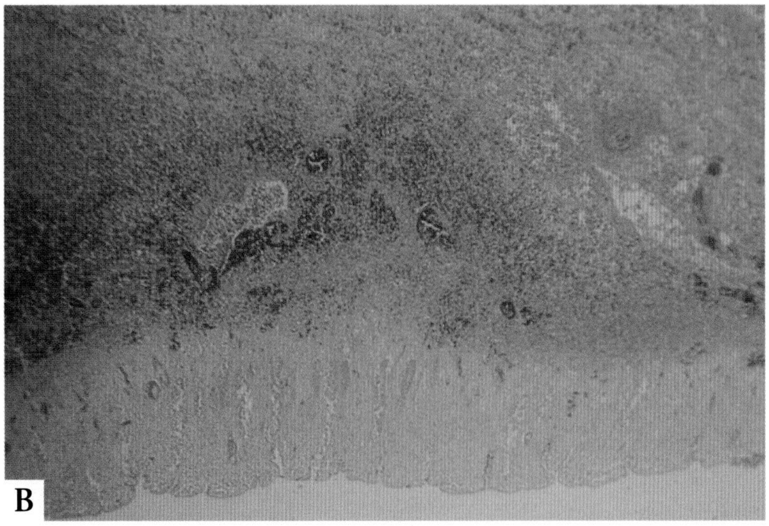

FIGURE 4-35.

Pathologic changes in colitis caused by enterohemorrhagic *Escherichia coli* infection (serotype O157:H7). The endoscopic appearance of infection caused by enterohemorrhagic *E. coli* can mimic that of ischemic colitis or pseudomembranous colitis. **A**, On gross pathology, diffuse inflammation of the colonic mucosa is not confined to the distribution of a major mesenteric vessel. There are large areas of pseudomembrane formation and marked edema. **B**, Microscopically, diffuse mucosal necrosis with underlying submucosal inflammation and vascular congestion is detected. Ghosts of destroyed glands are seen.

CYTOMEGALOVIRUS COLITIS

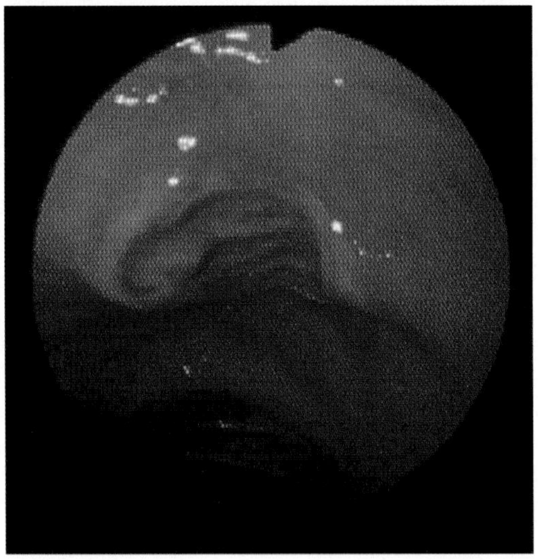

FIGURE 4-36.

Cytomegalovirus colitis. Cytomegalovirus may cause colitis, particularly in immunosuppressed hosts such as patients with AIDS or transplant recipients. Endoscopic findings may include diffuse colitis as well as solitary ulcers of the colon. As shown, the ulcer may be large with raised edges but the surrounding mucosa is normal.

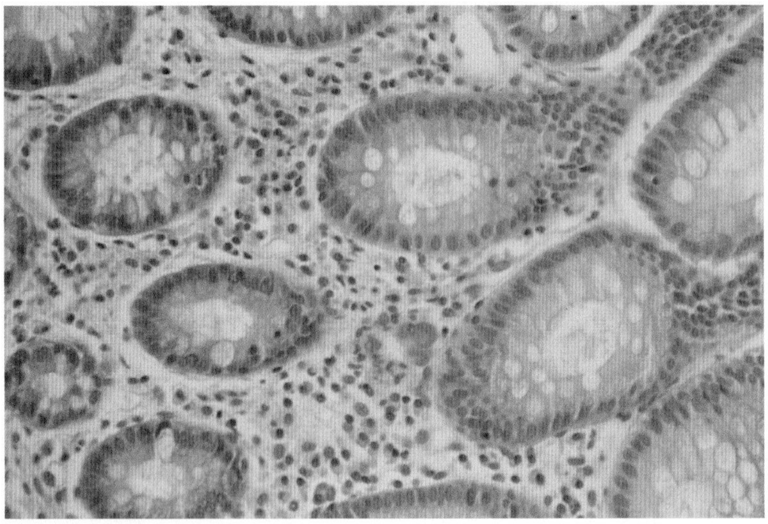

FIGURE 4-37.

Histologic features of cytomegalovirus colitis. In addition to mild nonspecific inflammation, characteristic cytomegalovirus inclusions may be seen in endothelial cells of small mucosal blood vessels.

MISCELLANEOUS DISORDERS

Solitary rectal ulcer syndrome

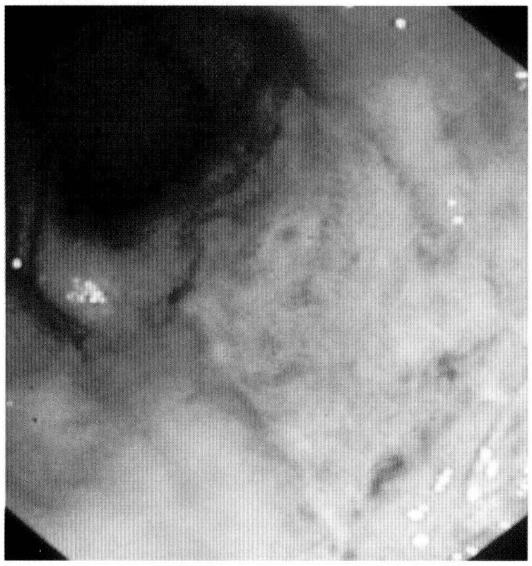

FIGURE 4-38.

Solitary rectal ulcer syndrome. A solitary ulcer in the rectum may represent solitary rectal ulcer syndrome when no other causes can be identified. The pathogenesis is related to the combination of prolonged straining at stool, resulting in mucosal prolapse, and inappropriate external anal sphincter and puborectalis muscle contraction during defecation. Anorectal pain and bleeding may result. Ulcers, which may be multiple, are usually on the anterior rectal wall. Occasionally a nodular elevation rather than an ulcer is observed. Characteristic histologic findings include fibrous obliteration of the lamina propria, thickening of the muscularis mucosa, regenerative changes in the crypt epithelium, and mucosal ulceration.

Tuberculous ileocolitis

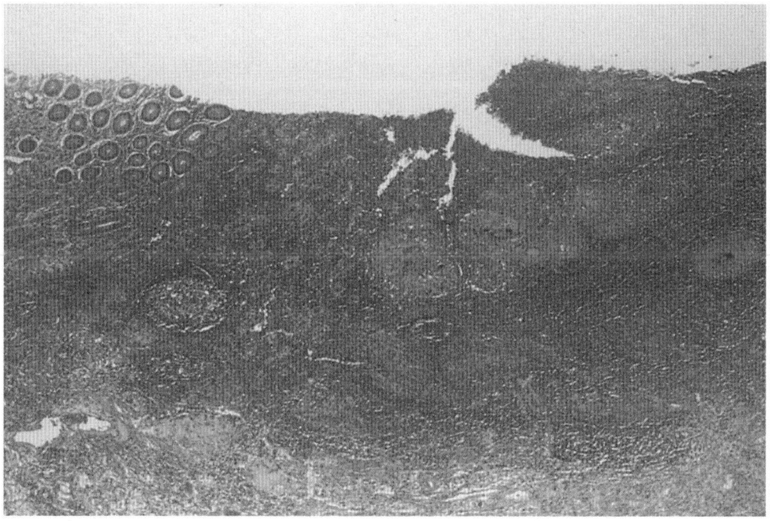

FIGURE 4-39.

Tuberculous ileocolitis. Occasionally, tuberculous ileocolitis enters into the differential diagnosis of Crohn's disease. Only half the patients have associated pulmonary tuberculosis. Histologically, extensive well-formed epithelioid granulomas, often with central (caseous) necrosis, are seen in association with a marked chronic inflammatory infiltrate through the bowel wall. Langhans-type giant cells may be seen in the granulomas. Stains for acid-fast bacilli and cultures confirm the diagnosis.

Small vessel vasculitis

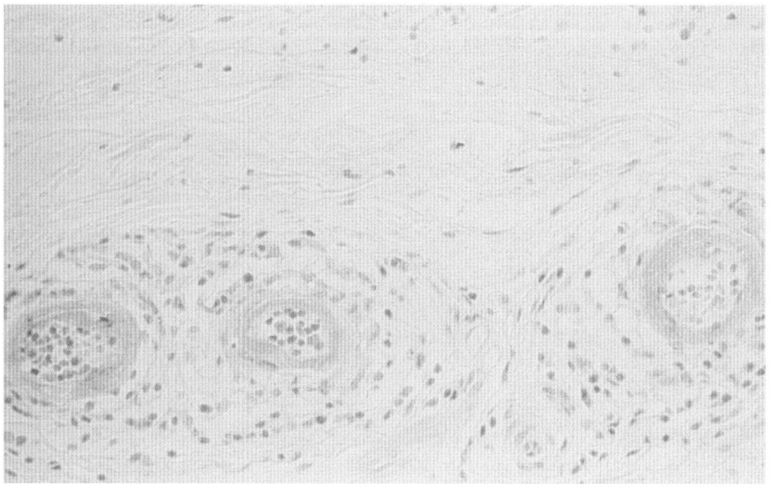

FIGURE 4-40.

Small vessel vasculitis. Occasionally, small vessel vasculitis, such as Henoch-Schönlein purpura, may involve the colon or small intestine and present as ulceration and occasionally intestinal perforation. The bowel appears edematous with subserosal and submucosal hemorrhage. Characteristic histologic findings include fibrinoid necrosis of vessel walls with a cuff of surrounding edema and mononuclear cells.

Graft-versus-host disease

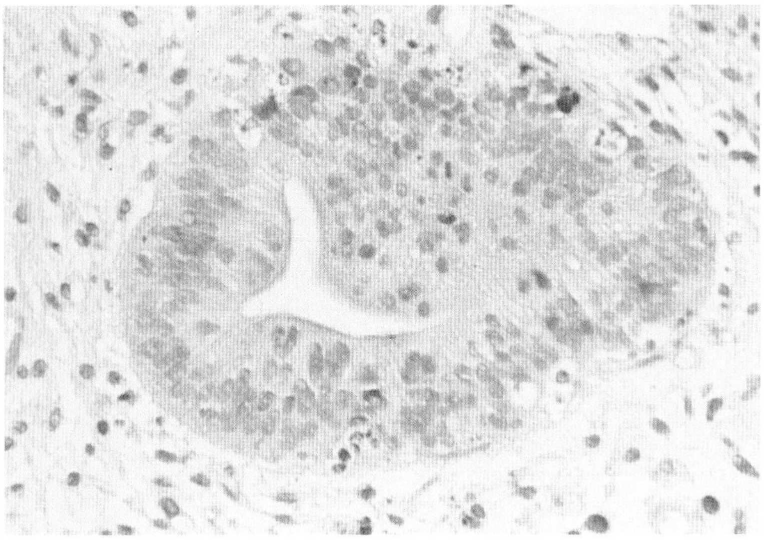

FIGURE 4-41.

Graft-versus-host disease. Graft-versus-host disease may involve the small intestine or colon in patients who have undergone bone marrow transplantation. Watery diarrhea may occur 3 weeks after transplantation, and in severe cases, intestinal bleeding and protein loss may occur. In some cases, diarrhea may be voluminous. Endoscopy may be normal or show patchy erythema or extensive mucosal sloughing, most commonly in the ileum, cecum, and ascending colon. Histologic changes are most likely to be diagnostic when biopsy specimens are obtained from endoscopically normal mucosa. A paucity of inflammation occurs in the lamina propria, and reactive colonic crypts are seen with necrosis of individual crypt epithelial cells.

Amyloidosis

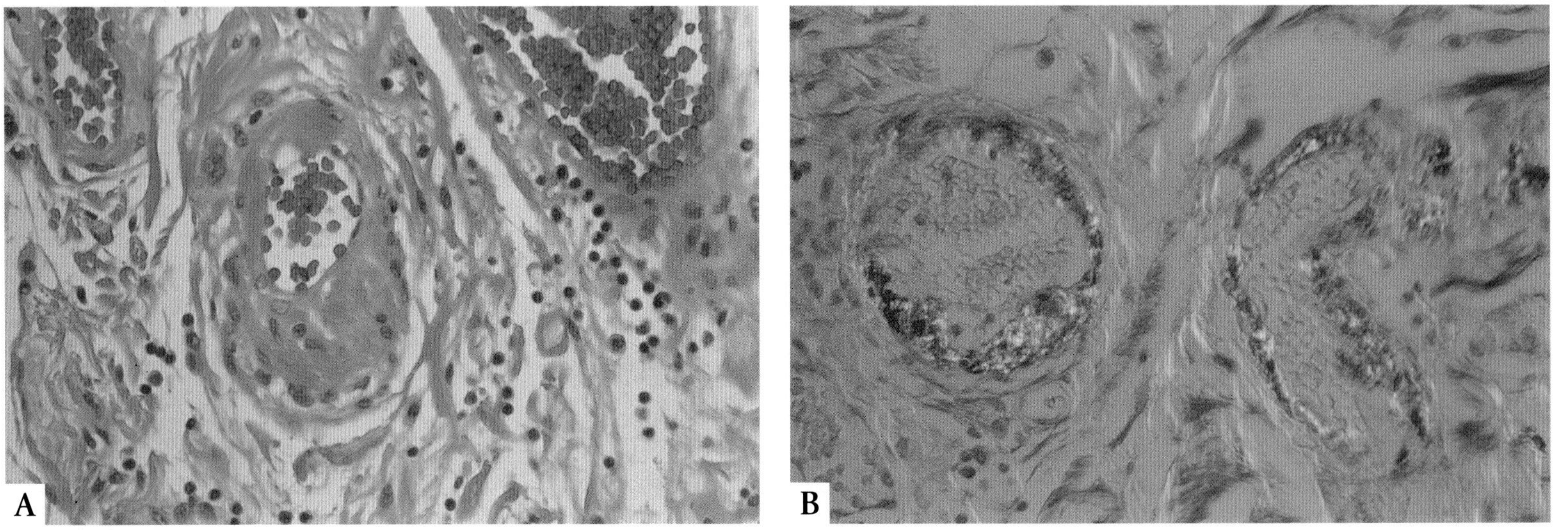

FIGURE 4-42.

Amyloidosis. **A**, Amyloidosis may involve the colon with characteristic deposition in the media or submucosal blood vessels. Rarely intestinal ischemia results, leading to enterocolitis, bleeding, and intestinal infarction. **B**, Characteristic apple-green fluorescence may be detectable with the use of a polarized lens.

Collagenous colitis

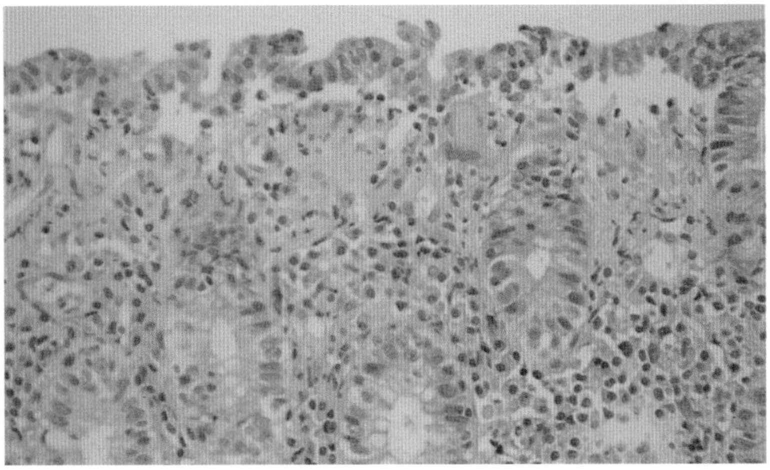

FIGURE 4-43.

Collagenous colitis. In the microscopic colidites, including lymphocytic colitis and collagenous colitis, the endoscopic appearance of the colon is normal. Diagnosis depends on histologic examination, which shows superficial epithelial injury associated with an acute and chronic inflammatory infiltrate of the surface and crypt epithelium and a bandlike mixed infiltrate of the superficial lamina propria. In collagenous colitis, there is also a thickened subepithelial collagen table.

Diversion colitis

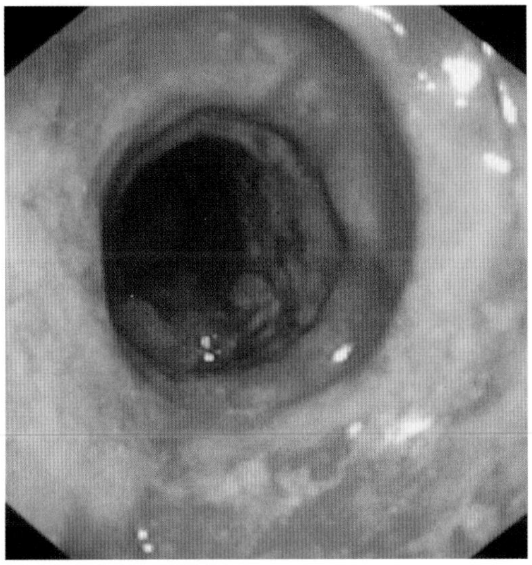

FIGURE 4-44.

Endoscopic appearance of diversion colitis. Diversion colitis occurs in 50% to 100% of cases in which the distal colon is excluded and the fecal stream diverted, depriving the distal colon of short chain fatty acids, the preferred metabolic substrate of colonic epithelium. Endoscopic findings are nonspecific and include edema, erythema, friability, granularity, erosions, and exudates. Histologically, the inflammation is limited largely to the mucosa but may be associated with fibrosis of the lamina propria and thickening of the muscularis mucosa. The findings may be indistinguishable from those of ulcerative colitis but reverse promptly when bowel continuity is reestablished or with topical short chain fatty acid therapy.

REFERENCES

1. Sartor RB: Roll of intestinal microflora in initiation and perpetuation of inflammatory bowel disease. *Can J Gastroenterol* 1990, 4:271–277.
2. Targan SR, Deem RL, Shanahan F: Immune-mediated cytotoxicity in inflammatory bowel disease. *Can J Gastroenterol* 1990, 4:278–284.

Chapter 5

Anorectal and Colonic Dysmotility

ARNOLD WALD

The major function of the colon is to reduce approximately 1500 mL of liquid residue that enters from the ileum daily into solid fecal material, which is then stored for variable periods of time until expelled. This function is achieved by coordinated motor activity and alterations in colonic wall tone, which allow water and unassimilated nutrients to be absorbed from fecal residue that is moved by intermittent propulsive motor activity towards the distal colon. The anorectum stores fecal wastes and eliminates them at an appropriate time; this function is coordinated by anorectal and pelvic floor mechanisms.

Disturbances of colonic and anorectal motility are expressed as constipation, diarrhea, visceral pain, or fecal incontinence. Some disorders represent primary motility disturbances, but disturbances of motility also arise as a consequence of inflammatory or infectious diseases or following exposure to noxious substances. Those colorectal disorders thought to be associated with primary motor disturbances include fecal incontinence, chronic constipation, idiopathic megacolon, colonic pseudoobstruction, defecatory dysfunction, and irritable bowel syndrome. Many techniques may be used to study colonic and anorectal motor activity, including radiologic and scintigraphic studies, anorectal and colonic manometry, anal endosonography, and neurophysiologic methods to evaluate striated pelvic floor muscles and pudendal nerve function.

NORMAL FUNCTION OF ANORECTUM

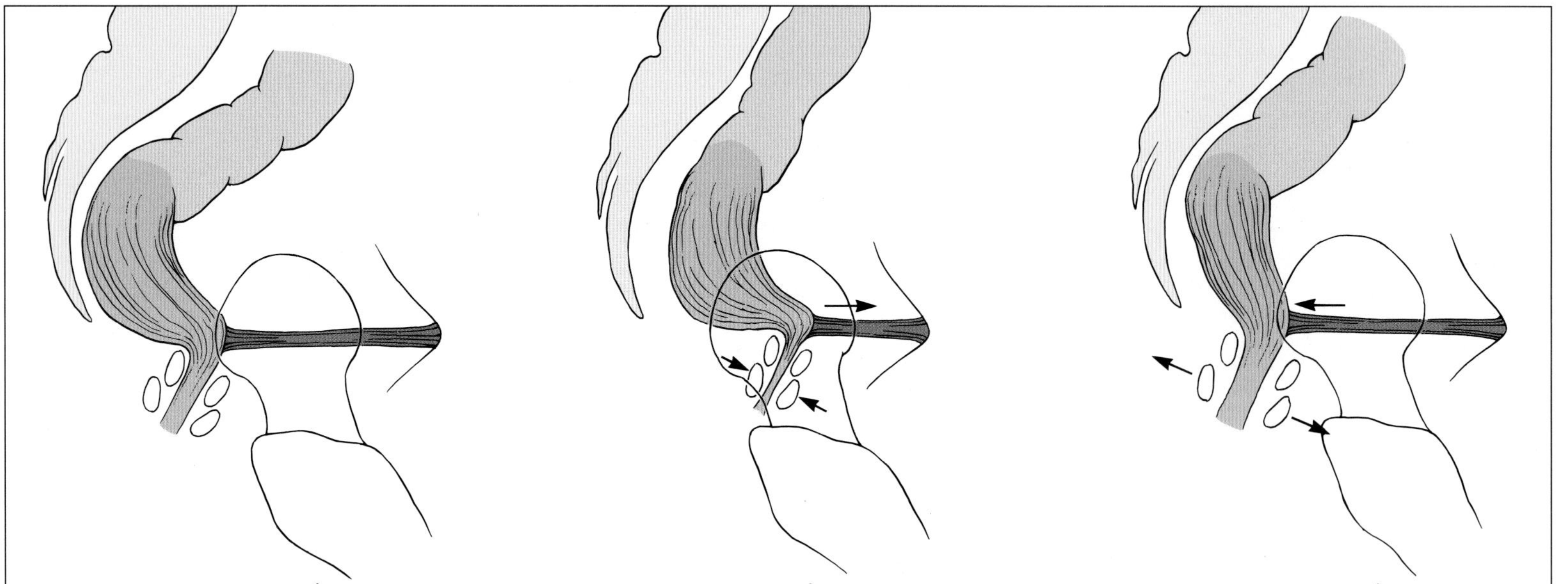

FIGURE 5-1.

The sagittal view of anorectal anatomy during continence and defecation. The major structures of the anorectum are the rectum, the puborectalis muscle which forms the anorectal angle, and the internal and external anal sphincters surrounding the anal canal. Sensory mechanoreceptors in the perirectal tissues allow perception of rectal filling or distension, whereas anal nerve endings permit discrimination of gas, liquid, and solid rectal contents. At rest (*left*), the anorectal angle of approximately 85° to 105° is at a line drawn from the symphysis pubis to the tip of the coccyx. Most of the resting pressure in the anal canal is derived from the internal anal sphincter and exceeds intrarectal pressure. The movement of fecal wastes to the rectum temporarily relaxes the internal anal sphincter; defecation is deferred (*center*) by contraction of the puborectalis muscle and external anal sphincter, the former narrowing the anorectal angle and the latter increasing pressures in the anal canal until the rectum accommodates to its increased contents and propulsive forces are diminished. During defecation (*right*), increased intra-abdominal pressures help to propel bowel contents toward the anal canal while relaxation of striated muscles results in perineal descent, widening of the anorectal angle, and decreasing pressures in the anal canal. After defecation is completed, anorectal structures return to their normal resting position. (*From* Wald [1]; with permission.)

TABLE 5-1. ANORECTAL CONTINENCE MECHANISMS

Reservoir elements
- Rectal compliance/accomodation
- Colonic compliance/accomodation

Sensorimotor elements
- Anorectal angle
- Rectal sensation
- Anal sensory nerves
- Internal anal sphincter
- External anal sphincter

TABLE 5-1.

Anorectal continence mechanisms. Anorectal continence mechanisms may be divided into reservoir elements and sensory and motor elements. Although fecal incontinence occasionally occurs because of behavioral disturbances (*ie*, social indifference) or voluminous diarrhea overwhelming the distal colon, most individuals with fecal soiling exhibit abnormalities of one or several of these continence mechanisms.

TABLE 5-2. DIAGNOSTIC STUDIES FOR FECAL INCONTINENCE

Tests	Information obtained
Sigmoidoscopy	Inflammation, strictures, tumors
Anorectal manometry	Sphincter pressures Rectal sensation, compliance External sphincter responses
Pelvic floor neurophysiology	External sphincter electromyography Puborectalis electromyography Pudendal nerve conduction
Proctography	Rectal capacity Anorectal angle Perineal descent Retention of contrast
Anal ultrasonography	Anal sphincter integrity

TABLE 5-2.

Diagnostic studies for fecal incontinence. Anorectal function can be studied by a variety of complementary techniques, each providing information concerning the various continence mechanisms. Of these, sigmoidoscopy and anorectal manometry are the most useful and are indicated in most patients; the other studies provide valuable information but are not necessary in all patients.

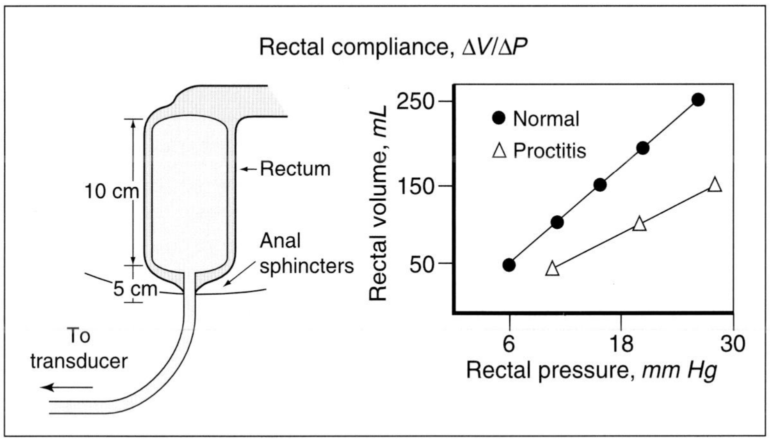

FIGURE 5-2.

Rectal compliance in health and proctitis with fecal incontinence. Rectal compliance is obtained by progressively inflating a cylindrical latex balloon (positioned in the rectum 5 cm from the anal verge) with air in 50 mL increments as illustrated. Pressures within the balloon are measured by an external transducer and are corrected by subtracting pressures obtained when inflated with the same volumes in ambient air. This corrects for pressures derived from the resistance of the balloon itself. A compliance curve is then constructed in which compliance equals Δ volume (V)/Δ pressure (P).

In inflammatory or ischemic diseases of the rectum, higher pressures are generated at all volumes of rectal distension of the compliance balloon, and intolerance to progressive distension occurs at lower volumes compared with normal subjects. Such patients may experience fecal incontinence associated with urgency despite normal anal sphincter function. (*From* Wald [1]; with permission.)

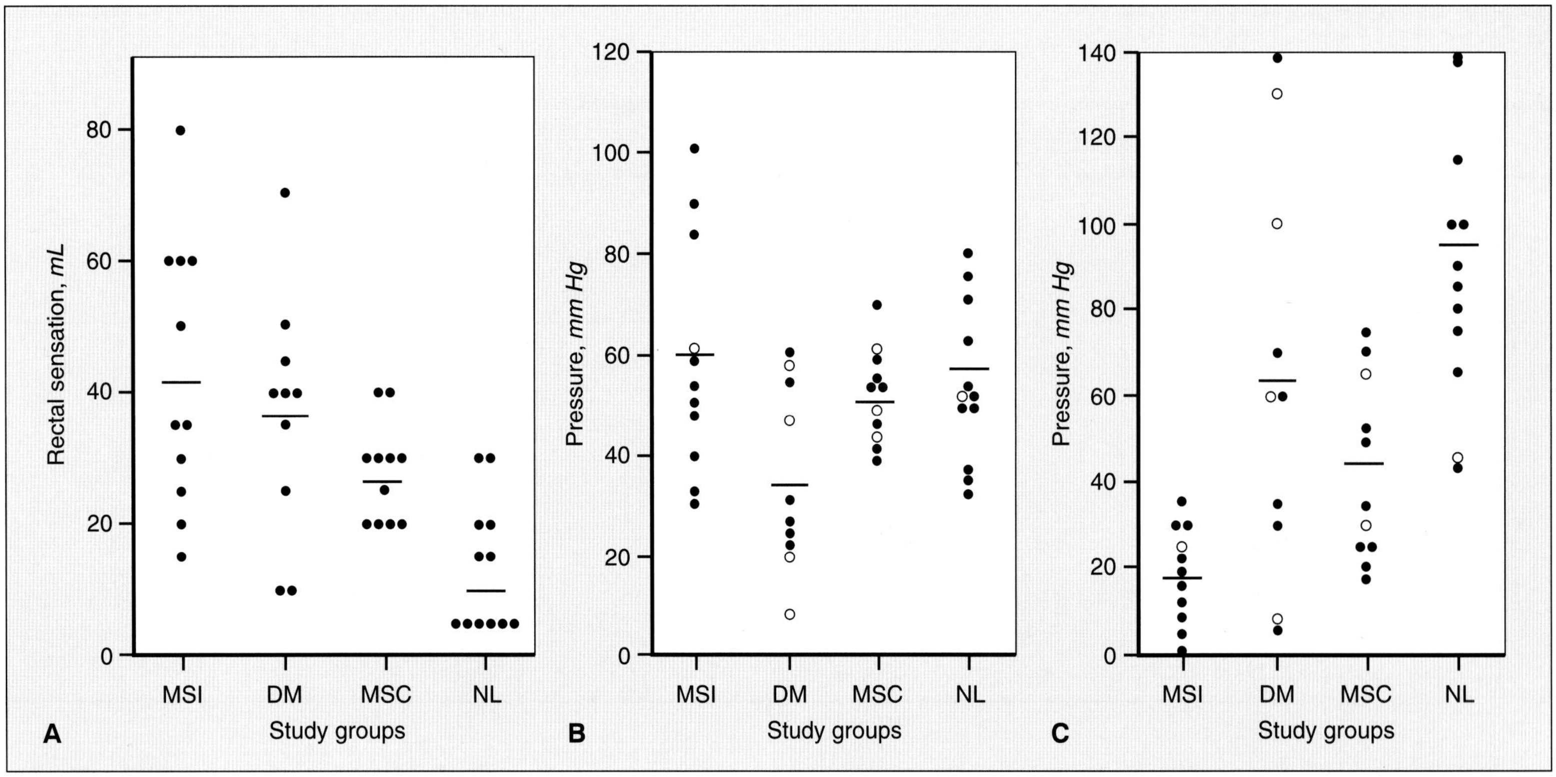

FIGURE 5-3.

Anorectal function in neurogenic disorders associated with fecal incontinence. **A**, Rectal sensory thresholds in patients with diabetes mellitus with fecal incontinence (DM), multiple sclerosis with fecal incontinence (MSI), continent multiple sclerosis patients (MSC), and normal control subjects (NL). Over 50% of DM and MSI patients have thresholds of rectal sensation exceeding 30 mL. All study groups have mean sensory thresholds that are significantly higher than that of the NL subjects. **B**, Resting anal sphincter pressures in the same groups of subjects. Patients with multiple sclerosis have normal pressures, whereas DM patients often have diminished pressures at rest, presumably reflecting autonomic nerve dysfunction. **C**, Anal squeeze pressures in the study groups. MSI patients uniformly have decreased squeeze pressures compared with NL subjects, whereas MSC patients have squeeze pressures that are modestly impaired. DM patients vary greatly with respect to squeeze pressures, making manometric studies important when assessing continence mechanisms. (*From* Caruana *et al.* [2]; with permission.)

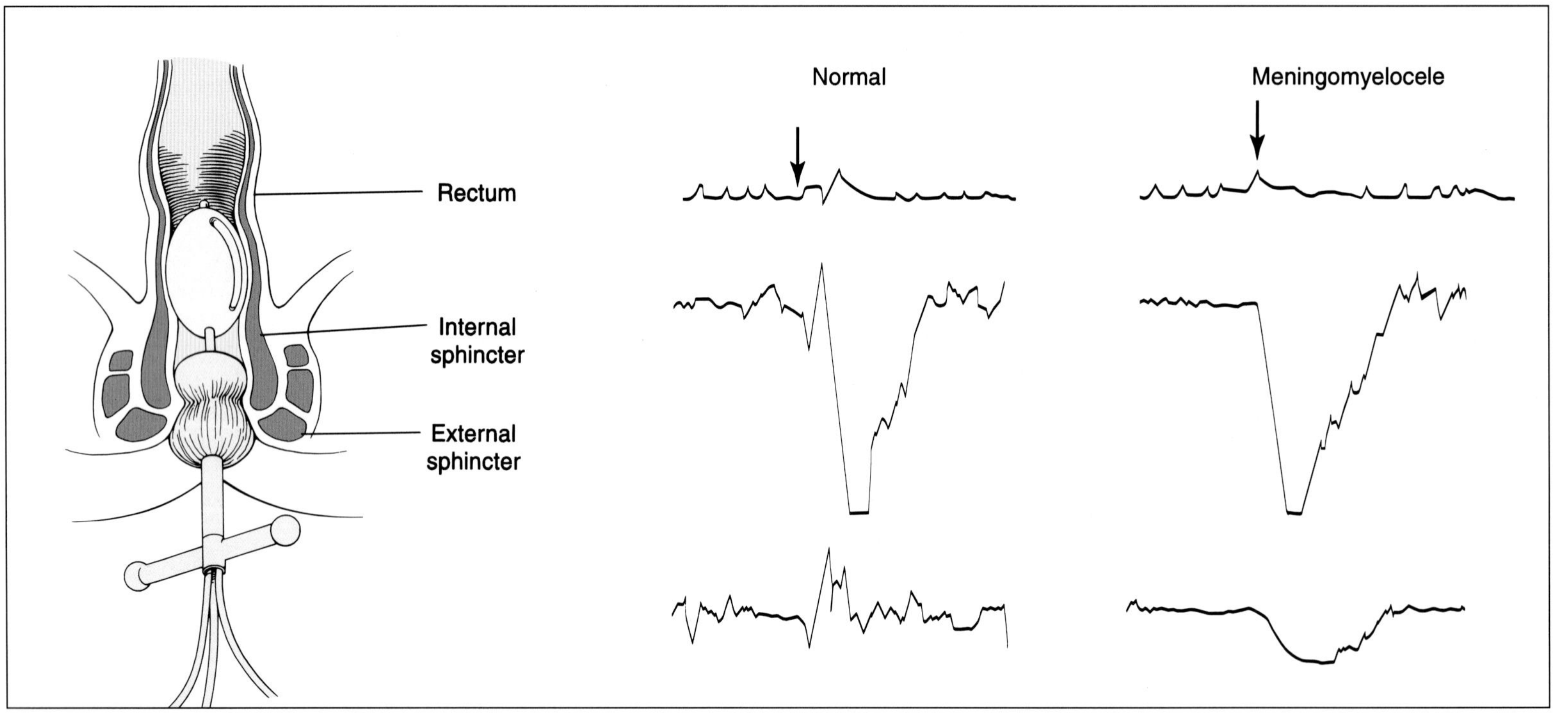

FIGURE 5-4.

Fecal incontinence associated with spinal cord injury. In a manometric study of a normal subject, rectal balloon distension (*arrow*) results in transient external anal sphincter contraction. In a patient with meningomyelocele and sacral denervation, rectal balloon distention (*arrow*) elicits normal internal anal sphincter relaxation, but there is no contraction response from the external anal sphincter; therefore, decreased pressures in the anal canal are recorded by the external anal sphincter balloon. Rectal sensation in these patients may be normal or impaired.

TABLE 5-3. ANORECTAL FINDINGS IN SPINAL CORD INJURIES

PARAMETERS	SACRAL	SUPRASACRAL
Rectal sensation	Usually absent	Absent
Basal anal pressure	Normal or low	Normal
Anal squeeze pressure	Probably absent	Absent
Reflex defecation	Usually absent	Present
Impending defecation	No warning, but occasionally abdominal pain is present	Often no warning; autonomic signs present

TABLE 5-3.

Anorectal findings in spinal cord injuries. Patients with sacral and suprasacral lesions have no rectal sensation or anal squeeze pressures, but basal anal sphincter pressures are generally preserved. Patients with suprasacral lesions can defecate in response to puborectalis or rectal stimulation, which helps in bowel management.

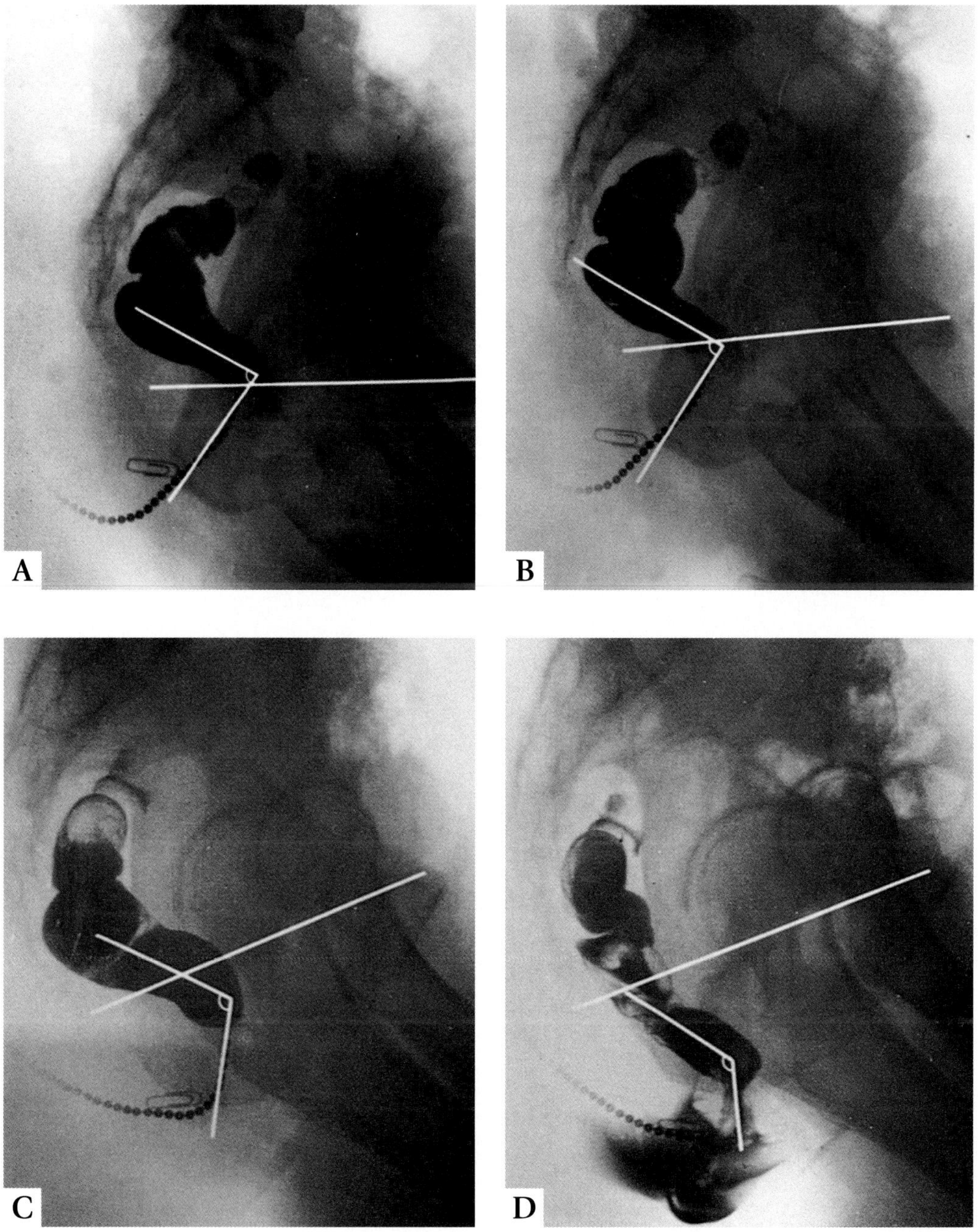

FIGURE 5-5.

Fecal incontinence associated with pudendal neuropathy. **A** and **B**, Barium proctography in a normal subject. With the patient in the left lateral recumbent position, 200 to 250 mL of barium contrast medium is instilled to fill the rectum and distal sigmoid colon. A small plastic lubricated sphere attached to a chain of radiopaque beads is inserted into the anal canal, and the chain is taped to the dorsal intergluteal cleft. Lateral radiographs are obtained at rest, when the patient squeezes, and when the patient strains while attempting to retain the barium. The anorectal angle is calculated from the intersection of a line drawn along the posterior rectal wall with a line drawn along the axis of the anal canal, as delineated by the beaded chain. The position of the pelvic floor is determined by the junction of the anorectal angle and compared with its normal position which approximates a line drawn from the symphysis pubis to the tip of the coccyx. This technique has been superseded by defecating proctography, in which 200 mL of thickened barium paste is administered into the rectum using a wide-tipped syringe. The paste consists of barium contrast mixed with a thickening agent such as hydrophilic psyllium colloid. This technique eliminates the need for a chain to outline the anal canal.

C and **D**, Fecal incontinence with perineal descent. In contrast to a normal subject, the anorectal angle in a patient with fecal incontinence is more obtuse and lies significantly below the pubococcygeal line at rest (*C*). When the patient strains (*D*), perineal descent is grossly apparent and there is loss of contrast material through a weakened anal sphincter musculature. (**A** and **B**, *Courtesy of* N.W. Read, Sheffield, UK)

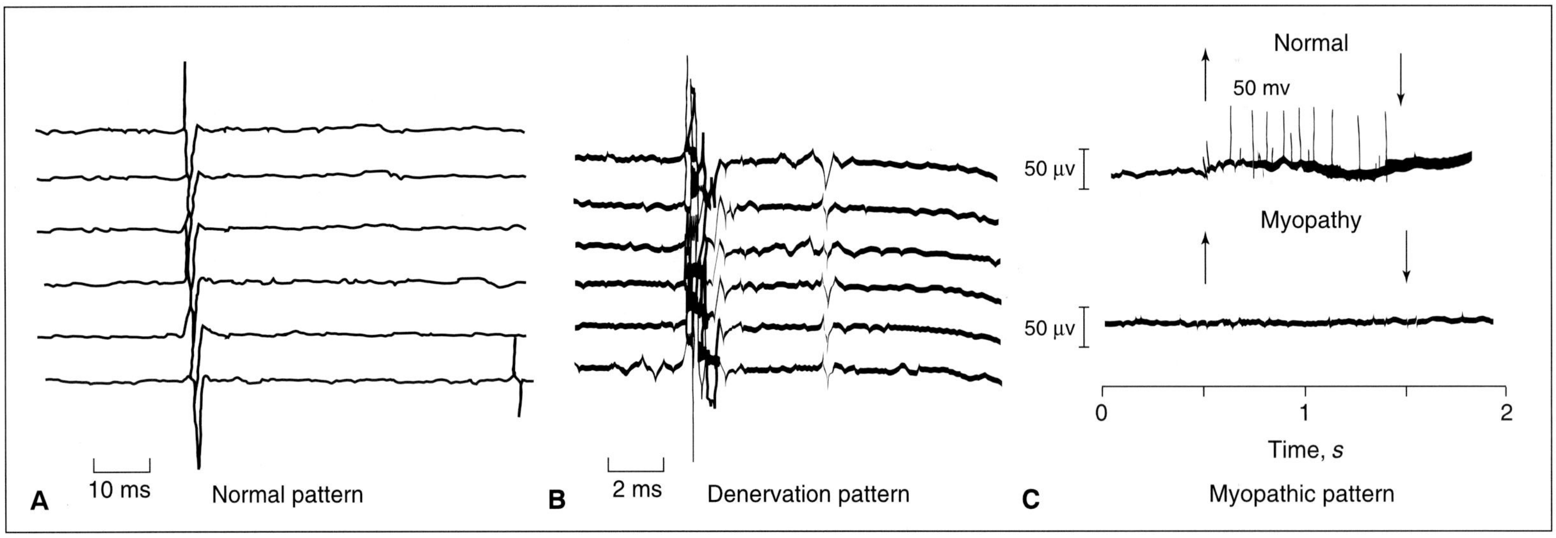

FIGURE 5-6.

External sphincter electromyographic patterns. **A**, An example of motor unit potentials of short duration that were obtained by a concentric needle electrode placed in the external anal sphincter of a normal subject. **B**, An example of a motor unit potential obtained by a concentric needle electrode inserted into the puborectalis muscle of a patient with neuropathic fecal incontinence. The first component of the motor unit potential shows prominent jitter (significant variation of the intervals between motor unit potentials) and intermittent blocking caused by failure of conduction across immature motor nerve end plates. The finding of prominent jitter and blocking using conventional electromyographic techniques implies recent and perhaps continuing injury of the motor nerve supplying the muscle. **C**, Concentric needle electromyographic recording in a normal subject and a patient with myopathy demonstrating normal and absent spike potentials in external anal sphincter during rectal distension (*arrows*). (**A** and **B**, *From* Bartolo *et al.* [3]; with permission.) (**C**, *From* Teasdall *et al.* [4]; with permission.)

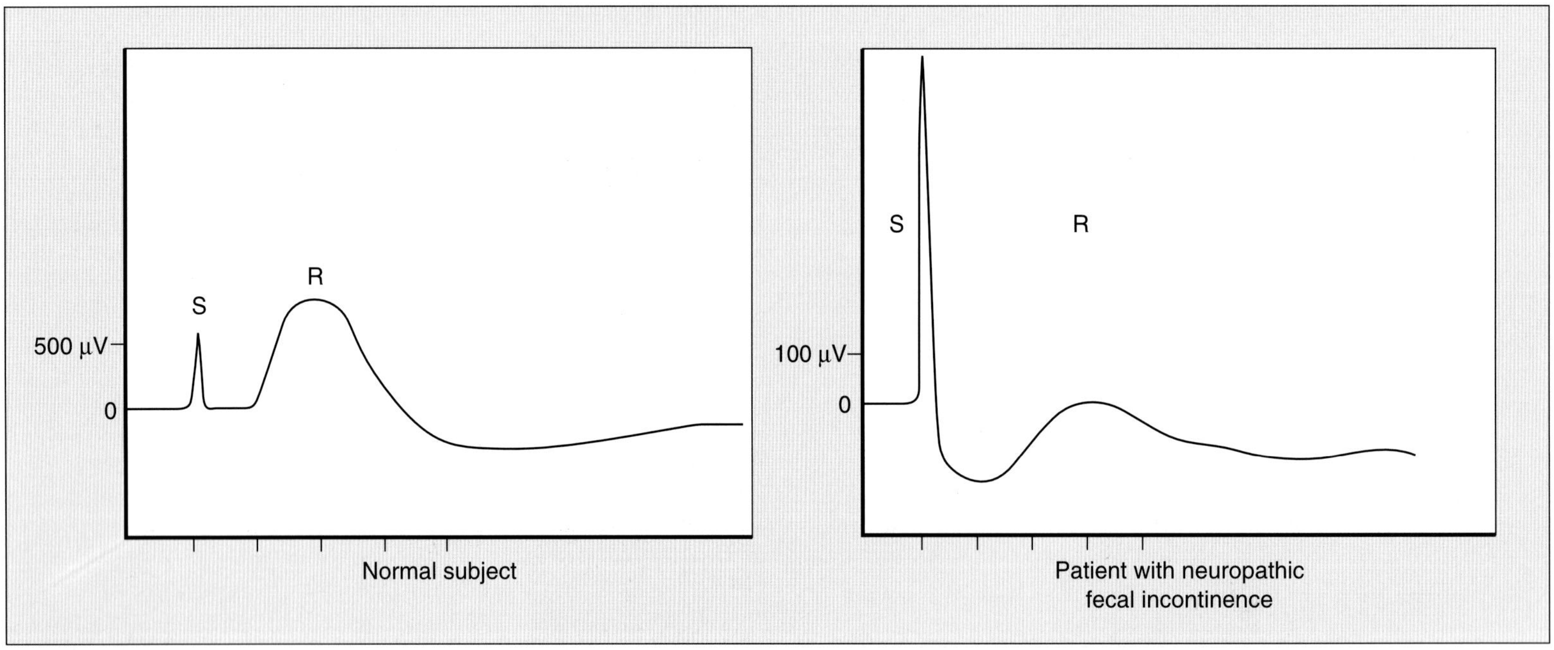

FIGURE 5-7.

Pudendal nerve latencies. Motor unit action potential in a normal subject (*left*) and a patient with neuropathic fecal incontinence (*right*) is shown. Latency period is measured from stimulus (S) to motor response (R). In normal subjects, latency periods range up to 2 ms, whereas in patients with peripheral neuropathic fecal incontinence, latencies often exceed these values. This longer latency indicates damage to one or both pudendal nerves, which leads to impaired function of the external anal sphincter muscles. Thus, patients with idiopathic fecal incontinence appear to have a form of neurogenic external anal sphincter or puborectalis dysfunction caused by injury to the pudendal nerves. (*From* Kiff and Swash [5]; with permission.)

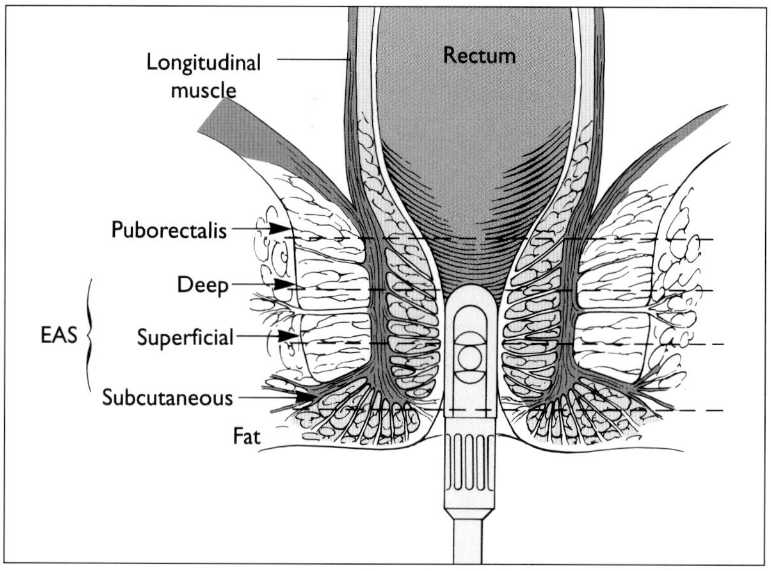

FIGURE 5-8.

Anal endosonography. A schematic representation of the anorectal muscles in the coronal section with a sonographic probe in situ. The subdivisions of the external anal sphincter (EAS) are indicated. (*From* Sultan and Kamm [6]; with permission.) (*Data from* Milligan and Morgan [7] and Gorsh [8].)

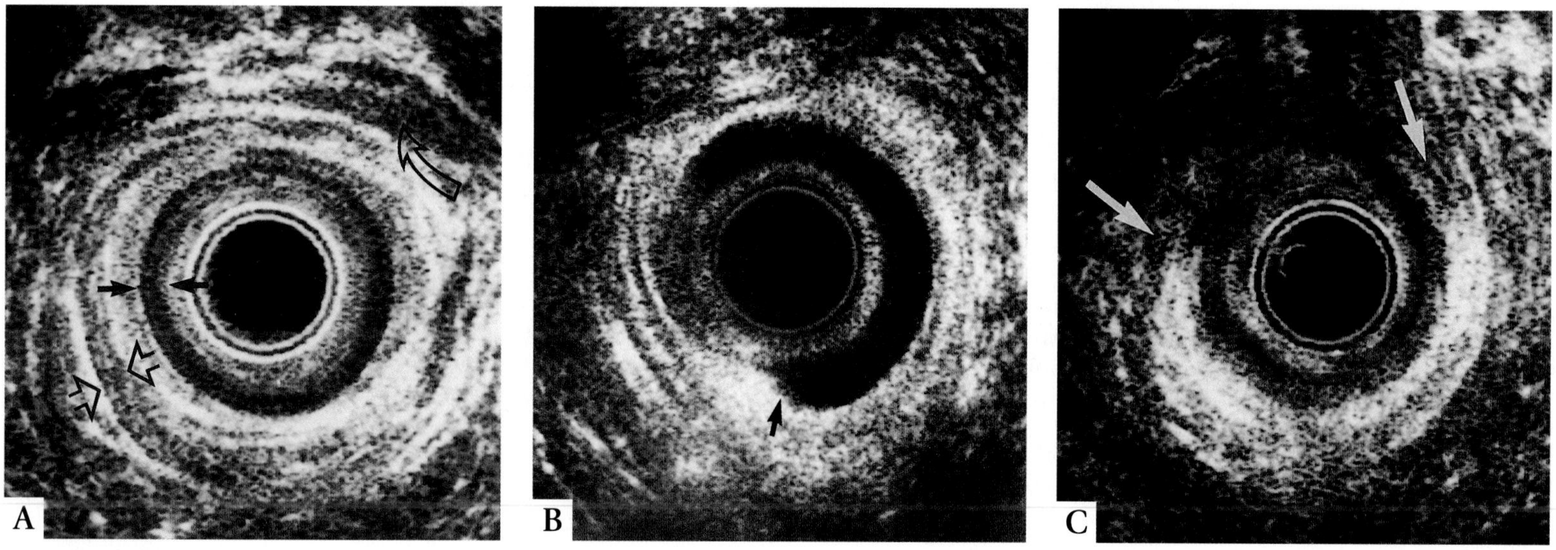

FIGURE 5-9.

A, Normal anatomy as viewed by anal endosonography. The cone around the sonographic probe creates two inner bright interfaces. Just outside the interfaces, the subepithelial tissues are seen to be slightly hyperechoic. The internal sphincter creates a well-defined hypoechoic ring (*closed arrows*). The hyperechoic longitudinal muscle surrounds the internal sphincter, and the external sphincter (*open arrows*) envelopes the longitudinal muscle. In this male patient, the external sphincter is hypoechoic relative to the longitudinal muscle. In most females, these sections are equally echogenic and cannot be identified separately. The transverse perineii are noted anteriorly (*curved arrow*). The image is oriented so that anterior is in the uppermost position. **B**, Lateral internal anal sphincterotomy within the 6 to 10 o'clock positions (*arrow*). The remaining internal anal sphincter has bunched up slightly and appears somewhat thickened. Surgical defects in the internal anal sphincter are usually clear-cut with well-defined ends. **C**, Obstetric trauma caused by forceps delivery with internal and external defects within the 9 to 1 o'clock positions (*arrows*). (*Courtesy of* C.I. Bartram, London, UK)

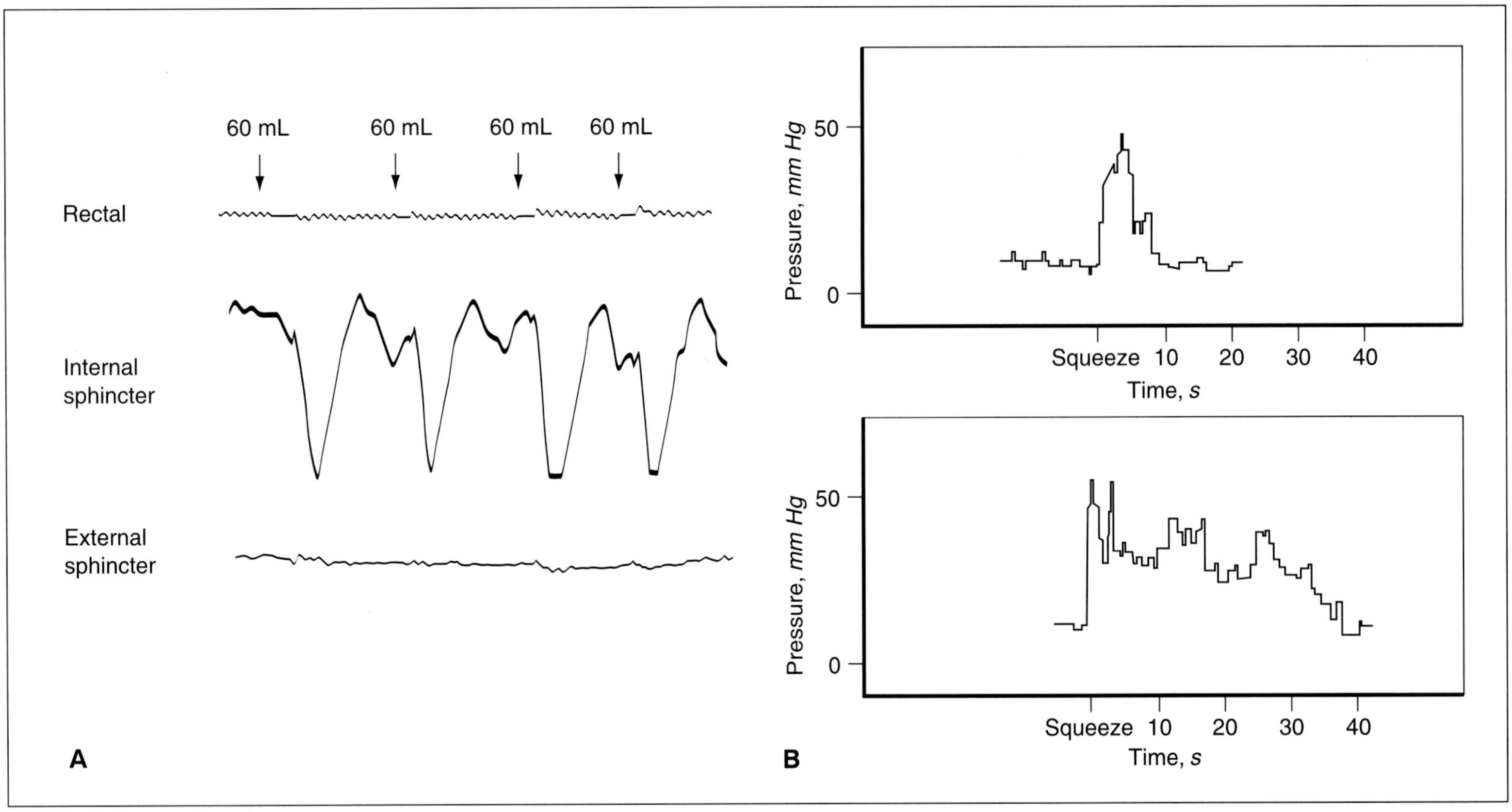

FIGURE 5-10.

Anorectal manometry in fecal incontinence. **A**, In many patients with fecal incontinence, external anal sphincter contraction following rectal distension is often absent or occurs only at much higher distending volumes than in normal subjects. In this tracing, rectal distension (*arrows*) induces relaxation of the internal anal sphincter, but no external sphincter contractions are observed. Reestablishing phasic contractions of the external anal sphincter is one aspect of sphincter muscle retraining using biofeedback techniques. **B**, Manometric tracing. The manometric tracings of a prolonged voluntary contraction from a healthy volunteer (*bottom*) is compared with a tracing from a patient with fecal incontinence (*top*). A rapidly fatiguing anal sphincter during an attempt of prolonged squeezing is illustrated in the patient with fecal incontinence. (**A**, *From* Engel *et al.* [9]; with permission.) (**B**, *From* Chiaroni *et al.* [10]; with permission.)

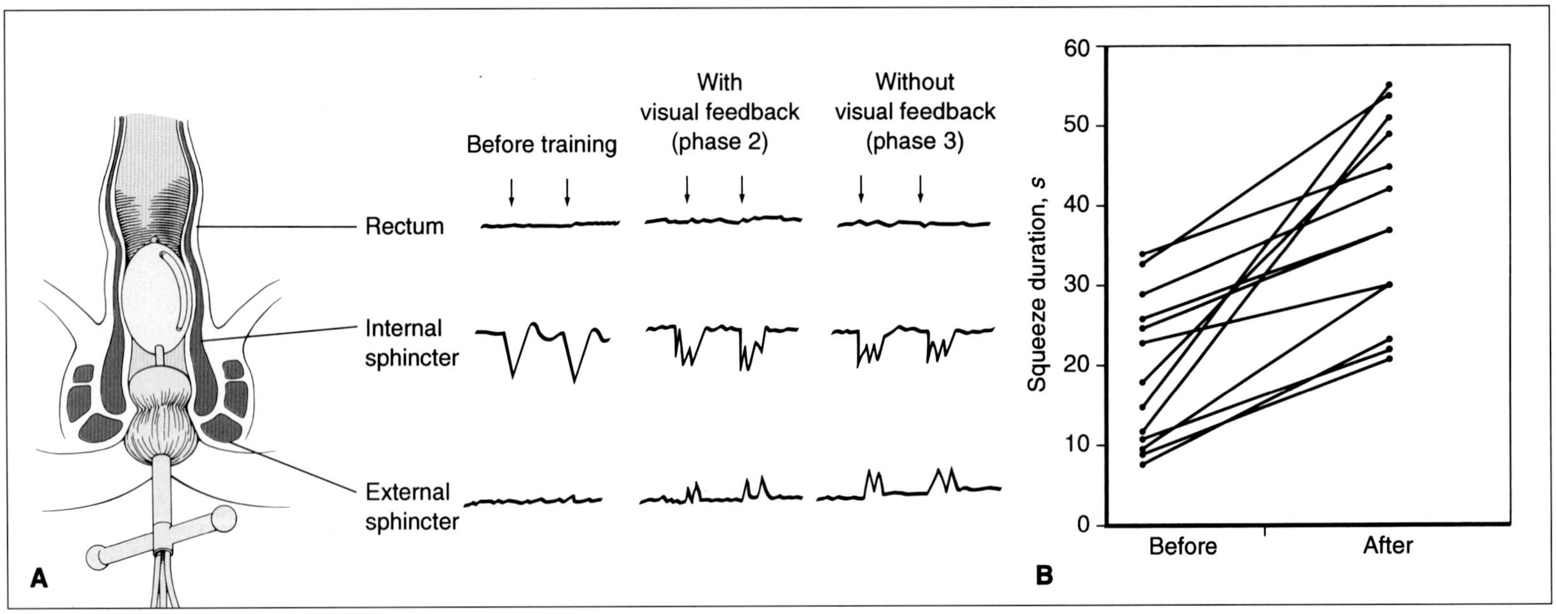

FIGURE 5-11.

Biofeedback. **A**, Biofeedback is a therapeutic modality involving external anal sphincter muscle retraining, using the anorectal manometric tracing to provide visual feedback to the patient with fecal incontinence. Before training, the patient is allowed to view the manometric tracing as it is being recorded. The abnormalities are pointed out to the patient who is then asked to correct the abnormality, *ie*, the absent external anal sphincter contraction following rectal distension (*arrows*). A normal response is drawn for the patient who then tries to duplicate it while sensing each rectal distension. Often thresholds of rectal sensation are lowered, and sphincter contractile responses are restored in successfully treated patients. This technique is often successful after only one to two sessions. **B**, Squeeze duration in 14 patients with fecal incontinence before and after sphincter retraining. A significant improvement in squeeze duration was demonstrated after biofeedback treatment. (**A**, *From* Wald [1]; with permission.) (**B**, *From* Chiaroni *et al.* [10]; with permission.)

Conceptually, idiopathic constipation may be viewed as a disorder of colonic motor activity, a disorder of anorectal function (defecation), or a combination of the two. These disorders can be studied by a number of techniques such as colonoscopy, barium radiographs, colonic transit using radiopaque markers or scintigraphic techniques, barium or scintigraphic defecography, anorectal and colonic manometry, and anal sphincter electromyographic studies.

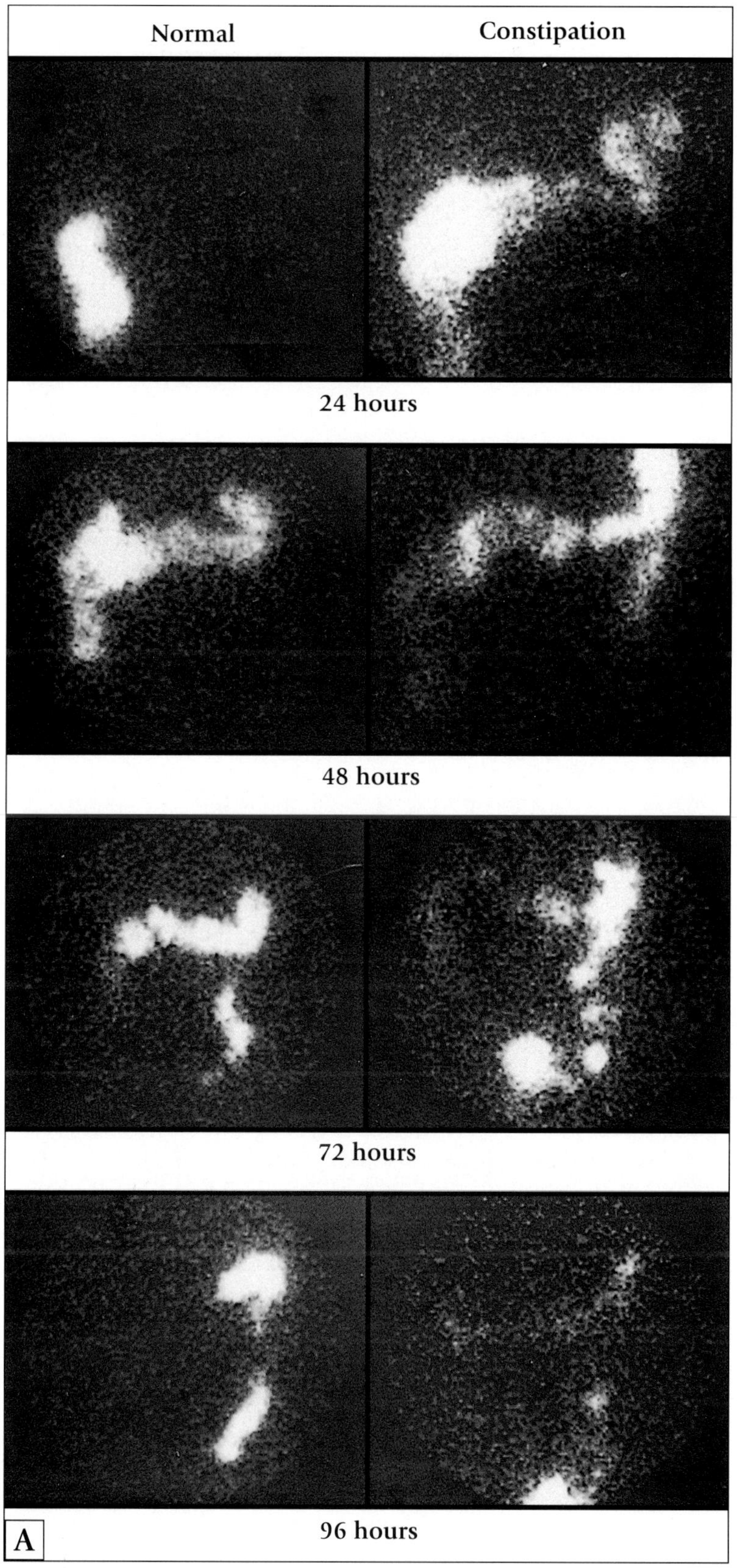

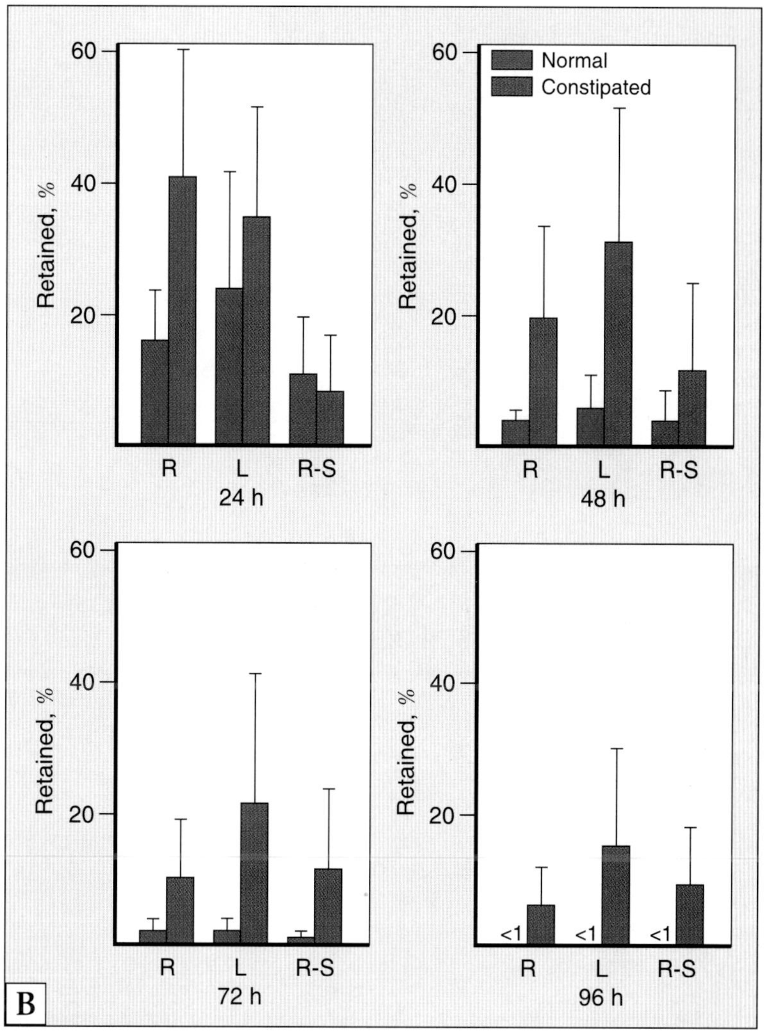

FIGURE 5-12.

Colonic scintigraphy. In these studies, a capsule coated with a pH-sensitive polymer releases radiolabeled particles into the ileocecal area where they are propelled into the cecum. Abdominal scans are obtained at fixed intervals using a large field-of-view gamma-camera, and standard regions of interest are defined. Using appropriate corrections for radioisotope decay and background, total and regional colonic transits are calculated. **A**, Representative images at 24 to 96 hours from a normal subject contrast with those from constipated patient **B**, Mean segmental percent retention for normal subjects and constipated patients are shown for the right colon (R), left colon (L), and rectum and sigmoid colon (R-S). (Reprinted by permission of the Society of Nuclear Medicine from McLean *et al.* [11]: Colon transit scintigraphy in health and constipation using oral iodine-131-cellulose. *Journal of Nuclear Medicine* 1990, 31:985–989. Figures 1, 3, and 4.)

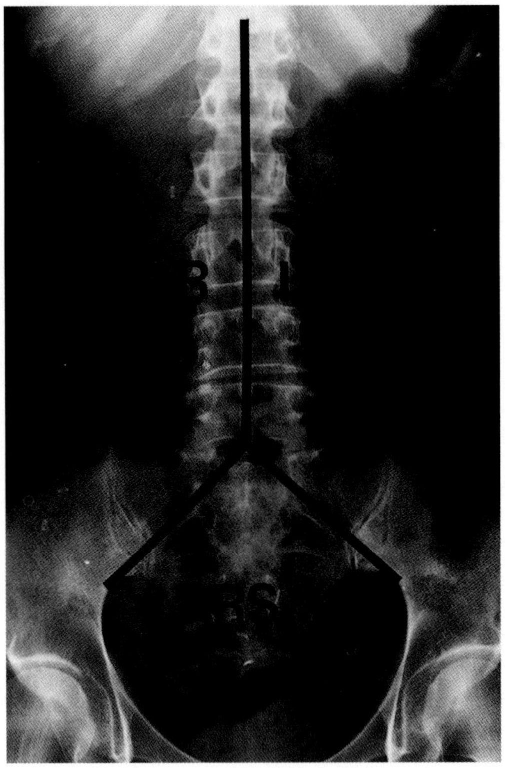

FIGURE 5-13.

Colonic transit of markers. In this technique, radiopaque markers are taken per os, and abdominal radiographs are taken at specific intervals to locate the markers in the right colon (R), left colon (L), and rectosigmoid colon (RS). Transit times through these regions are calculated using a derived mathematical equation:

$$\text{Transit time} = \frac{\text{hours between radiographs}}{\text{number of markers given}} [n_1 + n_2 + n_3 \ldots \text{ (where } n \text{ equals radiographs obtained on day 1, 2, 3...)}]$$

This technique has been simplified by using three doses of markers and radiographs on the 4th and 7th days. (*From* Metcalf *et al.* [12]; with permission.)

TABLE 5-4A. NORMAL TRANSIT CONSTIPATION—WILLFUL DECEPTION

Complaint: 32-year-old female; infrequent defecation for several years; all tests normal

Colon transit study:

DAY	R	L	RS	TOTAL
1	10	9	1	20
2	0	2	7	9
3	0	0	0	0

Bowel diary: one stool in 14 days

TABLE 5-4B. SLOW TRANSIT CONSTIPATION—COLONIC INERTIA

Complaint: 22-year-old female; infrequent defecation for 4 years; increasingly disabled

Colon transit study:

DAY	R	L	RS	TOTAL
1	12	8	0	20
3	6	9	5	20
5	2	9	4	15
7	0	10	5	15

Bowel diary: two stools in 14 days

TABLE 5-4.

Colonic transit patterns in chronic constipation. **A**, This young woman was referred for chronic intractable constipation after an extensive workup. Despite a prospective bowel diary indicating one small stool passed during 14 days, colonic transit demonstrated normal passage of markers within 3 days. Behavioral studies indicated high scores for anxiety, depression, and somatization. **B**, This young woman presented with a history similar to that of the previous patient. In contrast, passage of markers was significantly delayed in all regions of the colon. This pattern is known as colonic inertia and is associated with significant alterations of colonic propulsive motor activity (*see* Fig. 5-15). R—right colon; L—left colon; RS—rectosigmoid colon.

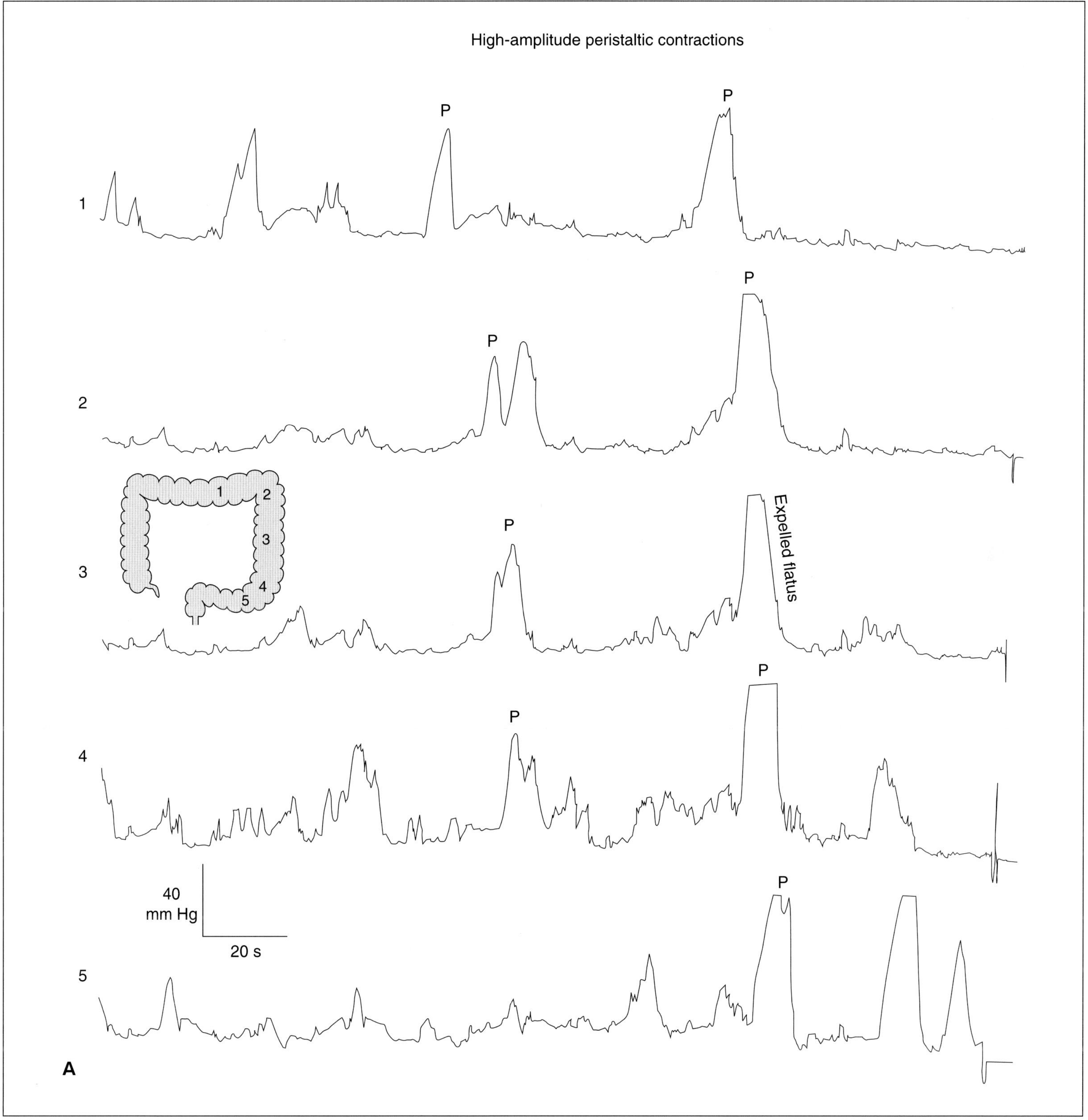

FIGURE 5-14.

Colonic motor activity can be studied using water perfusion manometry or solid state transducers that are placed by colonoscopic techniques. Although it is recognized that colon cleansing may alter colonic function and is not necessarily physiologic, one can study regional colonic motor activity at rest, after meals and pharmacologic stimuli, and can also study diurnal motor patterns.

Colonic motor activity. **A**, High-amplitude peristaltic contractions. Both high- and low-amplitude peristaltic contractions have been identified during prolonged recordings and are propagated over variable distances of the left and rectosigmoid colons. These contractions are responsible for mass movements of colonic contents. *(Continued on next page)*

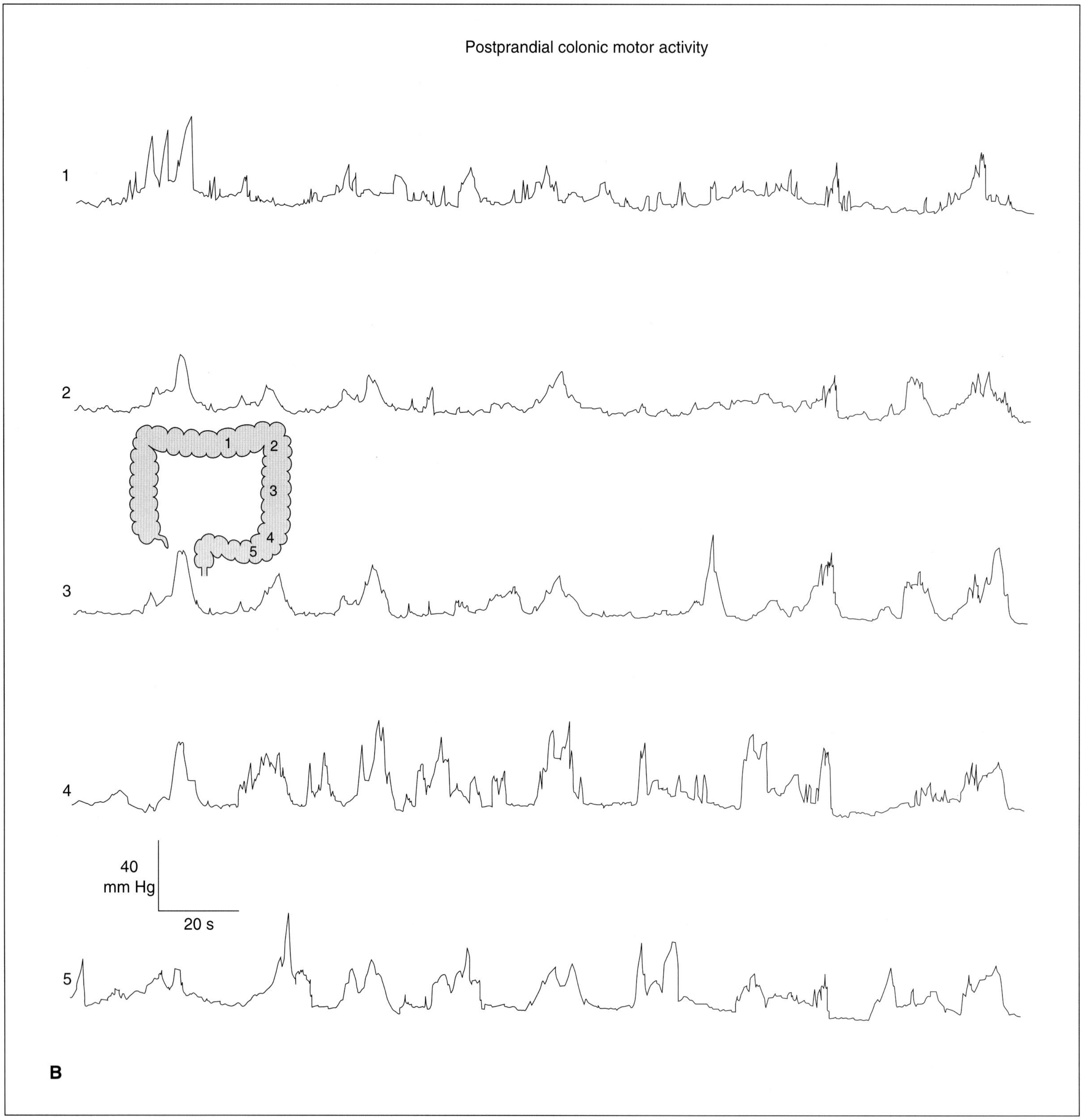

FIGURE 5-14. *(CONTINUED)*

B, Postprandial colonic motor activity. Following a meal or administration of a cholinergic agent such as edrophonium, increased motor activity is observed through the left colon. This activity may be nonpropagating or is propulsive over short distances in an orad or aborad direction.

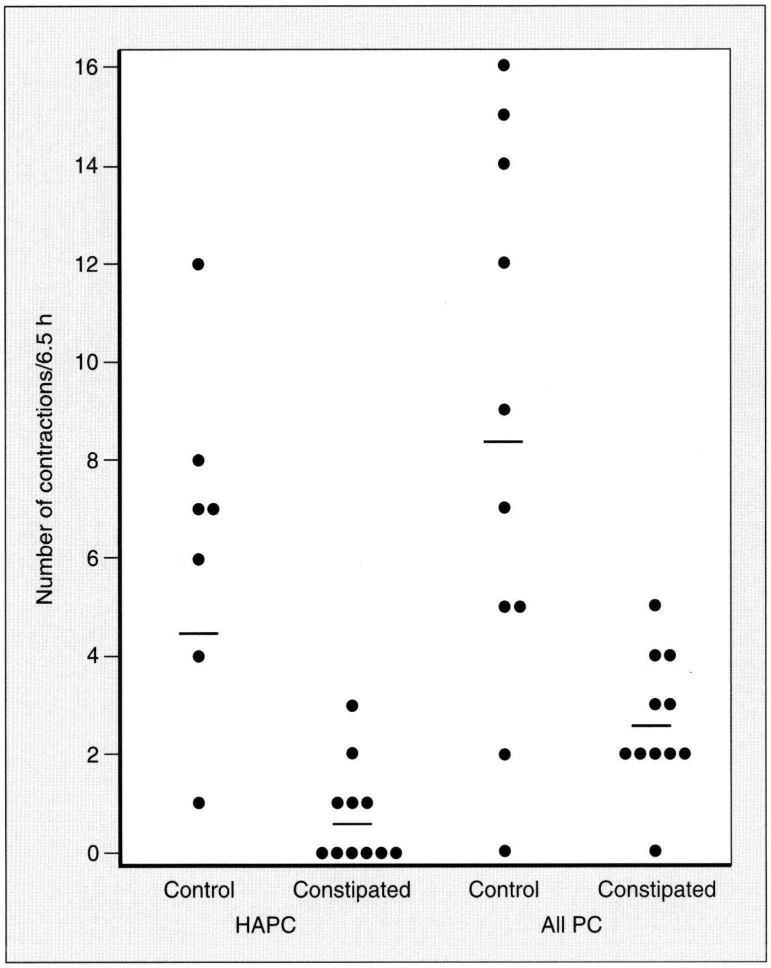

FIGURE 5-15.

Comparison of propagating contractions in healthy control subjects and patients with constipation associated with slow colonic transit. The number of high-amplitude propagating contractions (HAPC) ($P<0.03$) and low amplitude contractions. ($P<0.02$) are significantly lower in the patients with constipation. PC—propagating contractions.

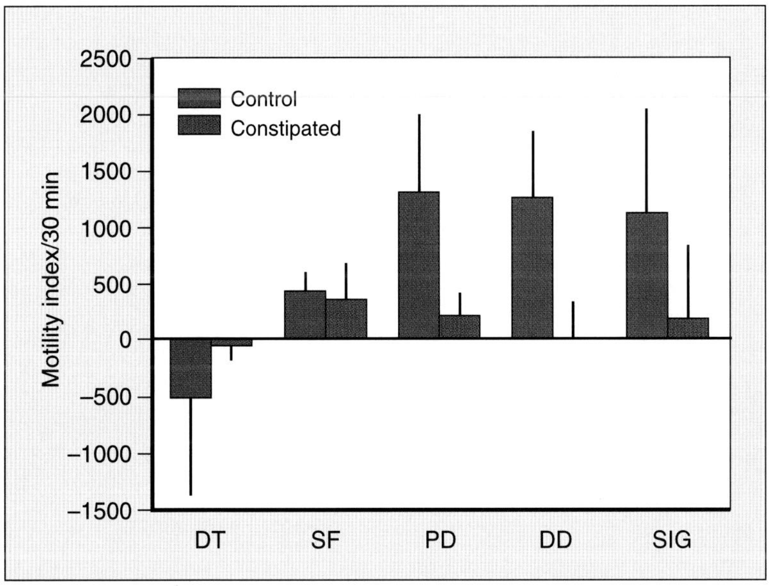

FIGURE 5-16.

Colonic motility within the first 30 minutes after breakfast. Postprandial motor activity in the left and sigmoid colons is reduced in chronically constipated patients compared with healthy controls. A similar reduction is observed following administration of edrophonium. DD—distal descending colon; DT—distal transverse colon; PD—proximal colon; SF—splenic flexure; SIG—sigmoid colon.

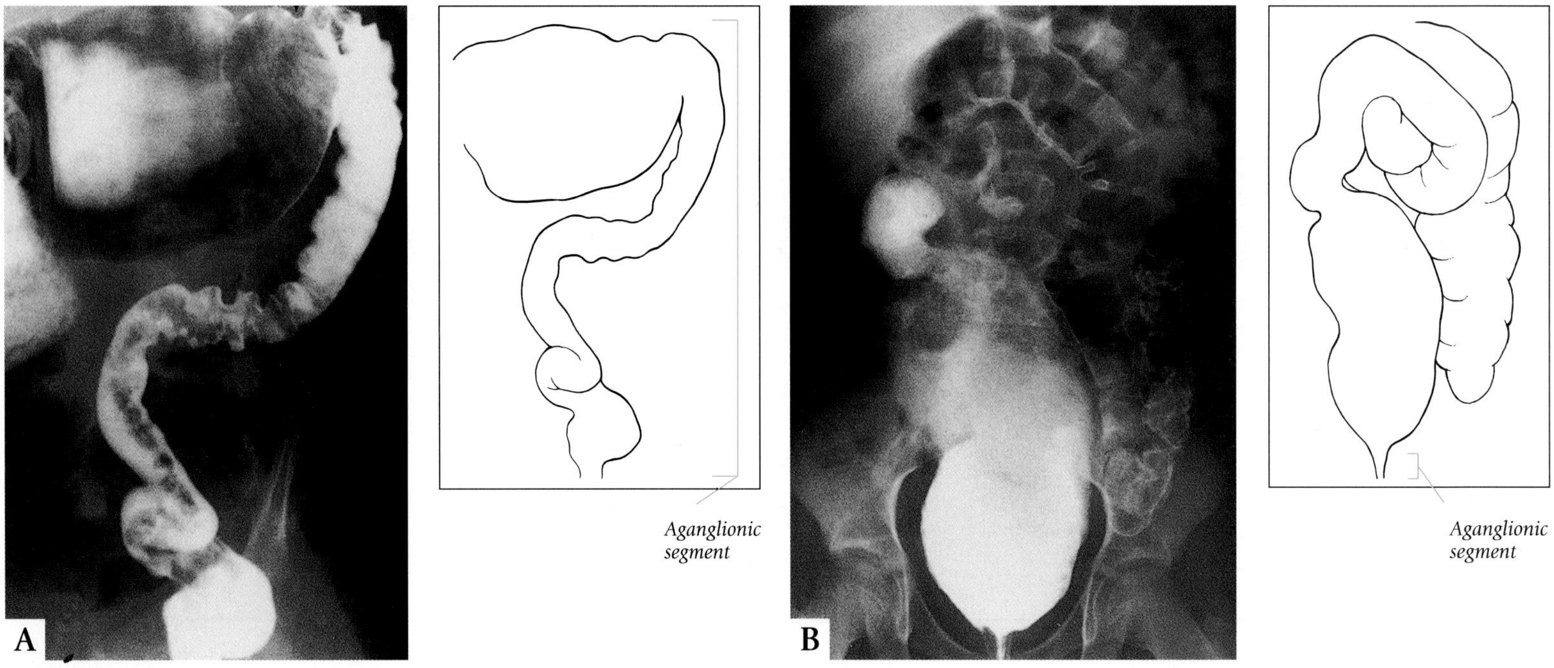

FIGURE 5-17.

In patients with Hirschsprung's disease (congenital aganglionosis), varying lengths of distal bowel receive no enteric innervation. The aganglionic bowel is narrowed and spastic, whereas the normally innervated proximal bowel is dilated and filled with fecal material. In cases of suspected aganglionosis, it is preferable not to cleanse the colon prior to barium studies in order to accentuate the transition zone from aganglionic to normally innervated bowel. **A**, Barium enema in a patient with aganglionosis to the splenic flexure. **B**, Patient with involvement of only the distal 1 to 2 cm of the rectum, *ie*, short segment disease. It is important to remove the insertion catheter used to instill barium in order to avoid missing short segment disease. (*From* Wald [1]; with permission.)

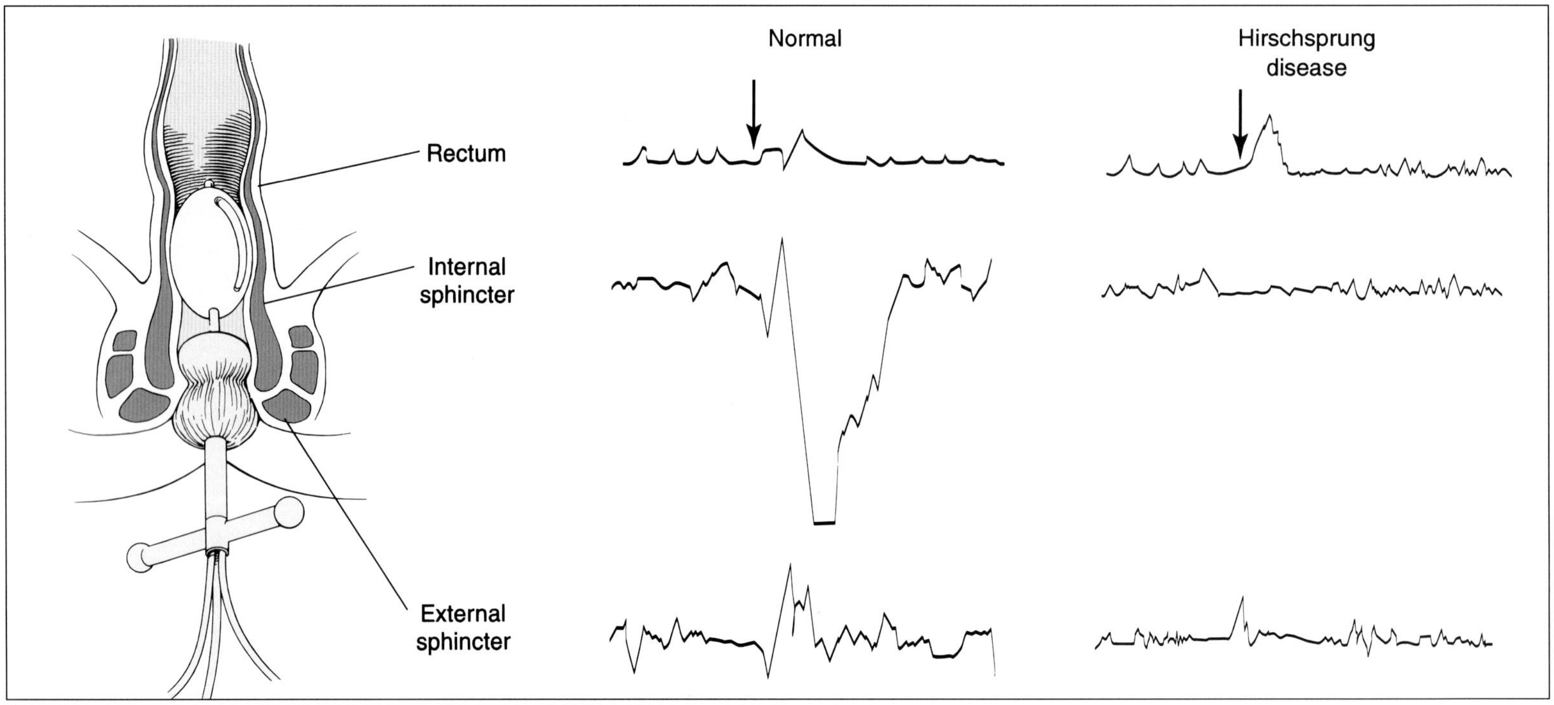

FIGURE 5-18.

Balloon manometry. Internal anal sphincter responses to rectal distension in a patient with Hirshsprung's disease are compared with those in a normal subject using the Schuster-type balloon manometer. In contrast to normal relaxation of the internal anal sphincter following rectal distension (*arrows*), no such relaxation occurs in a patient with Hirschsprung's disease. Thus, the presence of internal anal sphincter relaxation excludes Hirschsprung's disease from consideration. However, failure to detect internal sphincter relaxation is not specific for Hirshsprung's disease, and the diagnosis should be confirmed using histologic or neurohistochemical assessment of biopsy material. (*From* Wald [1]; with permission.)

IDIOPATHIC MEGACOLON AND MEGARECTUM

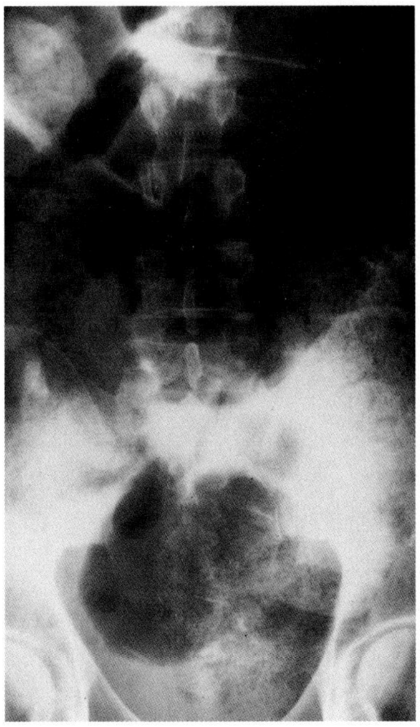

FIGURE 5-19.

Idiopathic megacolon. A large amount of retained stool in the distal colon and considerable distension with air of the transverse colon is depicted. The stool in the rectum suggests that this is not a mechanical obstruction, but an examination of the rectum to exclude a low-lying stricture would be wise.

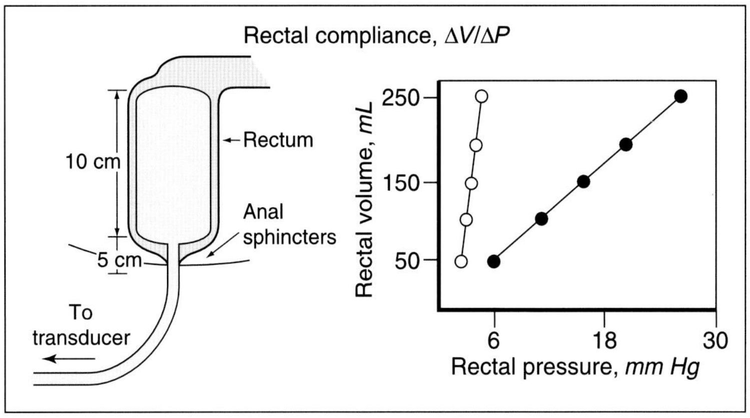

FIGURE 5-20.

Rectal compliance in idiopathic megarectum. The graph plots rectal pressures obtained by incremental distension of the compliance balloon in the rectum in a normal subject (*closed circles*) and a patient with megarectum (*open circles*). In patients with megarectum, rectal pressures at volumes of 50 to 250 mL are lower than normal subjects, and compliance curves (Δ volume [V]/Δ pressure [P]) are higher. In addition, a sense of rectal filling or urge to defecate occurs at much higher volumes of rectal distension (if at all) when compared with normal subjects. In our laboratory, a compliance of greater than 20 mL/mm Hg correlates well with the finding of megarectum as determined with radiologic studies. (*From* Wald [1]; with permission.)

PELVIC FLOOR DYSSYNERGIA

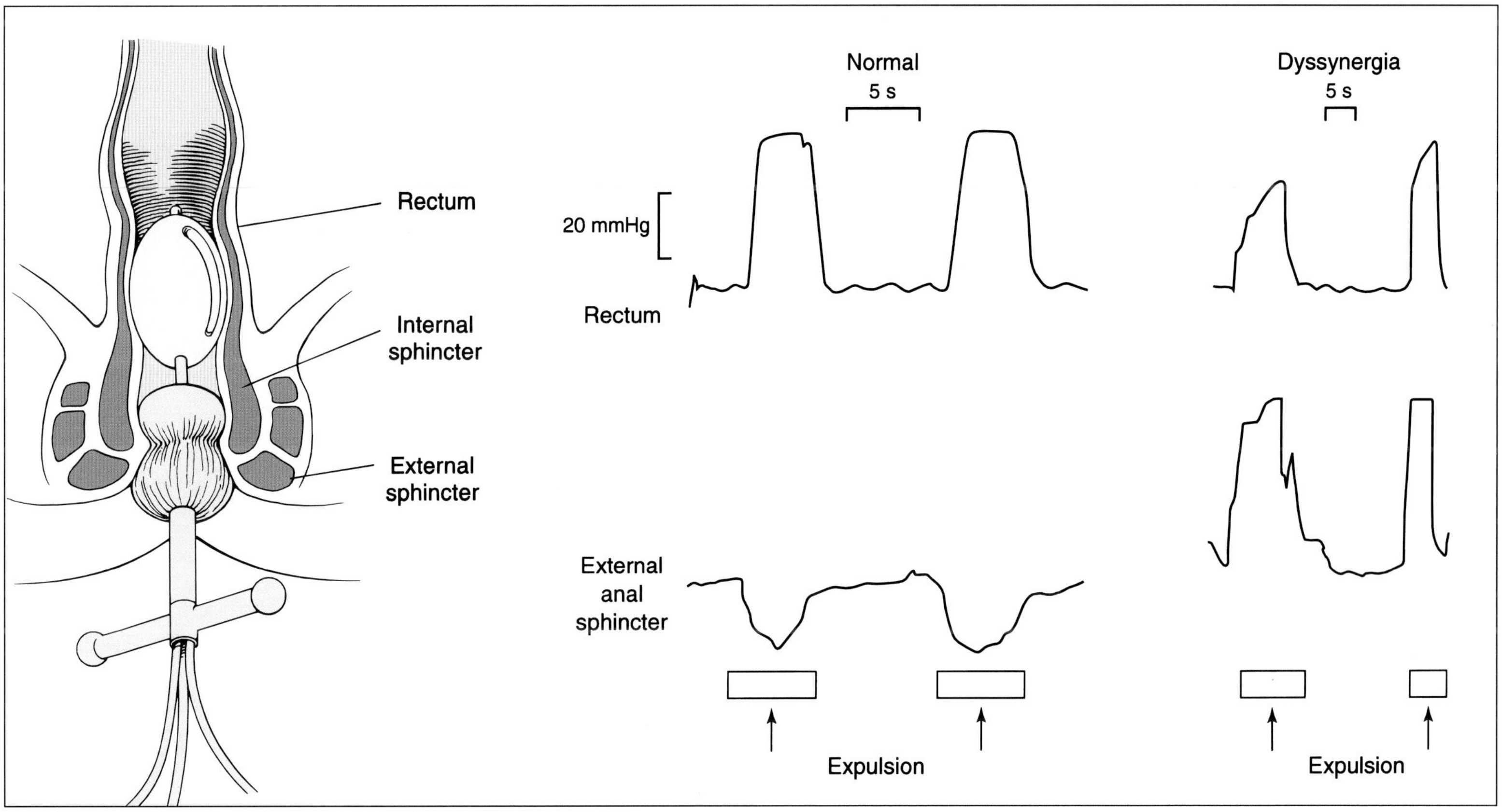

FIGURE 5-21.

Using the Schuster-type balloon manometer, the patient is asked to attempt to expel the manometer as they would when attempting to defecate. In contrast to the characteristic decrease in external anal sphincter pressure observed when a patient attempts to expel the balloon manometer, patients with pelvic floor dyssynergia unconsciously contract or fail to relax the external anal sphincter and puborectalis muscle, resulting in increased pressures on the external sphincter balloon. This manometric pattern can be distinguished from simple voluntary squeezing by observing the increased pressures in the rectal balloon as the patient bears down during pseudodefecation. However, such a study is not ideal, as patients lay on their side and false positives may occur if the buttocks are large. Diagnostic precision can be enhanced if simultaneous electromyographic recordings of the external anal sphincter are made during this maneuver. (*see* Fig. 5-24). (*From* Wald [1]; with permission.)

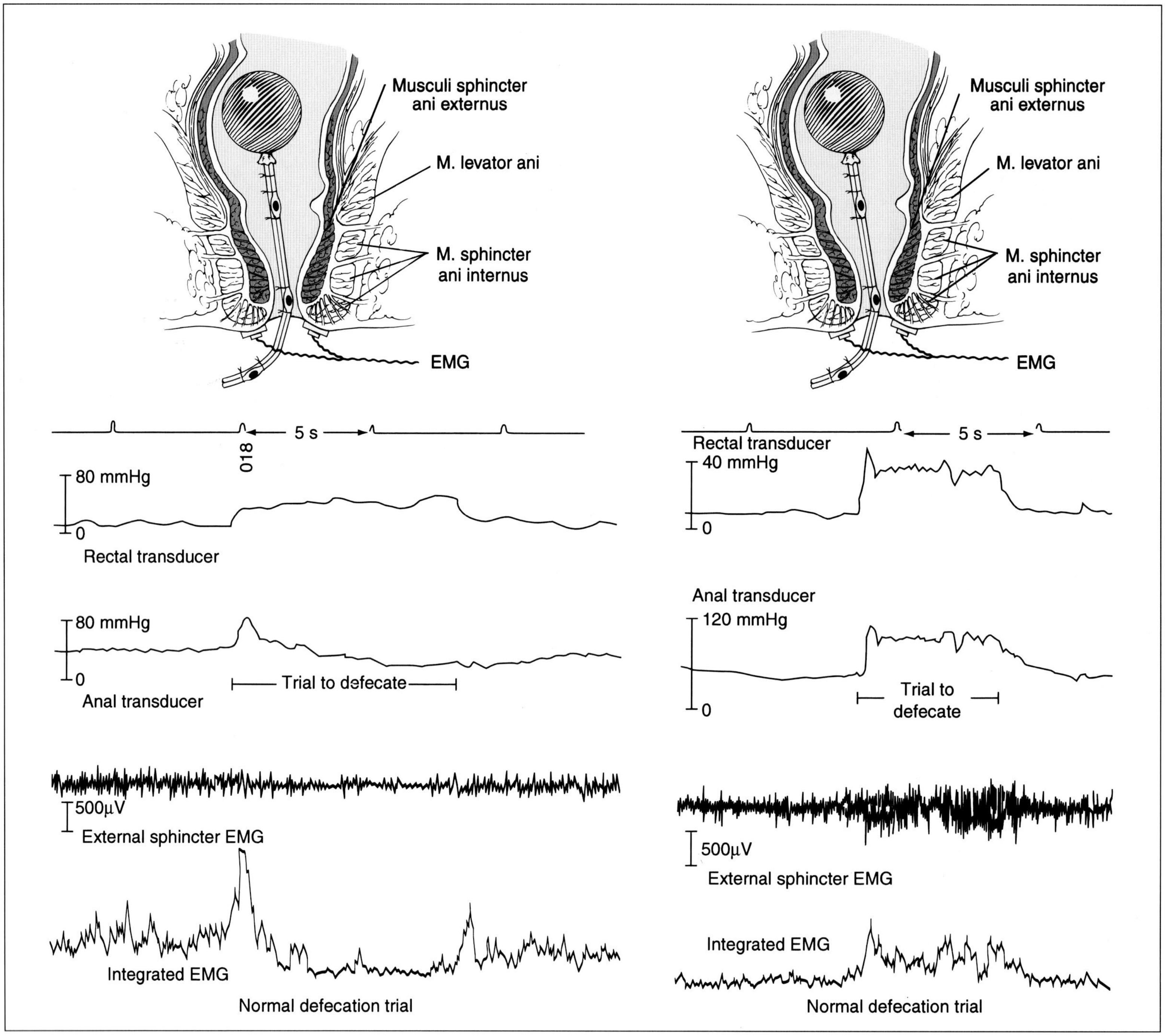

FIGURE 5-22.

Pressure changes in the rectum and anal canal and electromyographic (EMG) recordings from the external anal sphincter during pseudo-defecation. Normal defecation is characterized by increased rectal (intra-abdominal) pressure, decreased anal pressures, and decreased direct and integrated EMG activity as measured by surface electrodes (*left*). In a patient with pelvic floor dyssynergia (*right*), increased anal pressure and EMG activity of the external sphincter occurs during attempted defecation. (*From* Wald [1]; with permission.)

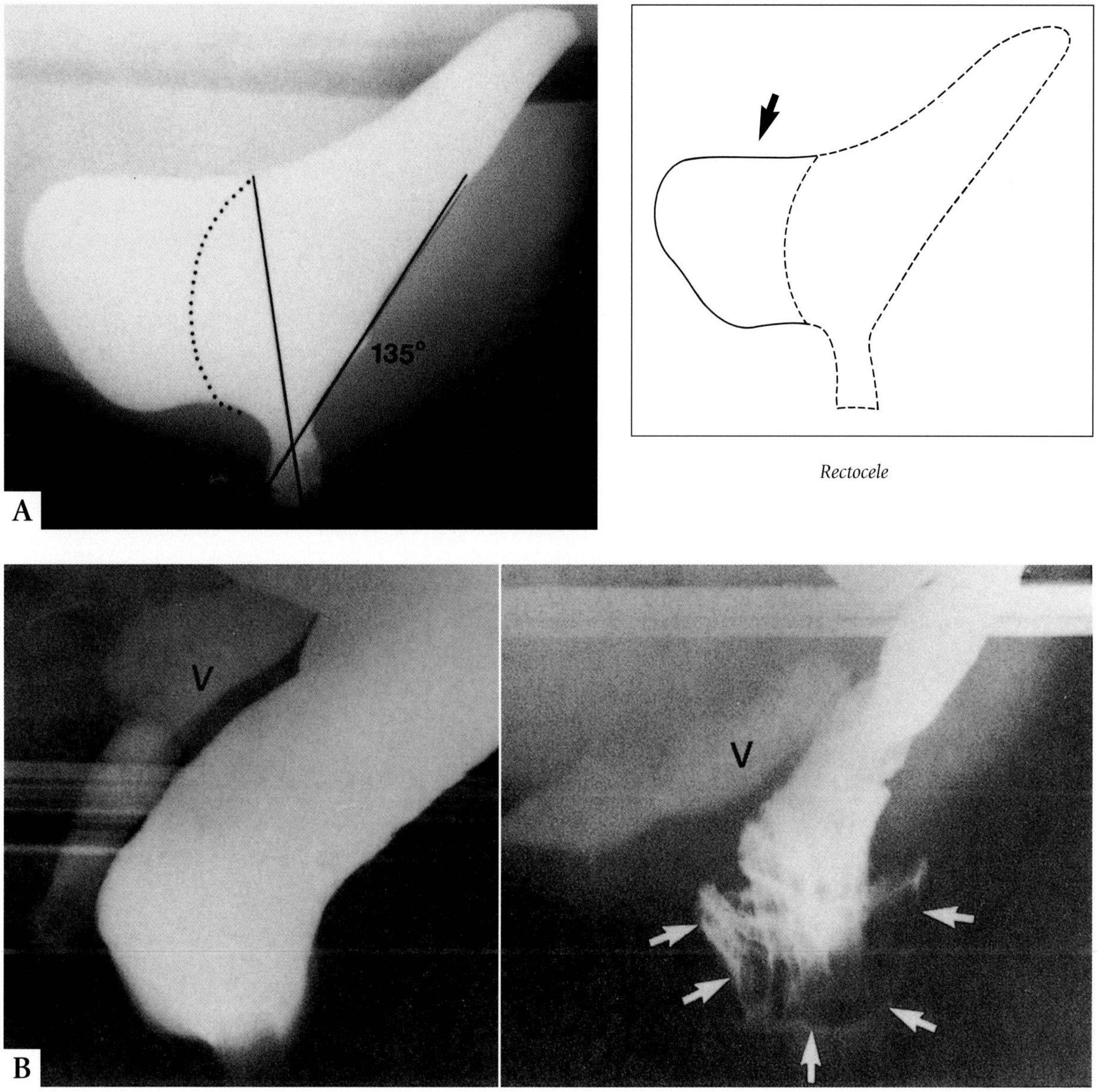

FIGURE 5-23.

A, Rectocele. During expulsion, a large anterior rectocele fills with barium (*arrow*), but expulsion of contrast appears normal. Several studies have demonstrated that rectoceles are common in women without defecation complaints so that caution is necessary before implicating a rectocele as the cause of defecation difficulty. **B**, Rectal intussusception. At *left*, the anorectum is filled with barium paste and appears normal. During attempted evacuation (*right*), inversion of the rectal mucosa occurs during maximal straining (*arrows*). No further emptying occurs in this patient. The vagina (V) is identified by a radiocontrast soaked tampon and lies anterior to the rectum. (**A**, *Courtesy* of D. Bauman, Pittsburgh, PA)

SUBTOTAL COLECTOMY WITH ILEORECTAL ANASTOMOSIS FOR CONSTIPATION

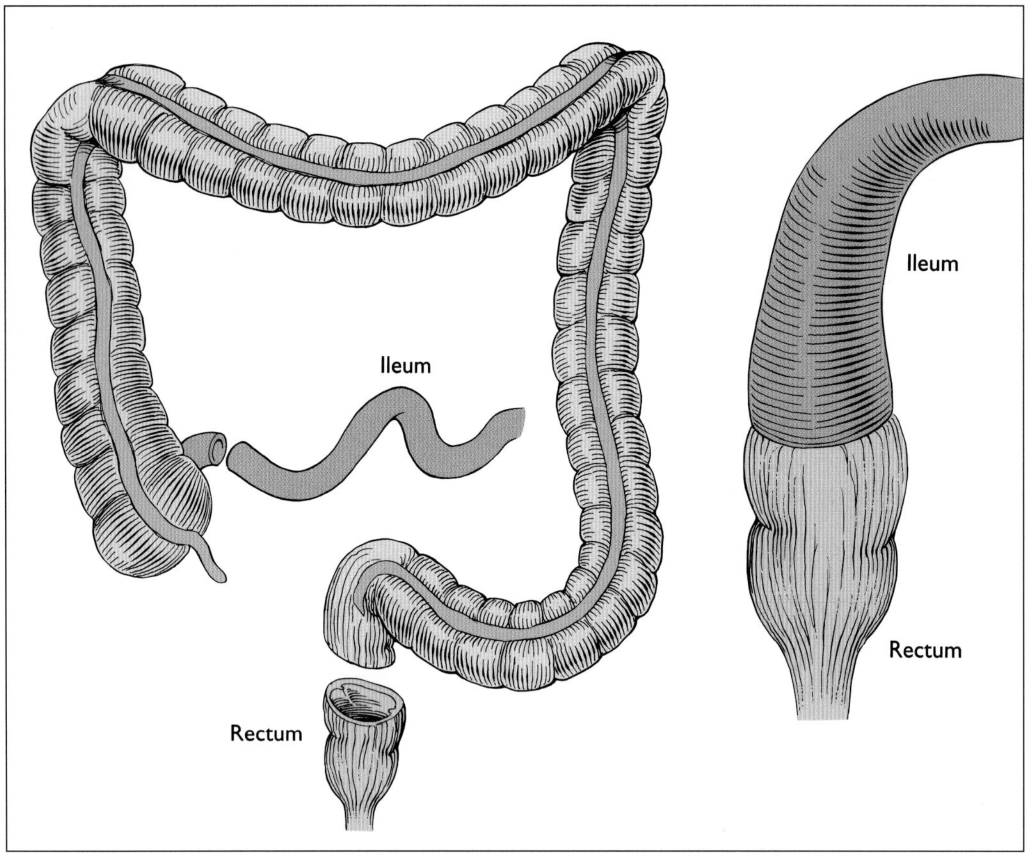

FIGURE 5-24.

Although somewhat controversial, subtotal colectomy with ileorectal anastomosis can dramatically ameliorate incapacitating constipation in carefully selected patients. Optimally, patients should exhibit colonic inertia without generalized intestinal pseudoobstruction or significant psychopathology.

IRRITABLE BOWEL SYNDROME

TABLE 5-5. DIAGNOSTIC OR ROME CRITERIA FOR IRRITABLE BOWEL SYNDROME

At least 3 months of continuous or recurrent symptoms of:

Abdominal pain or discomfort
- Relieved with defecation and/or
- Associated with change in stool frequency and/or
- Associated with change in stool consistency

Two or more of the following symptoms at least 1/4 of the time
- Altered stool frequency (<3/wk or >3/day)
- Altered stool form (hard or loose)
- Altered stool passage (staining, urgency, incomplete evacuation)
- Passage of mucus
- Bloating/abdominal distension

TABLE 5-5.

Irritable bowel syndrome is considered a disorder of gastrointestinal function manifested by abdominal pain and altered bowel habits that occur in chronic or recurrent fashion at times of life stress and emotional tension. Symptom patterns include lower abdominal (occasionally other locations) pain and altered bowel habits, *ie*, constipation, diarrhea, or both. The presence of organic disease that can produce similar symptoms must be excluded. However, a precise, reproducible, and objective definition of this syndrome remains elusive and is particularly problematic for clinicians and investigators. An international committee has put forth a definition of irritable bowel syndrome that uses symptomatic criteria, known as the *Rome Criteria* (shown). (*From* Drossman *et al.* [13]; with permission.)

The three major hypotheses put forth to explain the etiology of symptoms in irritable bowel syndrome are 1) patients have an underlying disorder of intestinal motility; 2) emotional tension and psychological factors lead to gastrointestinal symptoms and health seeking behavior; and 3) individuals with irritable bowel syndrome have a low tolerance for pain or an excessive response to normal signals from the gastrointestinal tract.

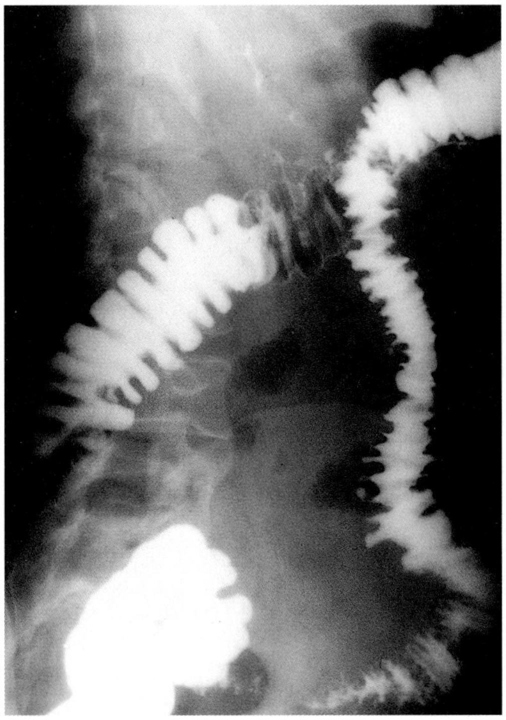

FIGURE 5-25.

Barium enema in an irritable bowel syndrome patient. The extreme hypercontractility of the left and sigmoid colon is indicative of excessive segmenting motor activity. Current evidence suggests that disordered basal motor activity is unlikely and that the exaggerated colonic motor responses to certain stimulants requires more rigorous analysis. Several studies report a high frequency of hysteria, somatization disorder, depression, and anxiety in patients with irritable bowel syndrome. Other studies suggest that laboratory stressors can alter gastrointestinal motility.

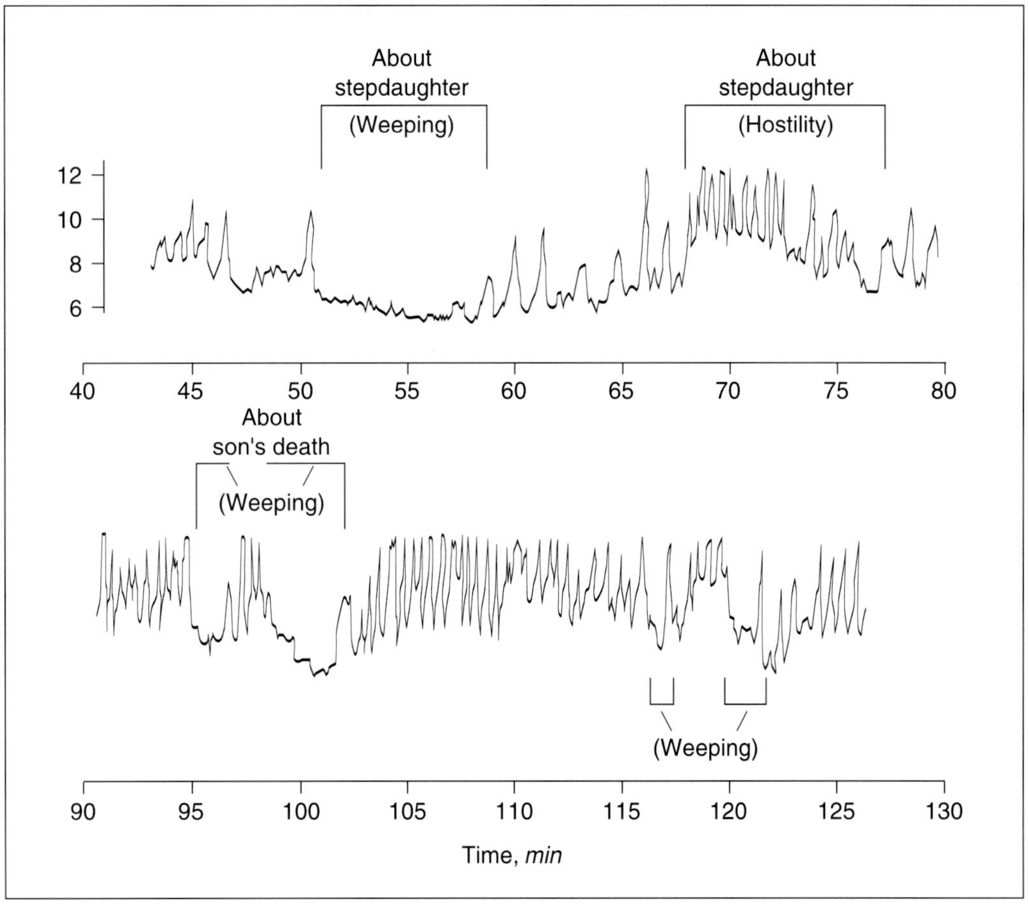

FIGURE 5-26.

Emotions and colon motility in irritable bowel syndrome. During a stressful interview, the mood of a 47-year-old woman with irritable bowel syndrome varied from weeping to mixed feelings of hostility and sorrow. Reactions characterized by feelings of helplessness and weeping were associated with inhibition of colon motility, whereas reactions characterized by anger and hostility were associated with increased motility and mucosal engorgement. Patients with constipation-predominant irritable bowel syndrome usually responded with irritability, whereas the opposite response generally occurred in irritable bowel syndrome patients with diarrhea as their main complaint. As shown in this patient, both response patterns can coexist in the same patient. (*From* Almy [14]; with permission.)

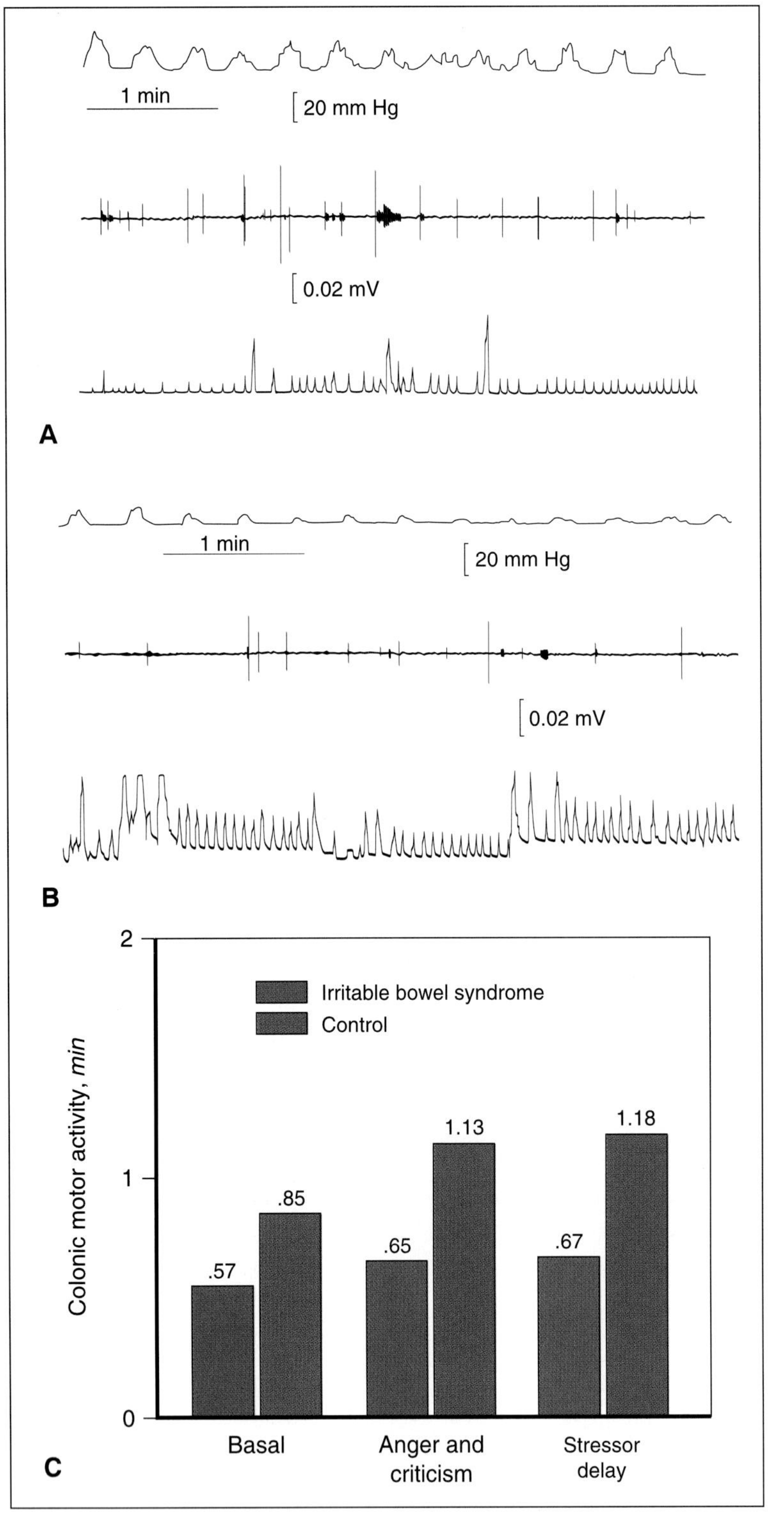

FIGURE 5-27.

Emotions and colonic motility in irritable bowel syndrome. **A**, An example of rectosigmoid motor and myoelectrical spike activity in a patient with irritable bowel syndrome. The upper tracing is rectosigmoid motor activity; the middle tracing is a spike potential activity; and the lower tracing is the respiratory pneumogram. These recordings occurred during the "delay stressor," which generated anger and hostility in the patient. In this stressor, the subject waited an unpredictable period of time for medical attention after being told that it was essential for a physician to remove or adjust the rectal catheter immediately because of a serious equipment malfunction. The experimenter left the room to locate a physician, returning four times at different intervals. Each time he criticized the physician, stating that he was either too busy to come or could not be found. This hoax continued for 30 minutes and evoked anger in all the irritable bowel syndrome subjects. **B**, Tracings from the same patient 30 minutes after the stressor was eliminated. As shown, the anger inducing stressor increased both rectosigmoid motor and spike activity over baseline values. These changes were significantly greater in irritable bowel syndrome patients than in age-matched control subjects. **C**, A graph demonstrating the effects of stressors on colonic motility in the group of 12 irritable bowel syndrome patients and 10 control subjects. (*From* Welgan *et al.* [15]; with permission.)

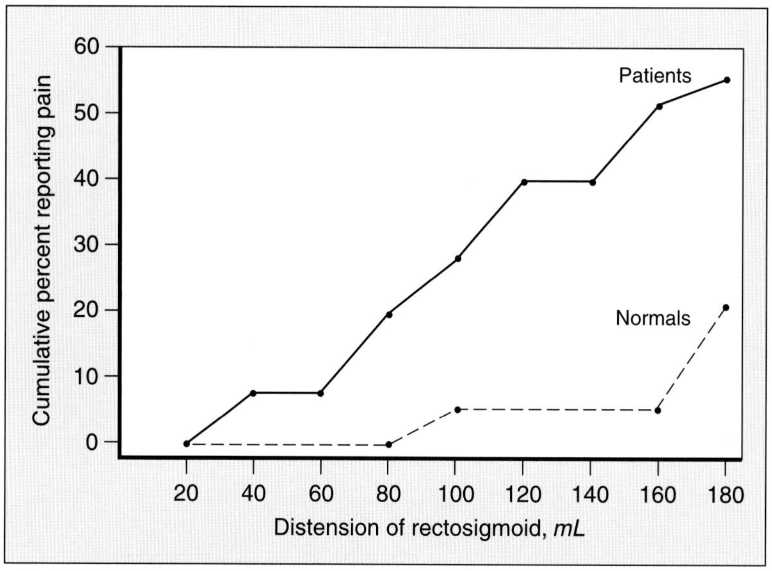

FIGURE 5-28.

Visceral sensations in irritable bowel syndrome. The graph depicts rectosigmoid balloon distension studies in 28 irritable bowel syndrome patients and 20 healthy control subjects. The rectosigmoid balloon was distended in a stepwise fashion by injecting an additional 20 mL of air every 2 minutes up to a total of 180 mL of air. Compared with the control subjects, the incidence of pain complaints was greater in irritable bowel syndrome patients. At maximum balloon distention, 60% of the irritable bowel patients compared with only 20% of the volunteers complained of rectal pain ($P<0.05$). This leftward shift of the pain curve confirmed the presence of an altered visceral pain threshold in the patients with irritable bowel syndrome. (*From* Whitehead *et al.* [16]; with permission.)

REFERENCES AND RECOMMENDED READING

1. Wald A: Anorectum. In *Atlas of Gastrointestinal Motility*. Edited by Schuster MM. Baltimore: Williams & Wilkins; 1993:29–249.
2. Caruana BJ, Wald A, Hinds JP, Eidelman BH: Anorectal sensory and motor function in neurogenic fecal incontinence: Comparison between multiple sclerosis and diabetes mellitus. *Gastroenterology* 1991, 100:465–470.
3. Bartolo DCC, Jarratt JA, Read MG, *et al.*: The role of partial denervation of the puborectalis in idiopathic faecal incontinence. *Br J Surg* 1993, 70:664–667.
4. Teasdall RD, Schuster MM, Walsh FB: Sphincter involvement in ocular myopathy. *Arch Neurol* 1964, 10:446–448.
5. Kiff ES, Swash M: Slowed conduction in the pudendal nerves in idiopathic (neurogenic) fecal incontinence. *Br J Surg* 1984, 71:614–616.
6. Sultan AH, Kamm MA: Ultrasound of the anal sphincter. In *Atlas of Gastrointestinal Motility*. Edited by Schuster MM. Baltimore: Williams and Wilkins; 1993:115–121.
7. Milligan ETC, Morgan CN: Surgical anatomy of the anal canal with special reference to anorectal fistulae. *Lancet* 1934, 2:150–156, 1213–1217.
8. Gorsh RV: The external anal sphincter muscle. In *Proctologic Anatomy*, edn 2. Baltimore: Williams and Wilkins: 1955:57–65.
9. Engel BT, Nikoomanesh P, Schuster MM: Operant rectosphincter responses in the treatment of fecal incontinence. *N Engl J Med* 1974, 290:646–649.
10. Chiaroni G, Scattolini C, Bonfante F, Vantini I: Liquid stool incontinence with severe urgency: Anorectal function and effective biofeedback treatment. *Gut* 1993, 34:1576–1580.
11. McLean RG, Smart RC, Gaston-Parry D, *et al.*: Colonic transit scintigraphy in health and constipation using oral iodine-131-cellulose. *J Nucl Med* 1990, 31:985–989.
12. Metcalf AM, Phillips SF, Zinsmeister AR, *et al.*: A simplified assessment of segmental colonic transit. *Gastroenterology* 1987, 92:40–47.
13. Drossman DA, Thompson WG, Talley NJ, *et al.*: Identification of sub-groups of functional gastrointestinal disorders. *Gastroenterology International* 1990, 3:159–172.
14. Almy TP: Experimental studies on the irritable colon. *Am J Med* 1951, 9:60–67.
15. Welgan P, Meshkinpour H, Beeler M: Effect of anger on colon motor and myoelectrical activity in irritable bowel syndrome. *Gastroenterology* 1988, 94:1150–1156.
16. Whitehead WE, Engel BT, Schuster MM: Irritable bowel syndrome. Physiological and psychological differences between diarrhea-predominant and constipation-predominant patients. *Dig Dis Sci* 1980, 35:404–413.

Chapter 6

Diseases of the Anus

JEFFREY L. BARNETT

The anorectal examination is part of the routine physical examination, but it should be performed with particular care and thoroughness in anyone with anorectal complaints. Careful explanation and a gentle manner will facilitate this awkward, uncomfortable portion of the examination. The patient is placed in the left lateral, or less often, the prone jackknife position. As the examination begins, one should have in mind a variety of conditions that may explain the symptoms offered by the patient. The buttocks, upper thighs, and sacral region are carefully inspected for signs of infection, dermatoses, and pilonidal disease. Next, the perianal region is inspected with the buttocks retracted apart. Mucous or fecal soiling, focal erythema, excoriations, scars, skin changes, and fistulous openings are important clues to underlying diseases. Anal inspection may demonstrate skin tags, thrombosed external hemorrhoids, prolapsed internal hemorrhoids, anal cancer, rectal prolapse, or traumatic focal sphincter injury. The anus is further examined by gentle eversion. This eversion may best expose anal fissures, internal hemorrhoids, and anal papillae. The digital examination is performed after adequate lubrication. Sometimes, even using a topical anesthetic, particularly painful lesions cannot be adequately examined because of patient discomfort, and evaluation under anesthesia is necessary. Palpable tenderness or areas of induration may be appreciated around the perineum. Palpation within the anal canal may identify the lump or tenderness of anal lesions previously described. Digital examination should also include the prostate (asymmetry, nodules), anterior wall (rectocele, fistula), sphincter musculature, posterior puborectalis impression, and rectal mucosa (polyps, tumors, foreign bodies). The sphincter tone and puborectalis impression should be appreciated at rest and during voluntary squeeze. Inappropriate contraction of the puborectalis muscle and prolapsing lesions are often best diagnosed during or just after bearing down.

A variety of metal and plastic disposable anoscopes are available for inspection of the anal canal. Metal anoscopes come in different lengths and with either built-in or external light sources. Internal hemorrhoids are usually best evaluated and treated through an anoscope. Primary fistulous openings, fissures, and other lesions may also been seen during slow withdrawal of the instrument. Rigid and flexible proctosigmoidoscopes are important tools for evaluation of the distal rectum. The flexible instrument has nearly replaced the rigid proctosigmoidoscope because of comfort, depth of passage, and accuracy of examination. Also, the flexible scope may be retroflexed 180° in the rectum to inspect the distal rectum and proximal anal canal.

EXTERNAL HEMORRHOIDS

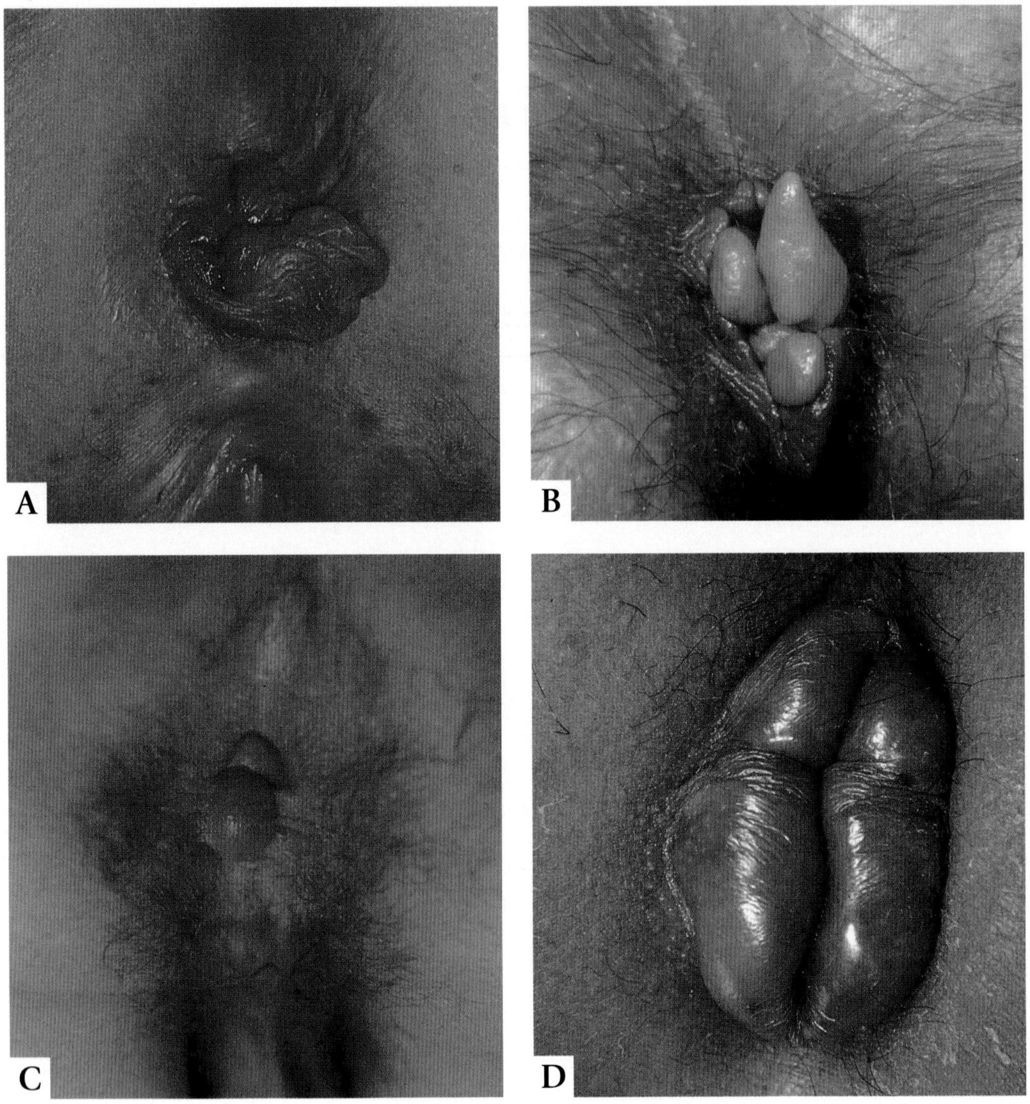

FIGURE 6-1.

External or perianal skin tags are soft, fleshy folds of fibrous connective tissue. They are often the sequelae after the clot from a thrombosed external hemorrhoid has resolved. External hemorrhoids arise from the inferior hemorrhoidal plexus and are located below the dentate line; they are covered by squamous epithelium. External hemorrhoids are usually asymptomatic unless thrombosis occurs. Internal hemorrhoids are submucosal vascular cushions arising from above the dentate line and are covered by rectal mucosa. Internal and external hemorrhoids may coexist as a mixed hemorrhoid. **A**, An external or perianal skin tag. Skin tags may interfere with adequate anal hygiene and may worsen anal irritation or pruritus. Surgical excision is rarely necessary. **B**, Prominent fibroepithelial anal canal tags. **C**, An acutely thrombosed external hemorrhoid. A thrombosed external hemorrhoid may be quite painful, and bleeding may occur if the overlying skin ulcerates and the hematoma is expressed. Most respond to conservative management, but if acute and painful, local incision and clot evacuation afford immediate relief. **D**, Acutely prolapsed large, bilateral external and internal (mixed) hemorrhoids. (*Courtesy of* R. Burney, Ann Arbor, MI)

INTERNAL HEMORRHOIDS

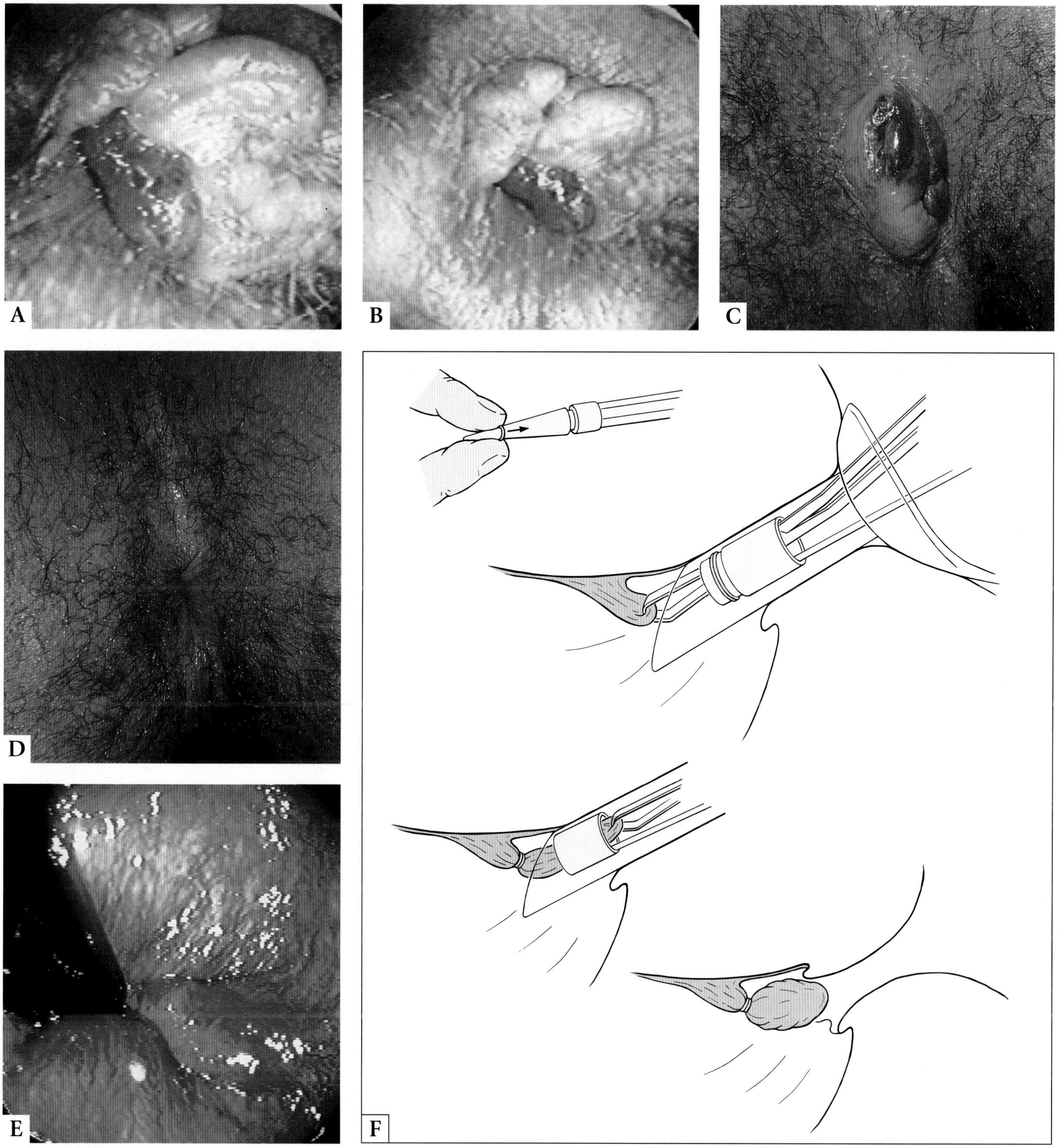

FIGURE 6-2.

Internal hemorrhoids may be associated with pruritus, fecal soiling, discomfort, or no symptoms at all. However, bleeding and prolapse are the most typical complaints and bring the patient to the physician. Internal hemorrhoids may be graded by bleeding and degree of prolapse. With first-degree hemorrhoids, the patient experiences painless, defecatory bleeding without significant prolapse of tissue. The hemorrhoids may be barely visible in the anal canal with straining, and they are best seen through the anoscope. Bleeding and prolapse occur at the time of defecation with second-degree hemorrhoids, but the hemorrhoid reduces spontaneously back into the rectum after straining. Bleeding and prominent prolapse

(Continued on next page)

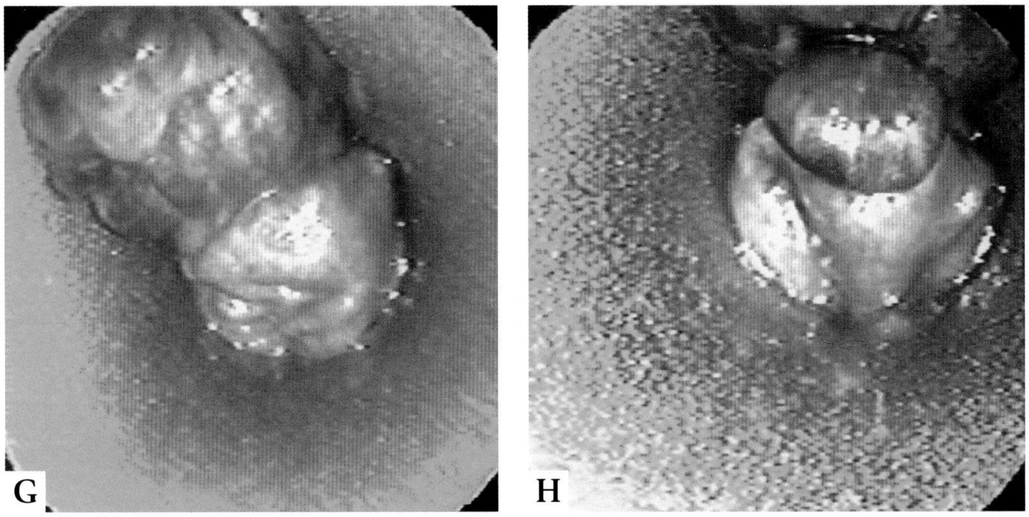

FIGURE 6-2. (CONTINUED)

after defecation or straining that require digital reduction characterize third-degree hemorrhoids. Large, usually acute, hemorrhoids that cannot be persistently reduced and are at risk for strangulation are considered fourth-degree hemorrhoids.

A and **B**, Prolapsed internal hemorrhoid. This friable internal hemorrhoid was the cause of hematochezia during defecation. External hemorrhoidal skin tags are also shown. Ulcerated, prolapsing internal hemorrhoids before (**C**) and after (**D**) reduction are depicted. **E**, This figure shows the view of internal hemorrhoids looking through the retroflexed sigmoidoscope. **F**, Rubber band ligation of an internal hemorrhoid. Banding is performed through a slotted anoscope using a simple Barron-type ligator and a grasping forceps. The O-ring rubber band is loaded using a removable cone. Then the ligator is advanced through the anoscope to the hemorrhoid, the tissue is grasped with the forceps and pulled into the chamber, and the ligator trigger is pulled to release the band. The band is placed on or just above (on the redundant rectal mucosa) the hemorrhoid. Care must be taken to remain well above the dentate line. Inflammation and ulceration will develop at the site of the sloughed tissue with resultant submucosal fibrosis and fixation of the prolapsing hemorrhoid. Other nonsurgical methods of treating internal hemorrhoids include infrared coagulation, bipolar coagulation, electrocoagulation, cryotherapy, sclerotherapy, and laser therapy. **G** and **H**, An internal hemorrhoid before and after rubber band ligation seen through a slotted, self-illuminated metal anoscope. The hemorrhoid and redundant rectal mucosa are visible (*G*). The band has been placed on the proximal portion of the hemorrhoid (*H*). Several sessions may be required depending on the number and size of hemorrhoids present. Eighty percent of patients will have good results and complications are rare. (**C** and **D**, *Courtesy of* R. Burney, Ann Arbor, MI) (**F**, *Adapted from* Goldberg and Buls [1] and Salvati and Eisentat [2]; with permission.)

ANORECTAL VARICES

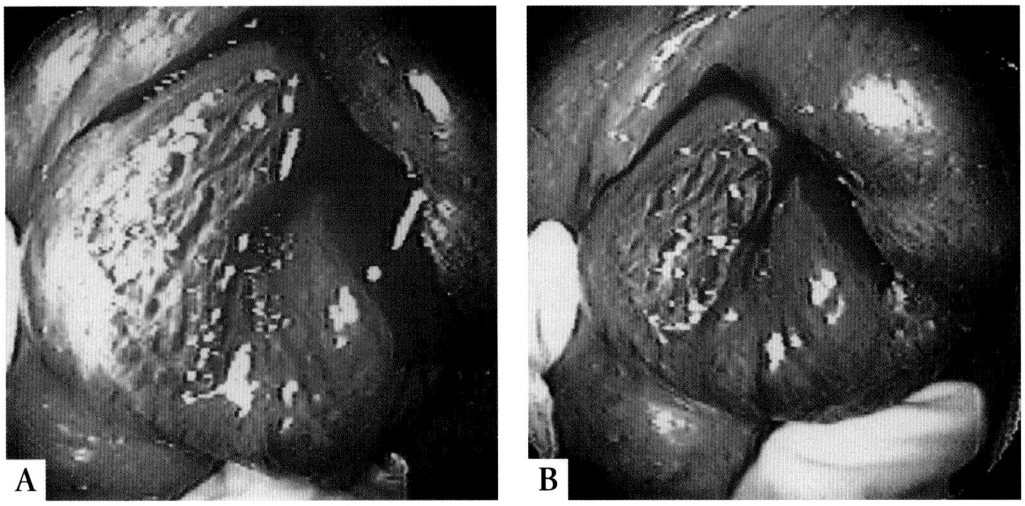

FIGURE 6-3.

A and **B**, Anorectal varices. These large vascular lesions may be mistaken for large external or mixed hemorrhoids. However, in contrast to external hemorrhoids, varices are compressible and refill rapidly. Hemorrhoids and anorectal varices are unrelated. The incidence of hemorrhoids is similar in those with and without portal hypertension, and hemorrhoids have no direct connection to the portal system. Bleeding may be massive. Nonsurgical means (banding, sclerotherapy, etc.) have been used to treat anorectal varices, but surgical ligation is probably safer and more effective.

PRURITUS ANI

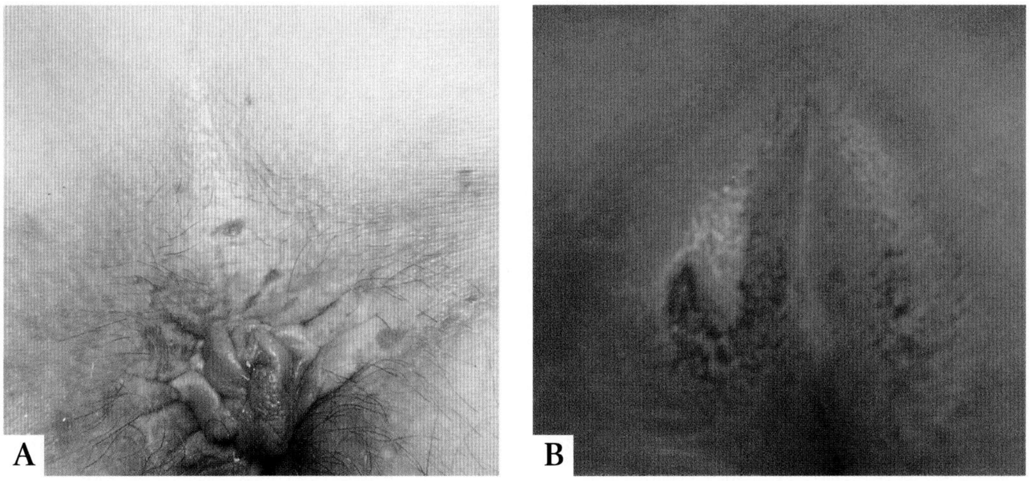

FIGURE 6-4.

Intense perianal itching and burning discomfort is called *pruritus ani*. Causes include local irritants or sensitivities, benign and malignant dermatoses, infections, and anorectal diseases that lead to fecal contamination or leakage. **A**, This excoriated perianal skin was a result of idiopathic pruritus ani. **B**, An erythematous, fissured perineum that was caused by *Candida albicans*. (*Courtesy of* R. Burney, Ann Arbor, MI)

ANAL FISSURE

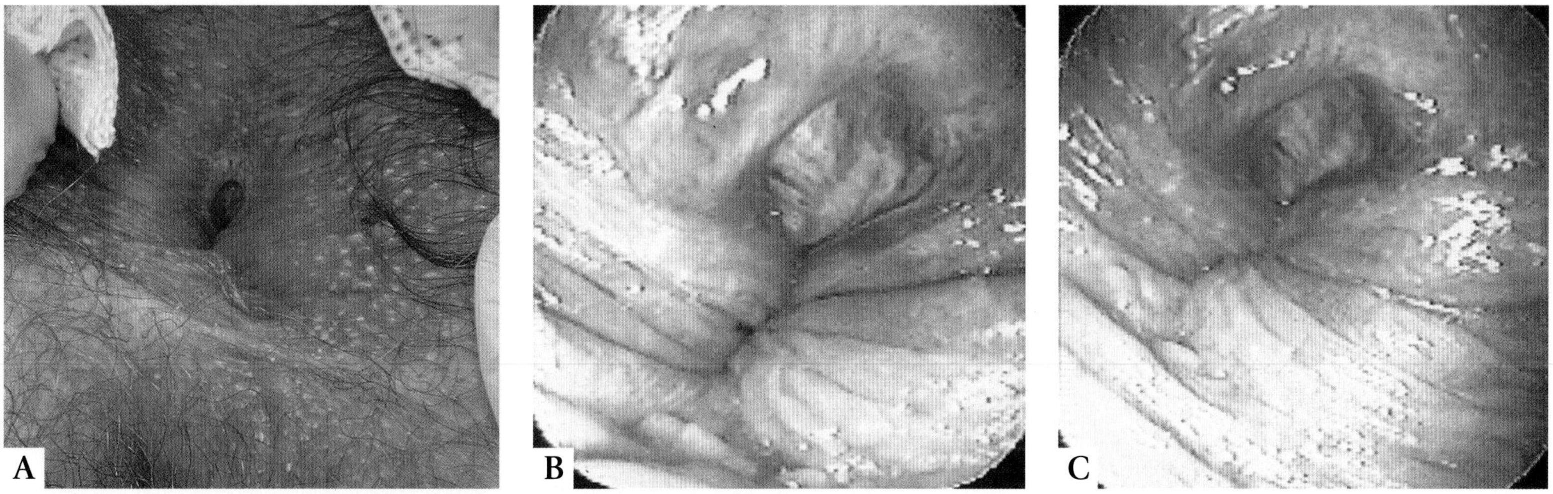

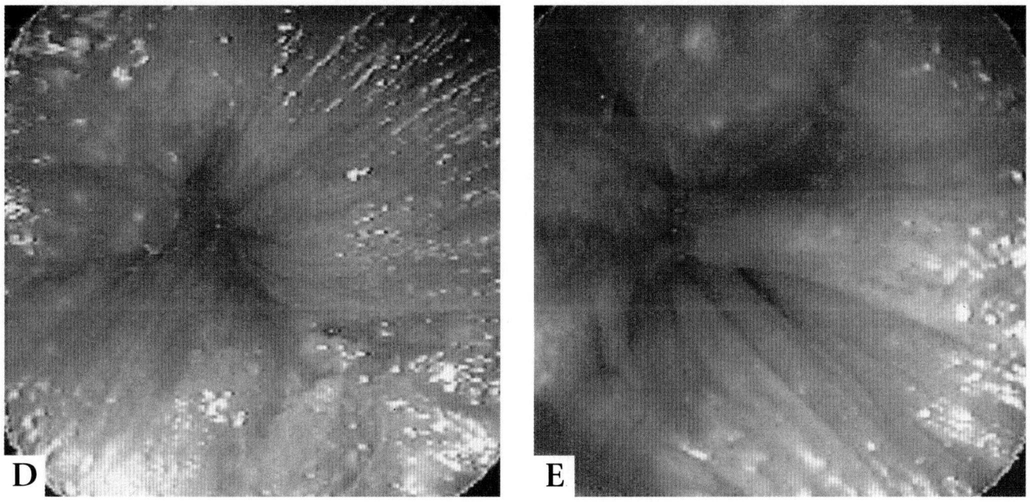

FIGURE 6-5.

An anal fissure is a painful, linear defect in the anal canal oriented perpendicularly to the dentate line. It is usually caused by a tearing that occurred during passage of a stool. The vast majority are located in the posterior midline; the remainder are anteriorly placed. A fissure located laterally should arouse suspicion of an underlying condition such as inflammatory bowel disease. An anal fissure is best identified by gentle but forceful lateral traction of the buttocks (after topical application of an anesthetic if necessary). Most acute anal fissures will heal with conservative medical

(Continued on next page)

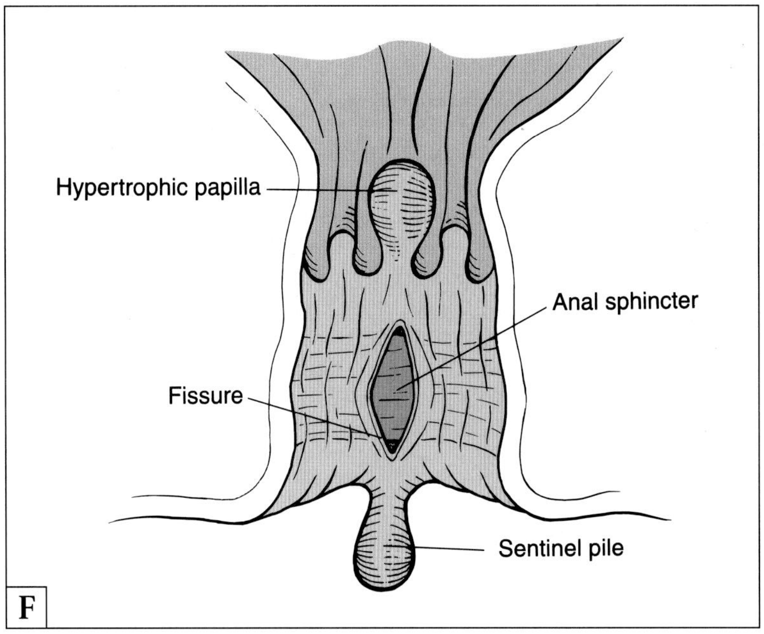

FIGURE 6-5. *(CONTINUED)*

management and time. Persistent acute fissures and most chronic fissures require definitive surgery, usually a lateral internal sphincterotomy to reduce resting sphincter tone. **A**, Typical fissure in ano located in the posterior midline. **B** and **C**, Large, painful anal fissure that failed to heal on medical therapy. **D** and **E**, The same patient a few weeks after lateral internal sphincterotomy; the fissure has nearly healed. **F**, The classic chronic anal fissure triad includes the hypertrophic anal papilla, anal fissure, and sentinel skin tag. The fissure margins may appear fibrotic and slightly undermined, and exposed internal sphincter muscle fibers may be visible. (**F**, *Adapted from* Hicks and Timmcke [3] and Barnett and Raper [4]; with permission.)

ANORECTAL ABSCESS AND FISTULA

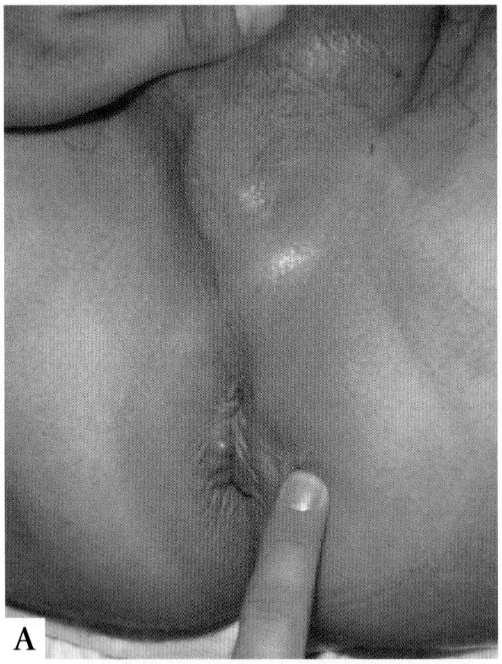

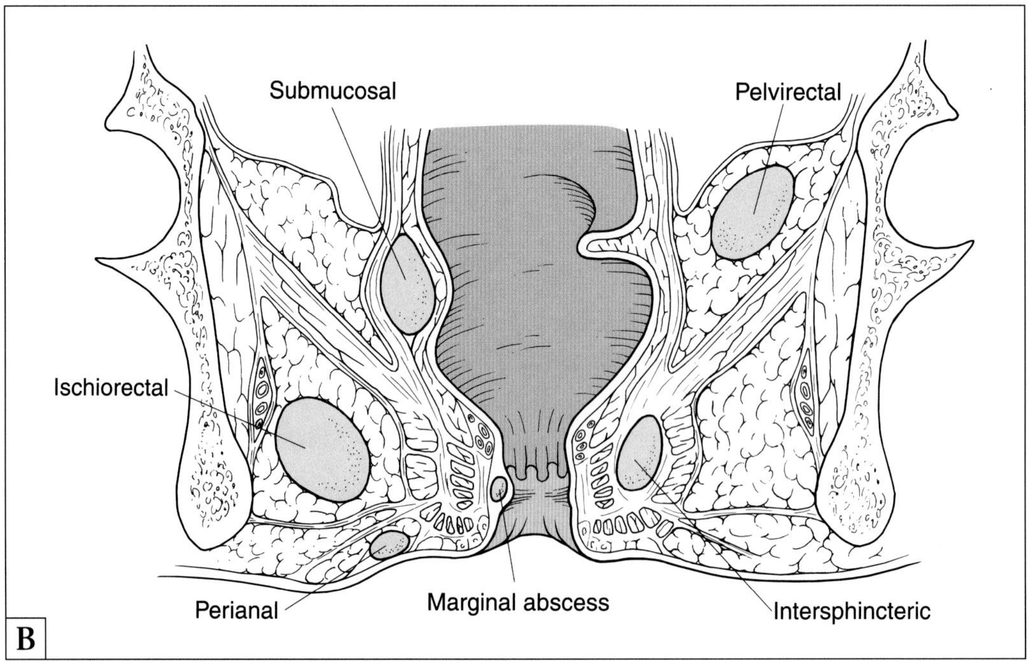

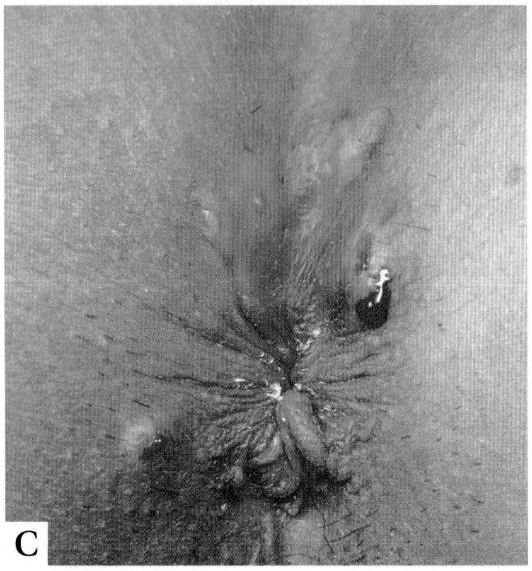

FIGURE 6-6.

Abscess is the acute manifestation and fistula is the chronic manifestation of suppurative anorectal infection. Fistulous disease and abscess are caused by infection of the anal glands, secondary to ductal obstruction caused by fecal material or anal trauma. The primary fistulous orifice is found at the level of the dentate line and the secondary opening at the anal verge or elsewhere in the perineum. Abscess typically presents as pain and swelling; fistula in ano usually causes discharge with occasional discomfort. **A**, Incision and drainage are indicated in this ischiorectal abscess with anterior extension. **B**, Typical anatomic locations of anorectal abscesses. **C**, Multiple perianal fistula sites from fistula in ano.

(Continued on next page)

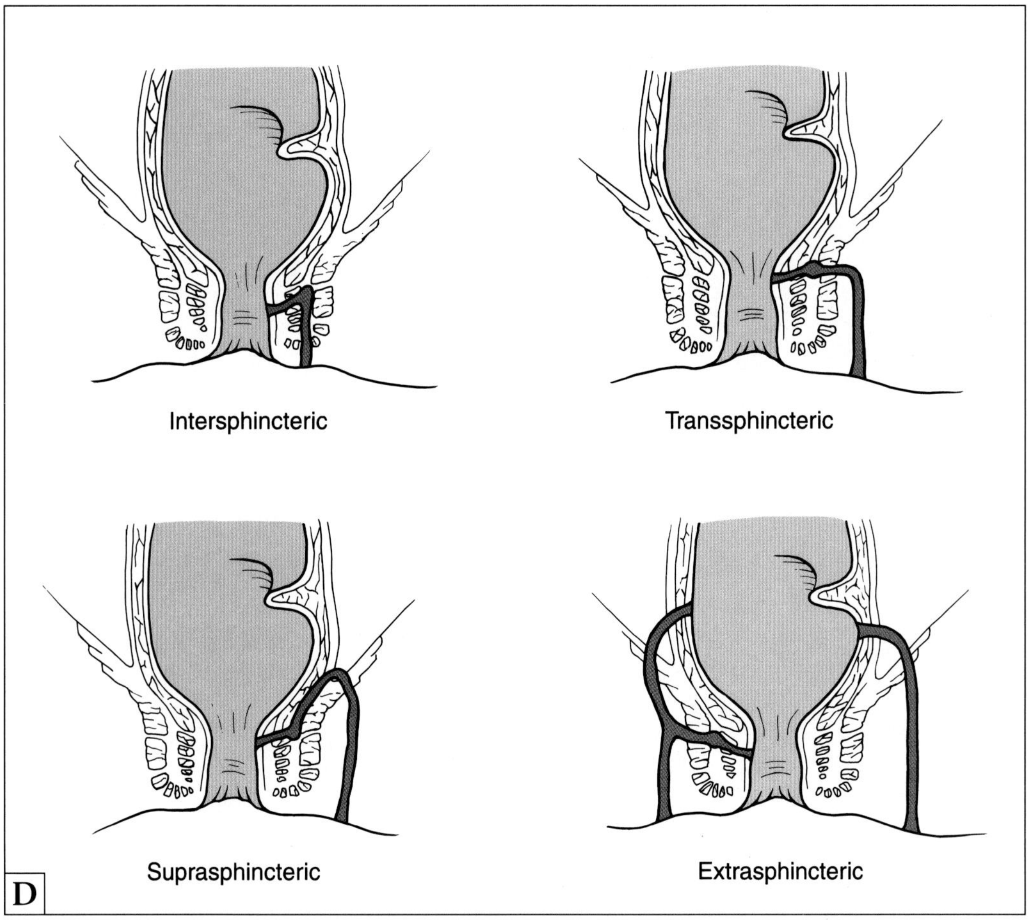

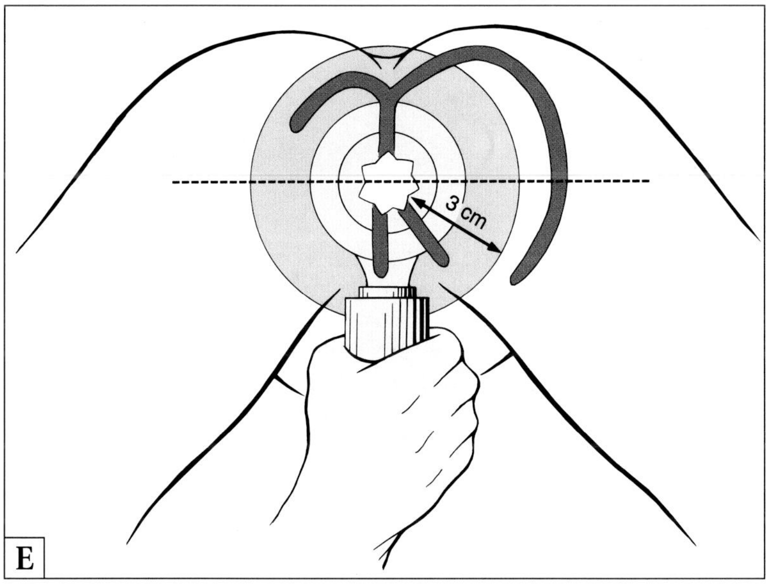

FIGURE 6-6. *(CONTINUED)*

D, Anatomic classification of anorectal fistulas. **E**, This figure is an example of Goodsall's rule. An external secondary fistulous opening located anterior to the transverse anal line (and located within 3 cm of the anal verge) usually runs directly into the anal canal. A secondary opening located posterior to this transverse line (or far from the anal verge) often takes a curved route prior to termination in the posterior midline. (**A** and **C**, *Courtesy of* R. Burney, Ann Arbor, MI) (**B**, **D**, and **E**, *From* Barnett and Raper [4]; with permission.)

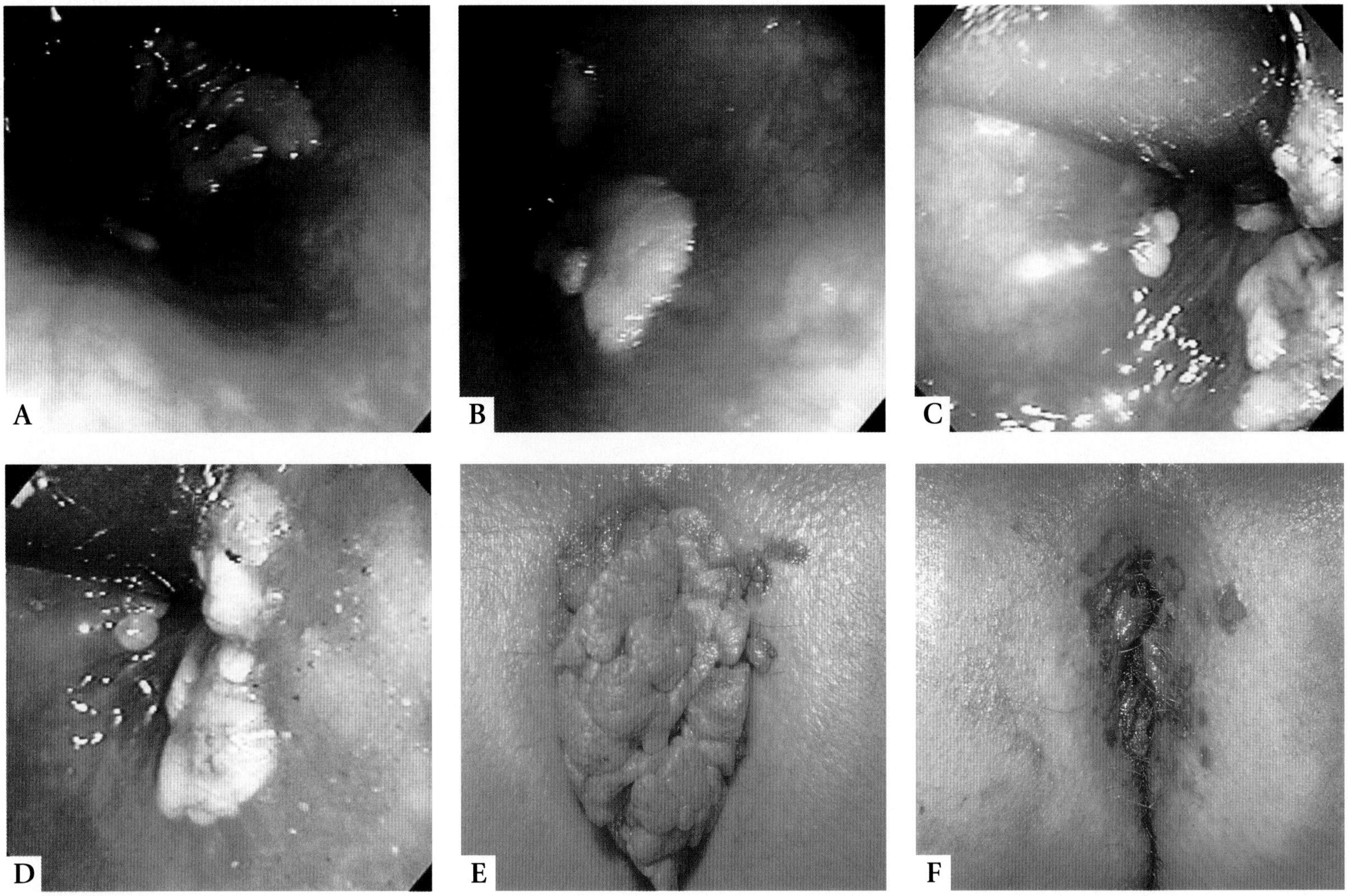

FIGURE 6-7.

Anal condylomata acuminata. Anal warts are caused by the human papilloma virus (HPV type 6). Spread is usually through anal intercourse, but autoinoculation from the genitals may also occur. Despite treatment with caustic agents or fulguration, recurrence and reinfection rates are high. **A–D**, Anal condyloma extending high up into the anal canal seen through the retroflexed sigmoidoscope. Recurrent perianal disease after adequate topical therapy may be secondary to repeated inoculation from undiagnosed lesions such as these in the anal canal. A biopsy specimen of this lesion also showed a focus of severe squamous dysplasia. Extensive, verrucous perianal condyloma before (**E**) and after (**F**) surgical excision. Bulky disease such as this disease may be confused with squamous cell carcinoma. Biopsy is required to make the distinction. (**A–D**, *Courtesy of* K. Turgeon, Ann Arbor, MI) (**E** and **F**, *Courtesy of* R. Burney, Ann Arbor, MI)

ANAL NEOPLASMS

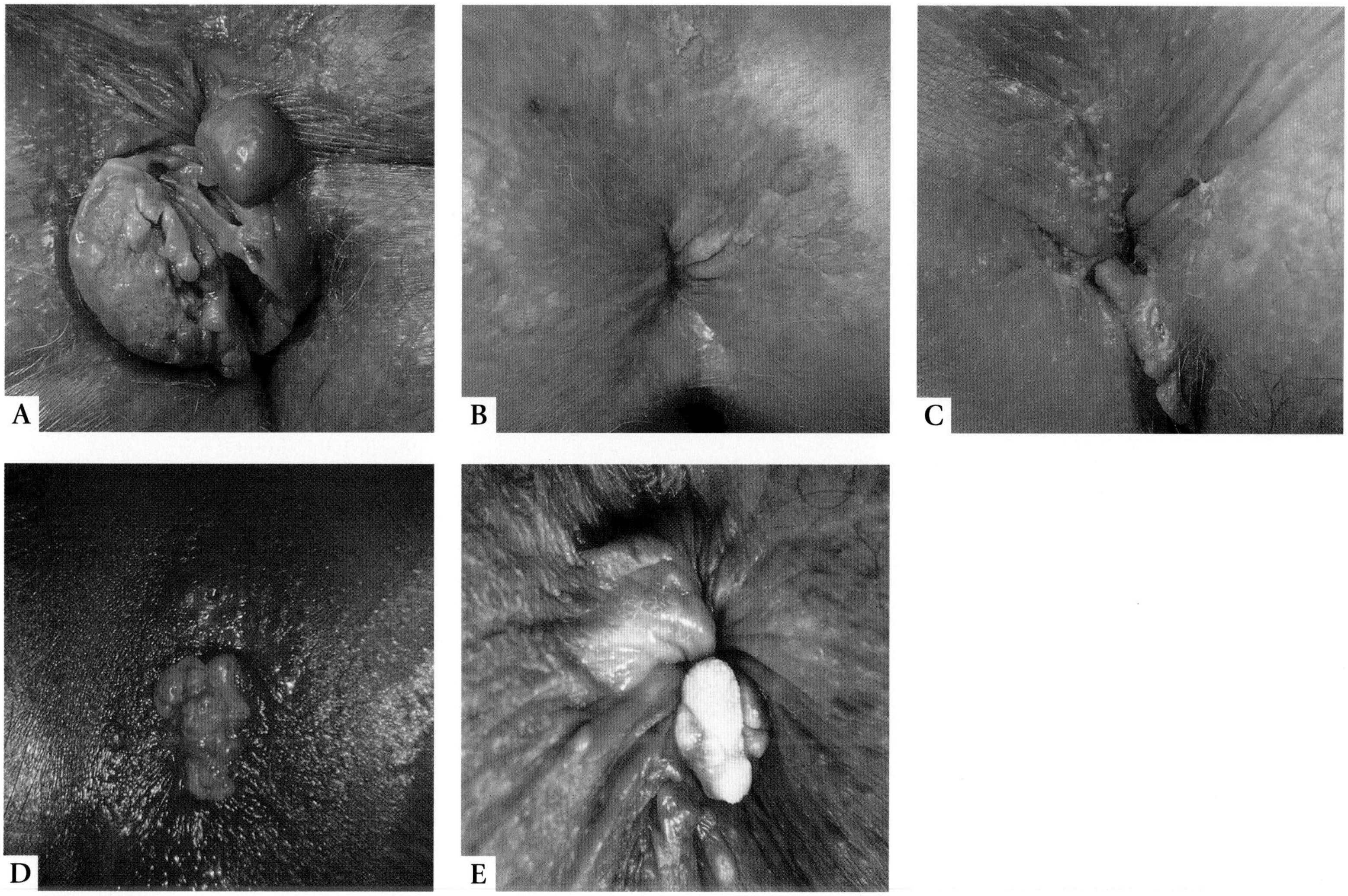

FIGURE 6-8.

Anal neoplasms. The most common malignancies of the anal margin and anal canal are of the squamous cell type. Presenting symptoms include bleeding and discomfort, but nearly 25% of malignancies are found incidently during routine examination. Occasionally, a surgical specimen for benign anorectal disease is found to contain previously unsuspected carcinoma. Risk factors for anal cancer include cigarette smoking, anal intercourse, genital warts and other venereal diseases, and chronic anal inflammation and scarring. Small lesions of the anal margin may be surgically excised, but extensive anal canal tumors are now usually treated with radiation and chemotherapy. Nonepidermoid anal malignancies are rare. They include adenocarcinoma of the anal canal, extramammary Paget's disease, Bowen's disease, basal cell cancer, and anal melanoma. **A**, Extensive, bulky squamous cell carcinoma of the anus. **B**, This figure is an example of Bowen's disease. This subtle, slow-growing lesion represents intradermal squamous cell carcinoma and may be mistaken for dermatitis or pruritus ani. Local excision is usually curative. **C**, This figure is an example of Paget's disease. This glandular tumor seen in the elderly appears as an eczematoid plaque. Similar to Bowen's disease, it is also easily mistaken for a benign anal condition. **D**, Protruding, cloacogenic polyp on a stalk is shown. This nonmalignant lesion was removed under local anesthesia. **E**, This firm, white, nodular growth was excised for fear of a small squamous cell carcinoma. However, the lesion was benign, revealing only thick hyperkeratosis and acanthosis. (*Courtesy of* R. Burney, Ann Arbor, MI)

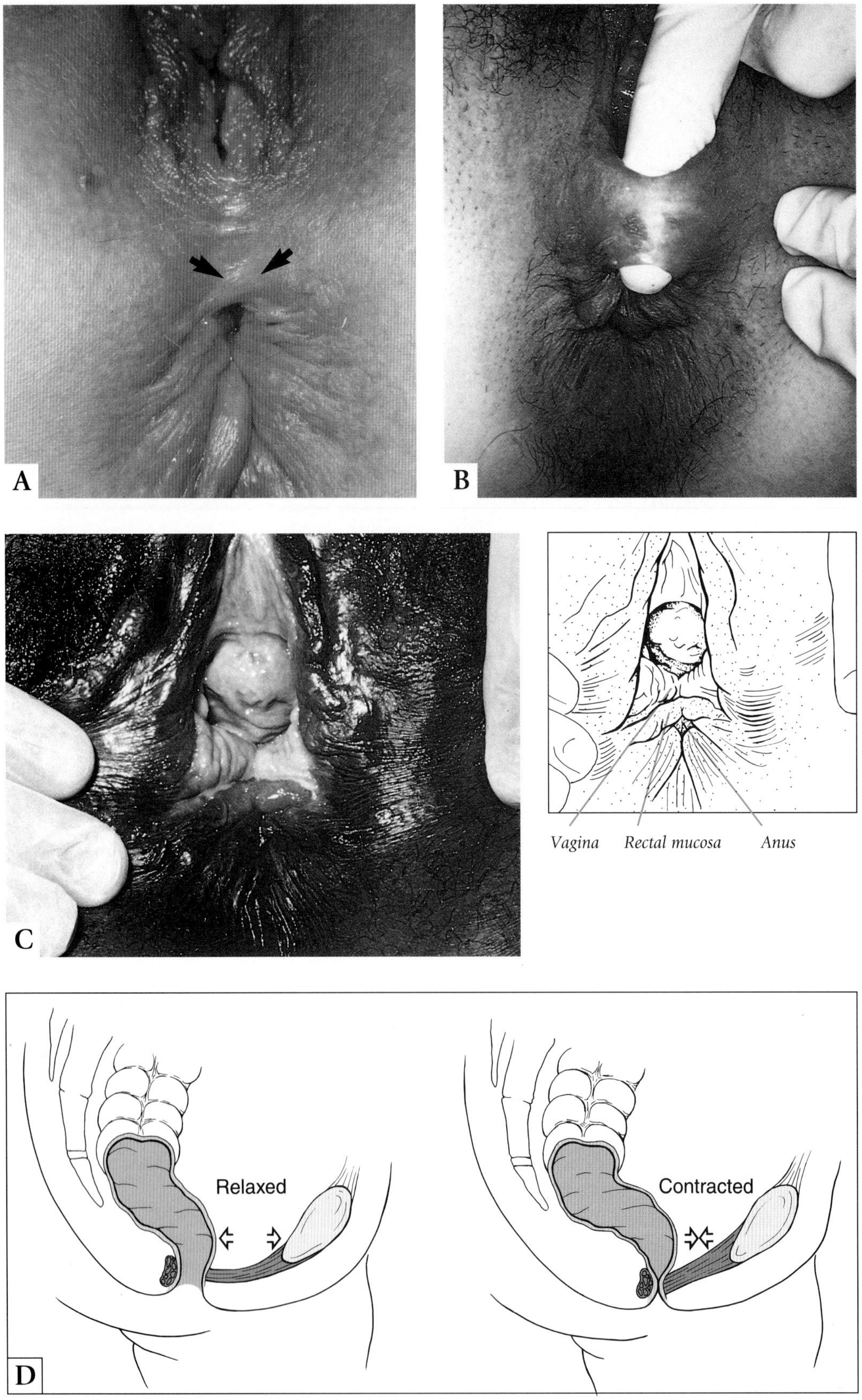

FIGURE 6-9.

The causes of fecal incontinence include irritable bowel syndrome, diarrheal illnesses, fecal impaction, neurologic diseases, rectal pathology, and a variety of anal pathologies. Idiopathic fecal incontinence is likely caused by chronic injury to the pudendal nerve from long-term straining at stool or childbirth injury. Once structural lesions of the anorectum have been eliminated, useful investigative tools include defecography, anorectal manometry, and electromyographic techniques. Many patients will respond to simple measures that prevent diarrhea and exercise the sphincter musculature. Biofeedback training is also a useful technique to improve sphincter function and rectal sensation. Mechanical injuries often require surgical repair. **A**, Subtle anterior anal sphincter separation after an obstetrical midline episiotomy in a woman with mild fecal incontinence is shown. Note loss of radiating sphincter folds along the anterior anal margin (*arrows*) where previous sphincter injury has occurred. **B**, Anterior anal sphincter injury and rectovaginal fistula that was caused by childbirth trauma. Only a bridge of skin caudally separates the anal canal from the vagina. **C**, A major (fourth degree) laceration at the time of childbirth produced this free communication between the vagina and the anal canal. **D**, The puborectalis muscle attaches to the symphysis pubis and wraps around the posterior aspect of the anorectal junction to form a sling. It tonically contracts to maintain the anorectal angle, and in concert with the external sphincter, it plays a major role in fecal continence. Sudden increases in intra-abdominal pressure (except during defecation) and voluntary withholding of stool cause additional contraction of the puborectalis muscle to sharpen the anorectal angle and maintain continence. Flexing the hips and pushing to defecate relax the puborectalis and straighten the angle to facilitate passage of stool. Traumatic or neuropathic injury to this muscle predisposes it to major problems with fecal incontinence. (**A–C**, *Courtesy of* J. Delancey, Ann Arbor, MI) (**D**, *Adapted from* Fleshman *et al.* [5]; with permission.)

RECTAL FOREIGN BODY

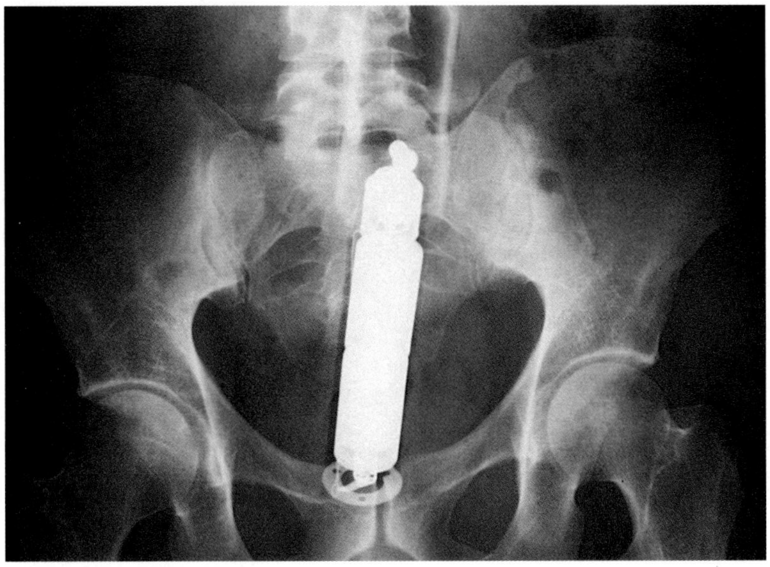

FIGURE 6-10.

This abdominal radiograph shows a large vibrator trapped in the rectum. An amazing variety of foreign bodies have been reported recovered from the rectum including bottles, tools, sexual devices, and vegetables. Objects may be placed into the rectum for purposes of concealment, for attempts at self-treatment, during an assault, or most commonly for erotic purposes. Small objects are removed using an operative anoscope and grasping forceps. Large or bulky objects may require regional anesthesia and anal dilatation. Sometimes insertion of a Foley catheter past the object and balloon inflation allows traction removal of a bulky, low-lying foreign body. High-lying objects require spinal anesthesia and abdominal palpation to move the object distally. Sometimes laparotomy is required if abdominal distress develops, a high-lying object cannot be delivered, or a potentially sharp object breaks during attempted retrieval. After removal of a rectal foreign body, a follow-up flexible sigmoidoscopy is often necessary to rule out mucosal laceration or retained foreign material.

REFERENCES AND RECOMMENDED READING

1. Goldberg SM, Buls JG: Perianal disease and rectal prolapse. In *Surgical Treatment of Digestive Disease*, edn 2. Edited by Moody FC, Carey LC, Jones RS, *et al*. Chicago: Yearbook Medical Publisher; 1990:817–846.
2. Salvati EP, Eisenstat TE: Hemorrhoidal disease. In *Shackelford's Surgery of the Alimentary Tract*, edn 3. Philadelphia: WB Saunders; 1991:294–307.
3. Hicks TC, Timmcke AE: Fissure in ano. In *Shackelford's Surgery of the Alimentary Tract*, edn 3. Philadelphia: WB Saunders; 1991:286–293.
4. Barnett JL, Raper SE: Anorectal disease. In *Textbook of Gastroenterology*. Philadelphia: JB Lippincott; 1991:1813–1835.
5. Fleshman JW, Kodner IJ, Fry RD: Anal incontinence. In *Shackelford's Surgery of the Alimentary Tract*, edn 3. Philadelphia: WB Saunders; 1991:349–361.

Chapter 7

Lower Gastrointestinal Bleeding

CHRISTOPHER S. CUTLER
DOUGLAS K. REX

Lower gastrointestinal bleeding is defined as bleeding originating below the ligament of Treitz. It accounts for approximately 20% of cases of acute gastrointestinal bleeding. Bleeding severity ranges from occult blood loss to massive hemorrhage and shock. The average age at presentation of acute lower gastrointestinal bleeding is 65 years.

Patients may present with occult blood not apparent in stool specimens but found on routine screening. Occult bleeding is identified in 2% to 4% of adults on prevalence screening. It may originate anywhere from the oropharynx to the rectum. The only established clinical application of fecal blood testing is as a screening tool for colorectal carcinoma. Melena is defined as black, tarry, sticky, malodorous stool caused by degraded blood in the gut. This melena usually signifies an upper gastrointestinal source of bleeding but may originate from the small bowel or right colon. Hematochezia is the passage of bright red blood per rectum. This blood usually indicates a lower gastrointestinal tract lesion, however, 10% of patients with upper gastrointestinal bleeding may have a massive hemorrhage presenting as hematochezia.

Eighty percent of acute lower gastrointestinal bleeding stop spontaneously; bleeding recurs in 25% of patients. The mortality rate for acute lower gastrointestinal bleeding ranges from 5% to 10%. Mortality is highest among patients with recurrent or persistent bleeding. Mortality has decreased over the past 20 years, presumably because of improved diagnostic techniques and earlier therapeutic intervention.

This chapter reviews the approach to the patient with overt lower gastrointestinal bleeding as well as the patient with occult blood loss. Diagnostic algorithms, diagnostic techniques, and the differential diagnosis of lower gastrointestinal bleeding is discussed. The significance of occult blood in the stool with special emphasis on its relationship to colorectal cancer is reviewed.

TABLE 7-1. CAUSES OF OVERT LOWER GASTROINTESTINAL BLEEDING

Cause	Percent
Upper gastrointestinal tract	10%
Small intestine	5%
Angiodysplasia	
Neoplasms	
Crohn's disease	
Drugs (NSAIDs)	
Aortoenteric fistula	
Meckel's diverticula	
Jejunal diverticula	
Duplication cysts	
Hemangiomas	
Colon	85%
Diverticulosis	
Angiodysplasia	
Neoplasms	
Hemorrhoids	
Inflammatory bowel disease	
Ischemia	
Radiation colitis	
Infectious colitis	
Anal fissures	
Iatrogenic (postpolypectomy)	
Solitary rectal ulcer syndrome	
Herditary hemorrhagic telangiectasia	
Dieulafoy's lesion	
Portal colopathy	
Ecotopic varices	
Drugs (NSAIDs)	
Hemangiomas	
Rectal trauma	
Aortocolonic fistula	
Diversion colitis	
Vasculitis	
Intussusception	
Endometriosis	

TABLE 7-1.

The causes of lower gastrointestinal bleeding are myriad. Approximately 10% of gastrointestinal bleeds presumed to be lower, based on the history and initial clinical findings, actually originate in the upper gastrointestinal tract, and 5% originate in the small bowel. Five percent to 8% remain undiagnosed despite aggressive diagnostic modalities. The causes of overt lower gastrointestinal bleeding are age specific. In infants and young children, the most common lesions include anal fissures, Meckel's diverticula, and juvenile polyps. This fact holds true for adolescents and young adults, with the addition of hemorrhoids and inflammatory bowel disease. In the elderly, diverticulosis, angiodysplasia, neoplasms, and hemorrhoids constitute the most common etiologies of lower gastrointestinal bleeding [1]. Careful consideration is needed before attributing bleeding to hemorrhoids because 25% of patients who present with rectal bleeding have serious pathology combined with anal disease [2]. NSAIDs—nonsteroidal anti-inflammatory drugs. (*Adapted from* Marshall [3]; with permission.)

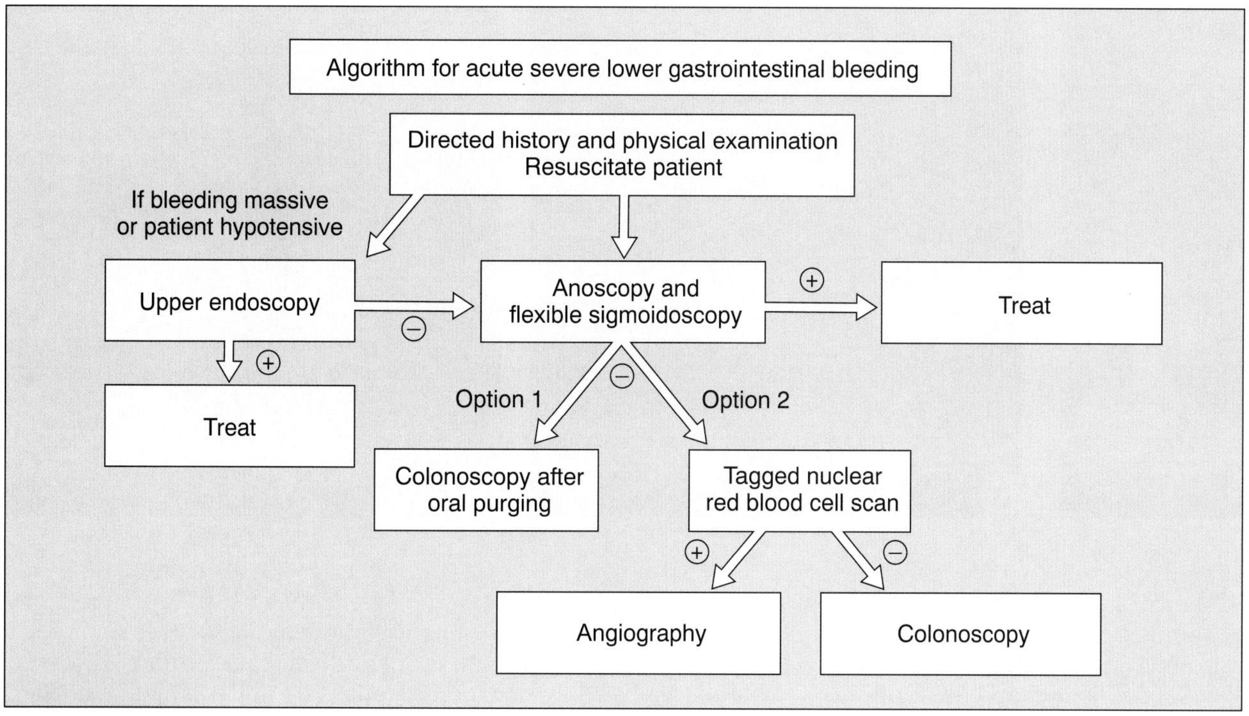

FIGURE 7-1.

The diagnostic approach to the patient with acute lower gastrointestinal bleeding must be individualized. The first steps in the management of these patients is a directed history and physical examination, assessment of the severity of the bleeding, and volume restoration. If bleeding is massive or the patient is hypotensive, an upper endoscopy should be performed to rule out an upper gastrointestinal source of bleeding. If suspicion for an upper gastrointestinal source is low, the patient should undergo anoscopy and flexible sigmoidoscopy to rule out a distal bleeding source. If these studies are not diagnostic, the next appropriate step depends on local preferences and expertise. Some expert endoscopists advocate colonoscopy after oral purging [4]. Another approach uses the radionuclide bleeding scan. A radionuclide-tagged red blood cell scan, prior to an attempt at angiography, can have several benefits. First, if the scan is negative, the bleeding has likely stopped and the patient can be prepared for colonoscopy. If the radionuclide scan is positive, it can direct the angiographer to a particular abdominal vessel, reducing the intravenous contrast load. If the scan is positive but the angiography shows no extravasation or lesion, the scan can direct the angiographer as to which vessel to leave a catheter in for subsequent infusion of vasopressin.

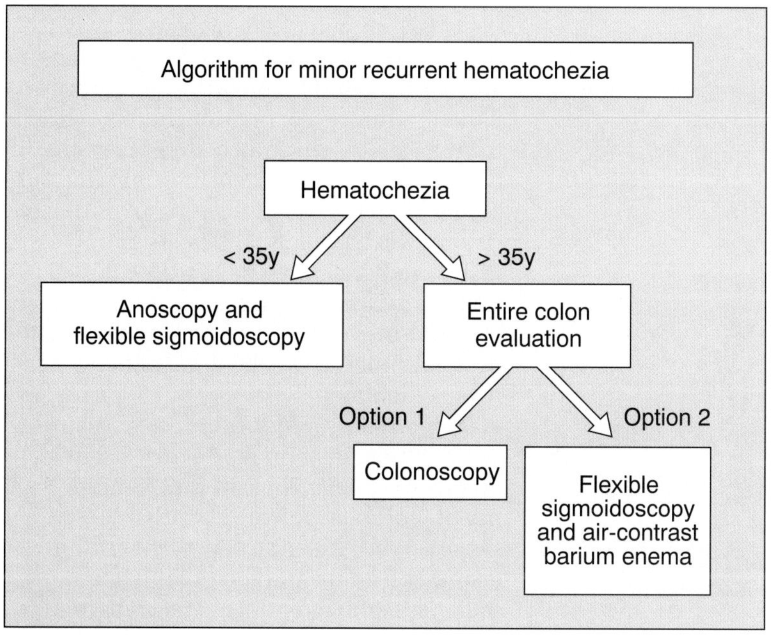

FIGURE 7-2.

Patients frequently present with recurrent minor hematochezia. This presentation may be spotting on the toilet paper, blood dripping into the toilet bowl, or red blood coating or mixed into the stool. The evaluation of these patients is age specific. If the patient is young, anoscopy and sigmoidoscopy may be all that is warranted, because perianal disease and distal colitis are the most common etiologies. If the patient is over 35 years of age, the entire colon should be evaluated because of the increased risk of neoplasm. This evaluation may be accomplished with colonoscopy or flexible sigmoidoscopy plus air-contrast barium enema. In most patients, colonoscopy is preferable and is particularly cost-effective in older patients where there is a high background prevalence of colorectal polyps [5].

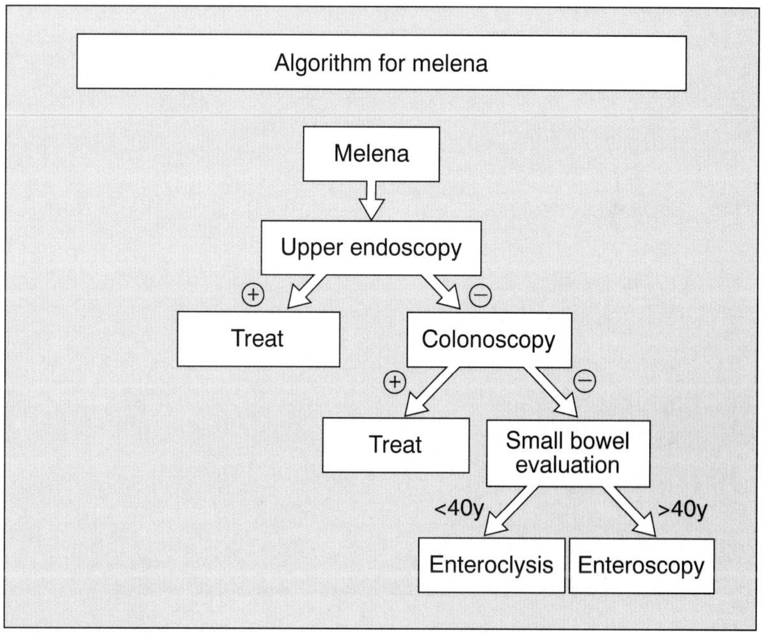

FIGURE 7-3.

The most common cause of melena is bleeding from the upper gastrointestinal tract, and thus the initial diagnostic step should be an upper endoscopy. If this outcome is negative, colonoscopy is performed. If the cause of bleeding is still unclear, the small bowel should be evaluated. If the patient is over 40 years of age, we would favor small bowel push enteroscopy as the first diagnostic test because of a high prevalence of small bowel angiodysplasia. For younger patients, enteroclysis would be an appropriate first option, because of a higher likelihood of small bowel tumors.

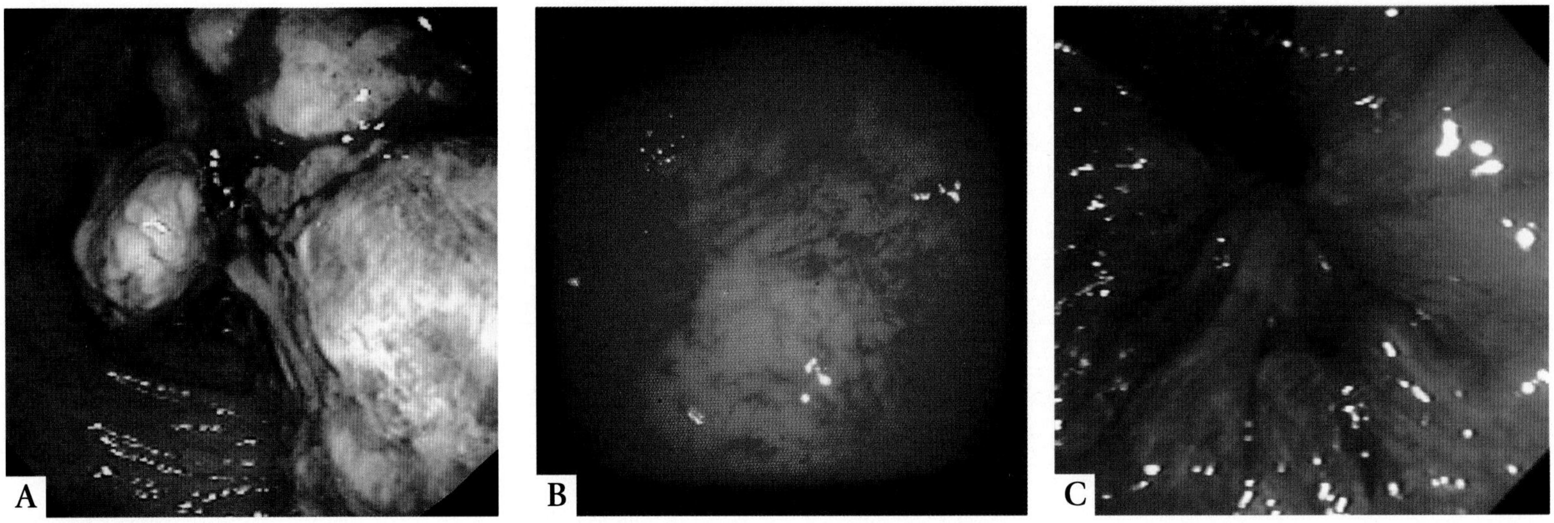

FIGURE 7-4.

After an upper gastrointestinal source of bleeding has been excluded, anoscopy and sigmoidoscopy should be the next diagnostic steps in the evaluation of lower gastrointestinal bleeding. Anoscopy is the most sensitive test to diagnose anal fissures and hemorrhoids. Sigmoidoscopy is used to evaluate the distal colonic mucosa for inflammatory bowel disease, polyps, or malignancies. Pictured are endoscopic photographs of patients undergoing flexible sigmoidoscopy for hematochezia. An exophytic rectal mass with oozing red blood (**A**), bleeding radiation proctitis (**B**), and internal hemorrhoids (**C**) are depicted.

TABLE 7-2. FINAL DIAGNOSIS FOR 80 PATIENTS WITH SEVERE HEMATOCHEZIA

LESION SITE	PATIENTS, *n (%)*
Colonic	59 (74)
Angiomata	24 (30)
Diverticulosis	13 (17)
Active bleeding	6 (8)
Adherent clot	7 (9)
Polyps or cancer	9 (11)
Focal colitis or ulcers	7 (9)
Rectal lesions	3 (4)
Bleeding polyp stalk	2 (2)
Endometriosis	1 (1)
Upper gastrointestinal	9 (11)
Small bowel*	7 (9)
No site found	5 (6)

**A diagnosis of presumed small bowel site of bleeding was made when the panendoscopy and colonoscopy were negative, but fresh blood, clots, or both were coming through the ileocecal valve.*

TABLE 7-2.

Colonoscopy during acute lower gastrointestinal bleeding may require considerable expertise. Some believe that the diagnostic yield is low in the setting of ongoing bleeding and that there is increased risk including perforation. Recent studies, however, have shown a very high sensitivity for colonoscopy following oral purging. Jensen and Machicado [4] studied 80 consecutive patients with severe ongoing hematochezia from an unknown source. All patients had upper endoscopies followed by purging and colonoscopy. Ninety-four percent of these patients had a potential bleeding source discovered, including 74% with colonic lesions, 11% with upper gastrointestinal tract lesions, and 9% with presumed small bowel lesions; only 6% of the patients had no site identified. Rossini *et al.* [6] performed 409 colonoscopies for acute lower gastrointestinal bleeding and reported a diagnostic accuracy of 76%. Thus, in experienced hands, colonoscopy offers both a high sensitivity for diagnosing lower gastrointestinal bleeding and the potential for therapeutic intervention. (*From* Jensen and Machicado [4]; with permission.)

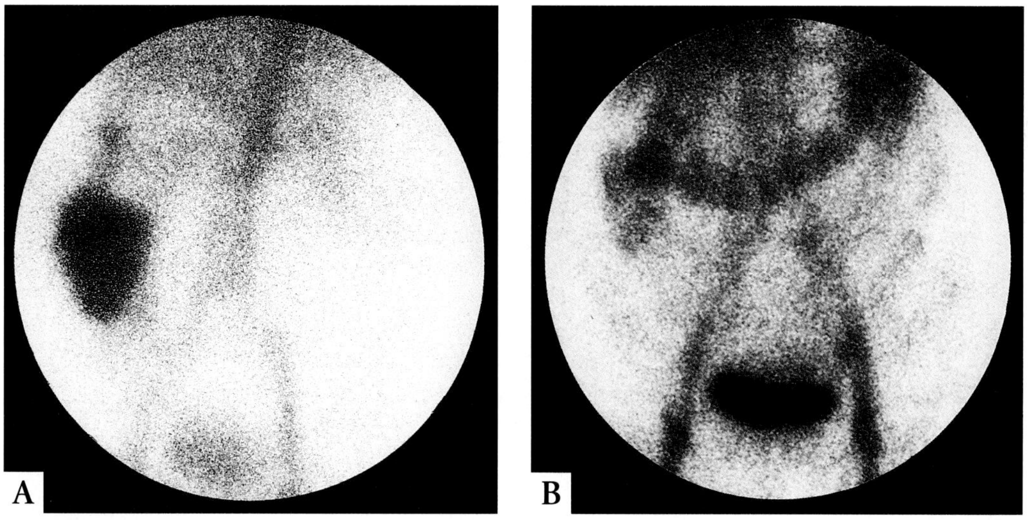

FIGURE 7-5.

Two radionuclide techniques are used for localization of gastrointestinal bleeding [7]. One technique is the technetium sulfur colloid scan. This radionuclide is injected intravenously and is rapidly cleared from the intravascular compartment by the reticuloendothelial system. Because of a very short half-life, positive scans are seen only with active bleeding at the time of injection. This method can detect bleeding at rates as low as 0.1 mL/min. Unfortunately, because of the prerequisite for activ

8% to 12%. A preferred radionuclide scan is the 99m technetium–labeled red blood cell scan. In this test, autologous red blood cells are labeled in vitro with technetium and injected into the patient. Images are obtained every 5 minutes for 30 minutes and then every few hours for 24 hours. The cells remain in the vascular pool for the life of the circulating red blood cells. Thus, this method is a sensitive test for diagnosis of intermittent gastrointestinal bleeding. Some studies have shown a sensitivity of 93% and a specificity of 95% for tagged red blood cell studies. As in the case of the sulfur colloid scan, tagged red blood cell scans can detect bleeding rates as low as 0.1 mL/min. A major deficit of this method is that delayed scans are often performed at wide intervals. Extravasation of radionuclide into the gut can be followed by considerable transit down the gut prior to the next scan, resulting in misleading information about the location of the bleed. Bleeding cecal diverticula (**A**) and ascending colon angiodysplasia (**B**) are shown.

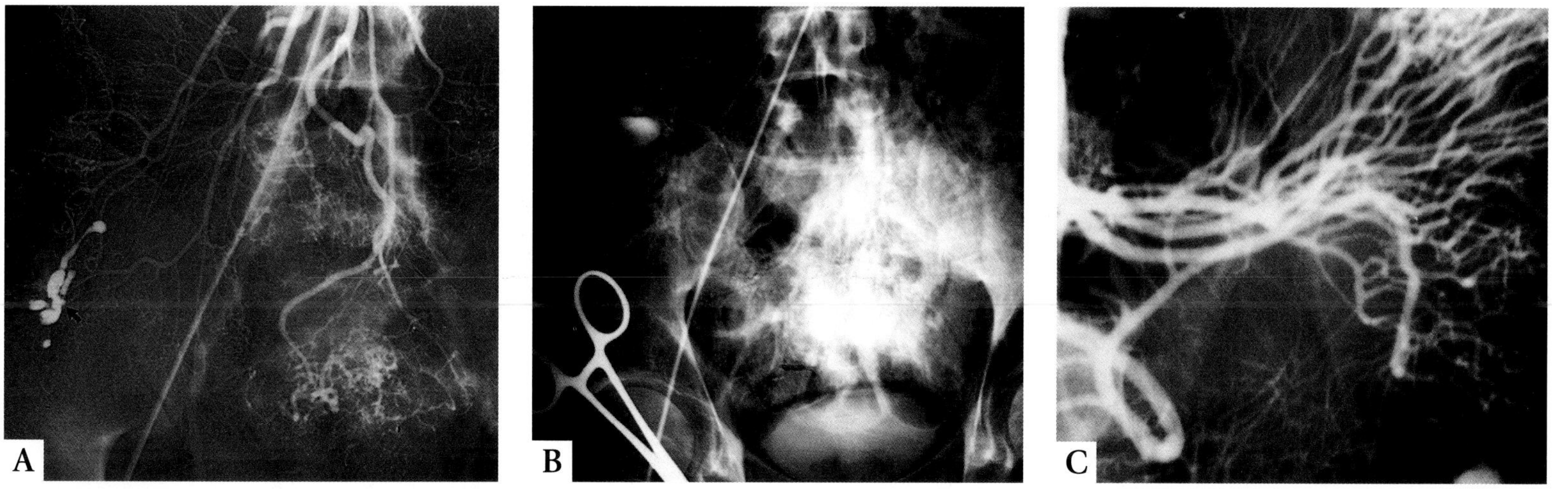

FIGURE 7-6.

Mesenteric angiography is sometimes useful for the diagnosis of lower gastrointestinal bleeding. It can provide precise anatomic localization of the bleeding site and requires no bowel preparation. Extravasation of contrast may be seen with arterial bleeding rates as low as 0.5 mL/min [7]. Sensitivities for diagnosing lower gastrointestinal bleeding range from 14% to 86% in various series. In most clinical practices, the actual sensitivity is near the lower end of this range. Because a considerable amount of diverticular bleeding and almost all angiodysplasia bleeding occurs in the superior mesenteric artery distribution, selective cannulation should begin with this vessel, followed by the inferior mesenteric artery and then the celiac artery. The complication rate ranges from 2% to 4%. Complications include arterial thrombosis, embolization, acute renal failure, and complications related to the catheter itself [8]. These figures represents an actively bleeding ileocolonic anastomosis in a patient with Crohn's disease (**A**), a bleeding ascending colon diverticula (**B**), and an activ

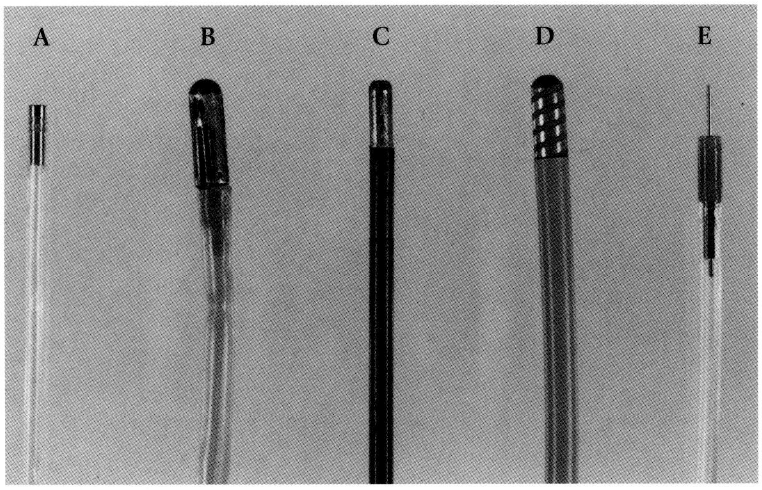

FIGURE 7-7.

The therapeutic endoscopist can use many tools for the treatment of lower gastrointestinal bleeding. These tools include Nd:YAG (neodymium:yttrium-aluminum-garnet) laser (**A**), heater probe (**B**), BICAP (bipolar electrocoagulation) electrocautery probe (**C**), multipolar electrocautery gold probe (**D**), injection therapy (**E**), and argon laser (not pictured). Angiography also offers therapeutic options [7]. Intra-arterial vasopressin may be infused at a rate of 0.2 units per minute and increased as necessary. If hemorrhage is controlled, the vasopressin dose is continued at 0.1 units per minute for 12 hours. This dose is 90% effective in stopping bleeding from diverticulosis or angiodysplasia. However, rebleeding occurs in up to 50% of patients following cessation of intra-arterial vasopressin therapy. Complications occur in 5% to 15% of patients treated with vasopressin and include cardiovascular toxicity. Angiography also permits selective arterial embolization, which is performed by injecting material such as gelfoam into the smallest and most distal artery leading to the bleeding site in order to minimize the risk of bowel infarction. Approximately 13% to 18% of patients will experience bowel infarction, and a much higher percentage of patients may develop colonic ischemia. Thus, this treatment is used only in very poor surgical candidates. For patients with massive hemorrhage or recurrent bleeding not responding to endoscopic or angiographic therapy, surgery must be considered. Progressive improvements in surgical technique and intensive care have resulted in decreased surgical mortality, which is now less than 5%. (*From* Rex [9]; with permission.)

CAUSES OF LOWER GASTROINTESTINAL BLEEDING

Diverticulosis

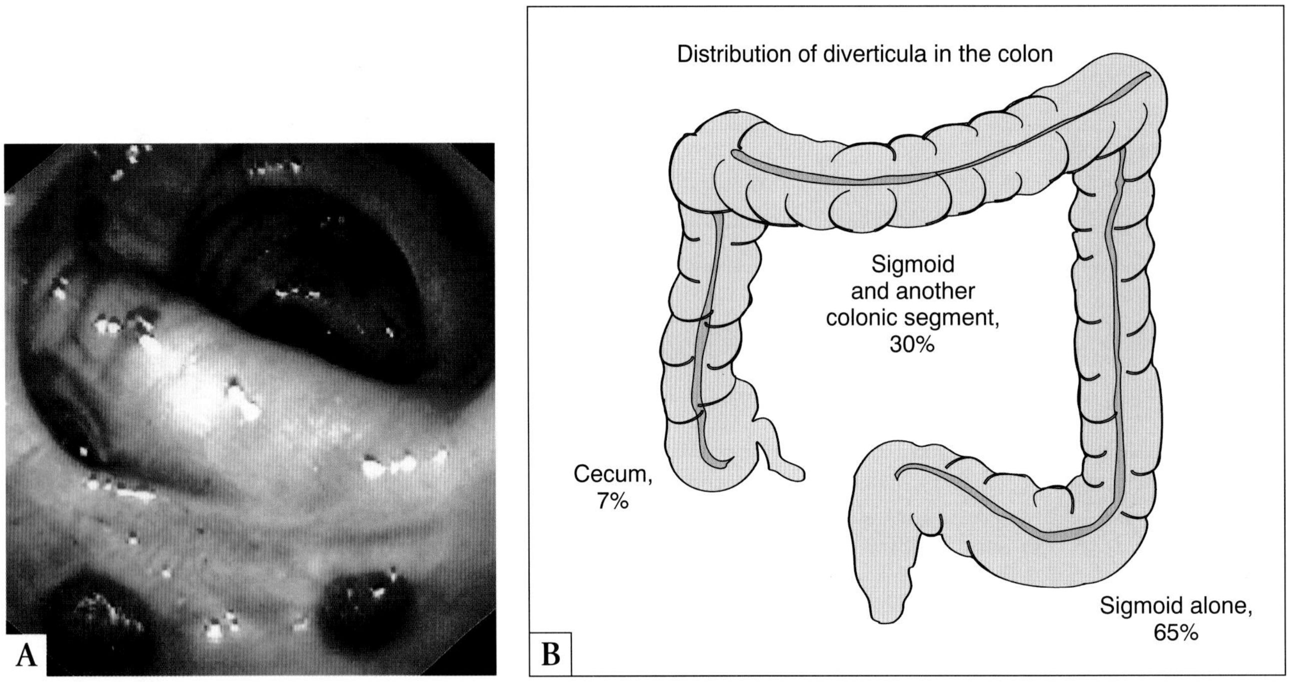

FIGURE 7-8.

In the western world, 33% to 50% of people over 50 years of age have colonic diverticula. Approximately 65% of these people have isolated sigmoid disease, 30% have involvement of the sigmoid colon and another area, and 5% have disease not located in the sigmoid colon [10]. Two-thirds of patients with diverticulosis have uncomplicated disease, however, 3% to 5% may have massive diverticular hemorrhage [11]. Interestingly, bleeding from diverticula is more often seen in the right colon and usually arises from a single diverticulum. Colonic diverticula are not considered a cause of chronic, occult loss of blood. Typically the patient will develop a sudden mild lower abdominal discomfort, rectal urgency, and the passage of large amounts of maroon, bright red, or melenic stool. Spontaneous cessation of bleeding occurs in 80% of patients, and 20% of patients will have recurrence after one episode. The chance of a second recurrence is approximately 50%. **A**, An endoscopic photograph of diverticula. **B**, The distribution of diverticula in the colon is represented. (*From* Rege and Nahrwold [10]; with permission.)

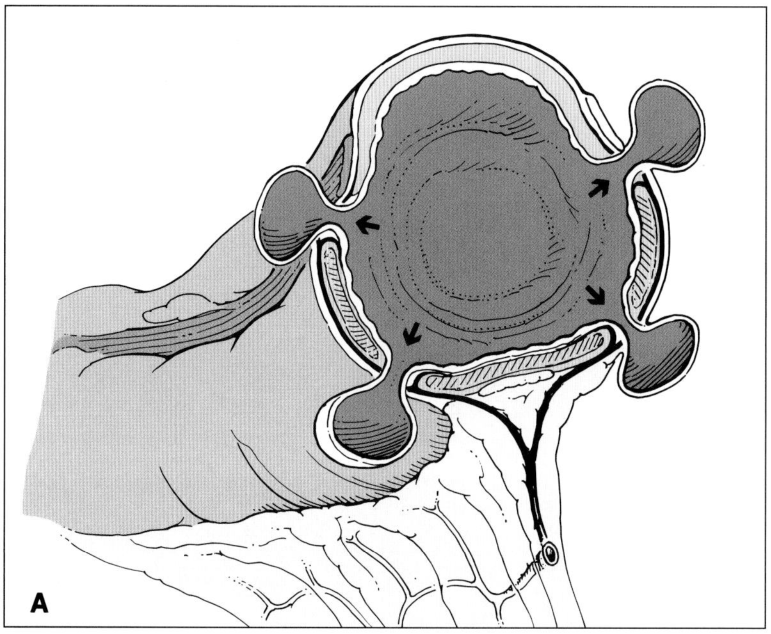

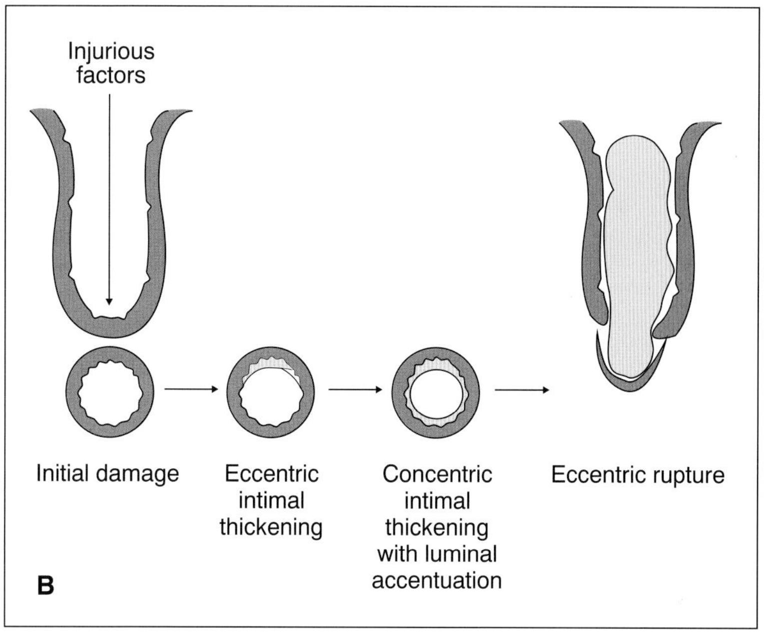

FIGURE 7-9.

The vasa recta, small branches of the marginal arteries supplying the colon, enter the wall of the colon through the connective tissue septa between fascicles of circumferential muscle. The points of entry of these vessels are sites of relative weakness through which diverticula develop. Thus, by virtue of their formation, diverticula are closely associated with the vasa recta (**A**). The factors responsible for the initiation of bleeding are unknown. Meyers *et al.* [12] demonstrated eccentric intimal thickening of the arteries, however, there is little inflammation. The artery ruptures eccentrically, always on the side of the vessel facing the lumen (**B**). (**A**, *From* Rex and Lewis [13]; with permission.) (**B**, *From* Meyers *et al.* [12]; with permission.)

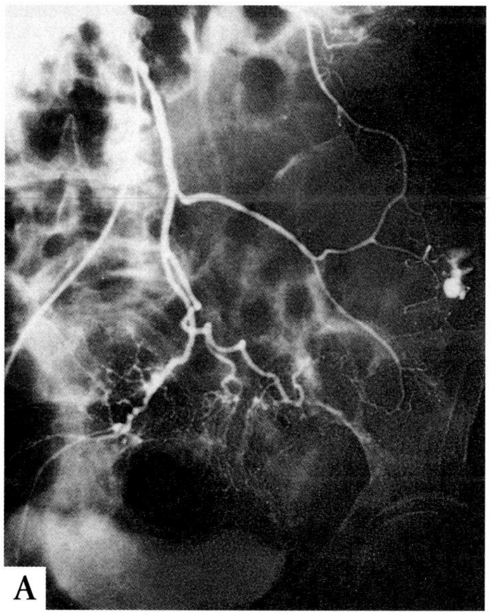

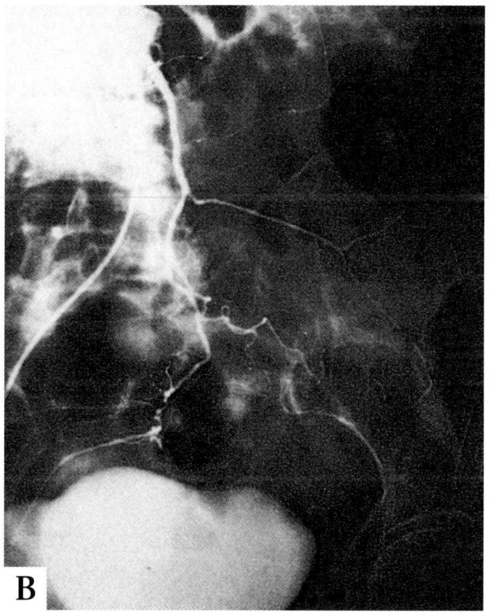

FIGURE 7-10.

Selective mesenteric angiography is effective in the diagnosis of active diverticular bleeding. Extravasation of contrast into a diverticula is the diagnostic radiographic finding. Angiographic infusion of vasopressors may halt diverticular bleeding in 80% to 90% of patients [14]. Typical infusion doses in the superior mesenteric artery range from 0.2 to 0.3 units per minute and in the inferior mesenteric artery from 0.1 to 0.2 units per minute. Fifteen percent to 25% of these patients rebleed and eventually require surgery. Angiographic embolization may also be used, but below the ligament of Treitz, there is a 30% incidence of bowel ischemia or infarction. Figures of a patient with an actively bleeding diverticula of the descending colon (**A**) and following intra-arterial vasopressin infusion (**B**) are shown. (*From* Dietzen and Pemberton [15]; with permission.)

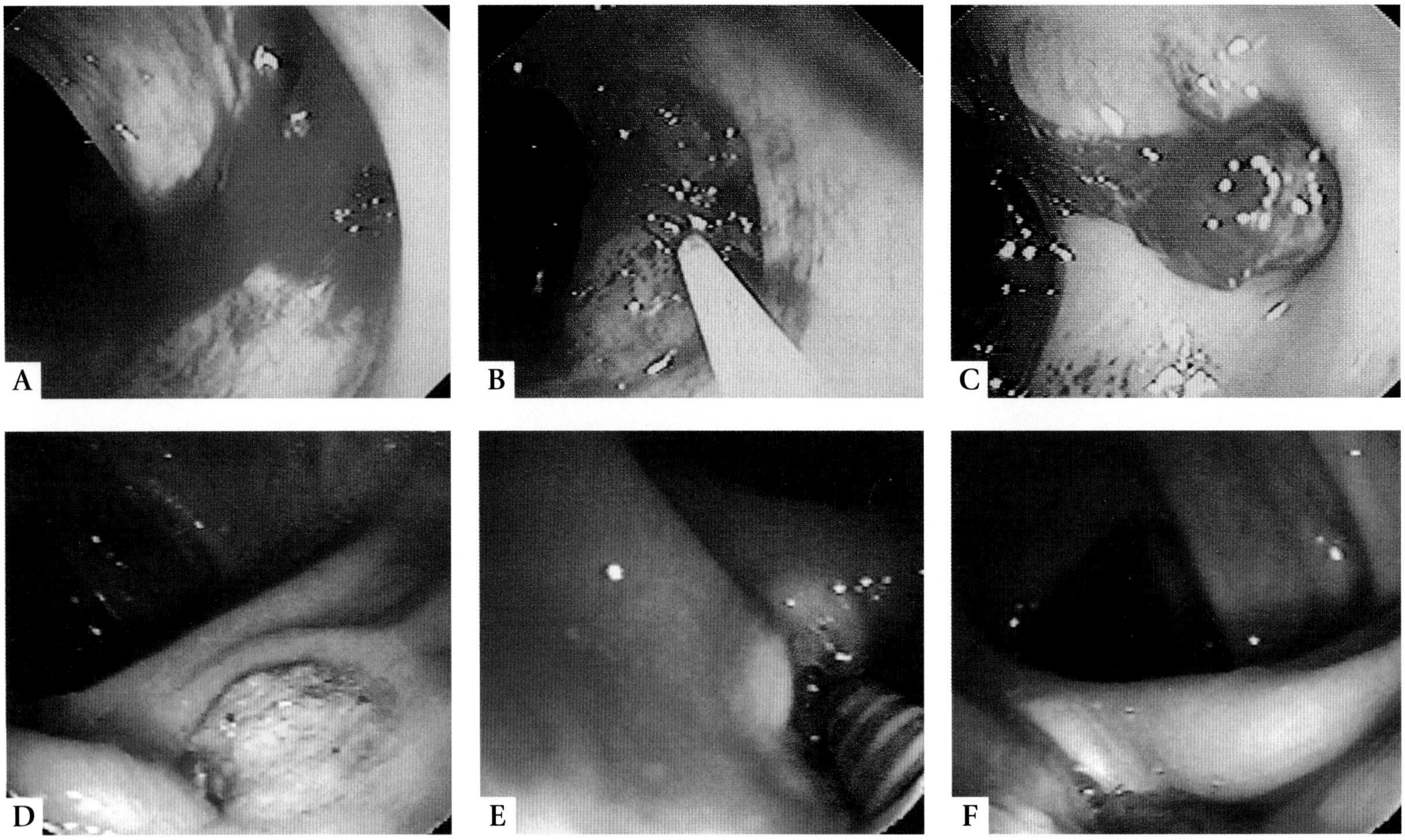

FIGURE 7-11.

Several recent reports have detailed a role for endoscopic treatment of diverticular hemorrhage. Endoscopic methods have included injection therapy with epinephrine 1:10,000 into the neck of the diverticulum [16,17]. Savides and Jensen [18] describe three cases of diverticular hemorrhage with a visible vessel on the edge of the diverticulum treated successfully with a gold probe. **A**, A bleeding diverticulum with an oozing fresh clot is discovered. **B**, The endoscopist injects epinephrine 1:10,000 into neck of diverticulum. **C**, Hemostasis is achieved. **D**, A visible vessel at the edge of a diverticulum is presented. **E**, The visible vessel is treated with the gold probe. **F**, The flattened visible vessel after coagulation is shown. (**A, B, and C**, *From* Bertoni *et al.* [16]; with permission.) (**D, E, and F** *From* Savides and Jensen [18]; with permission.)

Angiodysplasia

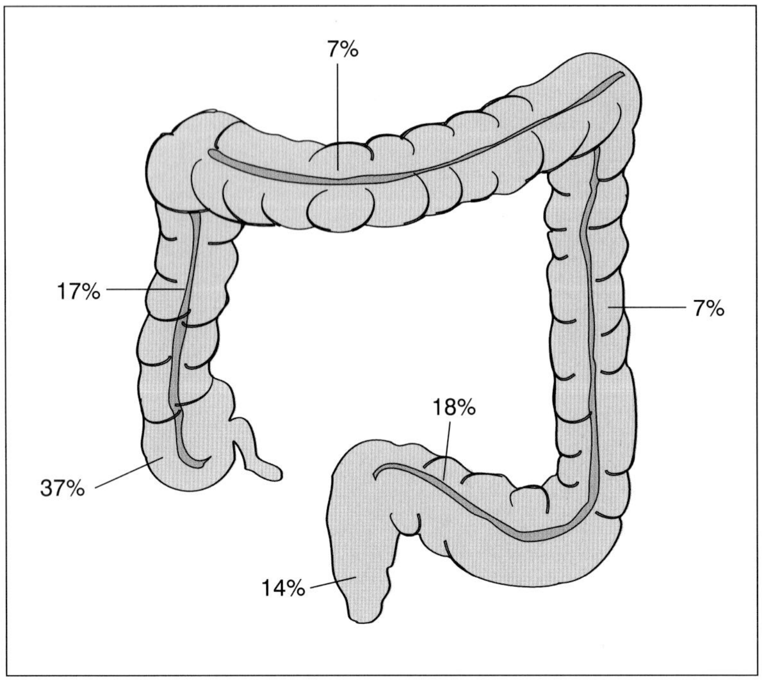

FIGURE 7-12.

Angiodysplasia are the most frequently encountered vascular abnormalities of the gastrointestinal tract and are a common etiology of lower gastrointestinal bleeding [14]. In patients with lower gastrointestinal bleeding, the prevalence of angiodysplasia ranges from 6% to 30%. Colonic angiodysplasia are most commonly found in the cecum and ascending colon. Pictured is the distribution of colonic angiodysplasia in one series of 59 patients. Multiple lesions are seen in 40% to 75% of patients. Bleeding is usually subacute and recurrent, but 15% of patients present with massive hemorrhage. In 90% of cases, bleeding stops spontaneously. With the advent of colonoscopy, angiodysplasia are often found in persons without evidence of bleeding. Of 964 asymptomatic patients undergoing colonoscopy for colorectal cancer screening, Foutch [19] found the prevalence of angiodysplasia to be 0.93%. (*From* Hochter *et al.* [20]; with permission.)

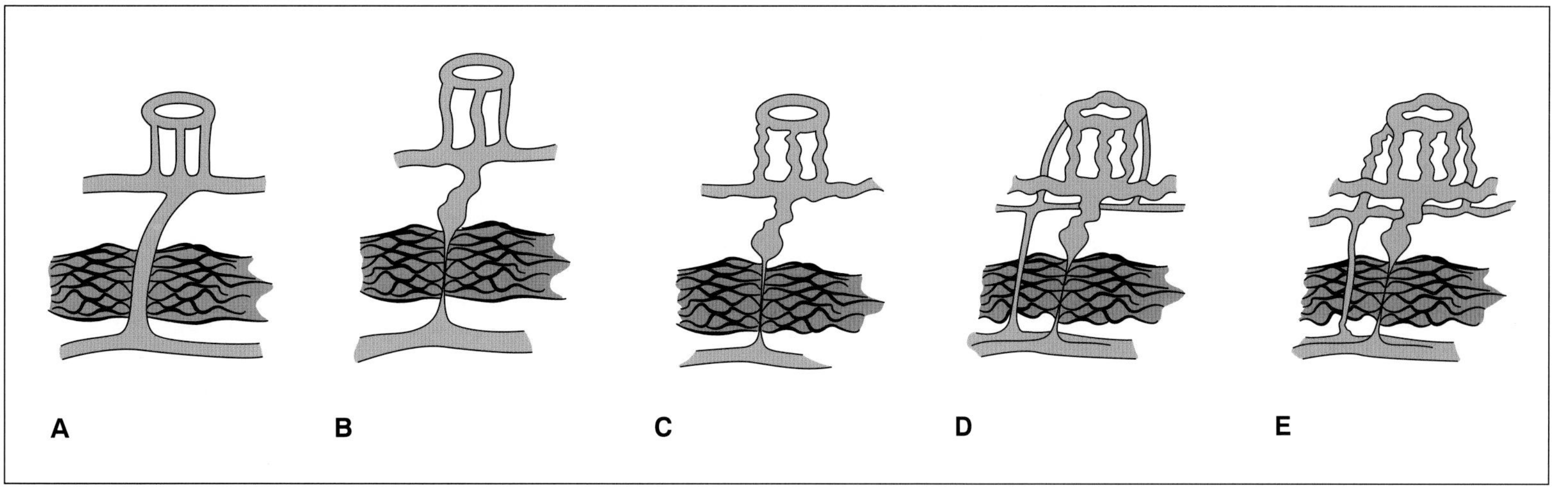

FIGURE 7-13.

Colonic angiodysplasia are thought to be acquired and associated with aging. Boley *et al.* [21] proposed that repeated intermittent low-grade obstruction of submucosal veins at the point where they crossed colonic muscle layers led to the development of angiodysplasia. A normal vein perforating the muscular layer is shown (**A**). The vein is partially obstructed because of muscular contraction or increased intraluminal pressure (**B**). Over a period of years, the submucosal vein becomes dilated and tortuous (**C**), the veins and venules draining into the submucosal vein become dilated (**D**), and the capillary ring becomes dilated, the precapillary sphincter becomes incompetent, and a small arteriovenous communication arises (**E**). Boley *et al.* [21] proposed that angiodysplasia were more prevalent in the right colon because of the increased diameter and wall tension. The factors responsible for the initiation of bleeding are unknown. (*From* Boley *et al.* [21]; with permission.)

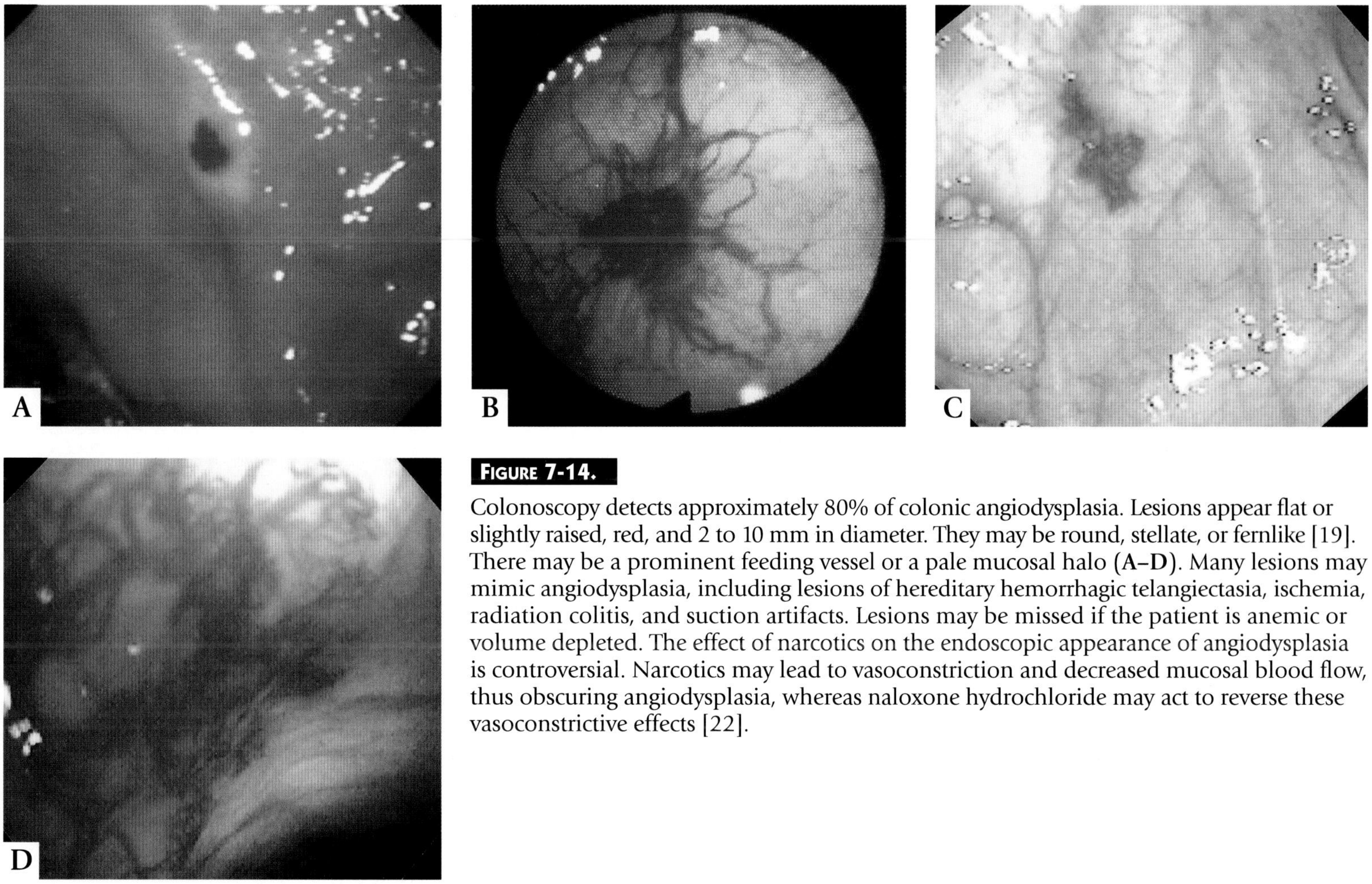

FIGURE 7-14.

Colonoscopy detects approximately 80% of colonic angiodysplasia. Lesions appear flat or slightly raised, red, and 2 to 10 mm in diameter. They may be round, stellate, or fernlike [19]. There may be a prominent feeding vessel or a pale mucosal halo (**A–D**). Many lesions may mimic angiodysplasia, including lesions of hereditary hemorrhagic telangiectasia, ischemia, radiation colitis, and suction artifacts. Lesions may be missed if the patient is anemic or volume depleted. The effect of narcotics on the endoscopic appearance of angiodysplasia is controversial. Narcotics may lead to vasoconstriction and decreased mucosal blood flow, thus obscuring angiodysplasia, whereas naloxone hydrochloride may act to reverse these vasoconstrictive effects [22].

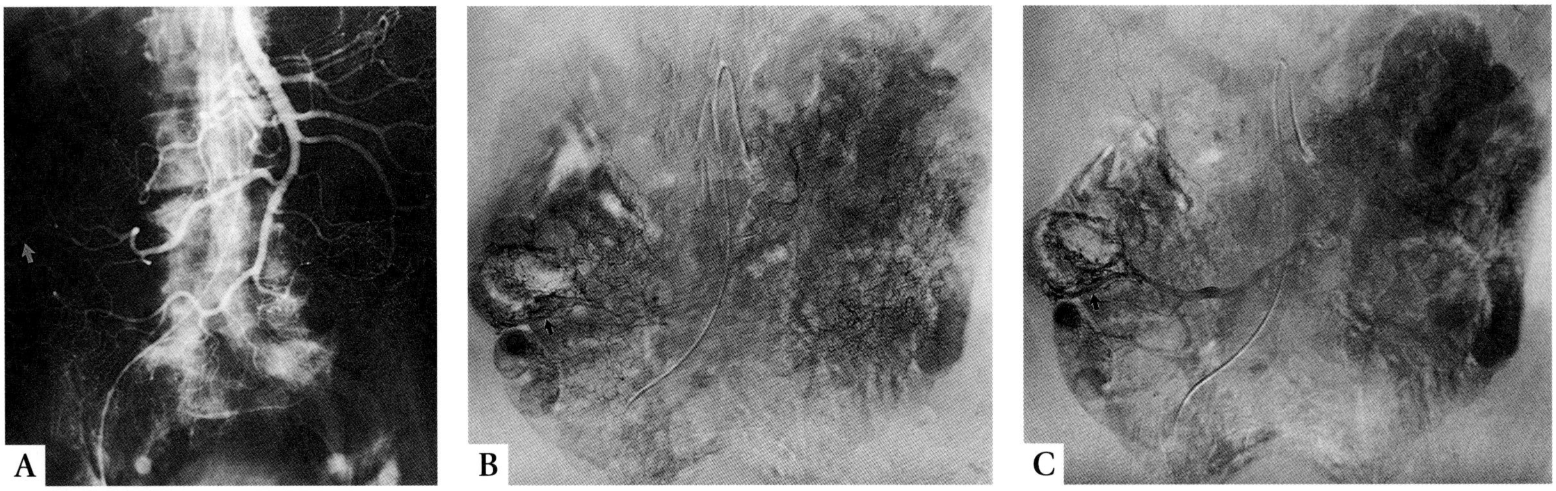

FIGURE 7-15.

The diagnostic yield of angiography for angiodysplasia is 17% to 20%. Classic findings include late draining veins (85% to 90%) representing obstructed submucosal veins (**A**), vascular tufts (70% to 75%) (**B**), early filling veins (60% to 80%) indicative of arteriovenous communication (**C**), and extravasation of contrast (6% to 20%)(not pictured) [19]. (*Courtesy of* N. Harris, Indianapolis, IN)

TABLE 7-3. RESULTS OF ENDOSCOPIC THERAPY FOR AD

				Treatments					
Study (*y*)	**Patients, *n***	**AD location***	**Number of AD per patient**	**Method**	**Mean, *n***	**Control bleed, %**	**Rebleeding, %**	**Morbidity†, %**	**Mean F/U, *mo***
Rogers [29]	27	Diffuse	?	HBF	?	81	19	0	?
Howard *et al.* [30]	23	Colon	3	HBF	1.2	48	52	9	17
Richter *et al.* [23]	19	Colon	?	HBF	1.0	47	53	5.2	36
Jensen and Machicado [24]	39	Colon	7	BICAP HP, AL	?	72	28	5.0	15
Roberts *et al.* [31]	13	Colon	?	BICAP HBF	1.2	46	31	15	24
Rutgeerts *et al.* [32]	59	Diffuse	17	Nd:YAG	2.7	71	29	10	12
Cello and Grendell [33]	43	Diffuse	18	AL Nd:YAG	1.2	84	51	2.3	13
Gostout *et al.* [34]	83	Diffuse	?	Nd:YAG	1–2 (median)	87	14	11	12
Mathus-Viegen [35]	107	Diffuse	?	Nd:YAG	1.9	78	34	7	18
Lanthier *et al.* [36]	26	Colon	5	AL HBF	1.1	88	19	0	29
Naveau *et al.* [37]	47	Diffuse	8	Nd:YAG	1	87	32	4.3	19

**Diffuse location refers to AD in the upper and lower gastrointestinal tract. †Mortality for all series was 0 except for Naveau et al. [37] which was 4.3%.*
AL—argon laser; HBF—hot biopsy forceps (monopolar electrocoagulation).

TABLE 7-3.

Asymptomatic patients with angiodysplasia (AD) will rarely bleed and do not require therapy. Richter *et al.* [23] followed 15 asymptomatic patients for up to 68 months and none bled. Thirty-six patients with lower gastrointestinal bleeding were managed with blood transfusions alone. At 1 year, 26% of the patients rebled, and at 3 years, 46% rebled. This high rebleeding rate justifies therapy in symptomatic patients. The therapy of choice for AD is endoscopic obliteration. Data comparing modalities is limited, however, contact probes (BICAP [bipolar electrocoagulation], gold probe, heater probe), Nd:YAG (neodymium:yttrium-aluminum-garnet) lasers, and argon lasers have all met with success. In a recent study, using BICAP, heater probe (HP), and argon laser, Jensen and Machicado [24] reported that at 15 months bleeding episodes decreased from 3.8 to 0.6, hematocrit increased from 25% to 36%, and rebleeding occurred in 18% of the patients. Therapeutic alternatives include intra-arterial vasopressin or transcatheter embolization for acute bleeding and surgical resection for acute or chronic bleeding. The hormonal therapy of AD is controversial. Proposed mechanisms of action include a reduction in the bleeding time, stasis of mesenteric microcirculation, and increased endothelial integrity. In a cross-over study of 10 patients with AD and hereditary hemorrhagic telangiectasia, van Cutsem *et al.* [25] found that nine patients receiving placebo required further transfusions compared with two patients receiving estrogen. Bronner *et al.* [26] described seven patients with chronic renal failure and AD who all stopped bleeding on hormone therapy. Lewis *et al.* [27] studied 30 patients with small bowel AD and found no difference in bleeding cessation between those receiving estrogen and historical controls. Recently a report of three patients with bleeding AD receiving octreotide showed a decreased need for subsequent transfusions [28]. (*From* Foutch [19]; with permission.)

Aortoenteric fistulas

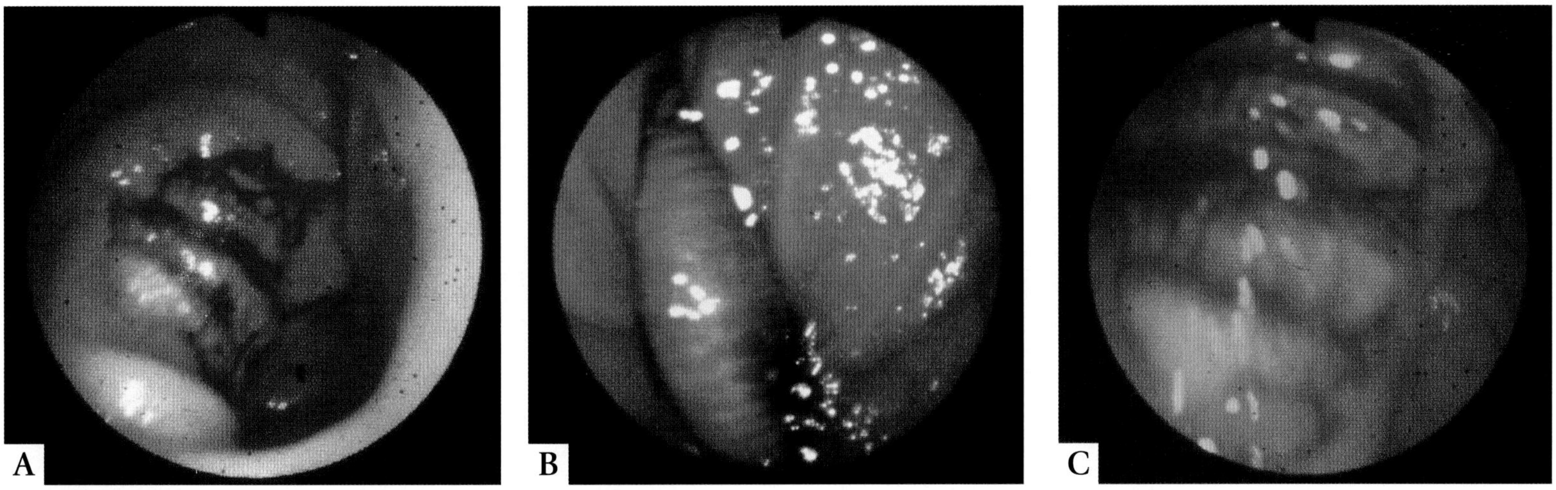

FIGURE 7-16.

Most aortoenteric fistulas are caused by prior aortic graft surgery but may rarely result from atherosclerosis, mycotic aneurysms, tuberculosis, or syphilis. The fistula usually involves the third portion of the duodenum but may rupture into any segment of the gastrointestinal tract, including the colon. Classically, patients present with a sentinel bleed that occurs and stops spontaneously hours to weeks before a massive hemorrhage. Pictured here are endoscopic photos of three patients with aortoenteric fistulas in the third portion of the duodenum (**A–C**). Treatment is surgical. (**A**, *From* American Society of Gastrointestinal Endoscopy; with permission.) (**B**, *From* SmithKline Beecham; with permission.)

Neoplasms

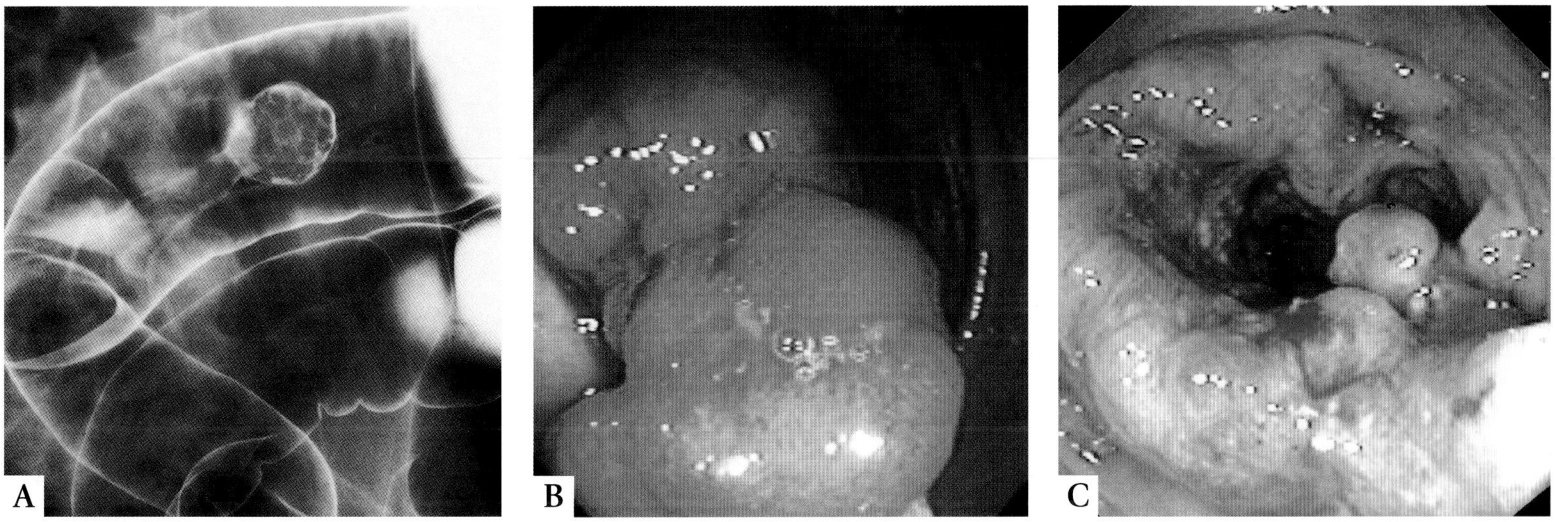

FIGURE 7-17.

Most bleeding from colorectal polyps and cancer is occult or mild and intermittent. Rarely polyps and cancer may cause significant lower gastrointestinal hemorrhage. Left-sided and rectal neoplasms are more likely to cause gross bleeding than right-sided lesions. Diagnosis is made by endoscopy or barium enema. Treatment for bleeding polyps or cancer is usually by colonoscopic removal or surgery. This figure depicts a pedunculated sigmoid polyp (**A**). A descending colon adenocarcinoma (**B**) and an annular rectal adenocarcinoma (**C**) are also shown. (**A**, *Courtesy of* J. Lappas, Indianapolis, IN)

Postpolypectomy bleeding

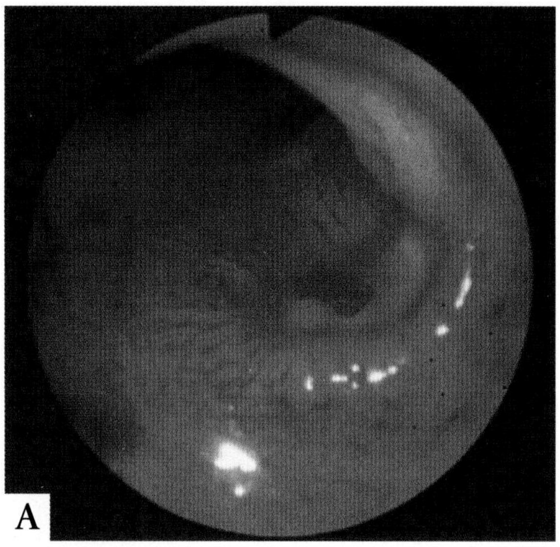

A

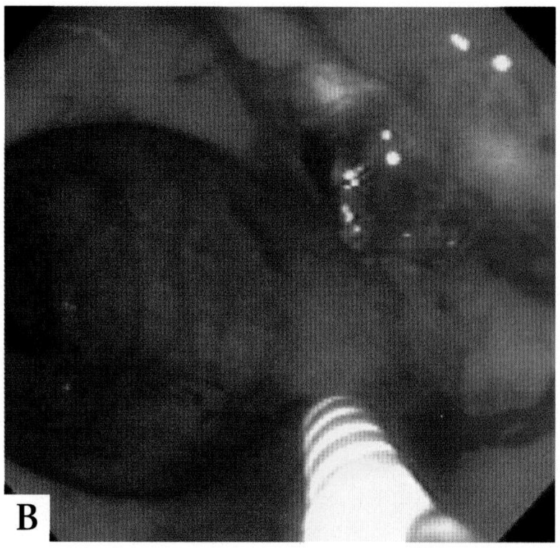

B

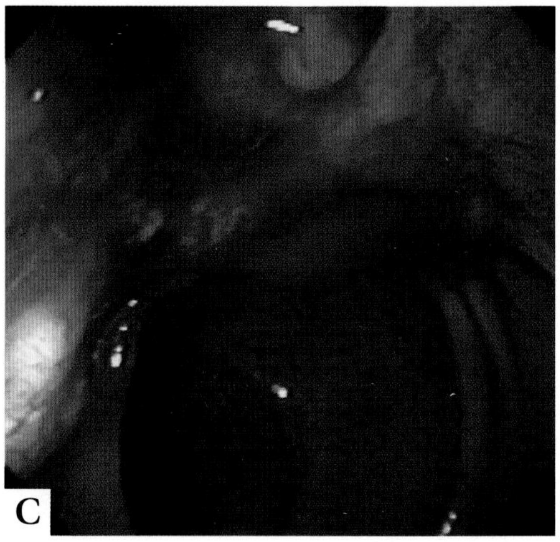

C

FIGURE 7-18.

The risk of postpolypectomy bleeding is approximately 0.3% to 0.5%. Most bleeding stops spontaneously, however, it may be massive. Acutely, endoscopic hemostasis may fail, and the polyp stalk may bleed after polypectomy. Bleeding may also be delayed for 1 to 21 days and probably occurs secondary to sloughing of a coagulum overlying a vessel in the ulcer base, created by the polypectomy. Drugs that interfere with coagulation should be stopped for 10 to 14 days following a polypectomy. The treatment of postpolypectomy bleeding is usually endoscopic in the acute setting. If there is a significant stalk remnant, snare strangulation of the stalk without additional application of cautery for 10 to 15 minutes will effectively stop the bleeding [38]. Injection of epinephrine into the base of the stalk or cautious electrocoagulation may also stop immediate bleeding from a polypectomy site. Delayed hemorrhage has been effectively and safely treated by repeat colonoscopy with epinephrine injection, electrocautery, or heater probe application. **A–C**, Endoscopic examples demonstrating postpolypectomy bleeding sites.

Ischemic colitis

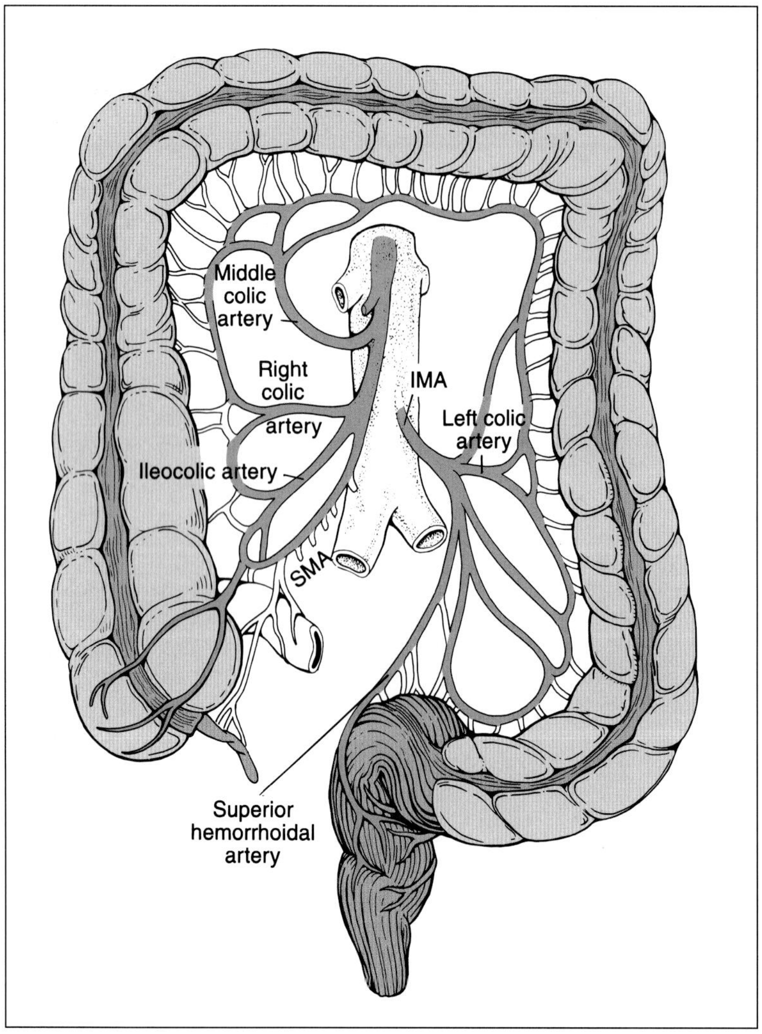

FIGURE 7-19.

The colon receives blood from branches of the superior mesenteric artery (SMA), inferior mesenteric artery (IMA), and internal iliac arteries. The right colon and the proximal half of the transverse colon are supplied by the middle, right, and ileocolic branches of the SMA. The distal transverse, descending, and sigmoid colons are supplied by the left colic and sigmoidal branches of the IMA. The rectum is supplied by the superior hemorrhoidal artery, which is a branch of the IMA, and the inferior and middle hemorrhoidal arteries that originate from the internal iliac arteries. Communications among the major arterial systems create an extensive collateral network. Ischemic colitis is most commonly a disease of the elderly. Patients often have preexisting coronary artery disease and peripheral vascular disease. Ischemic colitis may result from occlusive or nonocclusive events; it may develop following interruption of the IMA during aortic surgery. Other causes of occlusive ischemic colitis include trauma, thrombosis, or embolization usually from atrial fibrillation or a mural thrombus. Embolic disease affecting the colon usually results from an occlusion in the SMA at the origin of the middle colic artery. Because of the small size of the IMA, emboli are uncommon. Nonocclusive causes of ischemic colitis include cardiac failure, sepsis, dehydration, and other forms of shock. Ischemia results from vasoconstriction and shunting within the mesenteric circulation in response to decreased perfusion pressure. (*From* Bower [39]; with permission.)

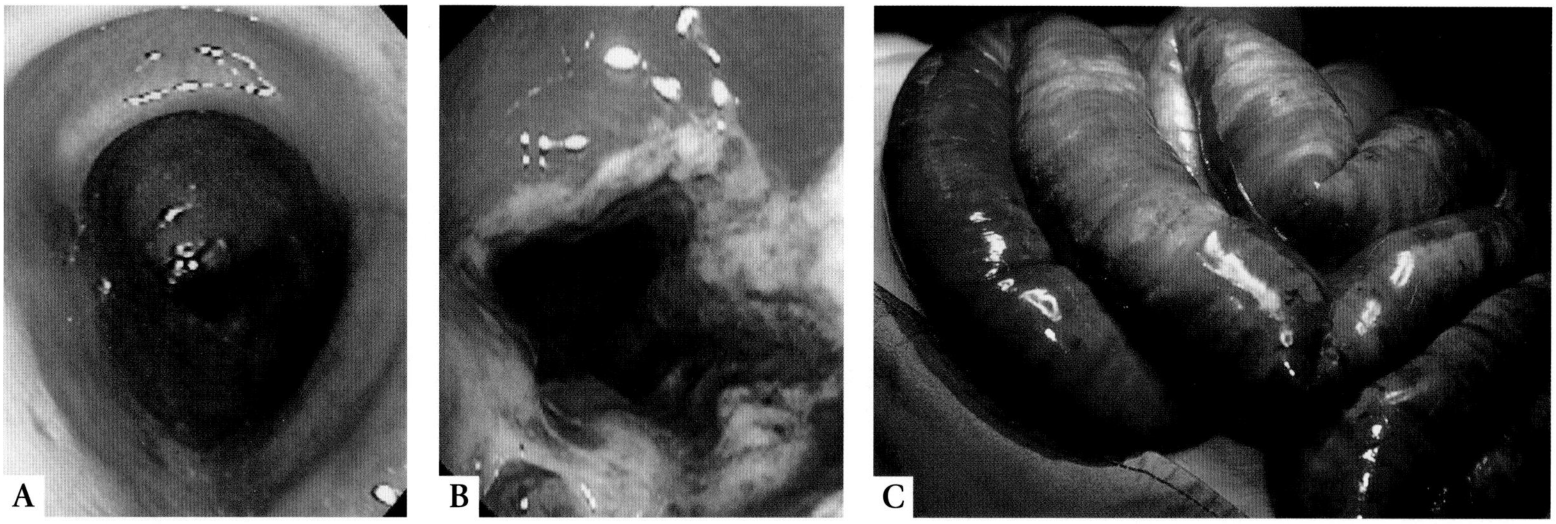

FIGURE 7-20.

Most patients with ischemic colitis present with abdominal pain, however, 15% to 25% of patients may present with overt rectal bleeding. Complete absence of bleeding, including occult bleeding, is uncommon. Bleeding is occasionally massive. Endoscopy is the diagnostic procedure of choice. Endoscopically, rectal sparing is typical because of the middle rectal artery collateral circulation. Ischemic proctitis has primarily been reported in patients with extensive pelvic surgery and presumed disruption of rectal blood flow. **A**, The mucosa may be pale, edematous, and friable in early disease. **B** and **C**, The mucosa may also show a blue-black discoloration signifying mucosal necrosis and submucosal hemorrhage if the disease is extensive. The areas most commonly affected are the watershed areas of the splenic flexure and sigmoid colon, which are at the periphery of the inferior mesenteric artery circulation. Most patients with ischemic colitis have a self-limited course with spontaneous recovery. However, transmural necrosis and peritonitis may develop, and this possibility necessitates careful clinical observation. In some cases, healing may occur with subsequent stricture formation. (**A**, *Courtesy of* D. Johnson, Norfolk, VA) (**B** and **C**, *Courtesy of* R. Goulet, Indianapolis, IN)

Perianal disease

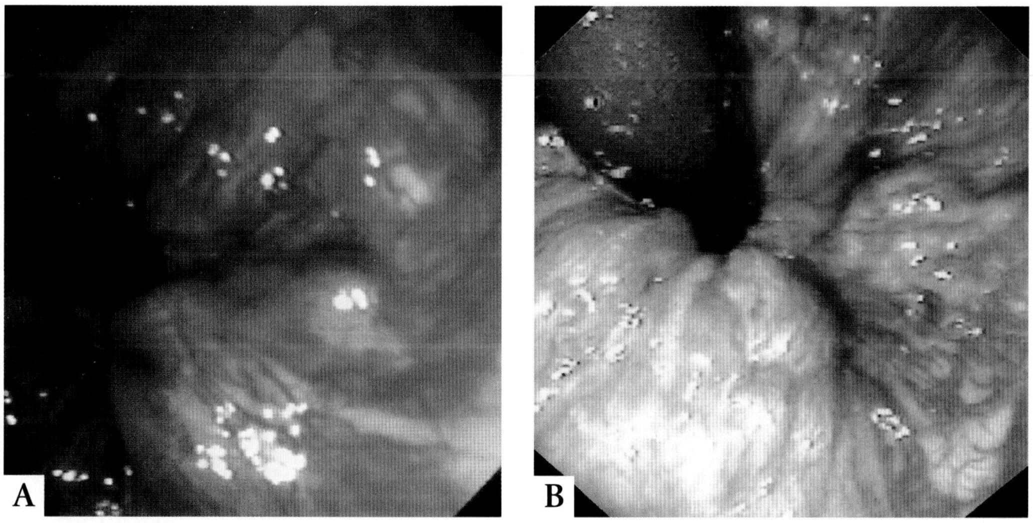

FIGURE 7-21.

Approximately 50% of adults over the age of 50 have hemorrhoids. Hemorrhoids are the most common etiology of lower gastrointestinal bleeding. Internal hemorrhoids arise from the superior hemorrhoidal plexus above the dentate line. These hemorrhoids are lined by rectal mucosa. The three primary locations of hemorrhoids are the right anterior, right posterior, and left lateral. External hemorrhoids arise from the inferior hemorrhoidal venous plexus below the dentate line. These hemorrhoids are lined by squamous epithelium. Internal and external hemorrhoids freely communicate to drain the lower rectum and anus through the internal pudendal vein and inferior vena cava. Internal hemorrhoids are graded on a 1 to 4 scale. Grade 1 hemorrhoids do not protrude from the anal canal. Grade 2 hemorrhoids protrude from the anal canal, however, they reduce spontaneously. Grade 3 hemorrhoids protrude from the anal canal, however, they need manipulation for reduction. Grade 4 hemorrhoids are completely prolapsed through the anal canal and cannot be reduced. Bleeding is the most common presentation of hemorrhoids, manifesting as bright red blood on the toilet paper or blood dripping into the toilet bowl. It is usually at the end of defecation and is separate from the stool. Patients may rarely have severe bleeding requiring transfusions or chronic blood loss leading to iron deficiency anemia. Hemorrhoids are not considered an explanation for occult gastrointestinal bleeding unless colonoscopy has first ruled out other causes. **A** and **B**, Endoscopic photographs of internal hemorrhoids that were seen at flexible sigmoidoscopy.

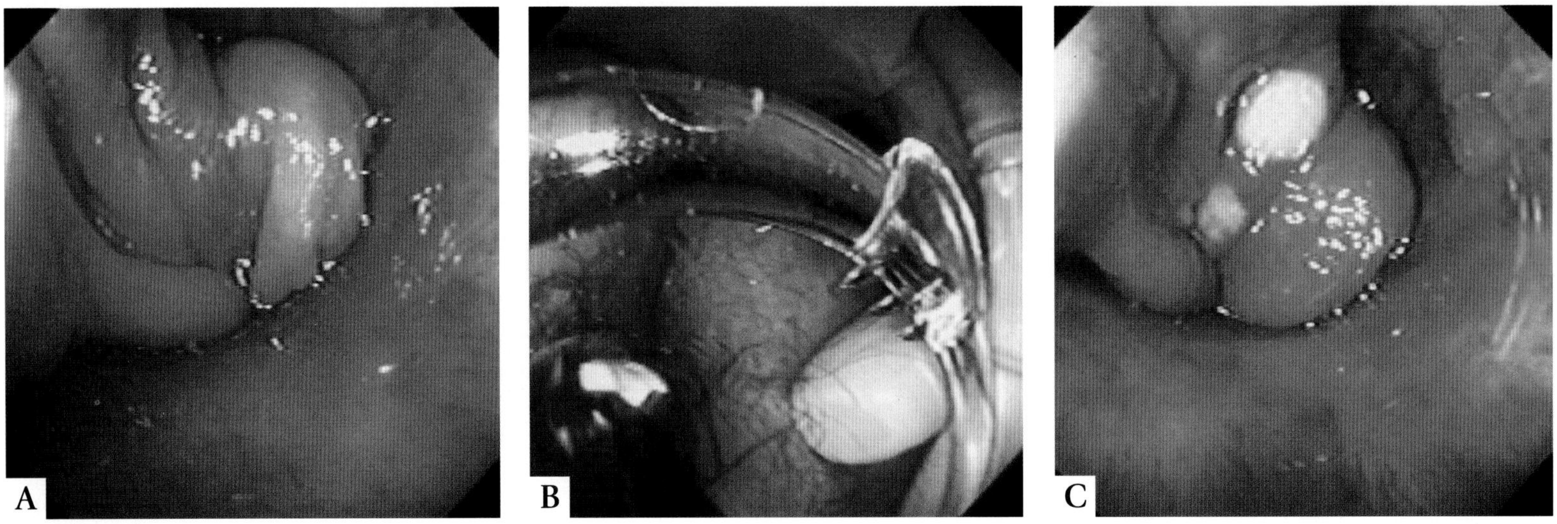

A B C

FIGURE 7-22.

There are many therapeutic options for hemorrhoids. The most conservative approach is the increase of fiber in the diet, the increase of fluid intake, the avoidance of straining, Sitz baths, and topical pharmacotherapy. Rubberband ligation of hemorrhoids is an alternative approach. This approach is used for first-, second-, and third-degree hemorrhoids with a 90% good, long-term result. Therapeutic alternatives include sclerotherapy, cryosurgery, and electrocoagulation using bipolar or direct current. Photocoagulation is performed using infrared light. **A**, An internal hemorrhoid discovered at anoscopy. **B**, Infrared photocoagulation of the hemorrhoid was performed. **C**, The same hemorrhoid after two applications of photocoagulation is shown. Hemorrhoidectomy is preserved for third- and fourth-degree hemorrhoids.

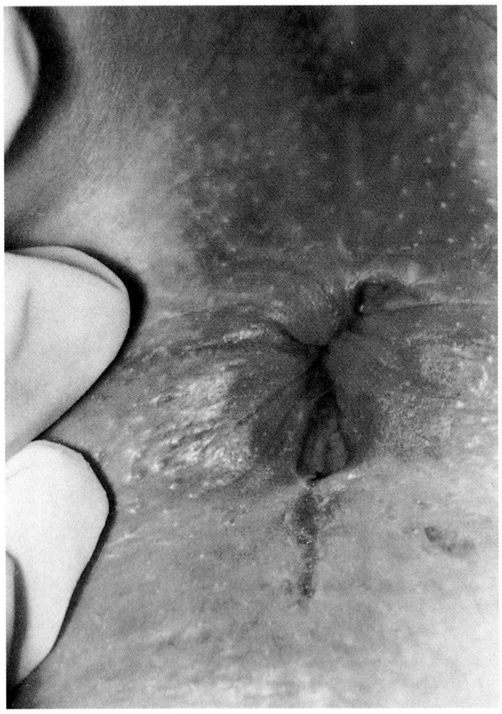

FIGURE 7-23.

Anal fissures are painful linear ulcers in the anal canal and can either be caused by straining or passage of hard stool or an underlying disease such as inflammatory bowel disease. Patients usually present with anal pain accompanied by bright red blood on the toilet paper or around the stool. Treatment consists of stool softeners and topical anesthetics. Chronic fissures may require surgical therapy. The procedure of choice is lateral internal sphincterotomy. (*From* Fleshman [40]; with permission.)

Radiation colitis

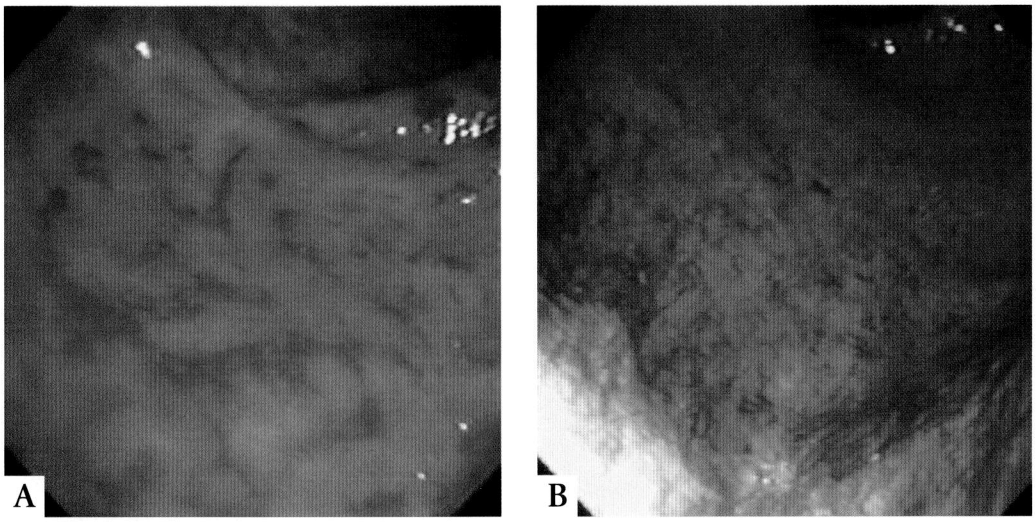

FIGURE 7-24.

Approximately 2% to 5% of patients receiving radiation therapy for gynecologic, prostate, bladder, or rectal cancer will develop chronic radiation injury to the rectum and sigmoid colon. The extent and severity of the injury depends on the total dose of radiation and the volume of the bowel exposed. The pathogenesis of the injury is believed to involve radiation-induced vascular changes of the bowel wall with resultant tissue ischemia. Because of its fixed position in the pelvis, the rectum is damaged in 70% to 90% of all patients with intestinal radiation injuries. Patients usually present with intermittent rectal bleeding, tenesmus, and altered bowel habits. The bleeding may be slow, resulting in iron deficiency anemia, or occasionally, massive. **A** and **B**, Endoscopically there is mucosal erythema, edema, friability, and diffuse telangiectasias. An effective therapy for hemorrhage from radiation proctitis is endoscopic laser ablation or electrocautery of telangiectasias. Decreased transfusion requirements can be achieved using the Nd:YAG (neodymium:yttrium-aluminum-garnet) laser or argon laser. Medical therapy of radiation proctitis has met with limited success. Oral or rectal steroids and sulfasalazine, sucralfate enemas, intrarectal formalin, and hyperbaric oxygen have all been used, but no controlled trials of these modalities have been performed. Surgery is seldom used for radiation injury because of a substantial risk of complications.

Inflammatory bowel disease

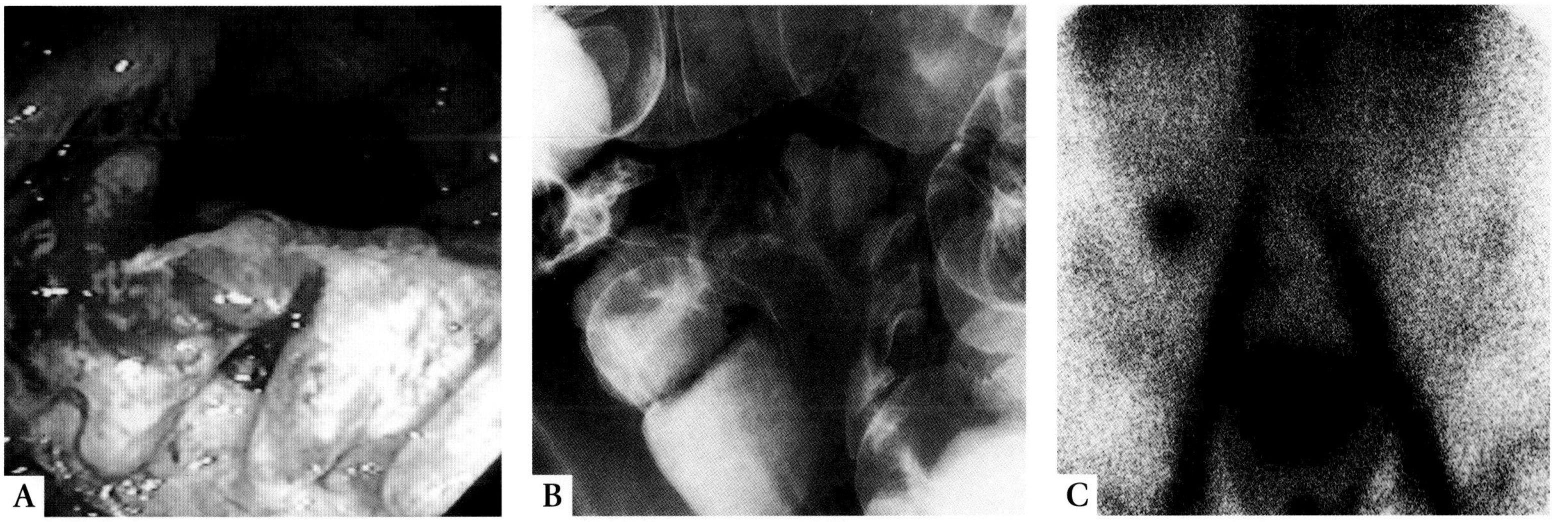

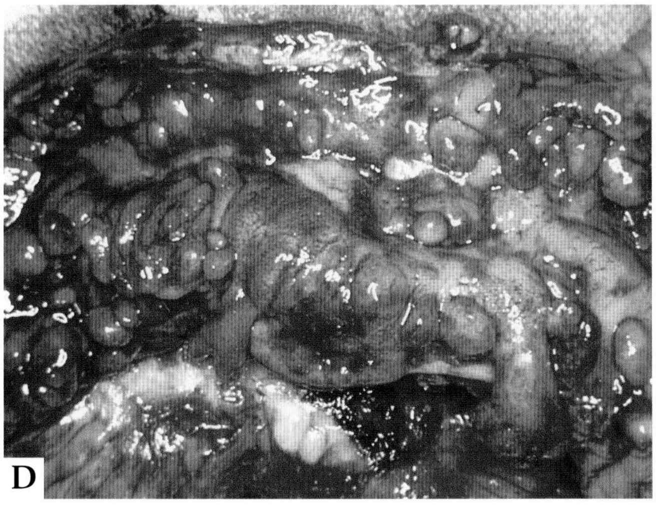

FIGURE 7-25.

Inflammatory bowel disease is a common cause of lower gastrointestinal bleeding in the younger patient. Rectal bleeding is a common manifestation of ulcerative colitis. Patients with Crohn's disease usually present with abdominal pain and diarrhea but may have bleeding. Bleeding in inflammatory bowel disease is usually recurrent and minor. Profuse bleeding develops in up to 6% of patients with ulcerative colitis or Crohn's disease. Robert *et al.* [41] evaluated 21 patients with Crohn's disease and severe gastrointestinal hemorrhage. They found that 66% of the patients had ileocolitis, 19% had enteritis alone, and 14% had colitis alone. The bleeding stopped spontaneously in 50% of the patients, but 33% had rebleeding. The authors advocated early surgical intervention in patients who have a high rebleeding rate. **A**, An endoscopic view of severe Crohn's colitis. **B**, Enteroclysis revealed terminal ileum involvement of Crohn's disease. **C**, A positive bleeding scan in a patient with Crohn's disease. **D**, Surgical resection specimen from a patient with Crohn's disease and severe bleeding. (**B** and **C**, *Courtesy of* J. Lappas, Indianapolis, IN) (**D**, *Courtesy of* R. Goulet, Indianapolis, IN)

Infectious colitides

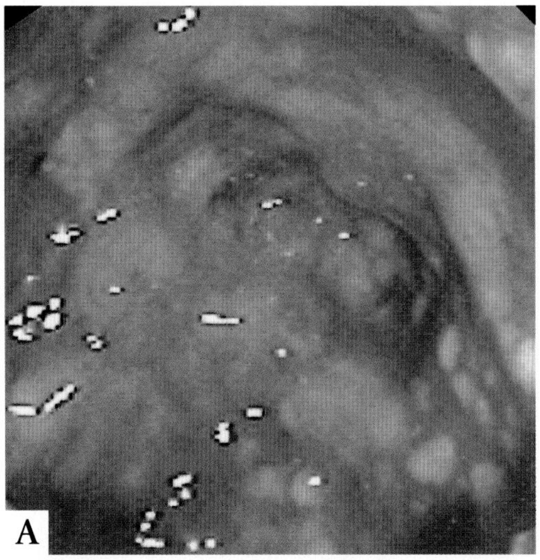

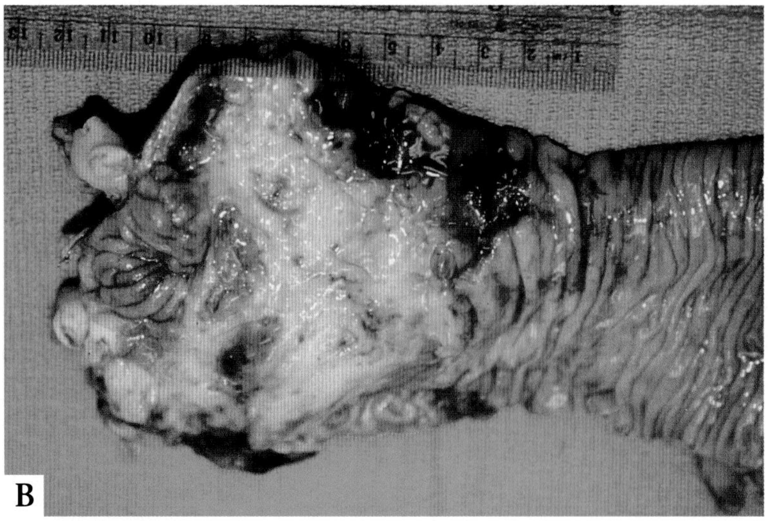

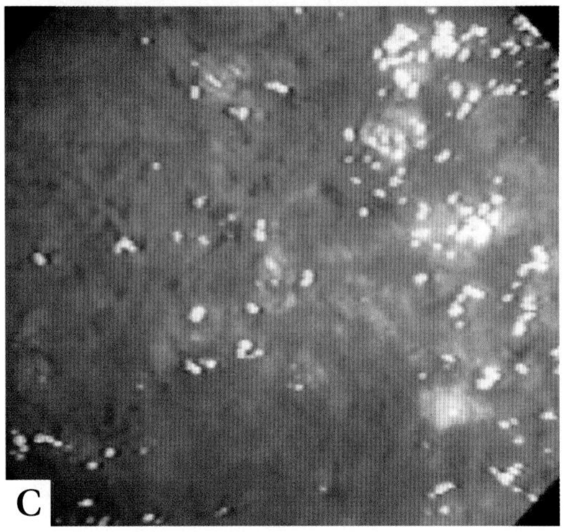

FIGURE 7-26.

Infectious colitides caused by *Escherichia coli* 0157:H7, *Clostridium difficile, Salmonella, Shigella, Campylobacter jejuni*, tuberculosis, ameba, and viruses including cytomegalovirus may present with rectal bleeding. The bleeding is usually part of a generalized symptom complex including diarrhea, abdominal pain, and fever and is usually of mild severity. The diagnosis is made by sigmoidoscopy and specific stool studies. Therapy is directed at the underlying infection, however, colonoscopic injection or cautery may be used for visibly bleeding lesions [42]. **A**, Endoscopic view of pseudomembranous colitis. **B**, Tuberculosis involving the small bowel. **C**, Endoscopic view of cytomegalovirus colitis. (**B**, *Courtesy of* R. Goulet, Indianapolis, IN)

Drug-induced colitis

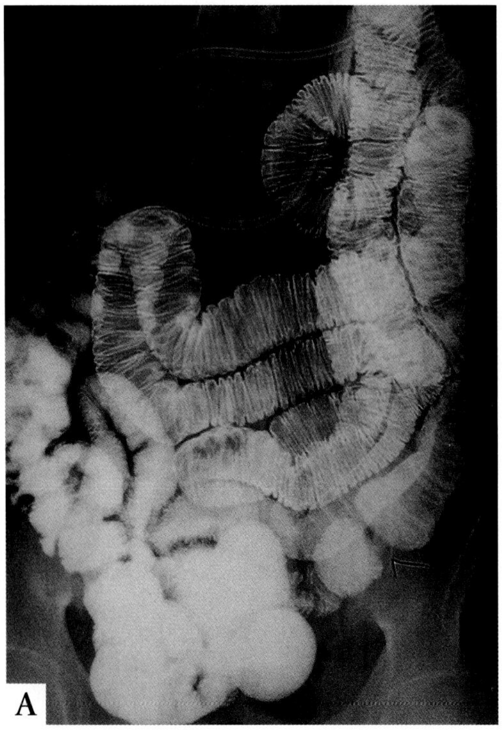

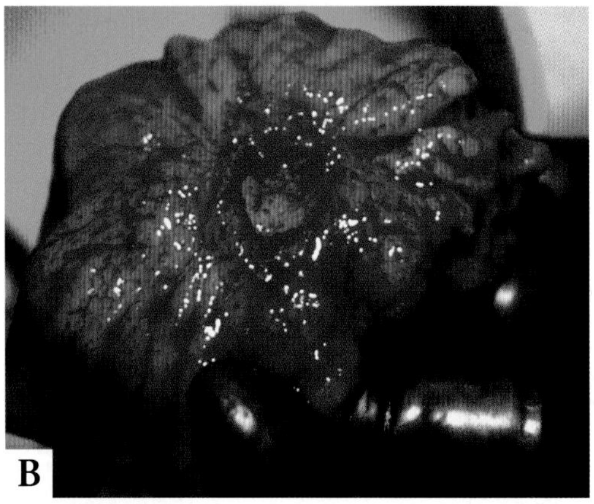

FIGURE 7-27.

Many drugs have been implicated as injurious to the gastrointestinal tract mucosa. The most common drugs that cause injury are the nonsteroidal anti-inflammatory drugs (NSAIDs). The major sites of injury are the stomach and duodenum. However, the esophagus, small bowel, and colon may be affected by ulceration, stricture formation, perforation, and bleeding. In addition, NSAIDs commonly are associated with gastrointestinal bleeding from lesions that are not self-NSAID induced. This effect is the result of the antiplatelet properties of NSAIDs. Lanas *et al.* [43] found that among patients with lower gastrointestinal bleeding, the prevalence of NSAID use was 86%. Patients with small bowel and colonic lesions caused by NSAIDs usually present with occult bleeding, however, they may present with massive hematochezia. Endoscopically, one sees submucosal hemorrhage, petechial eruptions, erosions, ulcerations, or diaphragm-like strictures [44]. Treatment of NSAID–induced enteropathy or colopathy usually requires simple discontinuation of the offending agent. However, bleeding, perforation, or obstructive symptoms may necessitate surgery. **A**, A diaphragm-like stricture of the small bowel seen on enteroscopy. **B**, Surgical resection specimen of an NSAID–induced small bowel ulcer is depicted.

Hereditary hemorrhagic telangiectasia

TABLE 7-4. PRESENTING MANIFESTATIONS OF HEREDITARY HEMORRHAGIC TELANGIECTASIA

Symptom	Patients, *n* (%)
Epistaxis	33 (51)
Gastrointestinal bleeding	16 (25)
Abnormal chest radiograph	3 (5)
Headache (brain abscess)	2 (3)
Seizure (CNS emboli)	2 (3)
Progressive skin lesions	2 (3)
Cyanosis	1 (< 2)
(large pulmonary arteriovenous malformation with emboli)	
Transient ischemic attacks	1 (< 2)
Abdominal pain, pulsatile right upper quadrant	
Mass (hepatic AVM)	1 (< 2)

TABLE 7-4.

Hereditary hemorrhagic telangiectasia is an autosomal dominant condition characterized by telangiectasias of the skin, mucus membranes, and various organ systems including the gastrointestinal tract. Approximately 13% to 44% of patients will develop gastrointestinal bleeding. Gastrointestinal bleeding is second only to epistaxis as the presenting symptom in these patients [45]. Gastrointestinal hemorrhage typically does not become manifest until the 4th or 5th decade compared with epistaxis that presents in childhood. Bleeding may originate anywhere throughout the gastrointestinal tract; however, patients usually present with melena. Treatment options include endoscopic obliteration with electrocoagulation or laser, hormone therapy, and surgery, which should be reserved for recurrent bleeding from localized sites. AVM—atriovenous malformation; CNS—central nervous system. (*From* Reilly and Nostrant [45]; with permission.)

Solitary rectal ulcer syndrome

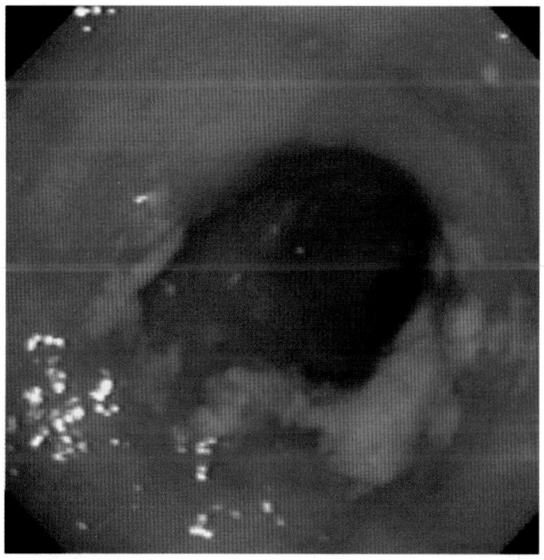

FIGURE 7-28.

Eighty-five percent to 95% of patients with solitary rectal ulcer syndrome present with hematochezia, usually of low volume and associated with mucus. Symptoms may also include anorectal pain, altered bowel movements, and straining with defecation. It is believed that solitary rectal ulcer syndrome is related to prolonged straining during bowel movements and difficulty initiating defecation. Classically, at sigmoidoscopy, there is a shallow, discrete 1-cm ulcer with hyperemic margins 7 to 10 cm from the anal verge on the anterior wall. Lesions, however, may be multiple or vary in size and location. These ulcers follow a benign course, and two thirds of patients improve with conservative measures, including a high-fiber diet, laxatives, and avoidance of straining. Diagnosis is histologic, and the characteristic histologic findings may be seen in patients whose endoscopic findings are only rectal polyps. Pictured is a solitary rectal ulcer seen during flexible sigmoidoscopy.

Dieulafoy's lesions

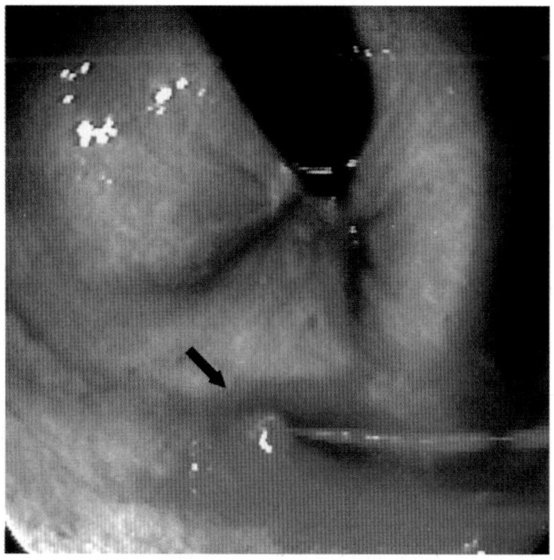

FIGURE 7-29.

Dieulafoy's lesions are usually seen in the proximal stomach, however, they may be found in the colon or small bowel. The pathologic defect is an abnormally large submucosal artery with a small mucosal defect overlying the artery. Bleeding occurs when there is rupture of the artery into the bowel lumen. For small bowel or colonic lesions, the diagnosis is usually made by angiography because bleeding is too massive for endoscopic visualization. Therapeutic options include endoscopic injection or cautery, intra-arterial vasopressin, angiographic embolization, or surgical resection. Pictured is a Dieulafoy's lesion in the rectum with an actively spurting vessel. (*From* Abdulian *et al.* [46]; with permission.)

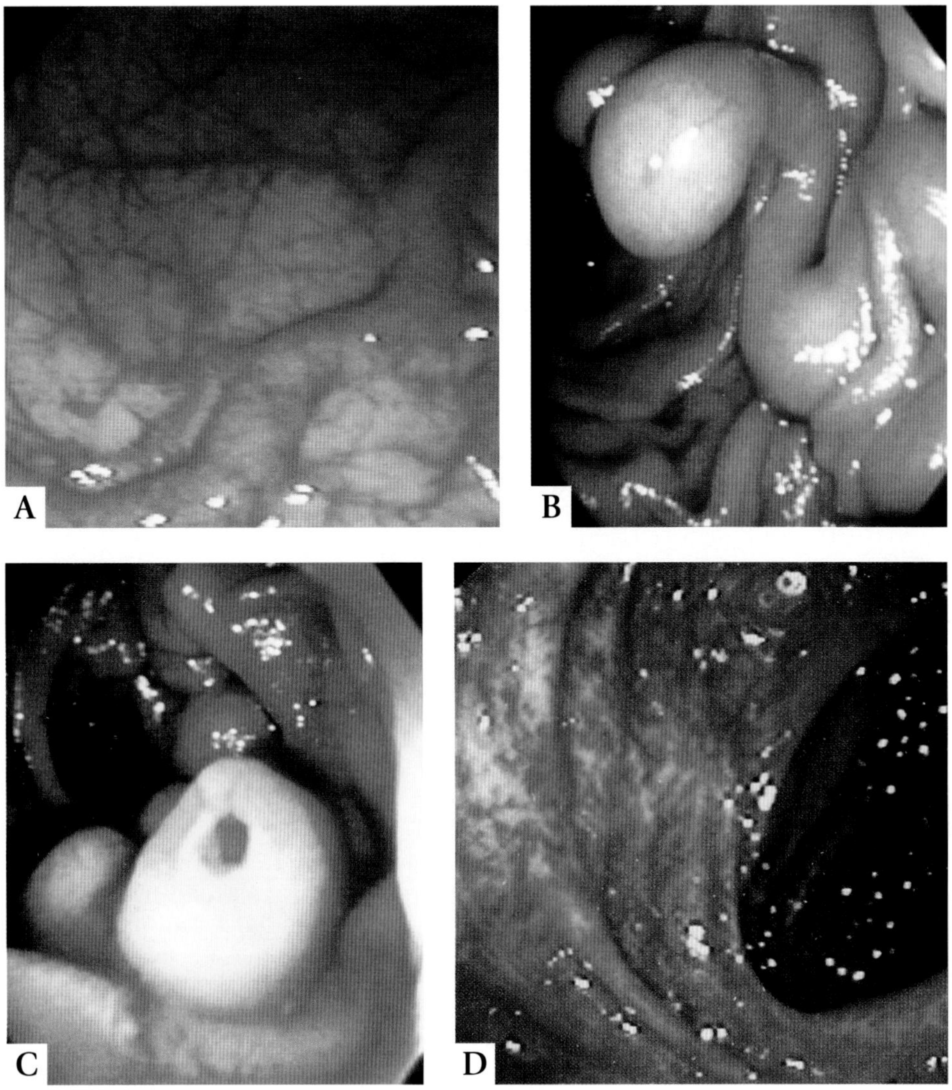

FIGURE 7-30.

Ectopic varices may occur in 1% to 3% of patients with cirrhosis and in 20% to 30% of patients with extrahepatic portal vein thrombosis [47]. They are most commonly located in the small and large intestine; however, extraintestinal sites have been reported. They are usually associated with prior abdominal surgery, the result of venous communications between portal and systemic circuits through postoperative adhesions. Patients present with melena or hematochezia with a negative nasogastric lavage. Ectopic varices may be diagnosed by angiography or endoscopy. Treatment is controversial. Some advocate segmental resection, whereas others advocate portosystemic shunting. Treatment alternatives include β-blockers, variceal sclerotherapy, or band ligation.

Kozarek *et al.* [48] recently described 20 patients with portal hypertension who underwent colonoscopy for hematochezia or occult blood in the stool. Seventy percent had mucosal lesions resembling multiple vascular ectasias, mostly in the right colon. A smaller subset of patients was found to have endoscopic findings resembling chronic colitis. There have been many case reports in the literature outlining similar endoscopic findings, now termed *portal hypertensive colopathy*, in patients with portal hypertension. No good randomized controlled trials have evaluated therapy for portal hypertensive colopathy. However, β-blockers or shunt surgery are options for patients with recurrent or persistent bleeding. Rectal varices (**A**) and small bowel varices (**B**) are shown. This figure depicts a small bowel varix with ulcer and red spot (**C**). Vascular ectasia-like appearance of portal hypertensive colopathy is presented (**D**). (**D**, *From* Kozarek *et al.* [48]; with permission.)

Gastrointestinal bleeding in athletes

TABLE 7-5. THE INCIDENCE OF BLEEDING IN RUNNERS

STUDY	METHOD	RACE (*n*)	RESULT, %
Porter (50)	Post-race Hemoccult	Marathon (39)	8
Keefe *et al.* (51)	Survey bright red blood/rectum	Marathon (707)	1.2–1.8
Halvorsen *et al.* (52)	Pre- and post-Hemoccult	Marathon (63)	13
McCabe *et al.* (53)	Pre- and post-Hemoccult	Marathon (125)	21
McMahon *et al.* (54)	Pre- and post-Hemoccult	Marathon (32)	22
Baska *et al.* (55)	Pre- and post-Hemoccult	Marathon (34)	85

TABLE 7-5.

Marathon runners frequently develop gastrointestinal blood loss and anemia [49]. Severe gastrointestinal hemorrhage has been reported but is rare. Various studies have shown a Hemoccult (SmithKline Diagnostics, San Jose, CA) positivity rate from 8% to 85% after competitive races. The most common source of blood loss is the stomach, followed by the colon. It is thought that blood loss results from ischemic injury caused by shunting of blood away from the gastrointestinal tract during vigorous exertion. Studies have shown the visceral blood flow falls from 20% to 50% of the baseline value with vigorous exercise. (*From* Moses [49]; with permission.)

Hemangiomas

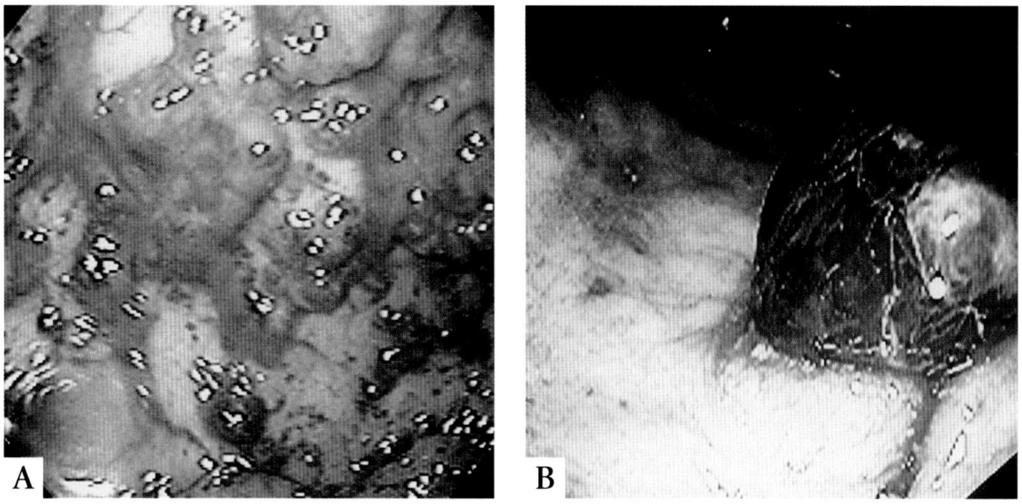

FIGURE 7-31.

Hemangiomas are hamartomatous vascular growths that can be found throughout the gastrointestinal tract including the colon. Most are discovered incidentally, but they may present with bleeding. Most symptomatic colonic hemangiomas are in the rectum and sigmoid colon. Capillary hemangiomas present usually with slow or occult bleeding. Ninety percent of cavernous hemangiomas will have overt bleeding, which may be massive. Diagnosis is by endoscopy, and therapy is usually surgical resection. **A**, Rectal hemangiomas. **B**, Hemangioma with clot. (*Courtesy of* D. Johnson, Norfolk, VA)

Small bowel bleeding

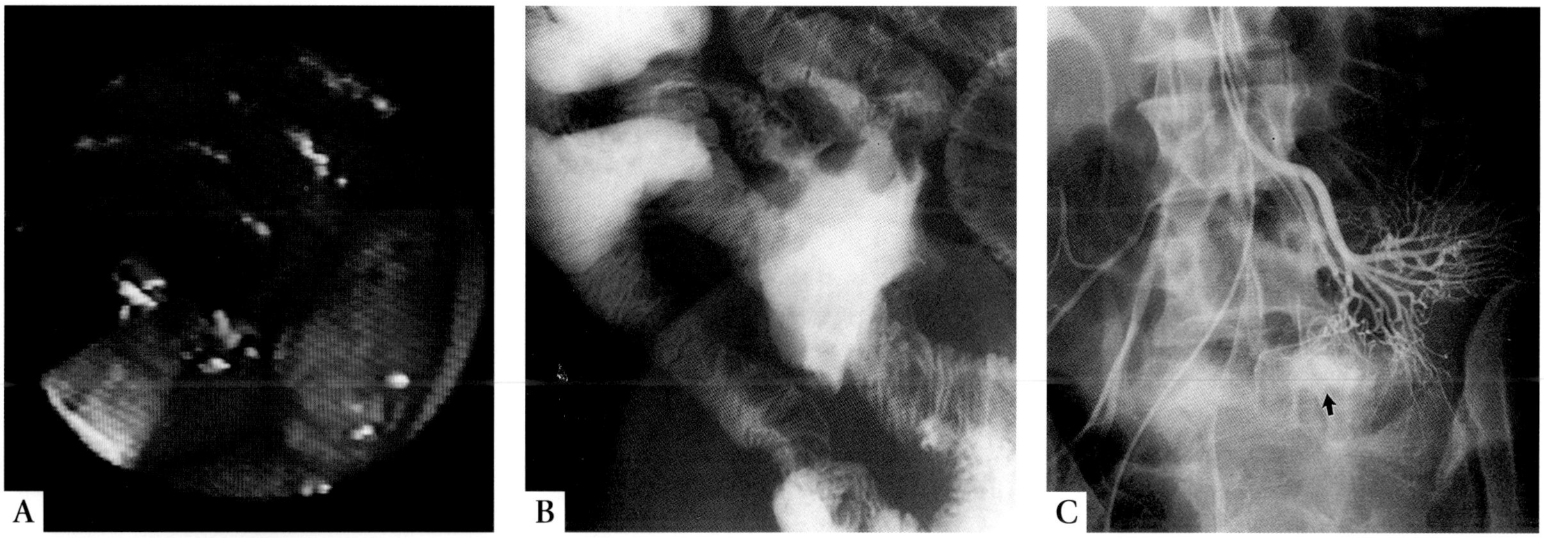

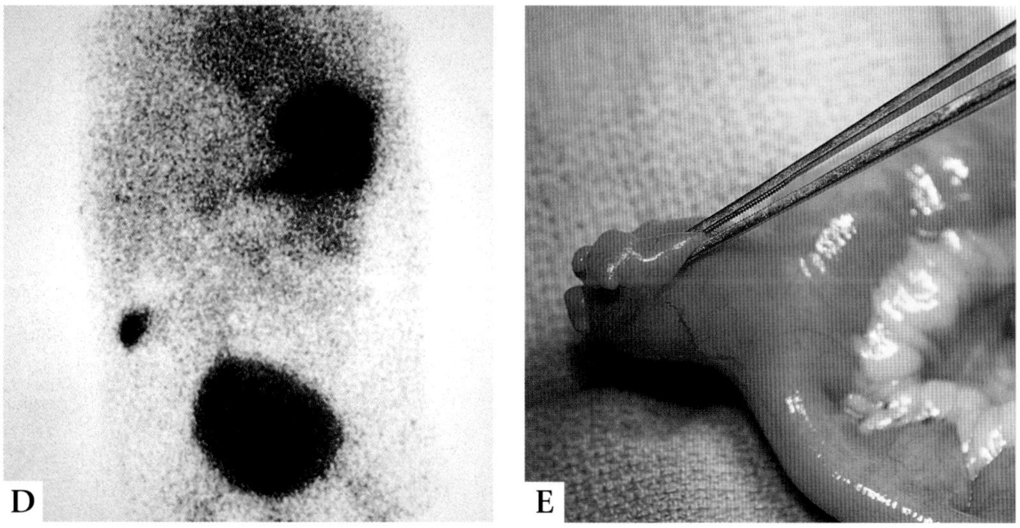

FIGURE 7-32.

Approximately 3% to 5% of cases presumed lower gastrointestinal bleeding originate in the small bowel. Diagnosis is made by enteroscopy, enteroclysis, angiography, tagged red blood cell scanning, or surgery. The yield of push enteroscopy varies from 13% to 38%, sonde enteroscopy from 26% to 33%, and intraoperative enteroscopy from 83% to 100% [56]. In the patient with obscure blood loss, small bowel follow-through detects an intestinal bleeding site in 5% of patients, and enteroclysis increases the yield to 10% [57]. The most common cause of small bowel bleeding is angiodysplasia, followed by small bowel tumors. Less frequent etiologies of small bowel bleeding include nonsteroidal injury, ectopic varices, jejunal diverticula, aortoenteric fistulas, and Meckel's diverticulum. Meckel's diverticulum is the most common congenital anomaly of the gastrointestinal tract and may present with massive hemorrhage. The treatment of choice is surgical resection. **A**, Metastatic lung cancer to the jejunum. **B**, Small bowel lymphoma. **C**, This angiogram reveals active bleeding from a small bowel tumor. **D**, A positive Meckel's scan. **E**, This figure shows surgical resection for bleeding Meckel's diverticulum. (**B** and **C**, *Courtesy of* J. Lappas, Indianapolis, IN) (**E**, *Courtesy of* R. Goulet, Indianapolis, IN)

Nonemergent rectal bleeding and colorectal cancer

TABLE 7-6. YIELD OF COLONOSCOPY FOR NEOPLASIA IN PATIENTS WITH NONEMERGENT RECTAL BLEEDING

Reference	Patients, *n*	Cancer, *n* (%)	Adenomatous polyps, *n* (%)
Goulston *et al.* [58]	145	15 (10)	25 (17)
Church [59]	174	18 (10)	51 (29)
Bat *et al.* [60]	101	29 (29)*	34 (34)*
Berkowitz and Kaplan [61]	123	11 (9)	15 (12)
Irvine *et al.* [62]	71	5 (7)	26 (37)
Thoeni and Venbrux [63]	215	27 (13)	29 (13)
Guillem *et al.* [64]	224	33 (15)	61 (27)
Brand *et al.* [65]†	221	16 (7)	51 (23)
Swarbrick *et al.* [66]†	239	23 (10)	39 (16)
Teague *et al.* [67]†	109	6 (6)	18 (17)
Total	1622	183 (11)	298 (18)

**Patients with lesion.*
†All had negative barium enema before colonoscopy.

Table 7-6.

Nonemergent rectal bleeding is a common symptom, and it is noted intermittently by about 15% of apparently well persons [58]. In patients without abdominal pain, the most commonly encountered etiologies are hemorrhoids, anal fissure, colorectal cancer, and large colorectal polyps. When diarrhea or abdominal pain are added to the clinical presentation, inflammatory diseases of the colon also become prominent in the differential diagnosis. In patients without abdominal pain or diarrhea, the principal goal of colonoscopy is to rule out colonic polyps and cancer. Patients with small amounts of blood on the toilet paper, blood dripping from the anus after bowel movements, or blood being passed without bowel movements have been generally considered to have an anal source of bleeding. Although this rule is helpful, prospective evaluations of family physicians and gastroenterologists found that neither are able to distinguish reliably anal from colonic bleeding by history alone [58]. Church [59] prospectively characterized bleeding as outlet type (bright red blood seen during or after defecation, on the toilet paper, or in the toilet bowel) or as suspicious (dark red blood, blood mixed with or streaked on stool, or blood associated with a change in bowel habit or mucus passage). Patients with suspicious-type bleeding were considerably more likely to have cancer (22%) than those with outlet type bleeding, but 4% of those patients with outlet-type bleeding also had colorectal cancer. Therefore, colonoscopy is generally indicated in patients with rectal bleeding. This fact appears true with persistent rectal bleeding, even if there is a previously negative barium enema. Likewise, two studies of colonoscopy in patients with melena and a negative upper endoscopy [65,68] found that 12% and 9%, respectively, of such patients had colorectal cancer.

Occult bleeding

TABLE 7-7. CAUSES OF PSEUDOBLEEDING

- Melena
  - Iron ingestion
  - Bismuth subsalicylate
- Hematochezia
  - Ingestion of beets

Table 7-7.

Blood that is present in feces but not evident on visual inspection of the feces is occult blood. Testing for the presence of occult blood is most commonly performed by using guaiac slide tests. Guaiac slide tests can also be used to test whether black or red stool actually contains blood. Thus, black stools may result from ingestion of iron or bismuth subsalicylate. Likewise, red stools can result from ingestion of beets. The use of guaiac slide tests in this circumstance is to distinguish melena or hematochezia from pseudobleeding. Under these circumstances, guaiac slide tests are not being performed as a test for occult blood, and a positive result may not have the same implications as when the tests are used to examine feces for occult blood.

A certain amount of occult bleeding is normal. Normal blood loss in the feces is 0.7 mL per day. Testing implies an attempt to detect a degree of occult bleeding that is abnormal. Guaiac-based slide tests cannot reliably differentiate abnormal from normal amounts of occult bleeding and demonstrate deficiencies in both sensitivity and specificity. In particular, the amount of occult blood in stool must be up to 10 times the upper limit of normal before guaiac-based slide tests positive in 90% of cases.

TABLE 7-8. TESTS FOR FECAL OCCULT BLOOD

TEST		REACTION		ADVANTAGES	DISADVANTAGES
Guaiac-based testing		Hydrogen peroxide (catalyst)		Inexpensive	Low sensitivity
	Phenol (guaiac) Coloress	→	Quinone (blue)	Simple	Low positive predictive value
		Peroxidase activity			
HemoQuant®		Step 1	Step 2		
		Stool heated → in reducing acid to remove heme iron	Purification by extraction to yield free prophyrin solution	Quantitative	Detects upper gastrointestinal bleeding Does not outperform guaiac testing in screening trials
Immunochemical testing HemeSelect®		Direct reaction of antibody with hemoglobin		Highly sensitive for blood Detects only intact hemoglobin	16–24 h Incubation period Not tested in screening trials

TABLE 7-8 AND FIGURE 7-33.

Fecal occult blood testing has only one purpose in clinical practice, *ie*, the detection of colorectal neoplasia. In clinical practice, fecal occult blood testing is sometimes used in evaluation of patients with upper gastrointestinal tract symptoms such as dyspepsia or to monitor patients ingesting nonsteroidal anti-inflammatory drugs. However, no study has defined the sensitivity, specificity, or clinical implications of fecal occult blood testing in these patients. In fact, fecal occult blood tests performed in these patients are actually still screening tests for colorectal cancer. Any positive fecal occult blood test should lead a patient to colonic imaging for colorectal cancer.

Clinical testing for occult blood can be performed using guaiac-based tests, quantitative tests for porphyrin derivatives such as HemoQuant (University of Minnesota) or immunochemical tests (Table 7-8). Only guaiac-based tests are used widely. Several tests employ guaiac-impregnated filter paper on a card. Of these, the best studied is the Hemoccult II Card (SmithKline Diagnostics, San Jose, CA). Hemoccult SENSA (SmithKline Diagnostics) is a newer guaiac-based test which is more sensitive and readable [69] than Hemoccult II (Fig. 7-33). Some guaiac-based tests have been developed that employ guaiac-impregnated paper that is dropped into the toilet bowel. These tests offer the theoretical advantage of improved patient compliance. However, improved compliance has not been proven in large clinical trials. Furthermore, the sensitivity and specificity of such tests has not been thoroughly studied, and it cannot be recommended for clinical practice. Guaiac is a natural occurring phenolic compound. In the presence of an oxidizing agent, guaiac is converted to a quinone, which is a blue color. The product should be unequivocally blue in order to be considered positive. In the guaiac reaction, hemoglobin supplies pseudoperoxidase activity, which permits oxidation. Addition of a developing solution containing hydrogen peroxide is usually necessary. Hydrogen peroxide serves as a catalyst for the oxidative reaction.

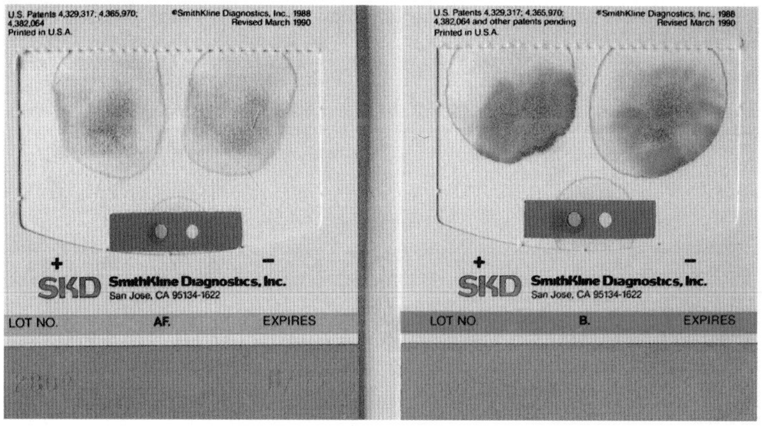

The HemoQuant test provides a quantitative measure of stool occult blood. The test measures not only intact heme but also biochemical breakdown derivatives of heme. Therefore, this test is more likely to detect occult bleeding from the upper gastrointestinal tract than other testing methods. In clinical practice, HemoQuant does not perform better than guaiac-based testing as a screening measure for colorectal cancer [70]. Unfortunately, there is a substantial overlap between the amount of bleeding that occurs in normal individuals and the amount that occurs in patients with colorectal cancer. This overlap is an insurmountable obstacle to the effectiveness of occult blood testing for colorectal cancer.

Immunochemical testing, which detects only intact hemoglobin, is probably the most sensitive and specific fecal occult blood test for colorectal cancer [69]. However, it is more expensive than guaiac testing, and major advantages in effectiveness and cost-effectiveness over guaiac testing have not been proven in clinical screening trials. (**Fig. 7-33**, *Courtesy of* SmithKline Diagnostics, San Jose, CA)

TABLE 7-9. FALSE GUAIAC REACTIONS

High peroxidase foods
Red meat
↓
False positive
False negative
↑
Vitamin C slide storage

TABLE 7-9.

False-negative guaiac reactions may occur in the presence of reducing agents, most notably vitamin C. Foods high in peroxidase activity may cause false-positive reactions [71]. This reaction is particularly important for red meat, which should be avoided if rehydration is used. Iron supplements, contrary to widely held beliefs, do not cause false-positive guaiac reactions. However, the dark color of feces in patients on iron supplements may confuse the card reader. Ingestion of aspirin or nonsteroidal anti-inflammatory drugs are very likely to cause a positive reaction that is not the result of colonic neoplasia and should be avoided if possible.

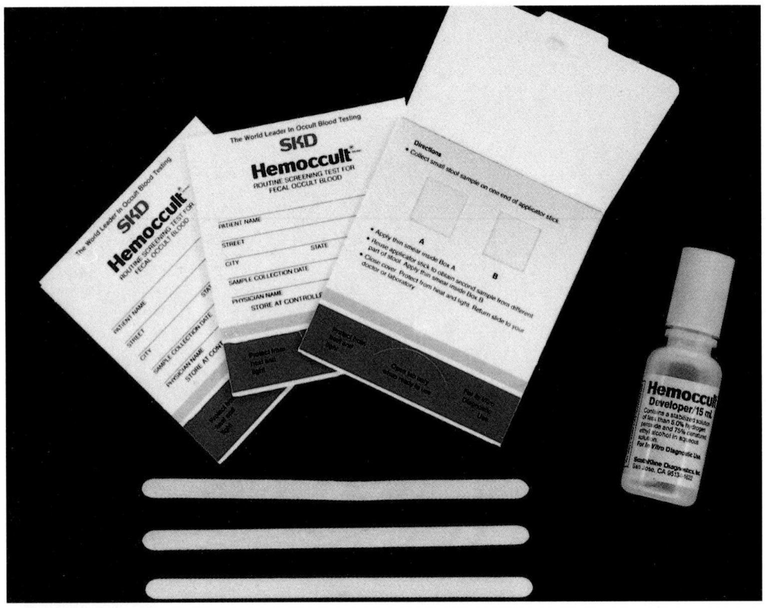

FIGURE 7-34.

Guaiac-based testing is typically performed at home. The patient collects stool samples using a small wooden stick from two different portions of the fecal sample on 3 consecutive days. Each of the six samples is wiped onto a separate guaiac-impregnated filter paper and the cards are enclosed and returned to the physician's office or screening center. In some centers, rehydration of the slides is performed, which refers to the practice of adding a drop of water to the slides before adding the developing solution. Rehydration improves the sensitivity for colorectal cancer detection but substantially decreases the positive predictive value. The sensitivity and positive predictive value of nonrehydrated guaiac-based slide tests for colorectal cancer is approximately 30% and 10%, respectively [71]. The sensitivity of rehydrated slides for colorectal cancer has been calculated at 90%, but this calculation is certainly an overestimate. The positive predictive value of rehydrated slides is approximately 2%. Only performance of annual occult blood tests with rehydration of slides and follow-up of positives by colonoscopy has been shown to reduce colorectal cancer mortality [72].

In clinical practice fecal occult blood tests are frequently performed on feces obtained during a digital rectal examination. Essentially, no data is available on the performance of fecal occult blood tests as a screening measure for colorectal cancer in asymptomatic patients when the test is performed on feces obtained by digital examination. Several studies examining patients with positive fecal occult blood tests obtained by digital examination, who were also frequently symptomatic, suggest that the yield of colorectal cancers is comparable with asymptomatic patients undergoing home testing [73–75]. At the present time, there is insufficient data available to justify ignoring a positive fecal occult blood test obtained by digital examination in an asymptomatic patient. Either the patient should be evaluated or the test should be repeated properly at home. (*From* Rex and Lewis [13]; with permission.)

TABLE 7-10. UNIVERSITY OF MINNESOTA FECAL OCCULT BLOOD TESTING TRIAL

Design	Results	Limitations
Prospective, randomized trial 46,551 People between 50–80 years of age Three arms Screened yearly Screened biennially No screening 83% Of slides rehydrated Positive tests → colonoscopy Endpoint → death from colorectal cancer Follow-up → 13 years	9.8% Tests positive Positive predictive value 2.2% for cancer 6% Reduction in death from colorectal cancer in biennially screened group (not significant) 33% Reduction in death from colorectal cancer in annually screened group	No effect from biennial screening 38% Of annual group had one or more colonoscopies Mortality reduction only 33%

TABLE 7-10.

The most important study on fecal occult blood testing in colorectal cancer yet published was performed at the University of Minnesota [72]. In this study, 46,551 people were randomly assigned to undergo annual, biennial, or no occult blood testing. Eighty-three percent of the slides were rehydrated. All people with a positive test underwent colonoscopy. The end point for the study was death from colorectal cancer. The interval of follow-up was 13 years. The results of the Minnesota trial were that colorectal cancer mortality was reduced by 33% in the annually screened group and 6% in the biennially screened group (not significantly different compared with controls). This study is a landmark study, as it is the first to prove the efficacy of occult blood testing in reducing colorectal cancer mortality.

This study, however, is open to several unenthusiastic interpretations. First, there was no reduction in mortality from biennial screening. Because compliance with annual screening may be difficult to achieve in the general population, some doubt can be cast on the applicability of the results to general population screening. Second, the percentage of positive tests in the study was 9.8%. This resulted in 38% of the annually screened group undergoing colonoscopy. A test that selects such a high percentage of the population to undergo a colonoscopy, a test with some risk and considerable expense, is less desirable. In addition, it has been argued that approximately one half of the mortality reduction in the annually screened group actually resulted from chance detection of neoplasia during colonoscopic procedures performed when the test was positive because of rehydration rather than abnormal amounts of occult bleeding. Finally, the mortality reduction in the annually screened group was only 33%. Universal application of these recommendations would reduce annual colorectal cancer deaths in the United States from approximately 60,000 to 40,000 per year. This reduction would still leave colorectal cancer as a major cause of cancer death in the United States. Some centers have discontinued the use of fecal occult blood testing based on this trial.

TABLE 7-11. COLONIC NEOPLASIA IN PATIENTS WITH POSITIVE FECAL OCCULT BLOOD TESTS (GUAIAC)

Test	Number of studies [references]	Total patients	Cancers, *n* (%)	Adenomas, *n* (%)
Nonrehydrated	6 [76–81]	1,591	163 (10)	552 (35)
Rehydrated	1[73]	>12,250	NS (2.2)	NS
Rehydrated positive Negative on repeat	1*[74]	108	1 (1)	NS (6)
Positive on repeat Neither rehydrated	2[83,84]	48	18 (38)	16 (33)
Rehydrated positive Positive on repeat	1*[82]	67	10 (15)	15 (22)

**This study evaluated patients by flexible sigmoidoscopy and double-contrast barium enema; all others used colonoscopy. NS—not significant.*

TABLE 7-11.

A positive fecal occult blood test is one of the strongest indications for colonoscopy. Not only is the positive predictive value for cancer high with a single nonrehydrated positive test (10%), but the distribution of Dukes' classes is shifted considerably towards Dukes' A and B tumors compared with tumors seen in symptomatic patients. The positive predictive value increases with age and decreases with subsequent repeat screenings in persons who are initially negative. The positive predictive value is lower for cancer when slides are rehydrated. Several small studies, all with limited numbers of patients, have examined the effect of repeating positive fecal occult blood tests in an effort to improve the predictive value. In at least one study, when patients had an initial positive rehydrated test and then had the test repeated and it was negative, the yield for cancer was low. However, if the initially rehydrated test was positive when repeated, the yield for cancer was substantial (15%). The authors argued that repeating positive rehydrated tests would cut down the number of colonoscopies needed, with little decrease in sensitivity. However, in clinical practice this repetition is probably not advisable. A positive nonrehydrated test that is positive when repeated has the highest yield for colonoscopy of any known indication.

TABLE 7-12. STUDIES EVALUATING POSITIVE FECAL OCCULT BLOOD TESTS BY BOTH ENDOSCOPY AND BARIUM ENEMA

Study	Patients with positive FOBT, *n*	Studies performed	Cancers detected, *n*	Sensitivity of barium enema for cancers, %	Sensitivity of barium enema for adenomas, %
Kewenter *et al.* [81]	127	C, ACBE	13	62	51
Winawer *et al.* [80]	873	C, FCBE	56	64	35
Sontag *et al.* [79]	76	C, ACBE	8	50	20++
Kronborg *et al.* [78]	32	C, ACBE	12	75	43
Frommer *et al.* [76]	609	C, ACBE	83	75	NS
Hardcastle *et al.* [77]	1831	FS, ACBE	60	75	74+

**Data for rectosigmoid colon only.*
†Sensitivity for adenomas ≥ 1 cm in size. ‡Sensitivity for polyps ≥ 0.5 cm in size.
ACBE—air-contrast barium enema; C—colonoscopy; FCBE—full-column barium enema; FOBT—fecal occult blood test; FS—flexible sigmoidoscopy; NS—not stated.

TABLE 7-12.

Evaluation of positive fecal occult blood tests is best performed by colonoscopy. Because occult bleeding is as common from right-sided as from left-sided tumors, it is essential that the entire colon be evaluated. Flexible sigmoidoscopy is inadequate as a single measure. Barium enema, particularly air-contrast studies, are not uncommonly performed in the evaluation of occult blood tests. However, it is erroneous to presume that the sensitivity of air-contrast barium enema for colorectal cancer in symptomatic patients can be matched in asymptomatic patients. This fact is because tumors in asymptomatic patients are more likely to be Dukes' A and B tumors and not uncommonly may be malignant polyps. Such lesions are more difficult for barium enema to detect than tumors in symptomatic patients, which are largely (60%) Dukes' C and D tumors. In fact, six studies have evaluated both barium enema and endoscopy for cancer and polyp detection in patients with positive fecal occult blood tests [79–82,84,85]. Five of the studies employed air-contrast barium enema, and one used single-contrast barium enema. Five of the six studies used colonoscopy, whereas one used flexible sigmoidoscopy in addition to air-contrast barium enema. The highest sensitivity of barium enema for cancer detection in these six studies is 75%, and polyp sensitivities have been as low as 20%. For this reason essentially all patients with positive fecal occult blood tests should be evaluated by colonoscopy rather than by air-contrast barium enema or flexible sigmoidoscopy plus air-contrast barium enema.

REFERENCES AND RECOMMENDED READING

1. Forde KA: Lower gastrointestinal bleeding: The magnitude of the problem. In *Gastrointestinal Bleeding*. Edited by Sugawa C, Schuman BM, Lucas CE. New York: Igaku-Shoin; 1992:13–25.
2. Waye JD: Diagnostic endoscopy in lower intestinal bleeding. In *Gastrointestinal Bleeding*. Edited by Sugawa C, Schuman BM, Lucas CE. New York: Igaku-Shoin; 1992:230–241.
3. Marshall JB: Acute gastrointestinal bleeding. A logical approach to management. *Postgrad Med* 1990, 87:63–70.
4. Jensen DM, Machicado GA: Diagnosis and treatment of severe hematochezia. The role of urgent colonoscopy after purge. *Gastroenterology* 1988, 95:1569–1574.
5. Rex DK, Weddle RA, Lehman GA, *et al.*: Flexible sigmoidoscopy plus air contrast barium enema versus colonoscopy for suspected lower gastrointestinal bleeding. *Gastroenterology* 1990, 98:855–861.
6. Rossini FP, Ferrari A, Spandre M, *et al.*: Emergency colonoscopy. *World J Surg* 1989, 13:190–192.
7. Shapiro MJ: The role of the radiologist in the management of gastrointestinal bleeding. *Gastroenterol Clin North Am* 1994, 23:123–179.
8. Gelfand DW, Routh WD, Cowan RJ: Diagnostic imaging in gastrointestinal hemorrhage. In *Gastrointestinal Bleeding*. Edited by Sugawa C, Schuman BM, Lucas CE. New York: Igaku-Shoin; 1992:205–221.
9. Rex DK: Instruments and equipment. In *Colonoscopy: Principles and Techniques*. Edited by Nord J, Raskin J. New York: Igaku-Shoin; 1995:17–32.
10. Rege RV, Nahrwold DL: Diverticular disease. *Curr Probl Surg* 1989, 26:133–189.
11. Cheskin LJ: Diverticular disease in the elderly. *Gastroenterol Clin North Am* 1990, 19:391–403.
12. Meyers MA, Alonso DR, Gray GF, Baer JW: Pathogenesis of bleeding colonic diverticulosis. *Gastroenterology* 1976, 71:577–583.
13. Rex DK, Lewis BS: Flexible sigmoidoscopy. Oxford: Blackwell Scientific; 1995.
14. Reinus JF, Brandt LJ: Vascular ectasias and diverticulosis. Common causes of lower intestinal bleeding. *Gastroenterol Clin North Am* 1994, 23:1–20.
15. Dietzen CD, Pemberton JH: Diverticulitis. In *Atlas of Gastroenterology*. Edited by Yamada T. Philadelphia: JB Lippincott; 1992:279–285.
16. Bertoni G, Conigliaro R, Ricci E, *et al.*: Endoscopic injection hemostasis of colonic diverticular bleeding: A case report. *Endoscopy* 1990, 22:154–155.
17. Kim Y, Marcon NE: Injection therapy for colonic diverticular bleeding. A case study. *J Clin Gastroenterol* 1993, 17:46–48.
18. Savides TJ, Jensen DM: Colonoscopic hemostasis for recurrent diverticular hemorrhage associated with a visible vessel: A report of three cases. *Gastrointest Endosc* 1994, 40(1):70–72.
19. Foutch PG: Angiodysplasia of the gastrointestinal tract. *Am J Gastroenterol* 1993, 88:807–818.

20. Hochter W, Weingart J, Kuhner W, *et al.*: Angiodysplasia in the colon and rectum. Endoscopic morphology, localization, and frequency. *Endoscopy* 1985, 17:182–185.

21. Boley SJ, Sammartano R, Adams A: On the nature and etiology of vascular ectasias of the colon. Degenerative lesions of aging. *Gastroenterology* 1977, 72:650–660.

22. Deal SE, Zfass AM, Duckworth PF, *et al.*: Arteriovenous malformation (AVMs). Are they concealed by meperidine [Abstract]? *Am J Gastroenterol* 1991, 86:1351.

23. Richter JM, Christensen MR, Colditz GA, *et al.*: Angiodysplasia: Natural history and efficacy of therapeutic interventions. *Dig Dis Sci* 1989, 34:1542–1546.

24. Jensen DM, Machicado GA: Bleeding colonic angioma: Endoscopic coagulation and follow-up [Abstract]. *Gastroenterology* 1985, 88:1433.

25. van Cutsem E, Rutgeerts P, Vantrappen G: Treatment of bleeding gastrointestinal vascular malformations with oestrogen-progesterone. *Lancet* 1990, 335:953–954.

26. Bronner MH, Pate MB, Cunningham JT, Marsh WH: Estrogen-progesterone therapy for bleeding gastrointestinal telangiectasias in chronic renal failure. *Ann Intern Med* 1986, 105:371–374.

27. Lewis BS, Salomon P, Rivera-MacMurray S, *et al.*: Does hormonal therapy have any benefit for bleeding angiodysplasia? *J Clin Gastroenterol* 1992, 15:99–103.

28. Rossini FP, Arrigoni A, Pennazio M: Octreotide in the treatment of bleeding due to angiodyplasia of the small intestine. *Am J Gastroenterol* 1993, 88:1424–1427.

29. Rogers BHG: Endoscopic diagnosis and therapy of mucosal vascular abnormalities of the gastrointestinal tract occurring in elderly patients and associated with cardiac, vascular, and pulmonary disease. *Gastrointest Endosc* 1980, 26:134–138.

30. Howard OM, Buchanan JD, Hunt RH: Angiodysplasia of the colon: Experience of 16 cases. *Lancet* 1982, 2:16–19.

31. Roberts PL, Schoetz DJ, Coller JA: Vascular ectasia: Diagnosis and treatment by colonoscopy. *Am Surg* 1988, 54:56–57.

32. Rutgeerts R, Van Gompel F, Gebos K, *et al.*: Long-term results of treatment of vascular malformations of the gastrointestinal tract by Neodymium-Yag laser photocoagulation. *Gut* 1985, 26:586–593.

33. Cello JP, Grendell JH: Endoscopic laser treatment for gastrointestinal vascular ectasias. *Ann Intern Med* 1986, 104:352–354.

34. Gostout CJ, Bowyer BA, Ahlquist DA, *et al.*: Mucosal vascular malformations of the gastrointestinal tract: Clinical observations and results of endoscopic neodymium-yttrium-aluminum-garnett laser therapy. *Mayo Clinic Proc* 1988, 63:993–1003.

35. Mathus-Viegen EMH: Laser treatment of intestinal vascular abnormalities. *Int J Colorectal Dis* 1989, 4:20–25.

36. Lanthier PH, D'Harveng B, Vanheuverzwyn R, *et al.*: Colonic angiodysplasia: Follow-up of patients after endoscopic treatment for bleeding lesions. *Dis Colon Rectum* 1989, 32:296–298.

37. Naveau S, Aubert A, Poynard T, *et al.*: Long-term results of treatment of vascular malformations of the gastrointestinal tract by neodymium Yag laser photocoagulation. *Dig Dis Sci* 1990, 35:821–826.

38. Williams CB, Price AB: Colon polyps and carcinoma. In *Gastroenterologic Endoscopy*. Edited by Sivak MV. Philadelphia: WB Saunders; 1987:921–945.

39. Bower TC: Ischemic colitis. *Surg Clin North Am* 1993, 73:1037–1052.

40. Fleshman JN: Fissure in ano and anal stenosis. In *Fundamentals of Anorectal Surgery*. Edited by Beck DE, Wexner SD. New York: McGraw-Hill; 1992:170–182.

41. Robert JR, Sachar DB, Greenstein AJ, *et al.*: Severe gastrointestinal hemorrhage in Crohn's disease. *Ann Surg* 1991, 213:207–211.

42. Rathgaber SW, Rex DK: Colonoscopy and endoscopic therapy of hemorrhage from viral colitis. *Gastrointest Endosc* 1993, 39:737–738.

43. Lanas A, Sekar MC, Hirschowitz BI: Objective evidence of aspirin use in both ulcer and nonulcer upper and lower gastrointestinal bleeding. *Gastroenterology* 1992, 103:862–869.

44. Halter F, Weber B, Huber T, *et al.*: Diaphragm disease of the ascending colon. Association with sustained-release diclofenac. *J Clin Gastroenterol* 1993, 16:74–80.

45. Reilly PJ, Nostrant TT: Clinical manifestations of hereditary hemorrhagic telangiectasia. *Am J Gastroenterol* 1984, 79:363–367.

46. Abdulian JD, Santoro MJ, Chen YK, *et al.*: Dieulafoy-like lesion of the rectum presenting with exsanguinating hemorrhage: Successful endoscopic sclerotherapy. *Am J Gastroenterol* 1993, 88:1939–1941.

47. Cutler CS, Rex DK, Lehman GA: Enteroscopic identification of ectopic small bowel varices. *Gastrointest Endosc*, 1995, 41:605–608.

48. Kozarek RA, Botoman VA, Bredfeldt JE, *et al.*: Portal colopathy: Prospective study of colonoscopy in patients with portal hypertension. *Gastroenterology* 1991, 101:1192–1197.

49. Moses FM: Gastrointestinal bleeding and the athlete. *Am J Gastroenterol* 1993, 88:1157–1159.

50. Porter AMW: Do some marathon runners bleed into the gut? *BMJ* 1983, 287:1427.

51. Keefe EB, Lowe DK, Goss JR, *et al.*: Gastrointestinal symptoms of marathon runners. *West J Med* 1984, 141:481–484.

52. Halvorsen FA, Lyng J, Ritland S: Gastrointestinal bleeding in marathon runners. *Scand J Gastroenterol* 1986, 21:493–497.

53. McCabe ME, Peura DA, Kadakia SC, *et al.*: Gastrointestinal blood loss associated with running a marathon. *Dig Dis Sci* 1986, 31:1229–1232.

54. McMahon LF, Ryan MJ, Larson D, *et al.*: Occult gastrointestinal blood loss in marathon runner. *Ann Intern Med* 1984, 100:836–837.

55. Baska RS, Moses FM, Graeber G, *et al.*: Gastrointestinal bleeding during an ultramarathon. *Dig Dis Sci* 1990, 35:276–279.

56. Lewis BS: Small intestinal bleeding. *Gastroenterol Clin North Am* 1994, 23:67–91.

57. Rex DK, Lappas J, Maglinte D: Enteroclysis in the evaluation of suspected small intestinal bleeding. *Gastroenterology* 1989, 97:58–60.

58. Goulston KJ, Cook I, Dent OF: How important is rectal bleeding in the diagnosis of bowel cancer and polyps? *Lancet* 1986, 261–265.

59. Church JM: Analysis of the colonoscopic findings in patients with rectal bleeding according to the pattern of their presenting symptoms. *Dis Colon Rectum* 1991, 34:391–395.

60. Bat L, Pines A, Shemesh E, *et al.*: Colonoscopy in patients aged 80 years or older and its contribution to the evaluation of rectal bleeding. *Postgrad Med J* 1992, 68:355–358.

61. Berkowitz I, Kaplan M: Indications for colonoscopy. An analysis based on indications and diagnostic yield. *S Afr Med J* 1993, 83:245–248.

62. Irvine EJ, O'Connor J, Forst RA, *et al.*: Prospective comparison of double contrast barium enema plus flexible sigmoidoscopy *v* colonoscopy in rectal bleeding. *Gut* 1988, 28:1188–1193.

63. Thoeni RF, Venbrux AC: The value of colonoscopy and double-contrast barium-enema examinations in the evaluation of the patients with subacute and chronic lower intestinal bleeding. *Radiology* 1983, 146:603–607.

64. Guillem JG, Forde KA, Treat MR, *et al.*: The impact of colonoscopy on the early detection of colonic neoplasms in patients with rectal bleeding. *Ann Surg* 1987, 206:606–611.

65. Brand EJ, Sullivan BH, Sivak MV, *et al.*: Colonoscopy in the diagnosis of unexplained rectal bleeding. *Ann Surg* 1980, 192:111–113.

66. Swarbrick ET, Revre DI, Hunt RH, *et al.*: Colonoscopy for unexplained rectal bleeding. *BMJ* 1978, 2:1658–1687.

67. Teague RH, Manning AP, Thorton JR, *et al.*: Colonoscopy for investigation of unexplained rectal bleeding. *Lancet* 1978, 1350–1352.

68. Tedesco FJ, Pickens CA, Griffin JW, *et al.*: Role of colonoscopy in patients with unexplained melena: Analysis of 53 patients. *Gastrointest Endosc* 1981, 27:221–223.

69. St. John DJB, Young GP, Alexeyeff MA, *et al.*: Evaluation of new occult blood tests for detection of colorectal neoplasia. *Gastroenterology* 1993, 104:1661–1668.

70. Ahlquist DA, Wieand HS, Moertel CH, *et al.*: Accuracy of fecal occult blood screening for colorectal neoplasia. *JAMA* 1993, 269:1262–1267.

71. Simon JB: Occult blood screening for colorectal carcinoma: A critical review. *Gastroenterology* 1985, 88:820–837.

72. Mandel JS, Bond JH, Church TR, *et al.*: Reducing mortality from colorectal cancer by screening for fecal occult blood. *N Engl J Med* 1993, 328:1365–1371.

73. Kim WR, Banerjee B: Outcome of endoscopic evaluation in patients with positive fecal occult blood test (FOBT) on digital rectal exam (DRE) without frank blood loss [Abstract]. *Gastrointest Endosc* 1993, 39:293.

74. Reilly JM, Ballantyne GH, Fleming FX, *et al.*: Evaluation of the occult blood test in screening for colorectal neoplasms. *Am Surg* 1990, 56:119–123.

75. Rex DK, Weddle RA, Lehman GA, *et al.*: Flexible sigmoidoscopy plus air contrast barium enema versus colonoscopy for suspected lower gastrointestinal bleeding. *Gastroenterology* 1990, 98:855–861.

76. Frommer DJ, Kapparis A, Brown MK: Improved screening for colorectal cancer by immunological detection of occult blood. *BMJ* 1988, 296:1092–1094.

77. Hardcastle JD, Chamberlain J, Sheffield J, *et al.*: Randomized controlled trial of fecal occult blood screening for colorectal cancer. *Lancet* 1989, 1160–1164.

78. Kronborg O, Fenger C, Søndergaard O, *et al.*: Initial mass screening for colorectal cancer with fecal occult blood test. *Scand J Gastroenterol* 1987, 22:677–686.

79. Sontag SJ, Durczak C, Aranha GV, *et al.*: Fecal occult blood testing for colorectal cancer in a Veteran's Administration hospital. *Am J Surg* 1983, 145:89–93.

80. Winawer SJ, Flehinger BJ, Schottenfeld D, *et al.*: Screening for colorectal cancer with fecal occult blood testing and sigmoidoscopy. *J Natl Cancer Inst* 1991, 85:1311–1318.

81. Kewenter J, Engarås B, Haglind E, *et al.*: Value of retesting subjects with a positive Hemoccult® in screening for colorectal cancer. *Br J Surg* 1990, 77:1349–1351.

82. Elliott MS, Levenstein JH, Wright JP: Faecal occult blood testing in the detection of colorectal cancer. *Br J Surg* 1984, 71:785–786.

83. Hobbs FDR, Cherry RC, Fielding JWL, *et al.*: Acceptability of opportunistic screening for occult gastrointestinal blood loss. *BMJ* 1992, 304:483–486.

84. Gilbertsen VA, McHugh R, Schuman L, *et al.*: The earlier detection of colorectal cancers. A preliminary report of the results of the occult blood study. *Cancer* 1980, 45:2899–2901.

85. Frühmorgen P, Demling L: Early detection of colorectal carcinoma with a modified guaiac test: A screening examination in 6000 humans. *Acta Gastroenterol Belg* 1978, 41:682–687.

Chapter

8

Colon and Rectal Surgery

Frederic E. Eckhauser
James A. Knol
Lisa M. Colletti

Colorectal diseases occur worldwide in medical and surgical practice and commonly result in complications that confound even the most experienced practitioner. Clinical manifestations can often be treated medically with good results. However, many complications of colorectal disease are potentially life threatening and require surgical intervention. Surgical strategy is generally based on sound surgical principles as well as an in-depth understanding of the relevant anatomy and the potential outcomes of treatment. Astute physicians are highly skilled in assessing the need for surgical evaluation and treatment, but they rarely understand the diverse factors that influence surgical decision making. This chapter provides a utilitarian review of colorectal anatomy as well as a summary of general surgical principles and treatment strategies for several common colorectal diseases, including carcinoma, diverticular disease, and ulcerative colitis. In addition, a section has been devoted to ostomies and their management. The goal is to facilitate physician-surgeon communication and thereby provide a sound basis for improved patient counseling.

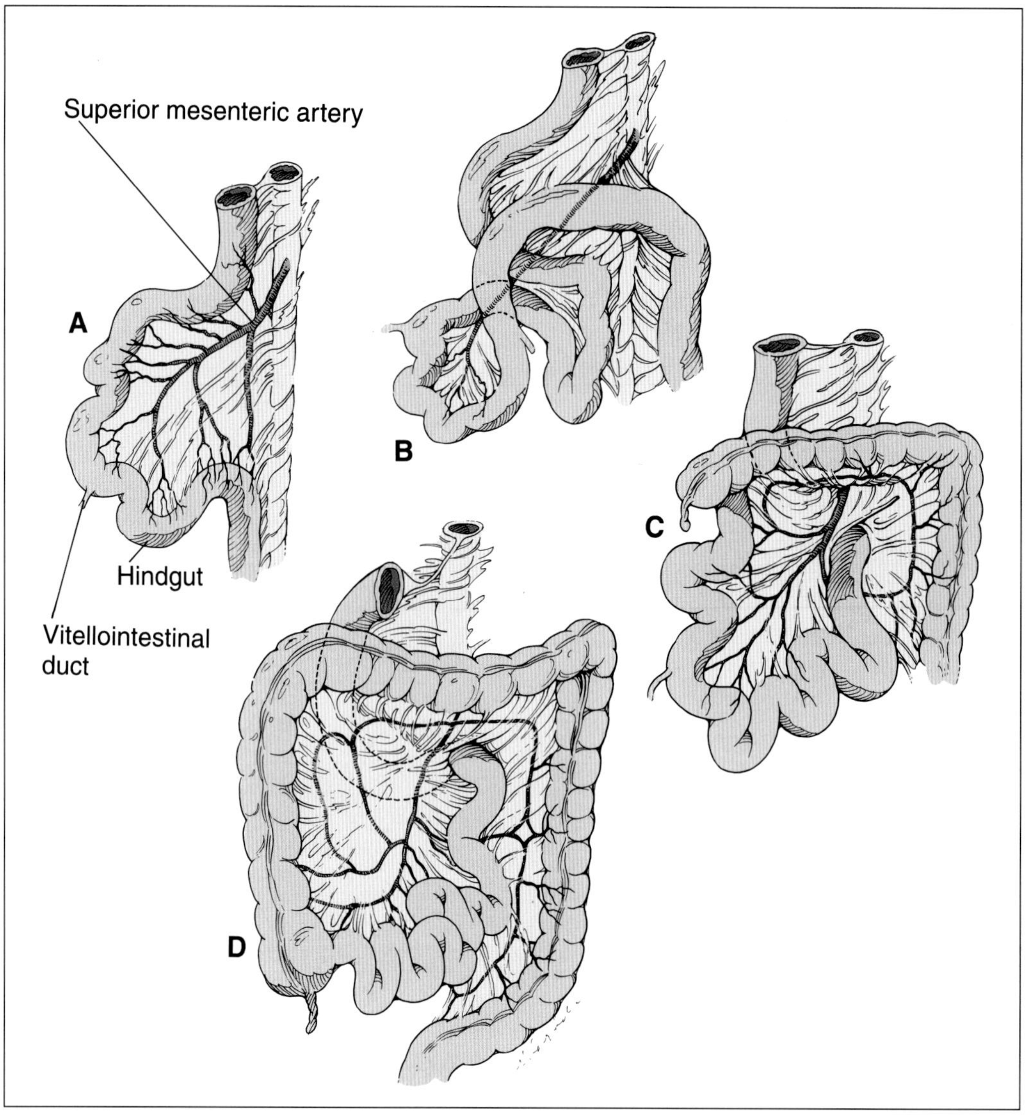

FIGURE 8-1.

The primitive intestinal tract. The primitive intestinal tract begins as a straight digestive tube suspended by a common dorsal mesentery. During embryologic development, the primitive digestive tube elongates on its mesenteric axis and bulges along the umbilical cord (**A**). As the midgut loop returns to the peritoneal cavity, it undergoes a counterclockwise rotation and ultimately becomes fixed to the posterior peritoneum (**B**). This figure illustrates the normal development sequence of midgut formation and extrusion into the coelomic cavity with subsequent return to the peritoneal cavity, followed by rotation and fixation (**C** and **D**). Anomalies of rotation and fixation frequently distort normal anatomical relationships and may give rise to internal hernias or bowel obstruction sometimes associated with vascular compromise and infarction [1]. Anomalies of blood supply may result in colonic atresia, which characteristically affects a distal site and may prove an elusive diagnosis with an associated high mortality. (*From* Zimmerman and Laufman [1]; with permission.)

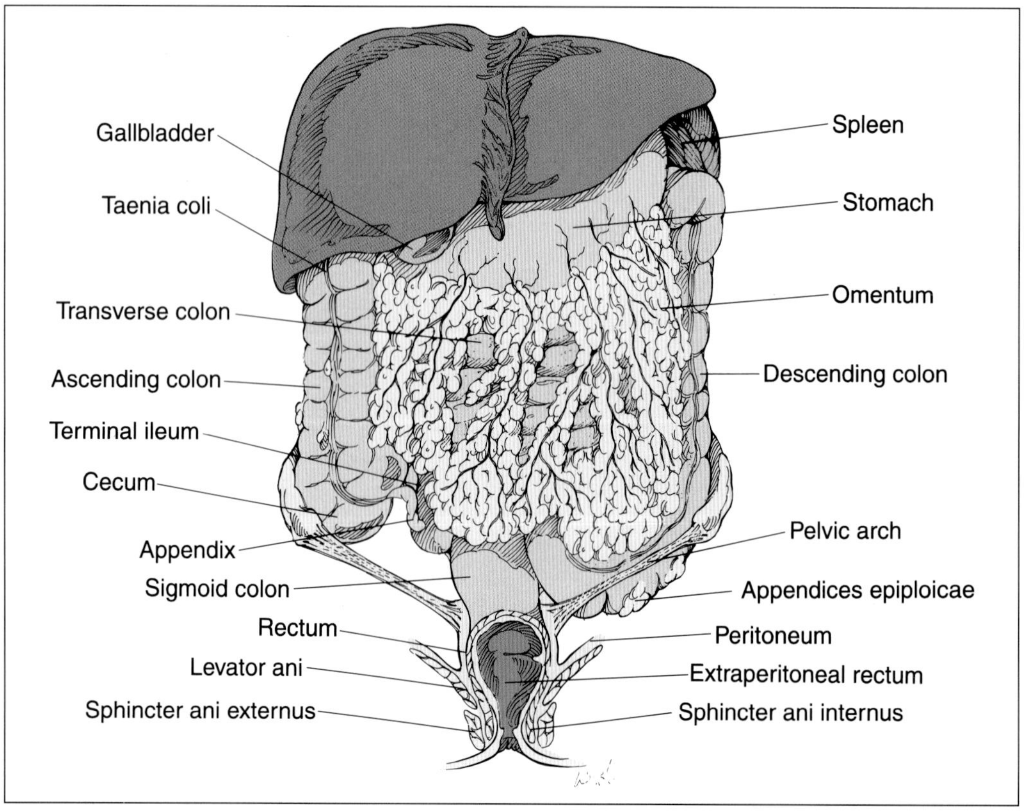

FIGURE 8-2.

The general position and relationship of the colon and rectum to other abdominal viscera. The colon is 120 to 200 cm in length and is highly distensible. This segment of bowel can be visually distinguished from the small intestine by the presence of longitudinal muscle bands called *taenia coli*, which extend from the cecum to the rectosigmoid, haustral sacculations or pouches created as a result of "bunching" of the colon by the taenia coli, and appendices epiploicae or fatty appendages that are most numerous along the taenia coli. The ascending and descending portions of the colon are fixed by peritoneum to the posterior and lateral abdominal wall. The transverse colon is highly movable and forms a natural partition between the supra- and inframesocolic compartments of the abdominal cavity. The sigmoid colon consists of fixed (iliac) and mobile (pelvic) segments and becomes continuous with the rectum below the sacral promontory. (*From* Keighley and Williams [2]; with permission.)

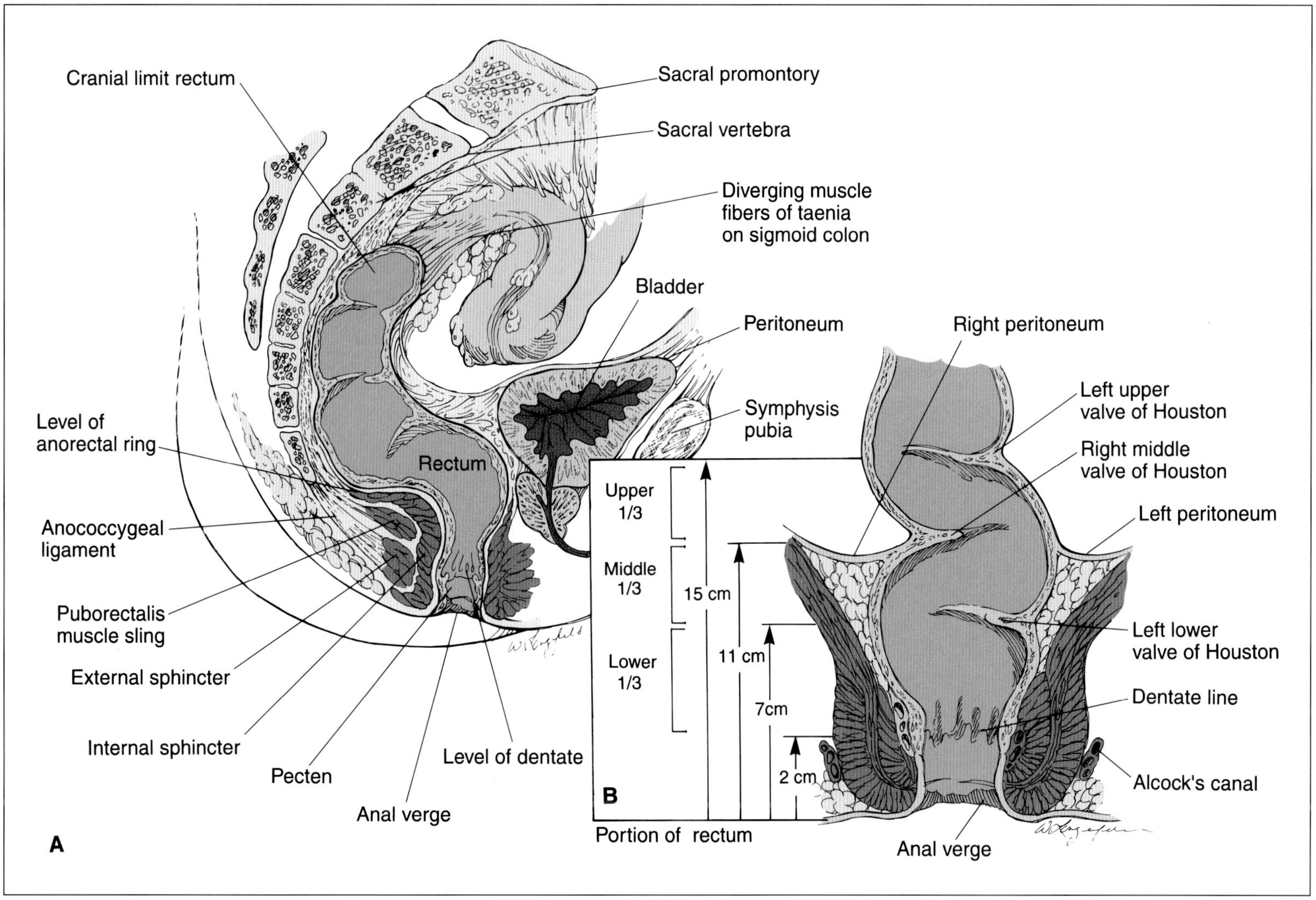

FIGURE 8-3.

Anatomy of the rectum. The rectum begins at the level of the sacral promontory at a point where the taenia coli fuse to form a continuous longitudinal muscle layer. It descends along the curve of the sacral hollow to the level of the levator ani and then turns downwards and posteriorly through the anorectal ring (**A**). The rectum is anatomically separated into upper, middle, and lower thirds based on approximate distances between the lower, middle, and upper valves of Houston and the dentate line (**B**). The vascular supply and lymphatic drainage of the upper one third of the rectum differs from that of the middle and lower two thirds and clinically influences treatment strategies for rectal cancer. (*From* Pemberton [3]; with permission.)

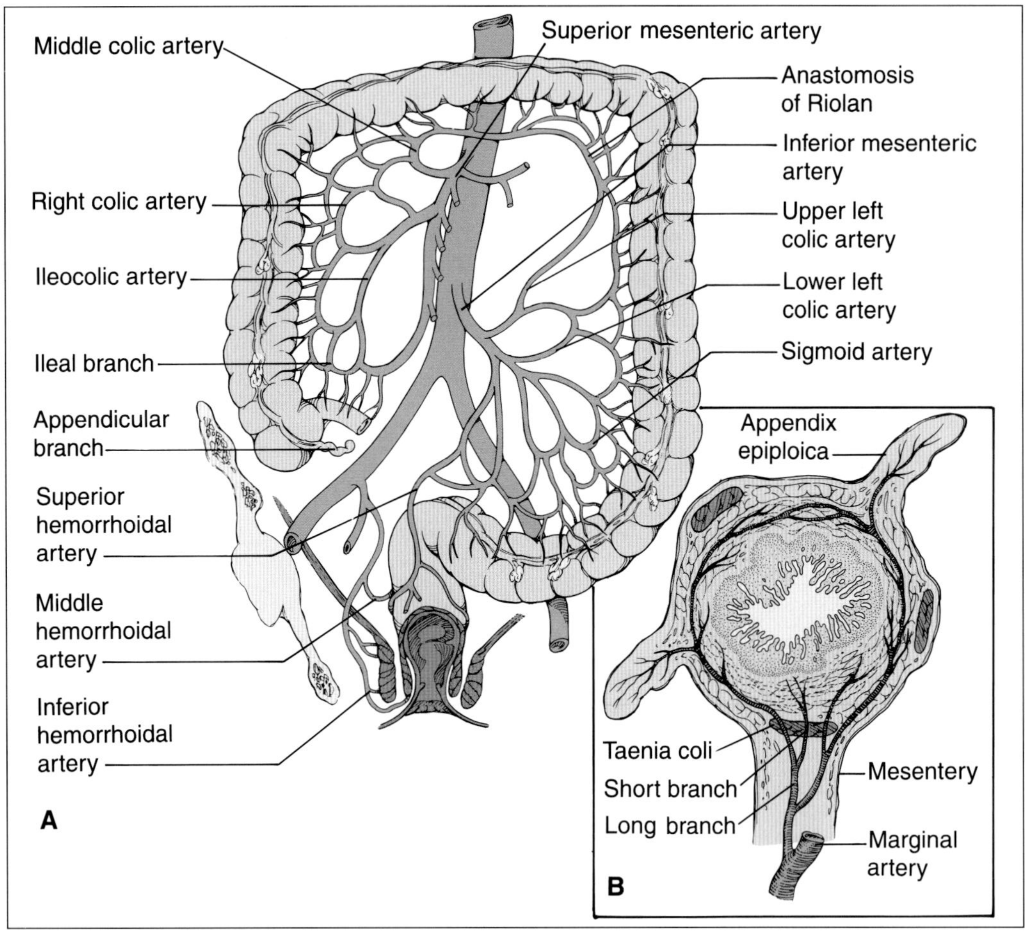

FIGURE 8-4.

Arteries of the colon and rectum. The colon and rectum derive their vascular supply from the superior and inferior mesenteric arteries (**A**). Branches of the superior mesenteric artery supply the territories of the cecum, ascending colon, and transverse colon to its midpoint. The inferior mesenteric artery supplies the left transverse colon as well as the descending and sigmoid portions of the colon and terminates as the superior hemorrhoidal artery to supply the upper one third of the rectum. The middle and lower two thirds of the rectum are supplied by branches arising from the internal iliac artery. The marginal artery of Riolan is formed by anastomozing vessels derived from both the superior and inferior mesenteric arteries and gives rise to terminal branches that run perpendicular to the bowel wall (**B**). These terminal branches in turn supply the adjacent colon wall and mucosa as well as the antimesocolic portion of the bowel wall and the appendices epiploicae. This artery is not usually critical but assumes much greater importance if the inferior mesenteric artery becomes occluded by atherosclerosis or is sacrificed during aortic aneurysmectomy. (*From* Keighley and Williams [2]; with permission.)

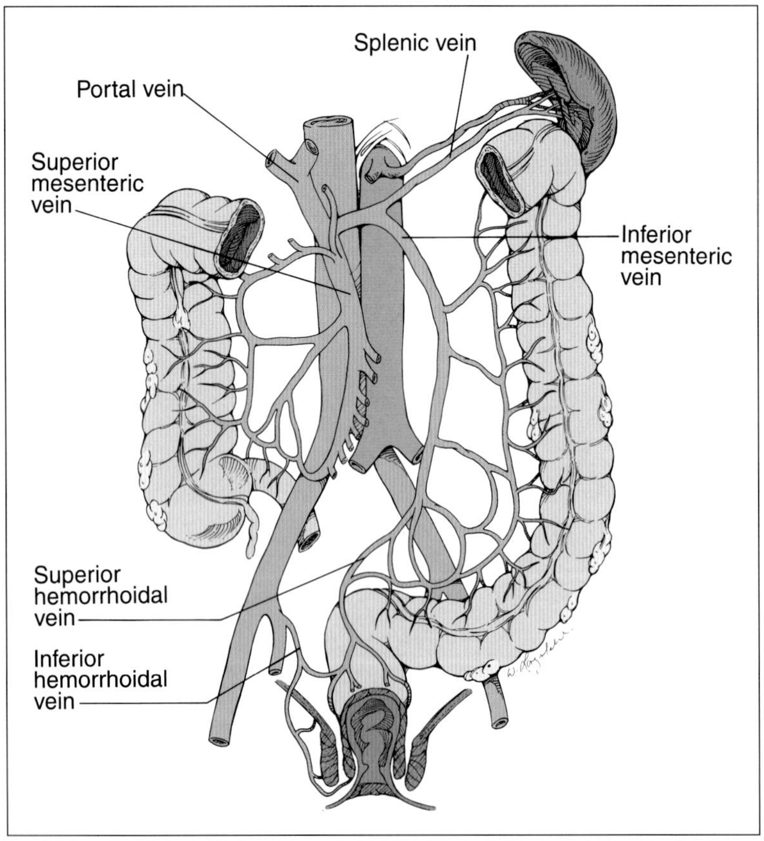

FIGURE 8-5.

Venous drainage of the colon. The venous drainage of the colon generally mirrors the arterial supply but differs with respect to the rectum. The superior hemorrhoidal plexus is submucosal in location and drains proximally into the inferior mesenteric and portal circulations. Because these veins are valveless, portal hypertension may be manifested by the development of internal hemorrhoids. The inferior hemorrhoidal plexus is extramuscular in location and originates from small vessels surrounding the anal canal. This plexus drains via the inferior and middle hemorrhoidal veins into the pudendal and hypogastric veins, respectively, and thereby enters the systemic venous circulation. Rich communications exist between these venous plexuses. (*From* Keighley and Williams [2]; with permission.)

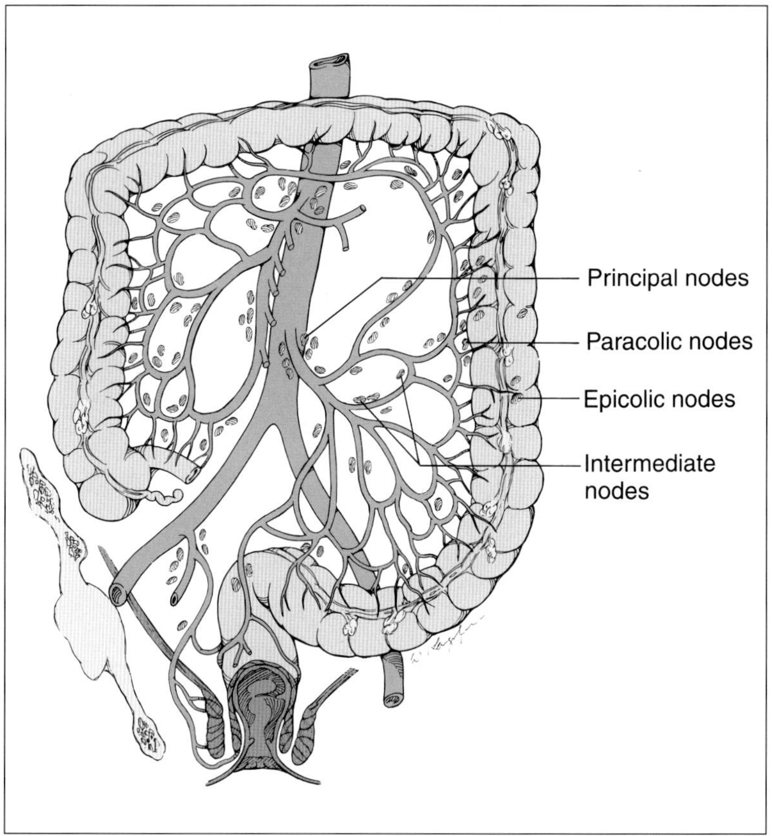

FIGURE 8-6.

Lymphatic drainage of the colon. The lymphatic drainage of the colon is uniform throughout and follows its vascular supply. Lymphatics located in the submucosa and subserosa communicate freely through the muscular layers and terminate in the epicolic nodes, which lie in the colon wall beneath the serosa. Epicolic nodes in turn drain to paracolic nodes, which are located along the mesial portion of the colon wall invested by peritoneum. Paracolic nodes then drain into intermediate nodes that correspond to the arteries supplying given territories of the colon. From the intermediate nodes, lymph from the entire colon proximal to the splenic flexure drains into the principal nodes surrounding the superior mesenteric vessels. Lymph from the colon distal to the splenic flexure drains into principal nodes along the inferior mesenteric vessels. Lymph from both groups of principal nodes ultimately drains into the iliolumbar chain, which empties into the thoracic duct. (*From* Keighley and Williams [2]; with permission.)

PRINCIPLES OF BOWEL ANASTOMOSIS

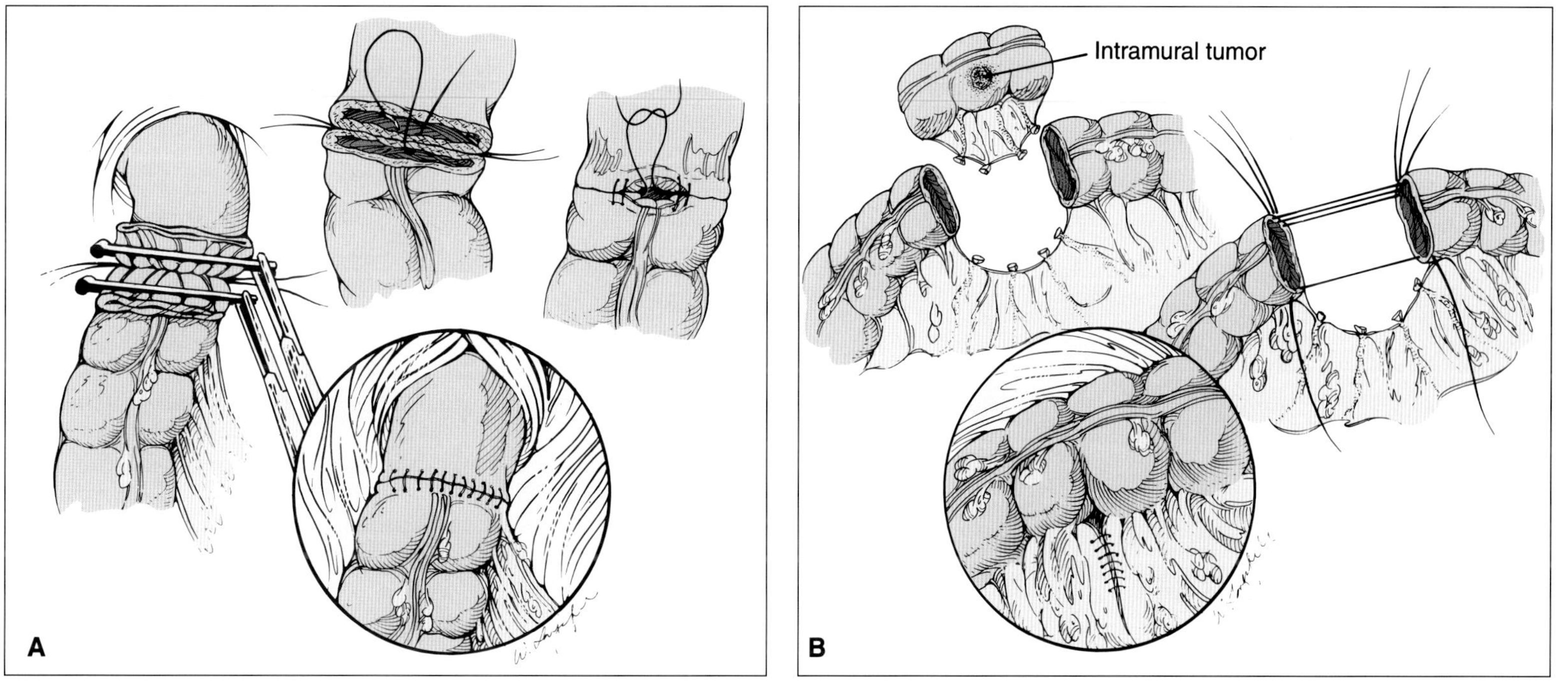

FIGURE 8-7.

Bowel anastomosis. To avoid postsurgical complications after large bowel anastomosis, certain principles must be adhered to at all times. These principles include adequate exposure of the two ends of the bowel to be reanastomosed, adequate blood supply, meticulous tissue apposition, and lack of tension on the anastomosis. The development of a leak following large bowel anastomosis substantially increases mortality and morbidity and results in significant prolongation of hospital stay [4].

The principles of manual or handsewn large bowel anastomosis have evolved significantly during the past century. Techniques that achieve serosal apposition and inversion of the mucosa result in lower anastomotic leak rates and are generally preferred worldwide. However, the issue of one-layer versus two-layer anastomoses remains controversial. Most experimental and clinical studies show no significant differences between the two techniques, despite

(*Continued on next page*)

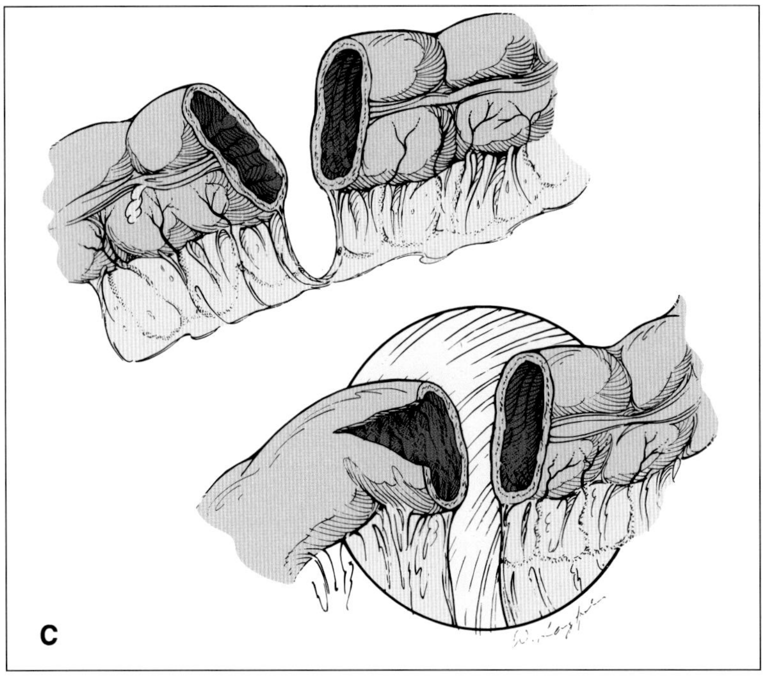

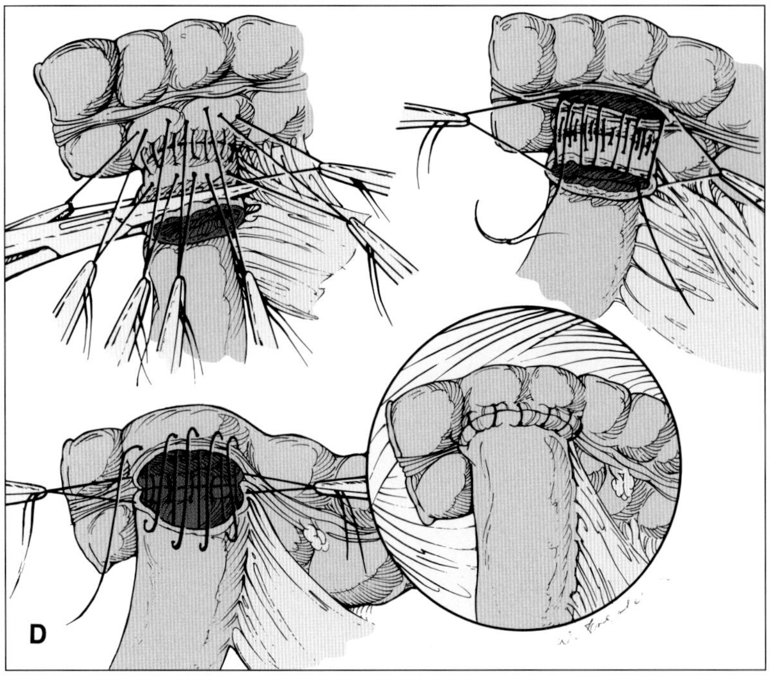

FIGURE 8-7. (CONTINUED)

theoretical concerns that a two-layer anastomosis will result in more tissue ischemia and narrowing of the colon lumen. One-layer anastomoses are easier to perform, have a dehiscence rate that is comparable with two-layer anastomoses, and are generally favored for low colorectal lesions.

Most surgeons favor an open technique for bowel anastomosis. This figure illustrates a traditional two-layer handsewn anastomosis (**A**). This type of anastomosis consists of front and back outer rows of interrupted seromuscular sutures and an inner row of continuous, full thickness sutures. Once the bowel ends have been opened and hemostasis has been achieved, redundant tissue is removed to avoid creating a large tissue ridge that could compromise luminal patency. For left-sided or low colonic anastomoses, many surgeons prefer to interrupt the inner row of sutures to avoid potential narrowing of the bowel lumen. Alternatively, a one-layer anastomosis can be employed (**B**). Using this technique, the divided bowel ends can be approximated with either full thickness or extramucosal sutures, which produce excellent inversion and may lessen the risk of tissue ischemia and dehiscence. Disparities in bowel diameter can be troublesome when constructing an end-to-end anastomosis. These difficulties can usually be overcome by dividing the bowel ends obliquely or enlarging one lumen by opening the bowel along the antimesenteric border (**C**). When bowel disparity prohibits end-to-end bowel anastomosis, an end-to-side or side-to-side anastomosis can yield satisfactory results (**D**). (**A** and **B**, *From* Condon [5]; with permission.) (**C** and **D**, *From* Keighley and Williams [2]; with permission.)

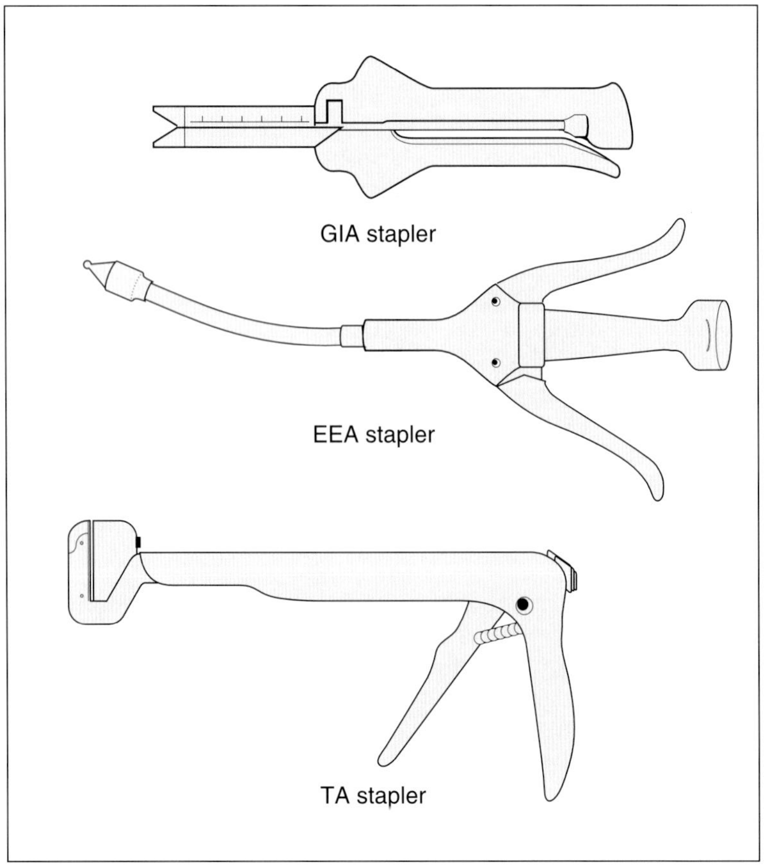

FIGURE 8-8.

Staplers. Stapling techniques were initially developed in Russia during the 1950s but were not introduced into Western surgical practice until the early to mid-1970s. These instruments facilitate closure and anastomosis of the colon, and the low colorectal anastomoses may reduce the risk of dehiscence compared with conventional handsewn or manual anastomic techniques. Currently linear staplers, linear cutters, and circular stapler or cutters are available for colorectal surgery. Each tool has different applications, and several tools are generally used in a complimentary manner to either close or anastomose bowel. EEA—End to End Anastomosis stapler; GIA—Gastrointestinal Anastomosis stapler; TA—Thoracic Abdominal stapler. (*From* Condon [5]; with permission.)

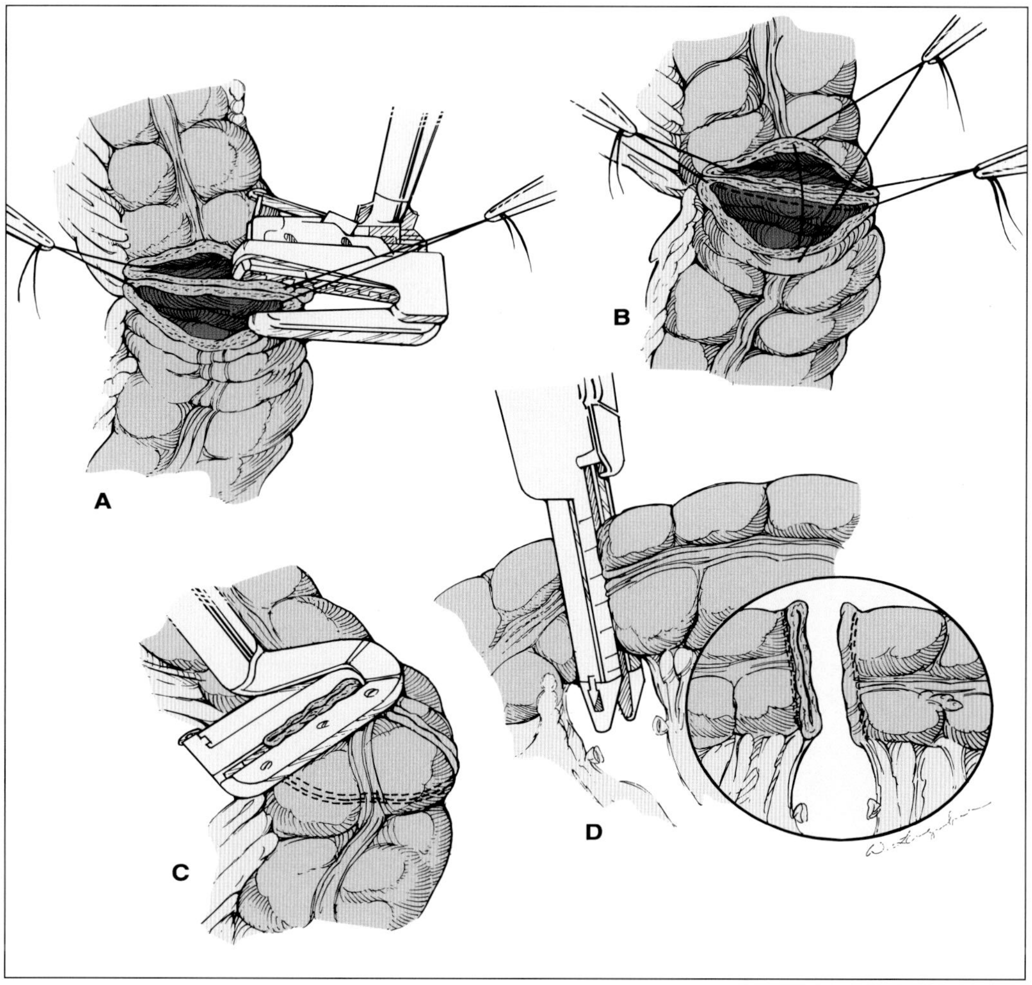

FIGURE 8-9.

Linear staplers. Linear staplers are designed to close a viscus by first apposing the two walls of the bowel without crushing them and then by inserting a double row of stainless steel staples (**A**). The staples are designed to provide firm tissue apposition without significant tissue ischemias that might predispose to anastomotic dehiscence. Stapled anastomoses are generally not as hemostatic as manual or handsewn anastomoses, and postoperative bleeding is a potential problem. To avoid this complication, most surgeons visually inspect all stapled anastomoses whenever possible. Sites of bleeding can be easily controlled with sutures or electrocoagulation. Linear staplers come in different lengths and staple heights. Larger staples (4.8 mm) are generally used for colorectal anastomoses. A linear stapler is generally used to close the divided end of the bowel but can also be used to construct an end-to-end bowel anastomosis. This method requires suture approximation of the divided bowel ends and closure of the bowel with three separate stapler applications to form a triangular anastomosis (**B**). Excess tissue is excised following insertion of each stapleline to avoid narrowing the bowel lumen, and hemostasis is achieved with sutures or cautery. Anastomotic integrity can be checked by immersing the bowel segment completely in sterile saline used for irrigation and compressing the normal bowel on either side of the anastomosis. An intact anastomosis should be airtight. The appearance of air bubbles in the irrigation fluid signifies a leak and should prompt careful inspection and repair of the anastomosis before returning the bowel to the peritoneal cavity and closing the abdomen.

Linear staple cutter instruments (**C**) come in various lengths and are useful for closing and dividing the bowel with a minimum of fecal spillage. All of these instruments work by inserting four rows of staples and dividing the bowel with a specially designed cutting blade (**D**). Prior to inserting the linear cutter, a small area devoid of blood supply is cleared along the mesial aspect of the bowel wall. Application and firing of this instrument across an area of well-vascularized mesentery can lead to troublesome bleeding. (*From* Condon [5]; with permission.)

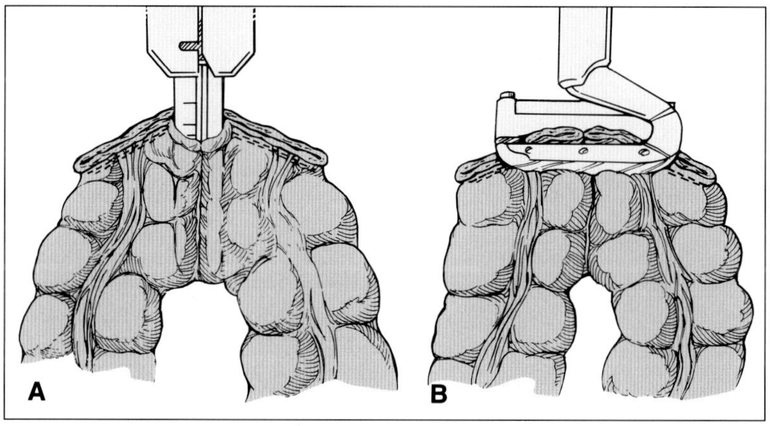

FIGURE 8-10.

Linear stapling and circular stapling instruments. A linear cutter instrument can also be combined with a linear stapler to construct a functional end-to-end bowel anastomosis (EEA) (**A**). The divided bowel ends are first approximated with several sutures placed along the antimesenteric border. A small hole is created in each segment of bowel for introduction of the forks of the linear cutter. The instrument is closed, and the cutting blade is advanced creating a side-to-side anastomosis (**B**). The stapleline is inspected to ensure adequate hemostasis. The opened corners are approximated and closed with a linear stapler that is positioned to slightly overlap the previously placed staplelines.

Circular stapling instruments differ from linear instruments by creating an inverted circumferential anastomosis. The device was initially developed in Russia and introduced into Western surgical practice in the mid- to late 1970s. The most recent generation of circular staplers are easy to use, are highly reliable, and have achieved widespread acceptance throughout the surgical community. The instrument consists of a removable anvil and a staple-containing cartridge with a movable shaft and compression handles for firing the device (*see* Fig. 8-12B). Although these instruments were originally designed for EEA and were aptly designated EEA, they can also be used in combination with linear staplers to construct end-to-side or side-to-side anastomoses. (*From* Condon [5]; with permission.)

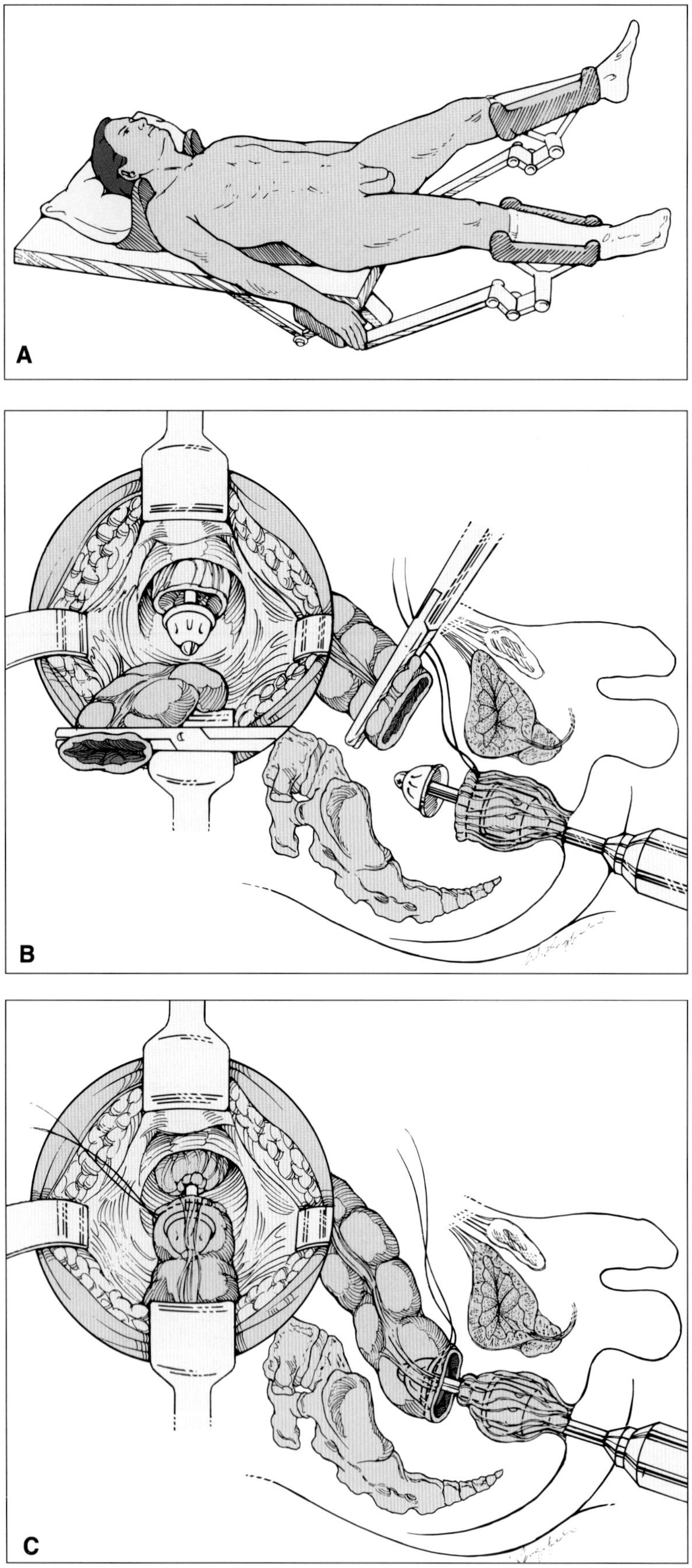
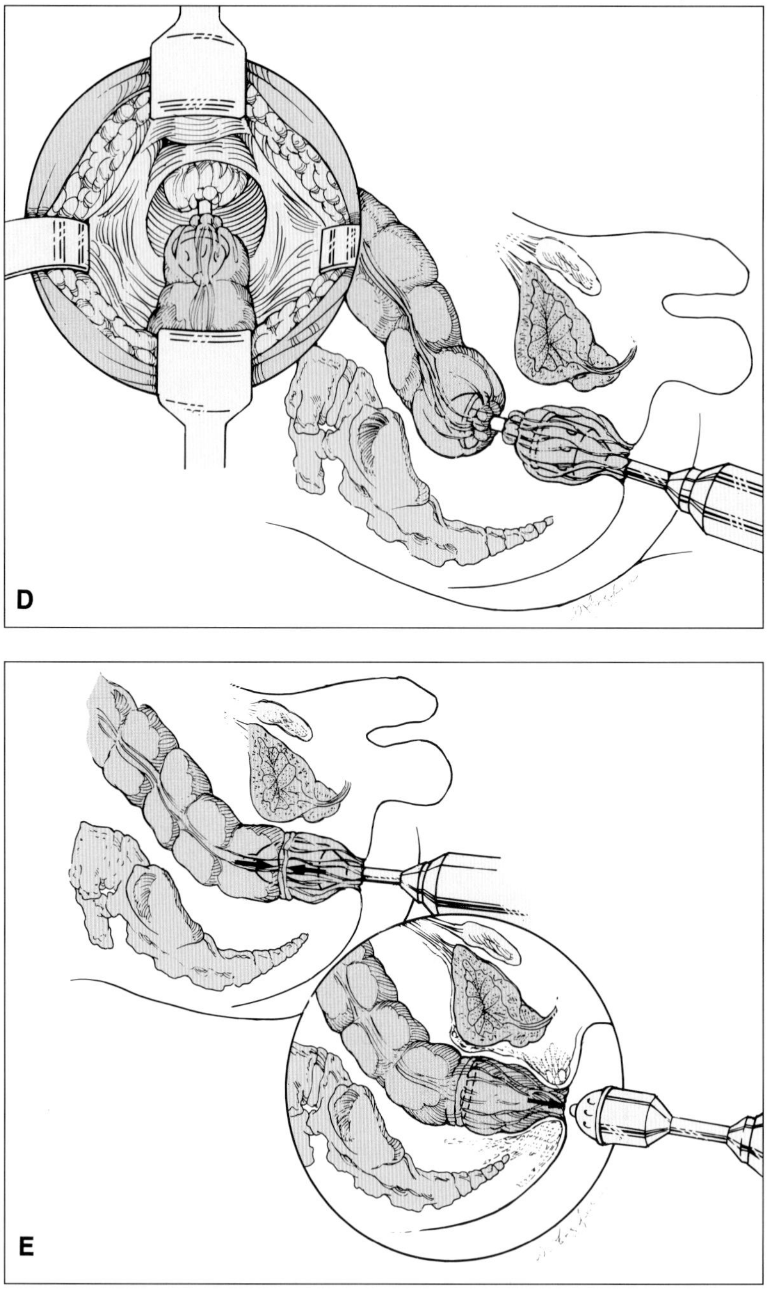

FIGURE 8-11.

Single-staple technique. The stapling devices are particularly useful for low colorectal, ileoanal, or coloanal anastomoses, which may not be technically feasible or safe using manual or handsewn techniques. End-to-end anastomosis with a circular stapler can be accomplished using either a single-staple technique or a double-staple technique. Both techniques can be best illustrated using low colorectal anastomosis as an example. The patient is placed in a modified lithotomy position to afford simultaneous access to the perineum and the peritoneal cavity (**A**). The single-staple technique requires placement of a circumferential pursestring suture of 2-0 polypropylene in the proximal colon and distal rectal remnants. This suture should include the full thickness of the bowel wall but should not include excessive tissue that would complicate securing the closed bowel end around the post of the stapler. The head of the stapler is introduced transanally, and the shaft is maximally extended separating the anvil from the cartilage (**B**). The rectal pursestring suture is tied securely and any gaps should be reinforced with additional sutures. Once the distal pursestring suture has been secured, the proximal colon is advanced over the anvil, and its pursestring suture securely tied (**C**). The stapler is slowly closed by rotating the shaft in a clockwise fashion, thereby approximating the proximal and distal bowel segments (**D**). Care must be taken to exclude extraneous tissue such as fat or mesentery from the anastomosis to insure correct tissue apposition and to minimize the risk of leakage. Once the stapler has been securely closed, the handles are compressed, thereby discharging a blade that cuts through the two bowel ends, producing "doughnuts" of tissue. The shaft of the stapler is rotated counterclockwise to slightly separate the anvil from the cartridge and the instrument is carefully removed using a rocking motion (**E**). (*From* Vernava and Goldberg [6]; with permission.)

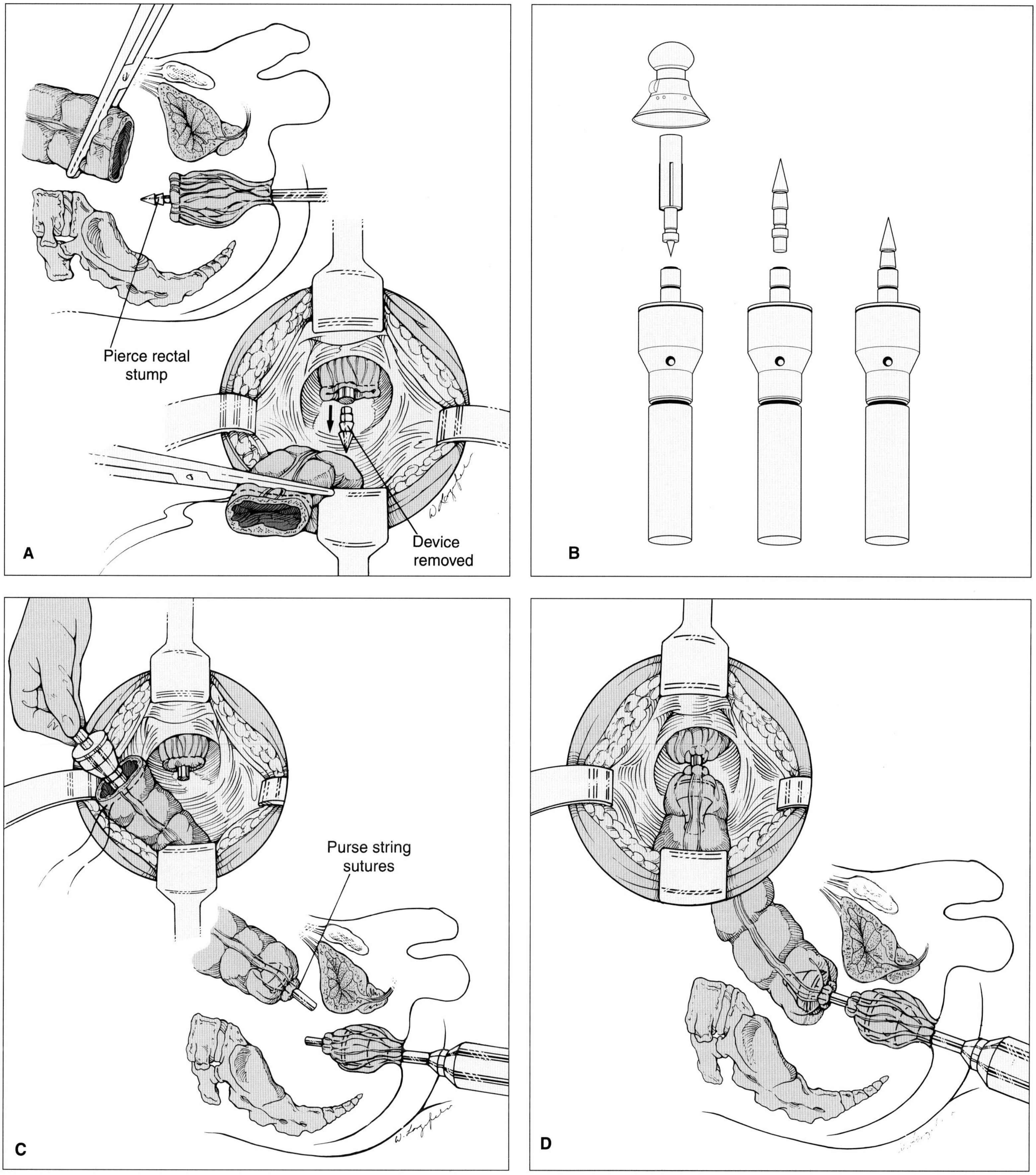

FIGURE 8-12.

Double-staple technique. This may be a useful option, especially for very distal rectal lesions where placement of a pursestring suture may be extremely difficult. This fact is especially true in men with a narrow, android pelvis and in morbidly obese patients in whom access to the pelvic is compromised. Prior to removing the diseased bowel segment, the distal rectum is closed with a linear stapling instrument. The integrity of the rectal closure is checked by insufflating air with the rectum submersed under sterile irrigation fluid. A pursestring suture of 2-0 polypropylene is placed in the divided proximal colon and left untied (**A**). A circular stapler with a removable center post is essential for this procedure. The post used ordinarily to secure the anvil to the stapler cartridge is removed and replaced with a plastic trochar (**B**). The shaft of the stapler containing the cartridge assembly is introduced

(Continued on next page)

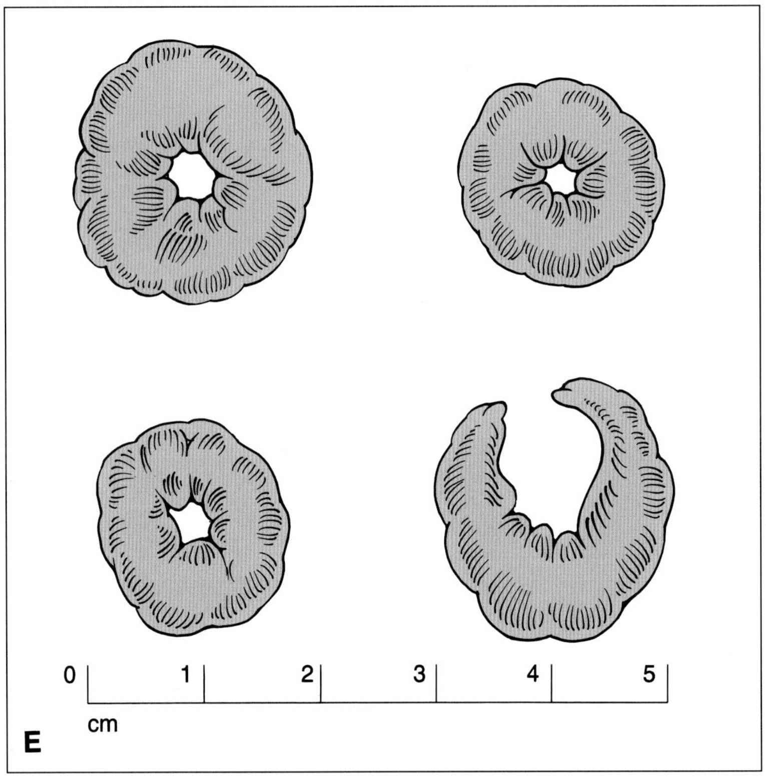

FIGURE 8-12. *(CONTINUED)*

transanally and advanced under direct vision to the level of the staple closure. Once the cartridge has been positioned near the center of the linear staple closure, the trochar is advanced through or immediately adjacent to the stapleline. The removable post and attached anvil is inserted into the proximal colon segment, and the previously placed pursestring suture is securely tied (**C**). The anvil post is inserted into a receptacle in the cartridge head and locked before closing the instrument. The stapler is closed under direct vision to insure that no extraneous tissue is trapped between the anvil and cartridge components and is then fired (**D**). The stapler is gently removed, and the doughnuts of tissue removed should be retrieved and inspected. An incomplete doughnut indicates a possible defect in the anastomosis (**E**). Before closing the abdomen, the integrity of the colorectal anastomosis should be checked by sigmoidoscopic inspection and air insufflation with the anastomosis submerged in sterile water. Small defects can be corrected with additional sutures. If the suture line is inaccessible for local repair, a diverting proximal colostomy should be considered to divert the fecal stream and prevent subsequent leakage and peritonitis. (**A–D**, *From* Vernava and Goldberg [6]; with permission.) (**E**, *From* Keighley and Williams [2]; with permission.)

SURGICAL TREATMENT OF COLORECTAL CARCINOMA

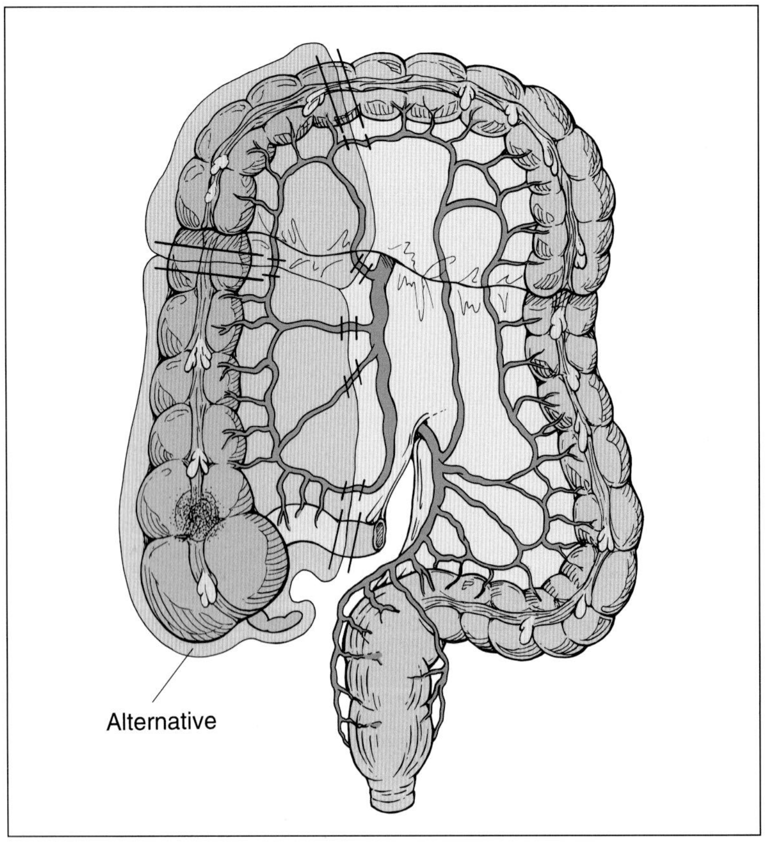

FIGURE 8-13.

Right hemicolectomy. The incidence of carcinoma of the colon and rectum continues to increase in the United States. It is estimated that each year approximately 150,000 new cases will be diagnosed and 60,000 patients will die of this disease. Certain groups of patients are predisposed to develop colon cancer during their lifetime. These identifiable, high-risk groups include patients with familial polyposis, other polyposis variants such as Gardner's syndrome and Turcot syndrome, and inflammatory conditions such as ulcerative colitis and Crohn's disease. In addition, ureterocolonic diversion and species-specific forms of endocarditis appear to increase the risk of colon cancer. Regardless of the underlying cause, the prognosis of large bowel cancer is related to multiple factors including the stage of disease at the time of diagnosis, the presence or absence of vascular or lymphatic invasion, the grade of histologic differentiation, and additional variables such as tumor size and DNA ploidy. Numerous schemes have been developed to stage colorectal cancer, but the simplest and most reproducible schemes are based on pathologic findings. Such systems have moderate prognostic value and facilitate study of adjuvant therapies by defining specific risk groups that can be compared with one another.

Surgery remains the mainstay of treatment for primary colon and rectal carcinoma. The mechanisms by which colorectal cancers spread include direct continuity within and through the bowel wall, dissemination into paracolic and regional lymphatics, spread via the bloodstream, and gravitational spread throughout the peritoneal cavity with implantation on contiguous and distant organs. The basic surgical principles of treating colorectal cancer include en bloc resection of the primary tumor including a margin of healthy tissue on either side of the primary lesion, in continuity resection of extramural and regional lymphatics, and efforts to minimize local implantation and venous embolization.

For carcinomas arising in the vermiform, appendix, cecum, and ascending colon, most surgeons recommend a right hemicolectomy dividing the ileocolic, right colic, and right branch of the middle colic vessels as close to their origin as possible. Some authors recommend more conservative resection for carcinoma of the cecum with sparing the hepatic flexure of the colon. For tumors of the hepatic flexure, both divisions of the middle colic vessels are divided, and the ileocolic vessels are spared. Bowel continuity is then restored using a variety of established stapled or handsewn techniques. (*From* Keighley and Williams [2]; with permission.)

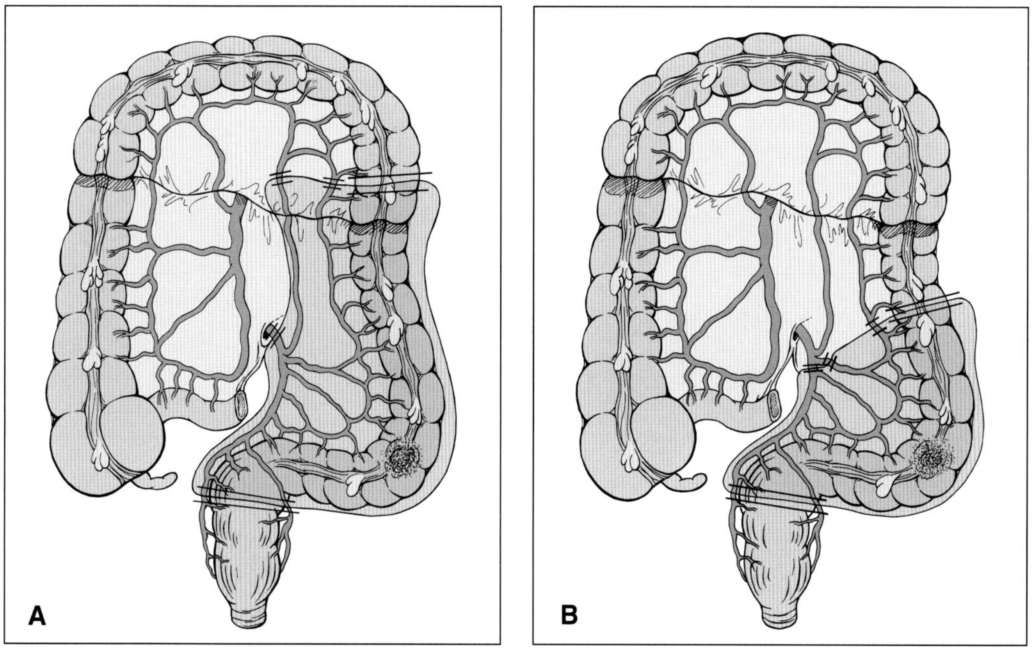

FIGURE 8-14.

Resections. The left colon includes left transverse, splenic flexure, descending, and sigmoid portions to the level of the sacral promontory or pelvic inlet. For cancers arising in the left colon, many prefer a classic left colectomy that includes division of the inferior mesentery vessels and incorporates adjacent mesentery and colonic attachments (**A**). Some authors advocate more selective, less radical resections, especially for elderly or infirm patients [7]. For example, a limited resection for a cancer arising in the sigmoid colon might include dividing the sigmoid vessels with sparing of the main trunk of the inferior mesenteric vessels (**B**). Because there are no prospective data demonstrating that the radical left colectomy confers better survival than more limited resections, the type of operation performed is likely to be influenced by the surgeon's training and personal bias. In addition to resection of bowel, mesocolon, and lymphatic tissues, it is sometimes necessary to excise a portion or all of an adjacent structure or organ that is adherent to the primary tumor. If the surgeon is well trained and versed in the principles and techniques of oncologic surgery, multivisceral resections can be lifesaving and should not be discouraged. (*From* Keighley and Williams [2]; with permission.)

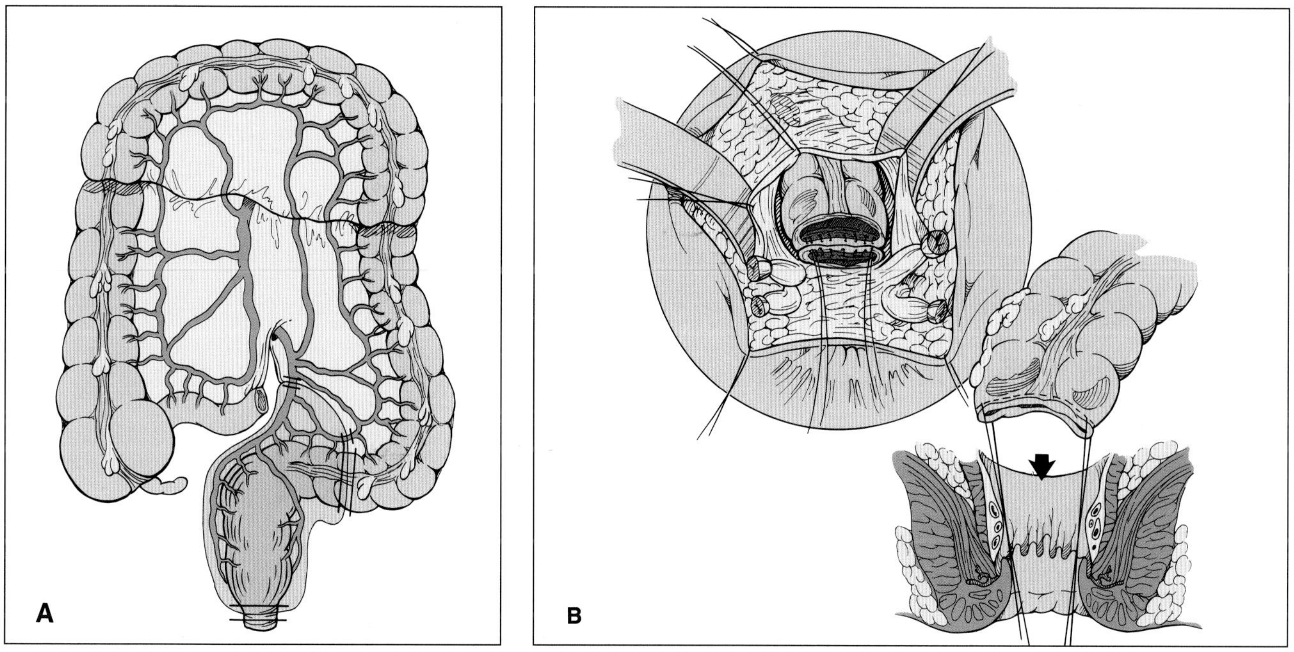

FIGURE 8-15.

Sphincter-saving procedures. Traditionally, carcinomas of the rectum have been treated by abdominoperineal resection with permanent end sigmoid colostomy. Improved understanding of the mechanisms of colorectal cancer spread and recent development of linear and circular stapling instruments have encouraged the use of sphincter-saving procedures that avoid the need for permanent colostomy. Anterior resections are appropriate for tumors arising in the mid- and upper portions of the rectum (**A**). Ideally, the resection should include a 2-cm margin of normal tissue beyond the tumor as well as the associated mesentery and draining lymphatics. Anatomic factors such as obesity and the boney margins of the pelvic may restrict the radical extent of the resection as one proceeds distally, especially in males. These limitations are more theoretical than practical because there is adequate published data to suggest that abdominoperineal resection confers no survival advantage over low anterior resection for cancers of the mid- and upper rectum [8]. It is now estimated that approximately two thirds of patients with rectal cancer can be treated with sphincter-sparing resections. However, sphincter-saving procedures should not be considered if the potential for curative resection would be compromised. As mentioned previously, deep pelvic dissection and removal of a relatively distal rectal cancer may be difficult in obese or male patients with a narrow pelvis. In these situations, alternative sphincter-saving resection techniques have included abdominotransanal resection and abdominotranssphincteric resection (**B**). However, introduction of staplers and improved stapling techniques has rendered both of these latter procedures relatively obsolete. (*From* Keighley and Williams [2]; with permission.)

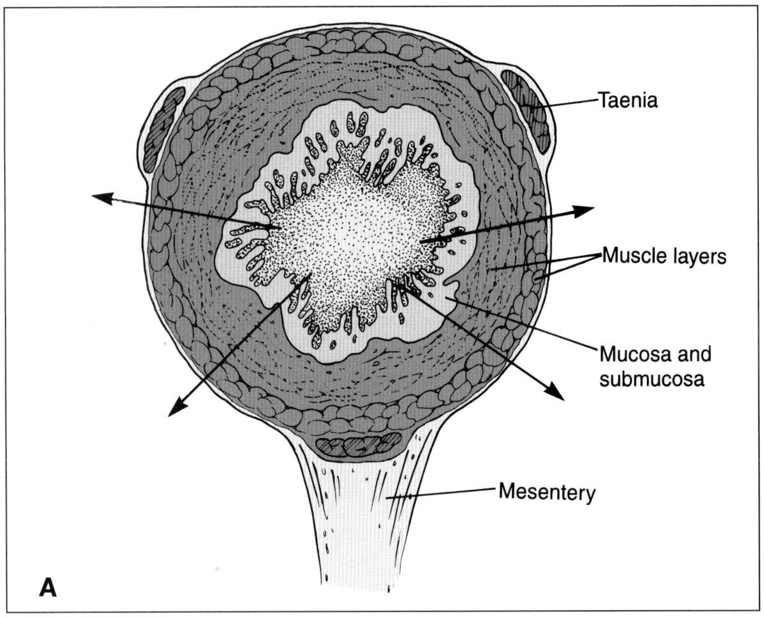

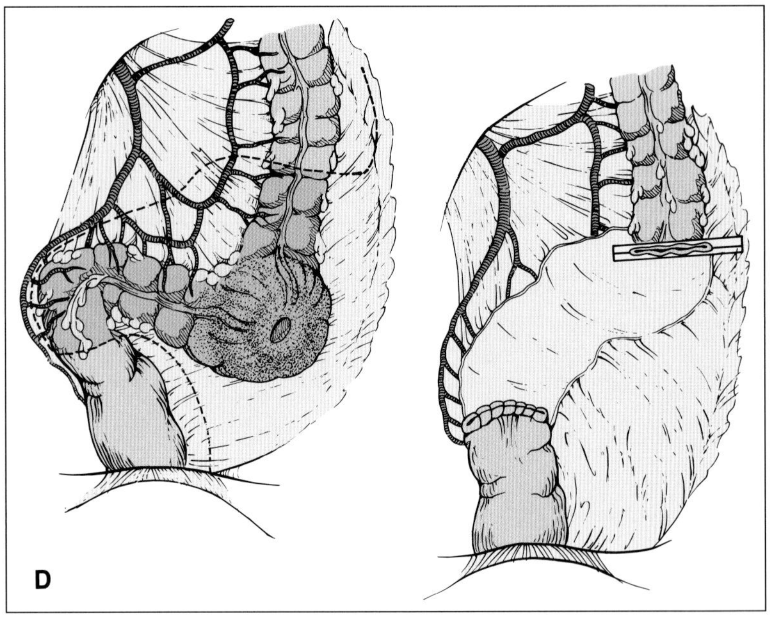

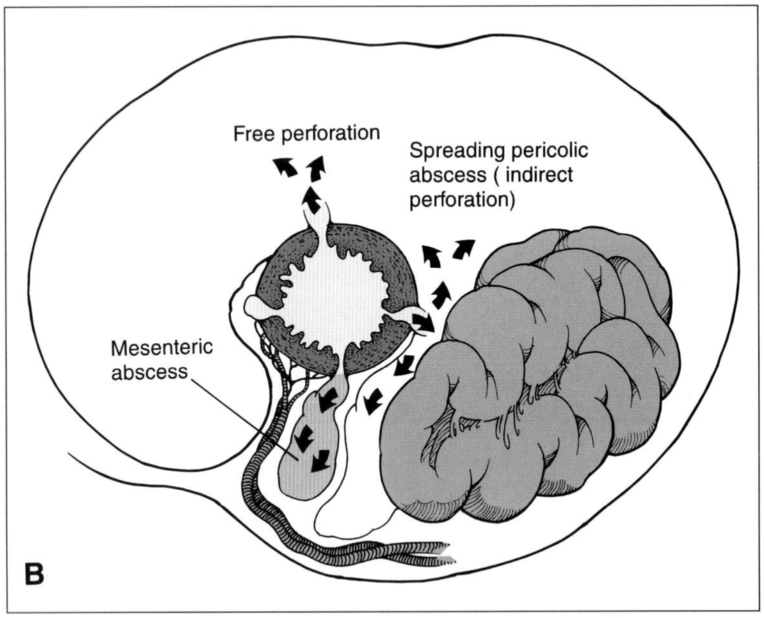

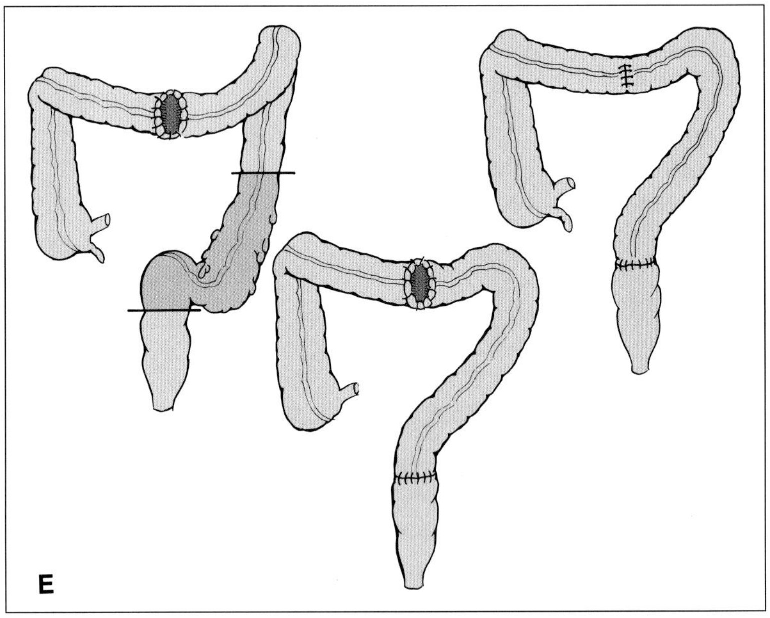

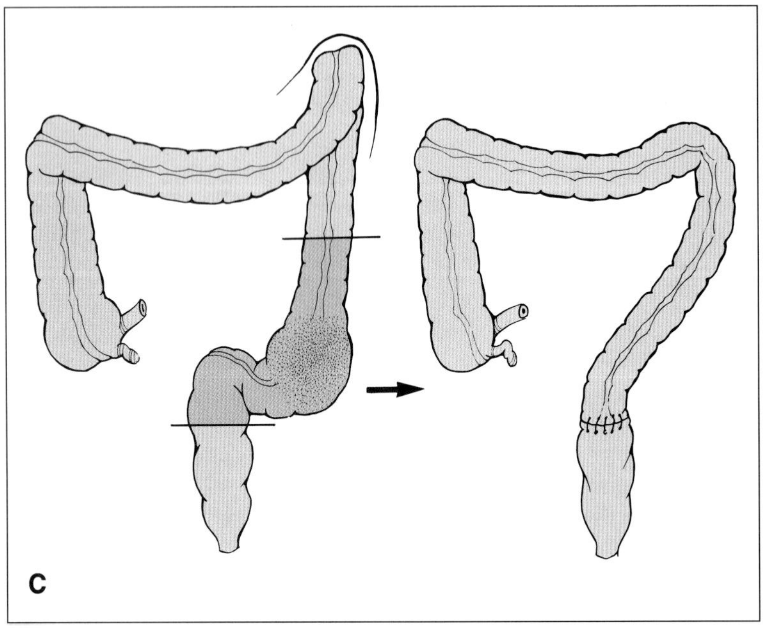

FIGURE 8-16.

Diverticular disease of the colon. It affects men and women with equal frequency. The incidence correlates with age and intake of nondigestible dietary fiber. Anatomic factors contribute to the development of colonic diverticulae, including relative weak points where the nutrient vessels penetrate the bowel wall, and a pressure gradient from the lumen to the serosa, which is highest in the distal portions of the colon. High-segmentation pressures cause herniation of colonic mucosa and submucosa through weak points in the bowel wall, resulting in the formation of pulsion or pseudodiverticuli (**A**). Concretions of stool can become impacted in these diverticula leading to erosion of nutrient arteries with lower gastrointestinal bleeding or inflammation with phlegmon or abscess formation. The principle complications of diverticular disease include phlegmon or abscess formation, obstruction, fistulization to the urinary bladder, vagina, or skin, free perforation, and hemorrhage (**B**). Patients with acute, uncomplicated diverticulitis may be treated medically. However, surgery is indicated for diffuse peritonitis, pneumoperitoneum indicating an

(Continued on next page)

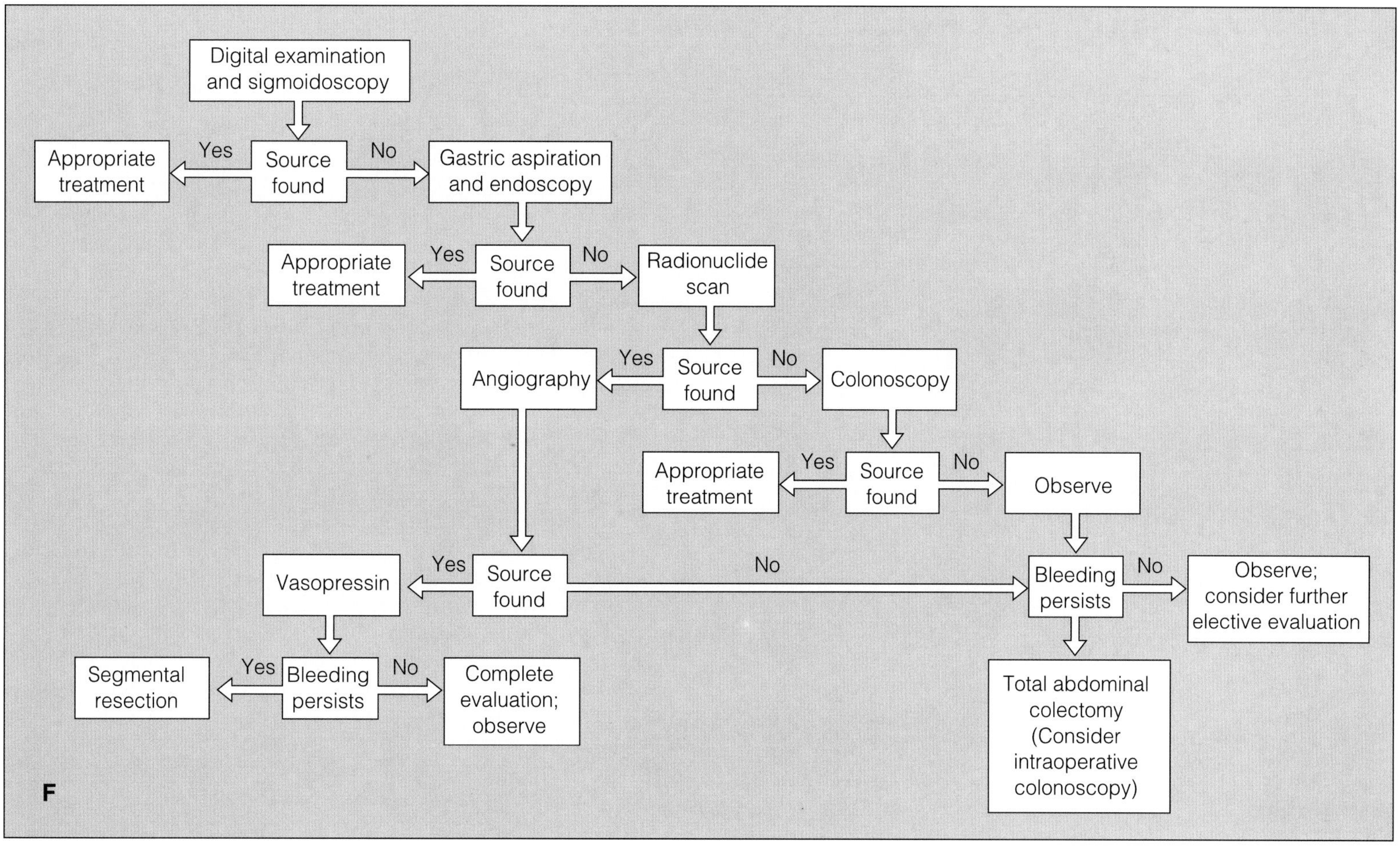

FIGURE 8-16. (CONTINUED)

uncontained perforation, or failure of medical therapy. The surgical strategy is influenced by the location of the inflammatory process, the extent and duration of fecal soilage, the degree of attendant inflammation and distortion of normal anatomic landmarks, and the general condition of the patient. One-stage procedures such as resection with primary anastomosis can sometimes be performed safely in patients with localized pericolic abscess or phlegmon. However, two-stage procedures are recommended in patients with localized purulent peritonitis or diffuse fecal peritonitis to reduce mortality and morbidity [9]. A typical two-stage resection includes initial resection of the perforated or inflamed bowel segment, creation of an end colostomy, and either exteriorization or closure of the distal rectal segment (**C**). The initial operation should be limited to removing only the perforated segment, especially if no anastomosis is intended. Limited mobilization of the colon decreases the risk of perioperative sepsis and makes it easier to restore bowel continuity at a later date. Frequently the distal colon segment is not long enough to be exteriorized as a mucous fistula, and a Hartmann's procedure or closure of the rectal stump must be performed (**D**). Restoration of continuity is usually performed 3 to 6 months after the initial resection and consists of pelvic dissection to identify and mobilize the rectal stump, mobilization of the splenic flexure of the colon to insure adequate bowel length for a tension-free anastomosis, and colorectal anastomosis using either handsewn or stapled techniques (**E**). Circular staplers have simplified these procedures, especially in patients with a short rectal stump. On rare occasion, a three-stage procedure is performed, especially when inflammation in the sigmoid fossa precludes a safe resection. A three-stage resection consists of initial diverting transverse colostomy with delayed sigmoid colectomy and later colostomy closure (**F**). Patients with diverticulitis complicated by colonic obstruction can usually be managed with a one- or two-stage resection, depending on whether luminal patency is adequate to complete a satisfactory bowel preparation.

Approximately 30% of patients with diverticulosis will develop lower gastrointestinal tract bleeding. The evaluation of such patients must be rapid and logical and is the same regardless of the presumed cause of bleeding. An upper gastrointestinal source of bleeding must be excluded. Radionuclide scintigraphy is quite sensitive for detecting slow rates of bleeding and should precede visceral angiography unless the rate of bleeding is life threatening. If the rate of bleeding exceeds 0.5 to 1.0 mL/min, angiography will frequently demonstrate the site of bleeding and provide access for infusion of vasopressin. If the source of bleeding can be localized preoperatively, segmental resection is adequate treatment and can be accomplished with low mortality. However, inability to localize the source of bleeding warrants subtotal colectomy as a "first" procedure. Blind segmental resection in this setting is associated with rebleeding and mortality rates of nearly 30%. *F* illustrates a proposed algorithm for treatment of lower gastrointestinal bleeding of presumed colonic origin. (**A**, *From* Hackford and Veidenheimer [10]; with permission.) (**B–F**, *From* Keighley and Williams [2]; with permission.)

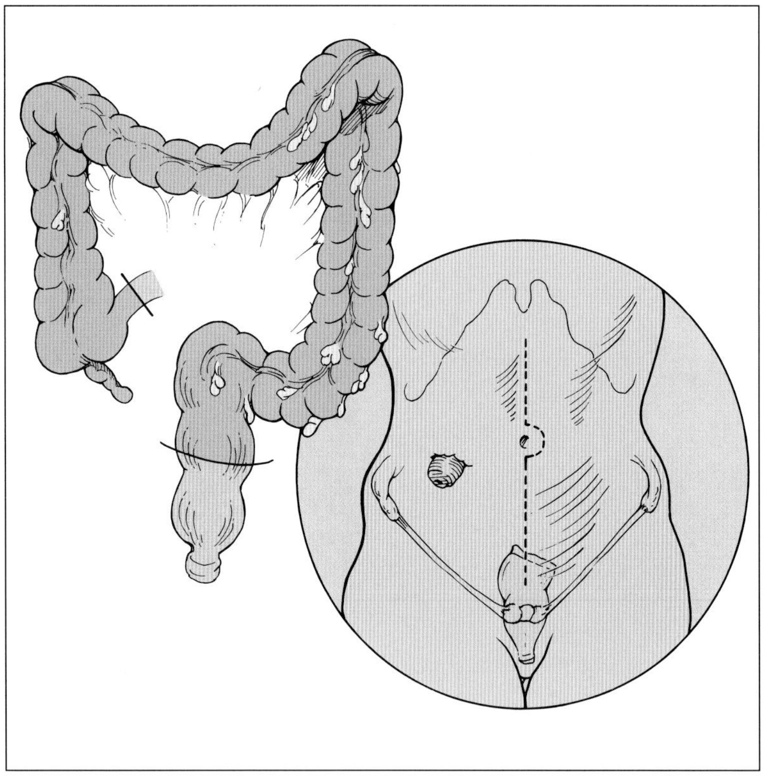

FIGURE 8-17.

Subtotal colectomy and ileostomy with Hartmann's closure of the rectum. Ulcerative colitis is an inflammatory disease of the colon that primarily affects the mucosa. The etiology of ulcerative colitis is unknown, but microbiological, immunological, dietary, psychological, and hereditary factors have all been implicated. Many patients with ulcerative colitis also have a demonstrable defect in glycoprotein mucous production. Ulcerative colitis has several presentations, of which the chronic, relapsing form is by far most common. Approximately 10% of patients present with acute, fulminant disease that must be differentiated from ischemic colitis. Long-term prognosis is determined by the risk of such complications as colon cancer and chronic hepatobiliary disease. The majority of deaths are associated with acute attacks and delayed surgical intervention.

The diagnosis of ulcerative colitis should be suspected in any patient with bloody diarrhea in whom an infectious etiology has been excluded. Radiology is helpful in patients with acute or quiescent disease. A carefully performed air-contrast barium enema may demonstrate pathognomonic features of ulcerative colitis but should never be obtained during an episode of acute colitis or immediately following a rectal biopsy. Colonoscopy is invaluable for documenting the extent and severity of colitis, for differentiating among the various etiologies of colitis, and for obtaining biopsies to monitor the development of dysplasia or neoplasia. Although colonoscopy is a highly accurate means of diagnosis, differentiation between ulcerative colitis and Crohn's disease may be impossible in up to 10% of patients.

The medical therapy for ulcerative colitis includes steroids for fulminating and active colitis and sulphasalazine and its derivatives to sustain periods of remission. High-dose steroids induce remission in the majority of patients with acute, fulminant colitis, but up to 25% of the patients will require an operation. The resection rate in patients with chronic, intermittent disease varies according to management philosophy but ranges from 5% to 15% at 5 years [11]. Factors that predict the likelihood of resection for ulcerative colitis include the severity of an attack and the extent and duration of the disease, the frequency of exacerbations, and the presence and severity of extracolonic complications such as pyoderma gangrenosum, monoarticular arthritis, and occasionally uveitis.

The prognosis of acute colitis depends on its severity and the extent of disease. Colonic dilation increases the risk of perforation and indicates a poor prognosis. The type of operation performed in this setting (subtotal colectomy or proctocolectomy and ileostomy) does not influence the prognosis. Although 30% of patients with toxic dilation will respond to intensive medical therapy, averting the need for emergency colectomy, inappropriate delays in surgical intervention are associated with mortality rates of 40% to 60%.

Early colectomy is perhaps the single most important factor in reducing the mortality rate of acute, fulminating colitis. Subtotal colectomy and ileostomy are considered by most surgeons to be the procedure of choice for acute colitis. One should never consider primary ileorectal anastomosis in this setting because of the prohibitive risk of anastomotic dehiscence, sepsis, and major complications. Subtotal colectomy removes all of the intraperitoneal colon but preserves the rectum for delayed restorative proctocolectomy if the patient wishes to avoid a stoma. However, in patients who chose not to undergo a second operation or have no interest in avoiding a permanent stoma, initial proctocolectomy and ileostomy should be considered. This figure illustrates subtotal colectomy and ileostomy with Hartmann's closure of the rectum. If the rectum is severely diseased and unsafe to close primarily, a short length of sigmoid colon should be retained and exteriorized as a mucous fistula. (*From* Keighley and Williams [2]; with permission.)

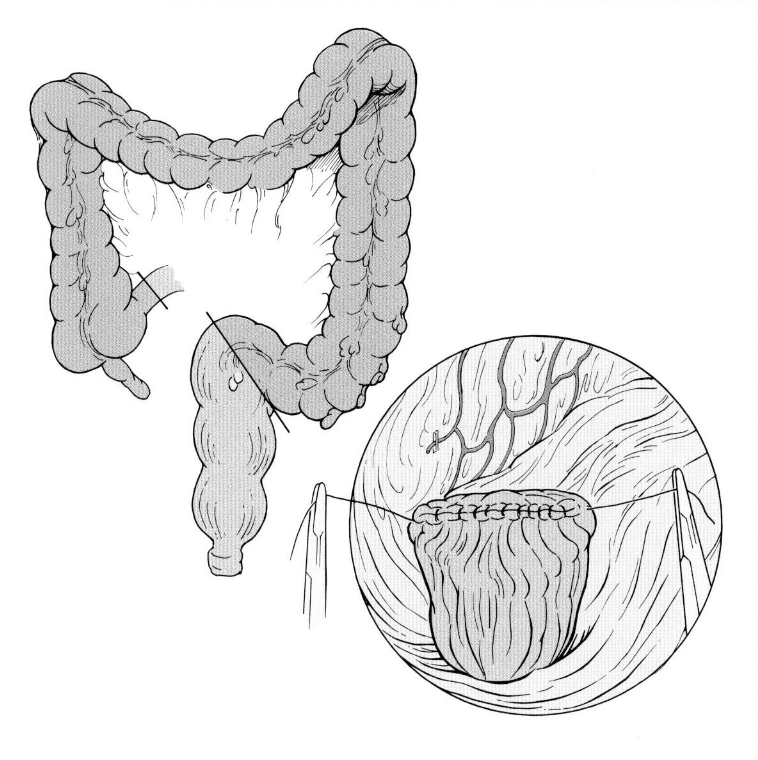

FIGURE 8-18.

Subtotal colectomy with ileorectal anastomosis. For patients with ulcerative colitis who require elective operation, proctocolectomy and ileostomy are the standard procedure against which other operations should be compared. This procedure removes all of the colon and rectum, thereby curing the disease and eliminating the need for further anti-inflammatory medications as well as the risk of developing colon cancer. The chief disadvantage is the presence of a permanent ileostomy stoma. However, the majority of patients adapt quite well to a permanent stoma.

In addition to proctocolectomy with ileostomy, three additional surgical options are currently available to patients with ulcerative colitis: abdominal colectomy with ileorectal anastomosis, proctocolectomy with construction of a continent ileostomy, and abdominal colectomy with mucosal proctectomy and ileoanal reconstruction using various types of intestinal reservoirs.

Subtotal colectomy with ileorectal anastomosis is the simplest procedure to perform and avoids the need for a permanent stoma. This option may be extremely useful for adolescents who do not wish to spend several months recovering from a two-stage pouch procedure, for older patients with relative rectal sparing and good sphincter tone, and for patients who require palliative resection for carcinomas of the colon complicating ulcerative colitis. This option should not be considered in patients with a nondistensible, fibrotic rectum that would compromise a good functional result or in patients with rectal dysplasia who are at increased risk of developing carcinoma. The procedure is straightforward, but the anastomosis must be performed below the sacral promontory to remove all of the colon. Reanastomosis with handsewn or stapled end-to-side or side-to-side techniques are equally acceptable. The recent development of pelvic pouch procedures has decreased the popularity of subtotal colectomy with ileorectal anastomosis. (*From* Keighley and Williams [2]; with permission.)

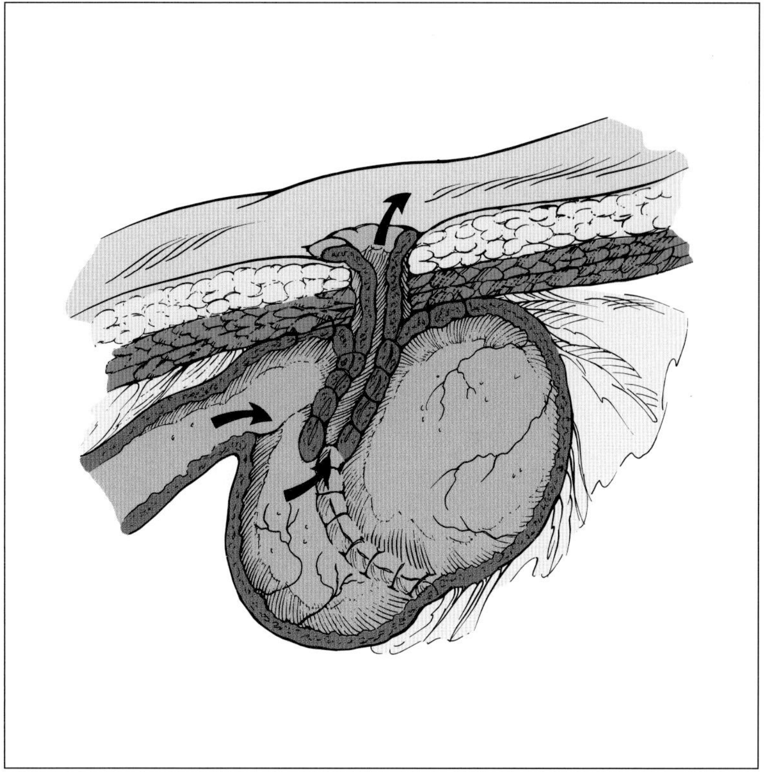

FIGURE 8-19.

Continent ileostomy. The continent ileostomy is another alternative for patients who find a conventional ileostomy unacceptable. This procedure is contraindicated in patients with Crohn's disease and in patients with a marginal length of small bowel who might need to undergo revision surgery with its increased morbidity. The concept of a reservoir ileostomy was introduced in the late 1960s. Early reservoirs were unsuccessful, but the creation of an intussusception valve to achieve continence revolutionized the procedure and increased its popularity. The essentials of a continent ileostomy include a J-shaped or S-shaped bowel reservoir and an intussuscepted nipple valve to achieve continence. The goals of a reservoir ileostomy include a moderate capacity pouch (800 to 1000 mL) that is continent of gas and stool, thereby avoiding the need for an external appliance that can be easily emptied by inserting a catheter several times each day. These procedures were initially associated with a complication rate of nearly 30% and a revision rate approaching 40% [12]. The most troublesome complications in order of decreasing frequency include desusception of the nipple valve leading to fecal soilage, fecal fistulas, and intestinal obstruction. Recent modifications, including the use of linear staplers to decrease valve slippage, have significantly decreased the complication rate to around 8% to 10% and have also reduced the need for revision surgery.

Despite what may seem to be a high incidence of complications and revision surgery, reservoir ileostomies achieve a highly acceptable level of continence. However, 10% to 20% of these patients develop nonspecific inflammatory changes within the reservoir ("pouchitis") with resulting megaloblastic anemia and steatorrhea. The exact etiology is unknown, but recent evidence attributes pouchitis to overgrowth of *Bacteroides fragilis* and possibly other obligate anaerobes. The diagnosis can be readily established endoscopically, and the condition usually responds to oral antibiotics such as metronidazole and a period of continuous catheter drainage to reduce stasis. Occasionally, it is severe enough to warrant excision of the pouch. (*From* Keighley and Williams [2]; with permission.)

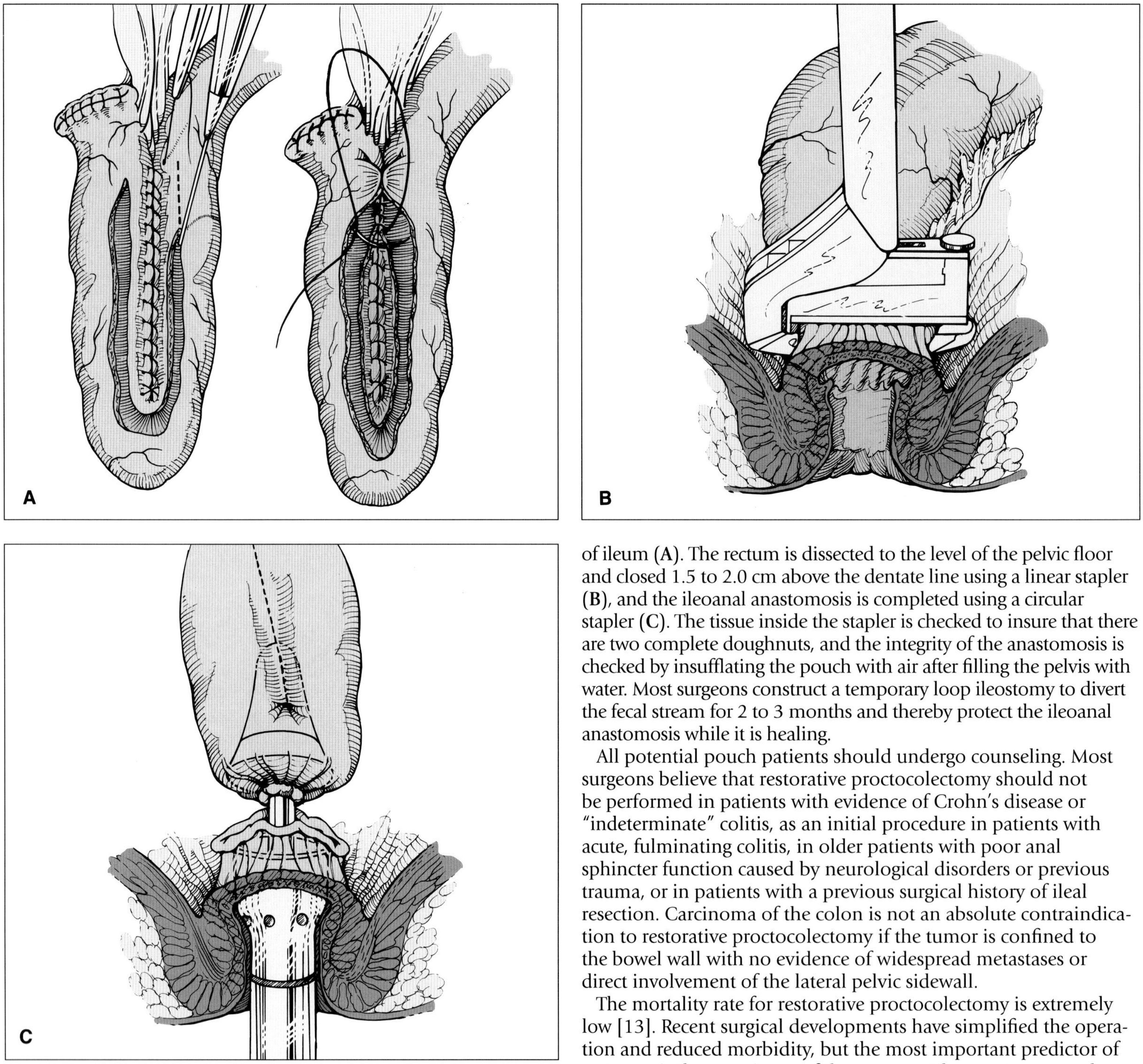

FIGURE 8-20.

Restorative proctocolectomy. Restorative proctocolectomy has become increasingly popular because it eradicates the disease and maintains continence. The technique of pelvic dissection avoids injury to the autonomic nerves and minimizes the risk of bladder denervation or sexual impotence in men. All of the colonic and rectal mucosa is excised to the level of the pelvic floor. Earlier techniques included rectal mucosectomy using a perioneal approach. However, most surgeons now leave 1 to 1.5 cm of anorectal mucosa to preserve the patient's sensitivity to gas and stool. A reservoir is constructed by anastomosing the ileal pouch to the anus using handsewn or stapled techniques. The techniques of pouch construction vary but the most widely used is the so-called J pouch. With this technique, a side-to-side anastomosis is constructed between two 15- to 20-cm segments of ileum (**A**). The rectum is dissected to the level of the pelvic floor and closed 1.5 to 2.0 cm above the dentate line using a linear stapler (**B**), and the ileoanal anastomosis is completed using a circular stapler (**C**). The tissue inside the stapler is checked to insure that there are two complete doughnuts, and the integrity of the anastomosis is checked by insufflating the pouch with air after filling the pelvis with water. Most surgeons construct a temporary loop ileostomy to divert the fecal stream for 2 to 3 months and thereby protect the ileoanal anastomosis while it is healing.

All potential pouch patients should undergo counseling. Most surgeons believe that restorative proctocolectomy should not be performed in patients with evidence of Crohn's disease or "indeterminate" colitis, as an initial procedure in patients with acute, fulminating colitis, in older patients with poor anal sphincter function caused by neurological disorders or previous trauma, or in patients with a previous surgical history of ileal resection. Carcinoma of the colon is not an absolute contraindication to restorative proctocolectomy if the tumor is confined to the bowel wall with no evidence of widespread metastases or direct involvement of the lateral pelvic sidewall.

The mortality rate for restorative proctocolectomy is extremely low [13]. Recent surgical developments have simplified the operation and reduced morbidity, but the most important predictor of outcome is the experience of the surgeon. The most commonly encountered postoperative complications include pelvic and wound sepsis, anastomotic strictures, small bowel obstruction, and fistulas to adjacent organs such as the urinary bladder and vagina. Failure, defined as removal of the pouch or construction of a secondary ileostomy, occurs in approximately 10% of patients and is usually caused by serious complications or dissatisfaction with functional results. Pouchitis occurs following restorative proctocolectomy in up to 30% of patients followed for 5 years or longer. The etiology is unclear but factors such as bacterial overgrowth, stasis, and ischemia have been implicated. Pouchitis occurs less frequently following surgery for familial polyposis and does not seem related to pouch design. Once diagnosed, pouchitis is generally responsive to metronidazole or topical 5-aminosalicyclic acid enemas. (*From* Keighley and Williams [2]; with permission.)

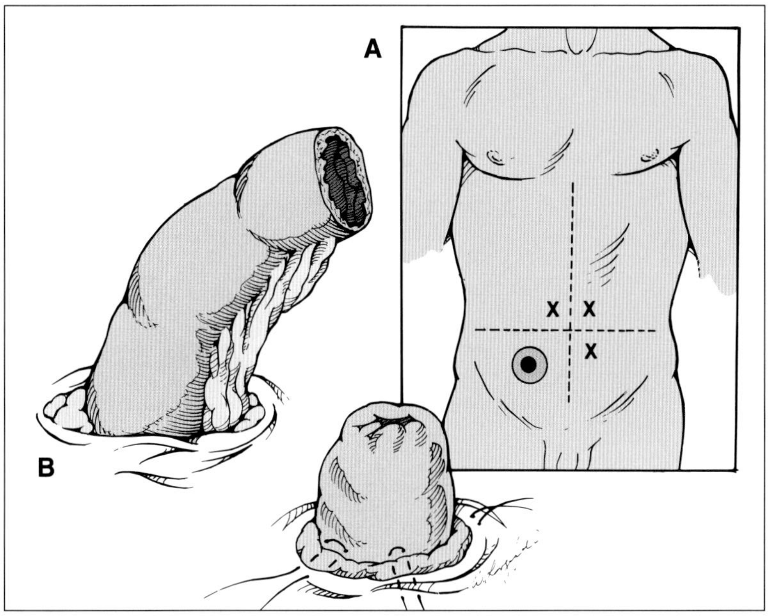

FIGURE 8-21.

Ileostomies. Any discussion of colorectal surgery would be incomplete without mention of ostomies and their management. Permanent ileostomy is inevitable in patients undergoing proctocolectomy for benign or neoplastic conditions that preclude preservation of the anal sphincter mechanism. Effluent from the ileum is liquid in nature, markedly alkaline because of pancreatic and biliary secretions, and highly corrosive to skin. An improperly sited or poorly constructed end ileostomy may produce skin irritation, maceration, and ulceration that is painful and prevents firm adherence of a stomal appliance. The optimum site for placement of an ileostomy stoma varies with the patient's body habitus and the presence of abdominal wall scars from previous operations. The stoma should be visible to the patient and readily accessible for pouch application. In general, an ileostomy should be exited through the rectus muscle and positioned in a relatively flat area away from the costal margin, iliac crest, abdominal folds or creases, previous scars, or the patient's beltline (**A**). Early ileostomies were sutured flush with the abdominal skin and resulted in severe excoriation and ulceration. In 1952, Brooke [14] largely solved this problem by designing an eversion ileostomy. With this technique, a 5- to 10-cm segment of ileum with an intact blood supply is delivered through a circular incision made at a preselected site on the abdominal wall. Several anchoring sutures are placed between the serosa of the bowel and the anterior rectus fascia or the rectus muscle (**B**). A 2- to 3-cm eversion ileostomy is made using mucocutaneous sutures that include a seromuscular bite placed several centimeters proximal to the divided end of the bowel. A pouch appliance can then be fitted snugly around the base of the ileostomy, minimizing the risk of effluent dermatitis and excoriation.

Ileostomies are not free of complications [15]. Prolonged ileus and mechanical bowel obstruction may develop following operation. Excessive swelling of the stoma may occur if the exit site through the abdominal wall is too small and compromises venous drainage. Patients can also develop a condition termed *ileostomy dysfunction*, which is characterized clinically by abdominal pain, ileostomy outputs that are highly variable but generally high, and vomiting. This condition is caused by partial obstruction of the stoma, occurs days or weeks following operation, and can generally be relieved by passing a soft-rubber catheter through the stoma. Progressive ischemia of an ileostomy stoma may lead to infarction or stenosis that requires later revision. Retraction of the ileostomy is a troublesome complication because it leads to skin excoriation and ulceration. In most cases, definitive correction requires revision of the stoma with placement of full thickness sutures or staples to maintain eversion. (*From* Smith and Heneghan [16]; with permission.)

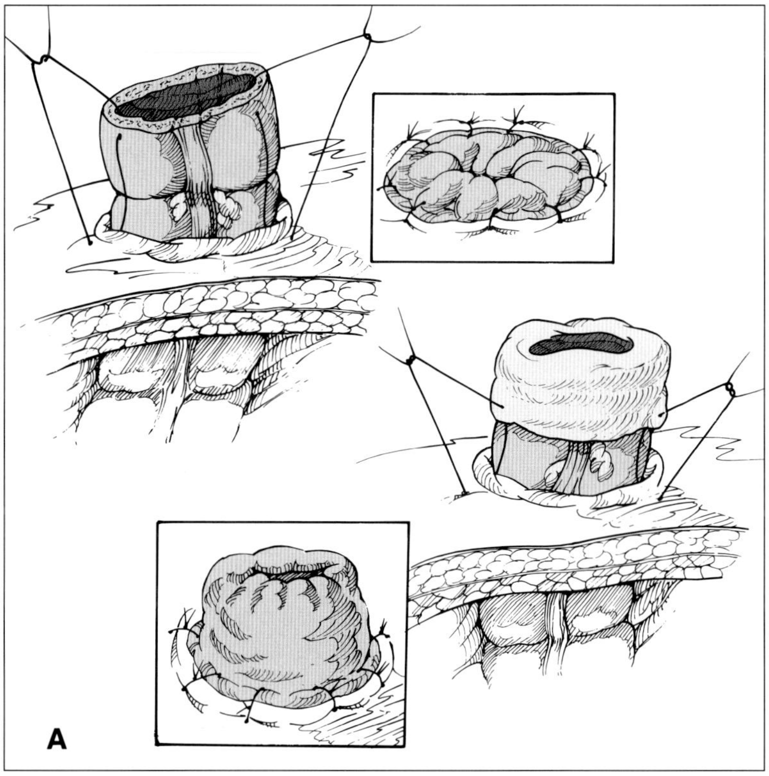

FIGURE 8-22.

Colostomies are either permanent or temporary depending on the indication for operation. Permanent colostomy is inevitable in patients undergoing proctectomy for rectal cancer or severe anorectal Crohn's disease unresponsive to conservative therapy; it is sometimes warranted in selected infirm patients with anal incontinence. Temporary colostomy is frequently indicated for complicated diverticulitis that precludes primary bowel anastomosis, for penetrating colorectal injuries, and for congenital disorders such as imperforate anus and Hirschsprung's disease. In general, a colostomy should be sited through the rectus muscle away from skin folds or creases, the iliac crest, the costal margin, previous scars, or the patient's beltline. Most permanent colostomies are constructed by exiting the divided end of a well-vascularized bowel segment through a preselected site in the abdominal wall and suturing the full thickness of the bowel wall to the surrounding skin to create a flush or everted stoma (**A**).

(*Continued on next page*)

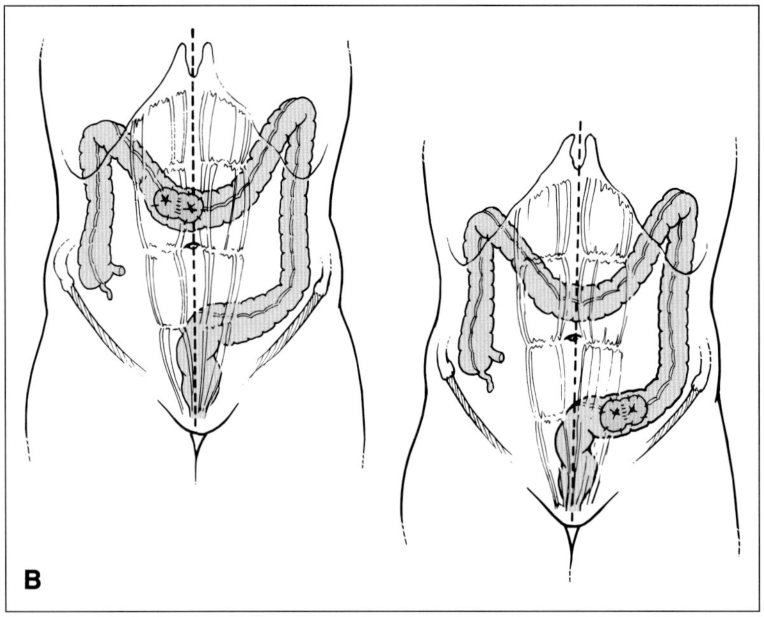

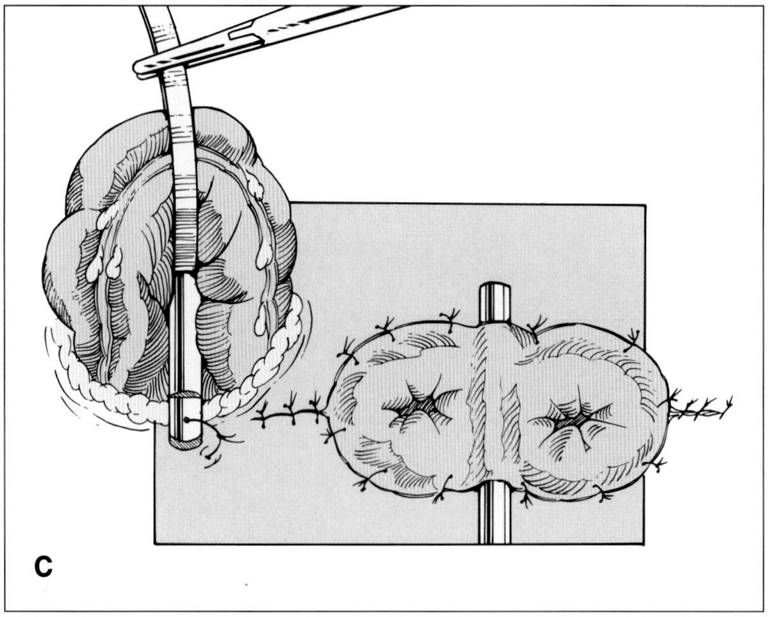

FIGURE 8-22. (*CONTINUED*)

A loop colostomy is usually sited in the right or left portions of the transverse colon or in the iliac fossa at the apex of the sigmoid loop (**B**). The mesentery is dissected off the colon to reduce bulk and facilitate delivery through the abdominal wall. A rod is inserted beneath the loop colostomy to prevent retraction, and the bowel is opened longitudinally and sutured full thickness to the surrounding skin (**C**). Loop colostomy may be lifesaving in patients requiring temporary fecal diversion. However, loop colostomy is associated with a high incidence of troublesome complications such as parastomal hernia, retraction, and prolapse and should be avoided if suitable alternatives are available [17]. (*From* Smith and Heneghan [16]; with permission.)

REFERENCES AND RECOMMENDED READING

1. Zimmerman LM, Laufman H: Intra-abdominal hernias due to developmental and rotational anomalies. *Ann Surg* 1953, 138:82–91.
2. Keighley MRB, Williams NS: *Surgery of the Anus, Rectum and Colon.* Philadelphia: WB Saunders; 1993.
3. Pemberton JH: Anatomy and physiology of the anus and rectum. In *Shackleford's Surgery of the Alimentary Tract.* Edited by Zuidema GD. Philadelphia: WB Saunders; 1991:242–274.
4. Fielding LP, Stewart-Brown S, Blesowsky L, Kearney G: Anastomotic integrity after operations for large bowel cancer: A multicentre study. *BMJ* 1980, 281:411–414.
5. Condon RE: Resection of the colon. In *Shackleford's Surgery of the Alimentary Tract.* Edited by Zuidema GD. Philadelphia: WB Saunders; 1991:179–197.
6. Vernava AM, Goldberg SM: Low anterior resection. In *Shackleford's Surgery of the Alimentary Tract.* Edited by Zuidema GD. Philadelphia: WB Saunders; 1991:198–212.
7. Bussitil RW, Foglia RP, Longmire WP Jr: Treatment of carcinoma of the sigmoid colon and upper rectum. *Arch Surg* 1977, 112:920–923.
8. Stearns MW Jr: The choice among anterior resection, the pull-through, and abdominoperineal resection of the rectum. *Cancer* 1974, 34:969–971.
9. Alexander J, Karl RC, Skinner DB: Results of changing trends in the surgical management of complications of diverticular disease. *Surgery* 1983, 94:683–690.
10. Hackford AW, Veidenheimer MC: Diverticular disease of the colon: Current concepts and managements. *Surg Clin North Am* 1985, 65:347–363.
11. Bonnevie O, Binder V, Anthonisen P: The prognosis of ulcerative colitis. *Scand J Gastroenterol* 1974; 9:81–91.
12. Goldman SL, Rombeau JL: The continent ileostomy: A collective review. *Dis Colon Rectum* 1978, 21:594–599.
13. Taylor BM, Beart RW, Dozois RR, *et al.*: The endorectal ileal pouch-anal anastomosis: Current clinical results. *Dis Colon Rectum* 1984, 27:347–350.
14. Brooke BN:The management of ileostomy including its complications. *Lancet* 1952, 2:102–104.
15. Phillips R, Pringle W, Evans C, Keighley MRB: Analysis of a hospital-based stomatherapy service. *Ann R Coll Surg Engl* 1985, 67:37–40.
16. Smith LE, Heneghan GM: Ostomy management. In *Shackleford's Surgery of the Alimentary Tract.* Edited by Zuidema GD: Philadelphia; WB Saunders, 1991:160–171.
17. Porter JA, Salvati EP, Rubin RJ, Eisenstat TE: Complications of colostomies. *Dis Colon Rectum* 1989, 32:299–303.

Chapter 9

Colonic Diverticulosis

DAVID A. ROTHENBERGER
CARLOS BELMONTE-MONTES
J. JAVIER PEREZ-RAMIREZ

Diverticular disease produces a wide spectrum of clinical presentations varying from minimal discomfort to life-threatening complications. The differential diagnosis of noninflammatory, functional, chronic diverticular disease with irritable bowel syndrome can be difficult. Caution must be exercised in attributing abdominal and intestinal symptoms, especially pain and bloating, to diverticular disease. There is often considerable discrepancy between clinical, radiologic, endoscopic, and pathologic findings. Diagnostic studies may underestimate or exaggerate the apparent significance of diverticular disease. Clinical expertise and mature judgment are required to avoid unnecessary surgery and conversely, to intervene before a catastrophic complication of diverticular disease develops.

Prophylactic resection to avoid complications of diverticular disease is not justified in minimally symptomatic individuals. Patients experiencing the early stages of diverticular disease, including a single episode of acute diverticulitis, may become totally asymptomatic and never have another problem. Repeated attacks of acute diverticulitis with localized peritoneal irritation are usually best managed by an elective resection after resolution of the acute inflammation. Chronic, refractory symptoms imply that the inflammatory focus has become irreversible and will eventually produce a major inflammatory complication. Operative intervention is advised.

This chapter focuses on inflammatory complications of diverticular disease including acute and chronic diverticulitis, perforation, abscess, fistula, stricture, and obstruction. Most elective resections for diverticular disease are performed for such complicated problems.

DIVERTICULOSIS OF THE LEFT COLON

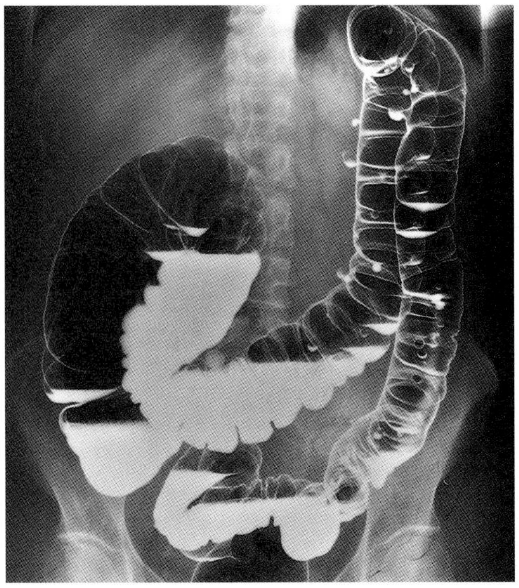

FIGURE 9-1.

An air-contrast barium enema demonstrates scattered diverticulosis of the left colon. Most of the 30 million Americans with diverticulosis have no symptoms [1,2]. The prevalence of diverticulosis increases from 5% in patients over 40 years of age to 50% in patients over 80 years of age [3]. Only 1% to 2% of the population under 30 years of age has diverticulosis [4].

PANCOLONIC DIVERTICULOSIS

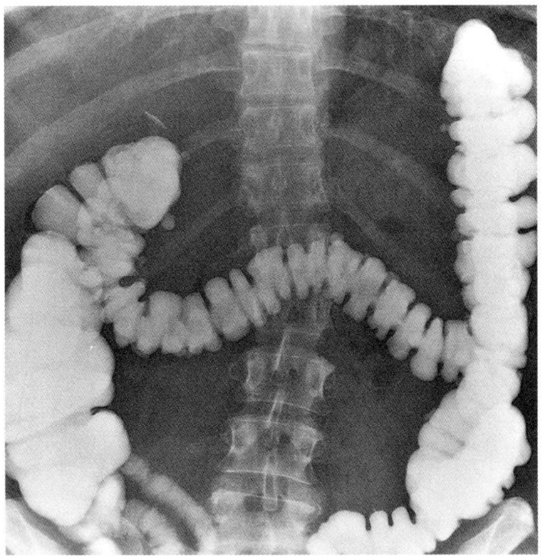

FIGURE 9-2.

Pancolonic diverticulosis is demonstrated in this barium enema and may occur in up to 10% of patients. Most often relatively few diverticula are present, as shown here. Occasionally a patient will have extensive pancolonic diverticulosis. Despite the diffuse location of the diverticula, inflammatory complications primarily occur in the left colon. The rectum is virtually never the site of pulsion diverticula.

NUMEROUS DIVERTICULA

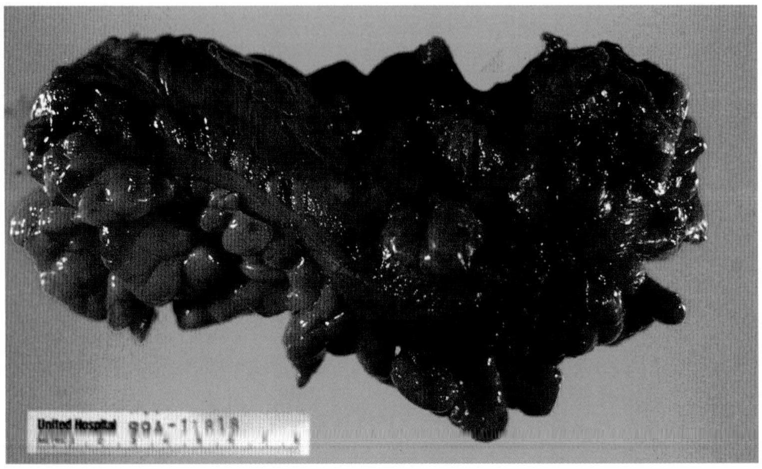

FIGURE 9-3.

This operative specimen demonstrates numerous diverticula. It is common to find two rows of diverticula, one on each side of the bowel wall between the mesenteric and antimesenteric taeniae. In about half the cases, a third row of diverticula is observed between the two antimesenteric taeniae. When present, the third row of diverticula are usually small and partially covered by muscle.

MUSCULAR HYPERTROPHY

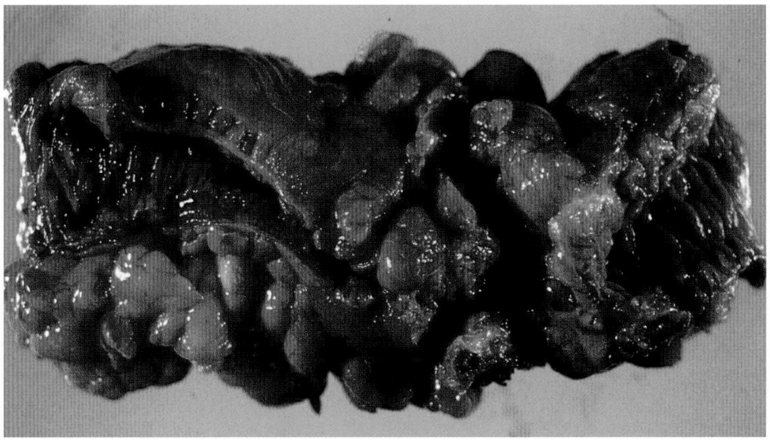

FIGURE 9-4.

Sigmoid diverticulosis may be additionally promoted because of sigmoid elastosis or muscle hypertrophy, which would raise intraluminal pressures. This operative specimen demonstrates the thickness of the bowel muscle wall and narrowing of the lumen. The higher intraluminal pressure that results promotes the development of additional diverticula and the perforation of existing diverticula, which produces the inflammatory complications of diverticular disease such as diverticulitis, abscess, and fistula formation.

WIDE-MOUTH DIVERTICULUM

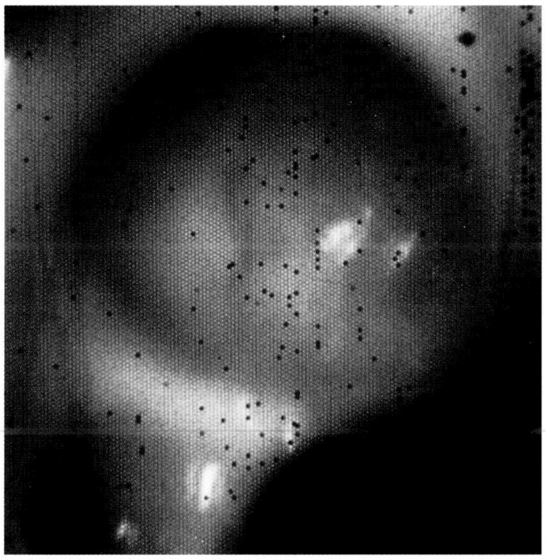

FIGURE 9-5.

A colonoscopic view of a wide-mouth diverticulum. Most colonic diverticula are pulsion or false diverticula, consisting of a herniation of mucosa (including the muscularis mucosa) and projecting through and beyond the circular muscle layer of the bowel wall to lie in the pericolic fat and appendices epiploicae. Diverticula are usually covered by a thin layer of longitudinal muscle externally and by colonic mucosa internally.

DIVERTICULOSIS OF THE SIGMOID COLON

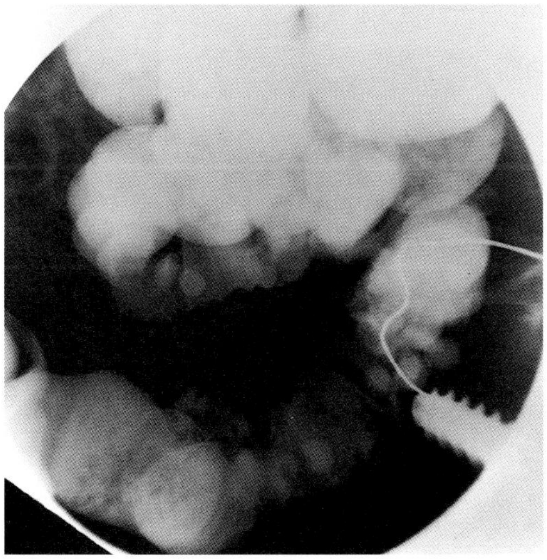

FIGURE 9-6.

In Western countries, the sigmoid colon is the primary site of diverticulosis, as noted in this barium enema. This fact may be explained on an anatomic and physiologic basis. Motor activity of the colon in conjunction with colonic segmentation causes pressure to be directed toward the bowel wall instead of causing distal propulsion. The law of LaPlace states that the tension in the wall of a hollow cylinder is proportional to its radius times the pressure in the cylinder. Thus, the intraluminal pressure would be expected to be greatest in the sigmoid colon because it is the most narrow portion of the colon. Pulsion diverticula result from herniation of the mucosa through the defects in the muscle layer of the sigmoid colon [5].

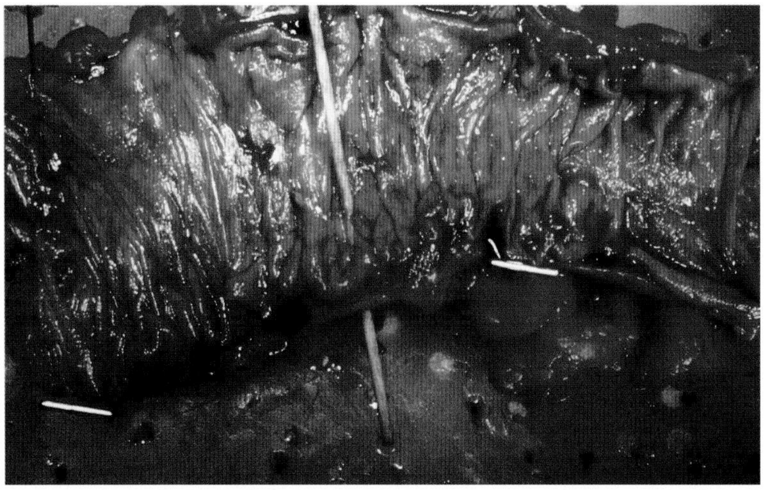

FIGURE 9-7.

This operative specimen demonstrates that perforation usually occurs through an isolated diverticulum to create the clinical picture recognized as diverticulitis. Often such perforations will seal and heal completely. The probe has been passed through the site of the perforation. Note that the mucosal surface of the colon is otherwise normal, despite the presence of numerous diverticula.

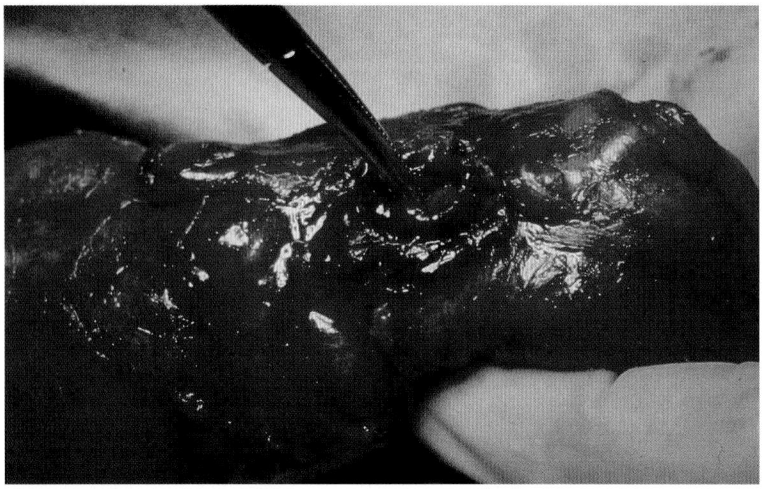

FIGURE 9-8.

This operative specimen demonstrates the serosal surface of the same segment of colon as depicted in Figure 9-7. The clamp points to the site of the diverticular perforation. Note the significant chronic inflammation and serosal thickening surrounding the site of perforation. This inflammation accounts for the usual operative finding of a thickened, sausagelike mass of colon with a phlegmonous reaction in the pericolic tissues.

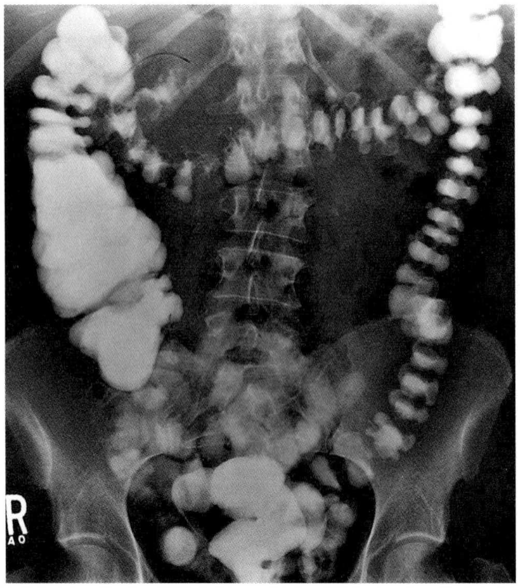

FIGURE 9-9.

This contrast study shows the unusual complication of a right-sided colonic diverticular perforation. Note the extravasation from the right transverse colon, which was locally walled off at the time of exploratory laparotomy.

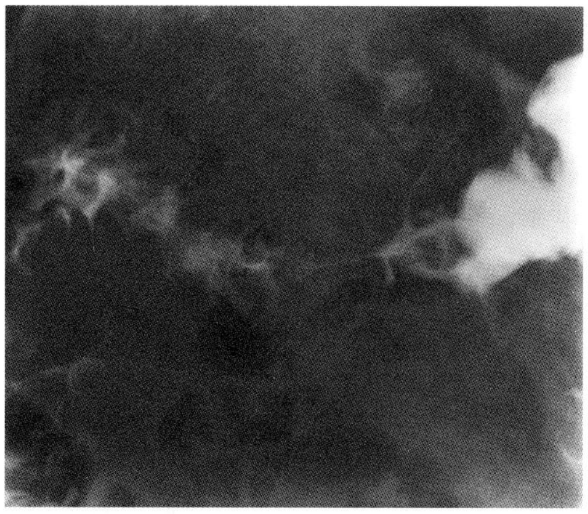

FIGURE 9-10.

This barium enema demonstrates a classic case of acute sigmoid diverticulitis. Note the long segment of colon involved in the inflammatory process and the luminal narrowing secondary to the inflammation. Endoscopic examination would reveal intense spasm and edema at the rectosigmoid junction.

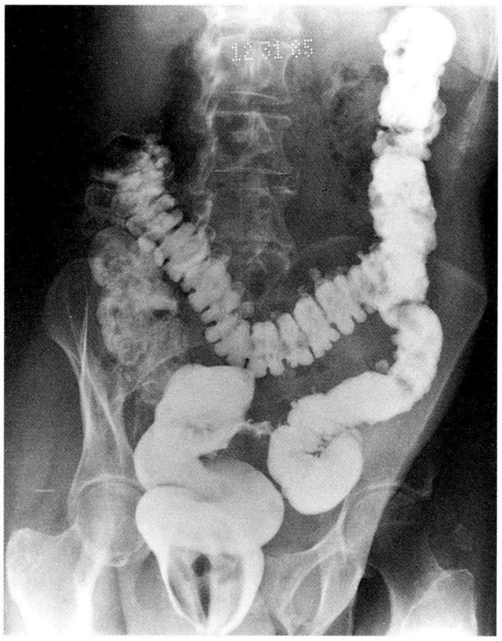

FIGURE 9-11.

Sigmoid diverticulitis can mimick a carcinoma. Careful endoscopic examination of the sigmoid after resection of the acute phase of the illness may be possible and is necessary to exclude carcinoma. If the stricture and obstructive symptoms resolve as the inflammation subsides and if other pathology can be excluded, nonoperative management is usually indicated, especially after the initial episode of diverticulitis. A high-residue diet supplemented with bulk agents may decrease the luminal pressure and the risk of perforation of diverticula. There is some evidence that a high-fiber diet can decrease recurrences of acute diverticulitis and prevent its complications [7].

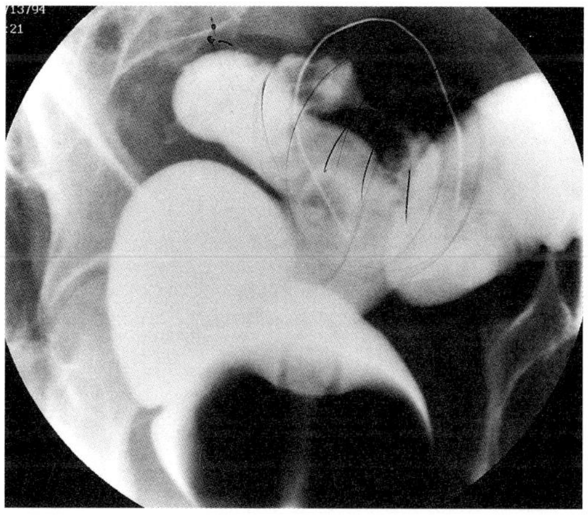

FIGURE 9-12.

This case of sigmoid diverticulitis has produced a stricture that causes obstructive symptoms and dilation of the proximal colon. After antibiotic treatment of the acute diverticulitis, the obstructive symptoms and dilation may resolve. If partial obstructive symptoms persist, if a recurrent pattern of diverticulitis develops, or if the patient develops another major complication of perforating diverticular disease, an elective resection is indicated. Today, this elective resection is almost always accomplished as a one-stage procedure with resection and primary anastomosis.

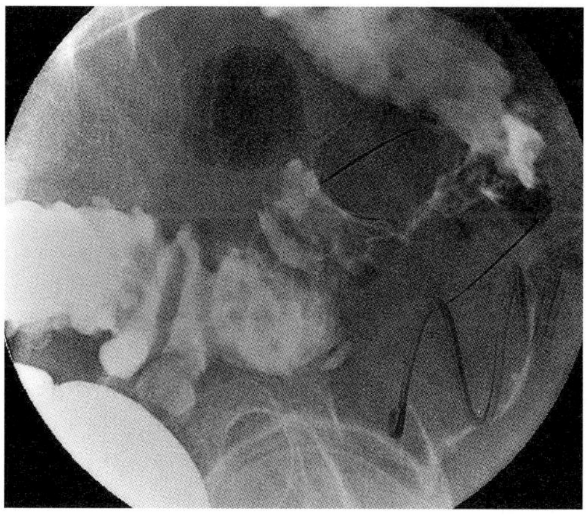

FIGURE 9-13.

This case of sigmoid diverticulitis produced a chronic stricture and persistent obstructive symptoms. A modified mechanical bowel preparation is usually possible in these circumstances, thus increasing the likelihood of a single-stage resection and colorectal anastomosis. If bowel preparation is impossible or inadequate, the surgeon can consider an on-table lavage preparation to enhance the safety of a primary anastomosis. Alternatively, a resection and primary anastomosis followed by lavage through the terminal ileum or appendical stump can be used. Occasionally, the obstruction is so severe that a primary anastomosis is contraindicated. In such cases, resection and diversion are necessary.

PERICOLIC EXTRAVASATION

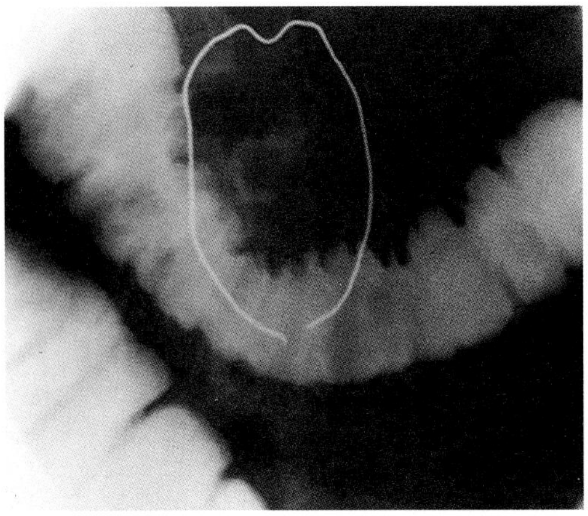

FIGURE 9-14.

Pericolic extravasation is noted in this contrast study. Diverticular disease rarely results in free perforation and diffuse peritonitis. Most often, as in this case, the perforation is contained and the infection is localized to the pericolic tissues. The degree of peritonitis has a major influence on the decision to perform a staged procedure. If diffuse fecal or purulent peritonitis is present, the operation of choice is almost always resection of the perforated segment of colon, including the distal sigmoid and construction of an end-descending colostomy with closure of the rectum as a Hartmann's pouch. With lesser degrees of peritonitis, other operative options including resection and anastomosis with or without proximal diversion are viable. The traditional three-staged delayed resection approach is almost never used today.

COMPUTED TOMOGRAPHIC SCANNING

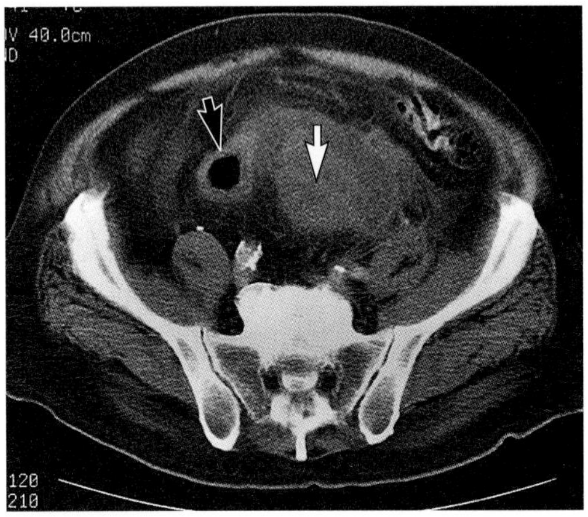

FIGURE 9-15.

A computed tomographic scan of a patient with acute diverticulitis and signs of sepsis demonstrates a large pelvic abscess. The abscess is indicated by the *open arrow* and the distended loop of bowel is indicated by the *closed arrow*. The computed tomographic scan is the most sensitive and specific test to diagnose the inflammatory complications of diverticular disease.

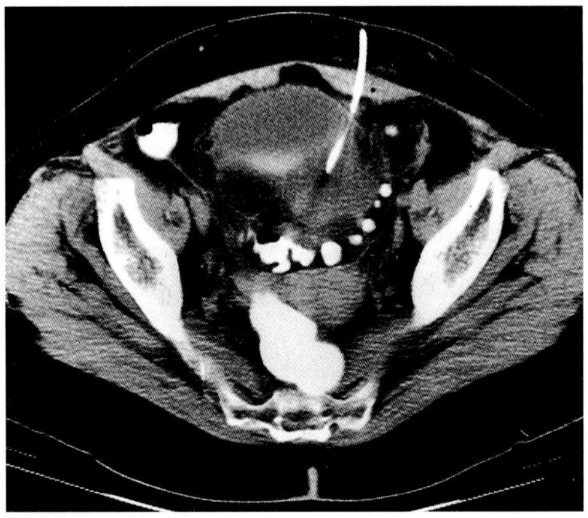

FIGURE 9-16.

Percutaneous drainage of diverticular abscesses under computed tomographic guidance has become a highly successful method of controlling sepsis. Drainage catheters are left in place until the drainage ceases and the patient's sepsis is controlled. Sinograms obtained by injection via the catheter can be used to demonstrate complete drainage and collapse of the abscess cavity. The drain can then be removed.

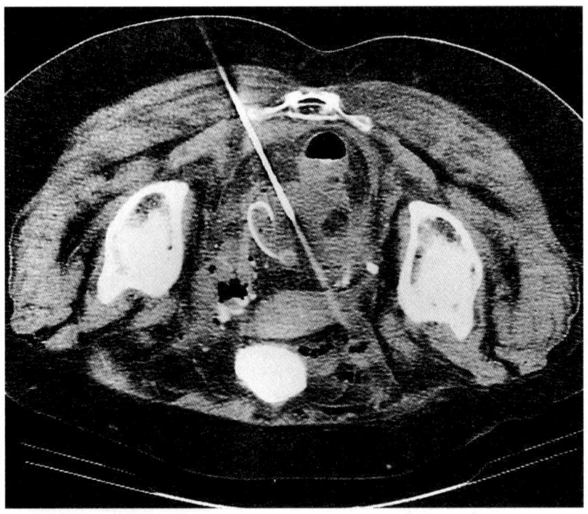

FIGURE 9-17.

Abscesses located deep within the pelvis can be drained by computed tomographic guidance. In this figure, a posterior approach is used to achieve abscess drainage. The patient is in a prone position. The needle enters the abscess from the left posterolateral approach.

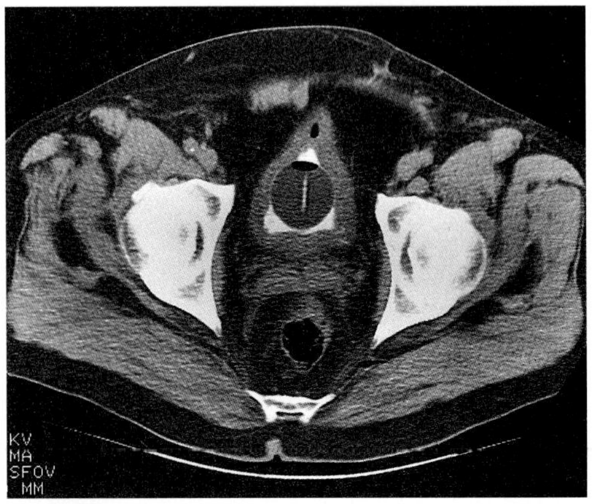

FIGURE 9-18.

Fistulas to other viscera are present in 8% to 42% of patients undergoing surgery for diverticular disease. Colovesical fistulas are the most common type of diverticular disease, accounting for approximately half of all such fistulas. Computed tomographic scanning is the best imaging procedure to establish the diagnosis of colovesical fistula. This computed tomographic scan demonstrates an air-fluid level within the bladder in a patient who presented with sepsis and pneumaturia. Systemic sepsis is usually controlled in such patients as the diverticular abscess drains itself into the bladder. Urosepsis is controlled with antibiotics until an elective colon resection is possible [8].

FISTULAS

Colovesical fistula

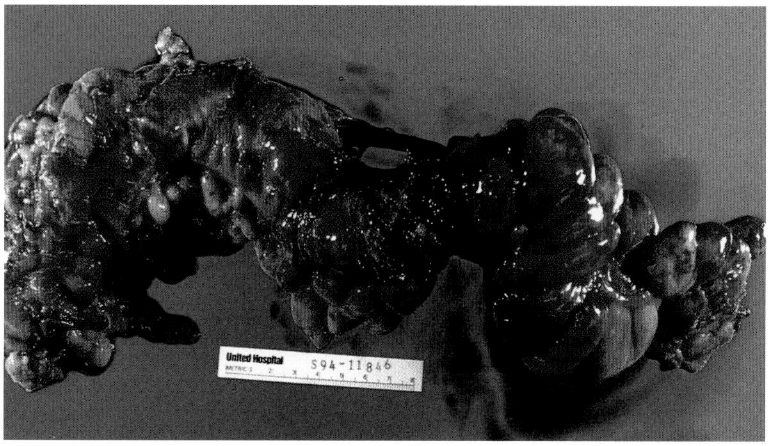

FIGURE 9-19.

The operative specimen from the same patient in Figure 9-18. Numerous diverticula are present. The colon is thickened and indurated at the site of origin of the colovesical fistula. Ureteral stents placed prior to laparotomy may help surgeons identify and avoid injury to the ureter, which often lies within the inflammatory reaction surrounding the diseased colon.

Complex fistula

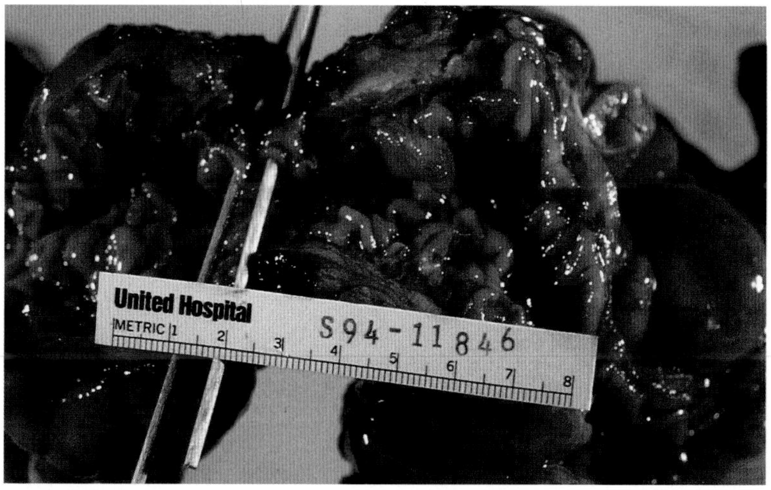

FIGURE 9-20.

This operative specimen demonstrates two adjacent sites of perforation. Note the thickened sigmoid colon and narrowing of the lumen at the sites of perforation. One fistula was to the bladder and the other to the vagina. Complex fistulas involving the sigmoid colon and at least two other organs occur in 10% to 25% of some surgical series [9].

Colovaginal fistula

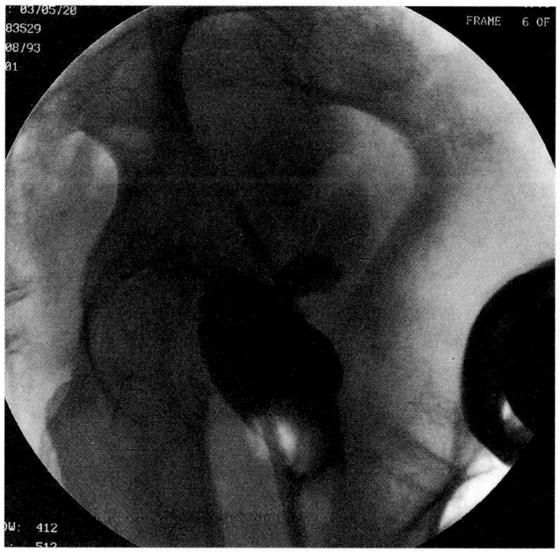

FIGURE 9-21.

This anterior-posterior reversed contrast study demonstrates filling of the vagina via a diverticular fistula from the sigmoid colon. Colovaginal fistulas are the second most common type of diverticular fistula.

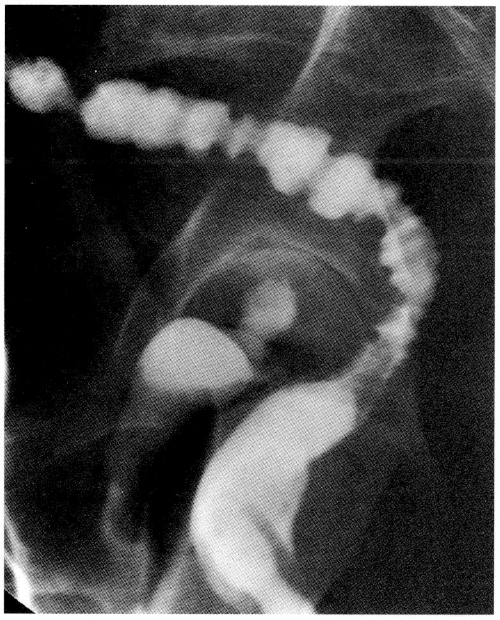

FIGURE 9-22.

This lateral contrast enema demonstrates a colovaginal fistula. Approximately half of colovaginal fistulas can be identified by barium enema. Vaginography can often confirm the presence of a colovaginal fistula, even if the barium enema shows no fistula.

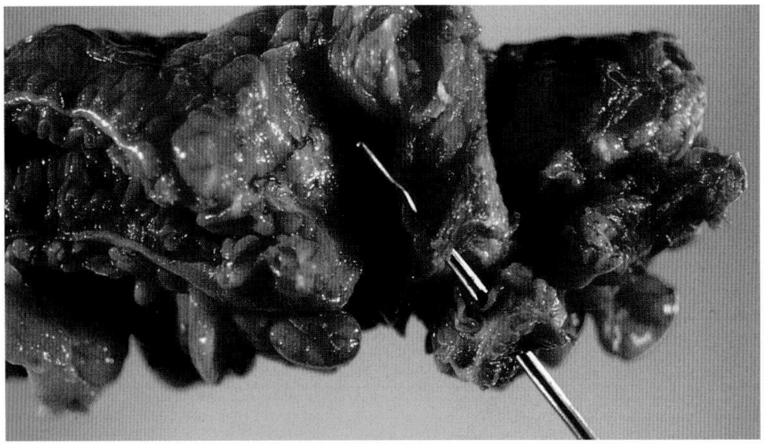

FIGURE 9-23.

The operative specimen from the same patient in Figure 9-22. The probe demonstrates the diverticular fistula that perforated into the vagina. Fifty percent of women with colovesical fistulas and 83% of women with colovaginal fistulas have had a prior hysterectomy.

Coloenteric fistula

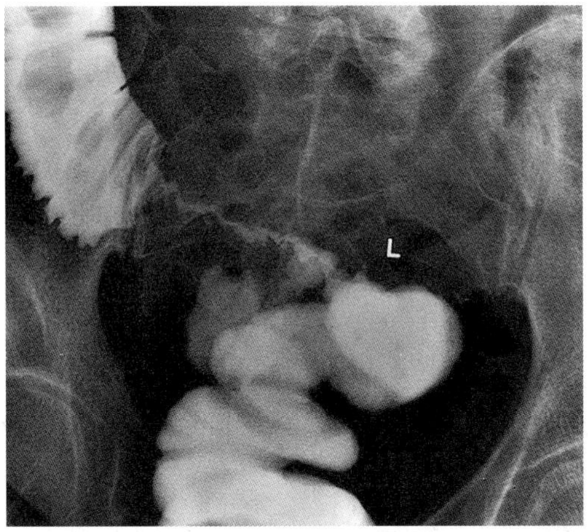

FIGURE 9-24.

A coloenteric fistula between the sigmoid colon near the rectosigmoid junction and the terminal ileum is noted on this barium enema. Differential diagnosis includes Crohn's disease. However, this contrast study shows a long segment of classic diverticulitis with a stricture. The limited amount of small bowel filled with contrast during this study is normal without any signs of inflammatory bowel disease.

Colocutaneous fistula

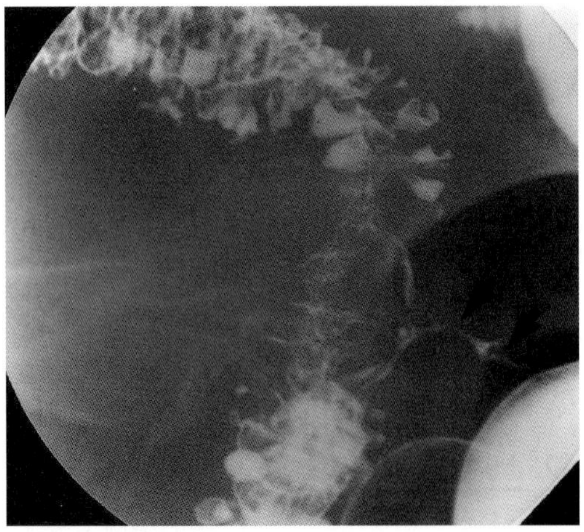

FIGURE 9-25.

A barium enema demonstrating a long fistula (*arrows*) originating in a segment of sigmoid diverticular disease. Although colovesical, colovaginal, and coloenteric fistulas constitute the vast majority of spontaneously occurring diverticular fistulas, unusual fistulas to the ureter, stomach, perineum, hip, thigh, buttocks, and inferior mesenteric vein have been reported. Colocutaneous fistulas usually develop in the immediate postoperative period. Most fistulas drain through the abdominal incision, and most originate from the anastomotic suture or staple line [10].

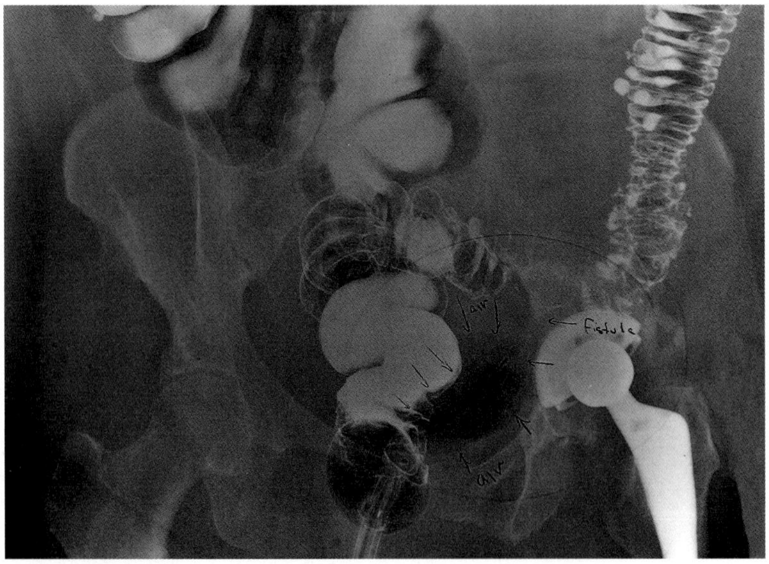

FIGURE 9-26.

A larger view from the same contrast study as in Figure 9-25 showing the fistula leading to a large confined pocket of gas. Further studies demonstrated that the pocket of gas was confined to the uterus. At laparotomy, a colouterine diverticular fistula was identified, and sigmoid colectomy was performed with a hysterectomy.

WATER-SOLUBLE ENEMA

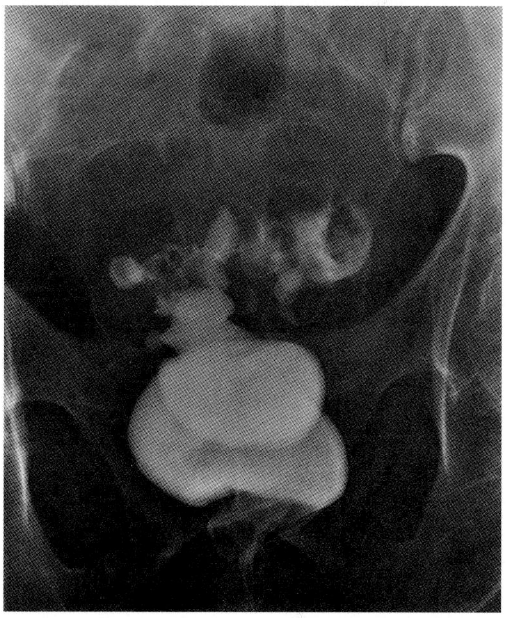

FIGURE 9-27.

A meglumine diatrizoate enema demonstrates scattered diverticula and complete midsigmoid retrograde obstruction in a patient with low-grade fever, left lower quadrant abdominal pain, bloating, and diarrhea progressing to obstipation. Examination revealed localized abdominal tenderness. A water-soluble enema, despite its limited ability to reveal mucosal detail, can complement the clinical assessment of such a patient. A water-soluble enema is preferred over a barium enema during an acute attack because it can be performed quickly on an unprepared bowel, may rapidly confirm the diagnosis, and is less dangerous than a barium enema if there is a perforation. Sometimes through its hydrophilic properties, a water-soluble enema can reduce edema at the site of obstruction and convert a complete obstruction to a partial one. This reduction and conversion allow a bowel preparation to be performed and may avoid emergency laparotomy.

COLONIC OBSTRUCTION

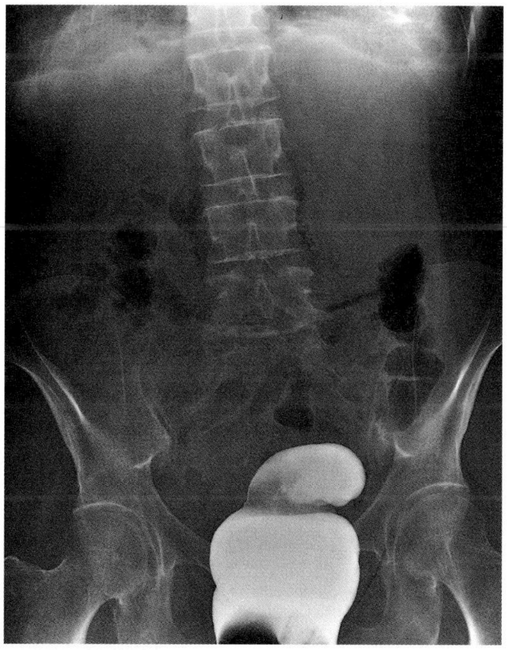

FIGURE 9-28.

A barium enema demonstrates complete retrograde obstruction at the rectosigmoid junction. No etiology is apparent. Usually, sigmoidoscopy (rigid or flexible) is deferred until the acute process has subsided with treatment, but in this case, sigmoidoscopy can help exclude a cancer and can assess the status of the distal rectum, which is essential information to obtain before proceeding with emergency laparotomy. When sigmoidoscopy is performed during the acute phase of diverticular disease, the endoscopist must be careful to use minimal or no insufflation of air to avoid colonic perforation.

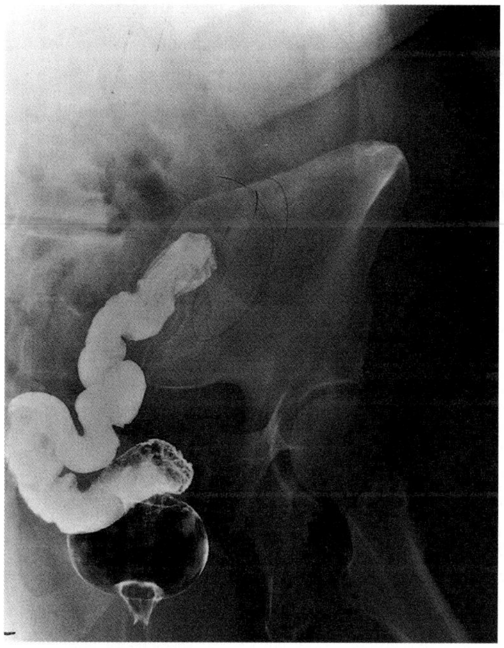

FIGURE 9-29.

This contrast study shows another example of complete obstruction to retrograde dye, but in this case, the sigmoid is relatively free of disease and the obstruction is at the level of the descending colon. At exploration, the etiology of the obstruction was severe diverticular disease of the descending colon. The surgeon must decide the extent of resection appropriate in such a case.

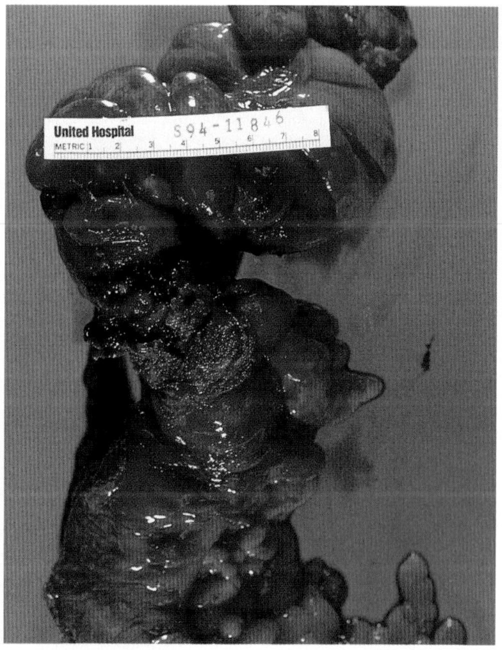

FIGURE 9-30.

This operative specimen from the patient described in Figure 9-29 demonstrates the site of the localized perforation, which created obstruction at the descending colon level. The surgeon resected not only the descending colon but also the sigmoid colon. This decision was based on data from the Mayo Clinic, which showed that a colosigmoidal anastomosis had a higher recurrence rate than a colorectal anastomosis (12.5% vs 6.7%, P=0.03). It is postulated that the higher recurrence rate is caused by a thickened muscle layer in the residual sigmoid colon [11].

REFERENCES AND RECOMMENDED READING

1. Almy TP, Howel DA: Diverticula of the colon. *N Engl J Med* 1980, 302:324–331.
2. Connell AM: Pathogenesis of diverticular disease of the colon. *Adv Intern Med* 1977, 22:377–395.
3. Parks TG: Natural history of diverticular disease of the colon. *Clin Gastroenterol* 1975, 4:53–69.
4. Rege RV, Nahrwold DL: Diverticular disease. *Curr Probl Surg* 1989, 26:133–189.
5. Connell AM: Applied physiology of the colon: Factors related to diverticular disease. *Clin Gastroenterol* 1979, 4:23–26.
6. Watters DAK, Smith AN: Strength of the colon wall in diverticular disease? *Br J Surg* 1990, 77:257–259.
7. Hyland JMP, Taylor I: Does a high fibre diet prevent the complications of diverticular disease? *Br J Surg* 1980, 67:771–779.
8. Woods RJ, Lavery IL, Fazio VW, *et al.*: Internal fistulas in diverticular disease. *Dis Colon Rectum* 1988, 31:591–596.
9. Edelman G: Surgical treatment of colonic diverticulitis: A report of 205 cases. *Int Surg* 1981, 66:119–124.
10. Smith HJ, Berk RN, James JV, *et al.*: Unusual fistulae due to colonic diverticulitis. *Gastroenterol Radiol* 1975, 2:387–392.
11. Benn PL, Wolff BG, Ilstrup DM: Level of anastomosis and recurrent colonic anastomosis. *Am J Surg* 1986, 151:269–271.

Chapter

10

Radiologic Images

EDWARD T. STEWART

Since the application of positive-contrast fluoroscopy became available in the early part of the 1900s, evaluation of the colon above the rectum fell into the hands of diagnostic radiologists. By the mid-1900s, radiologists had provided descriptions of many of the colorectal diseases encountered by physicians, especially those producing morphologic changes. Positive contrast using barium sulfate became one of the most commonly employed diagnostic examinations used by radiologists and gastroenterologists. Interest in gastrointestinal radiology has always been one of the major contributions of radiology to patient care. The initial employment of a "single-contrast examination" of the colon has now been augmented and, in many cases, replaced by double-contrast studies. The air-contrast examination of the colon or pneumocolon has resulted in improved visualization of the colonic mucosa. More recently, radiologists have been involved in describing the minute mucosal changes that are best seen using the double-contrast technique. This technique particularly influenced evaluation of inflammatory bowel diseases of the colon and the search for small polyps.

In the 1970s, endoscopy was introduced and became the yardstick by which positive contrast was to be measured. Unfortunately, the two technologies have been perceived by many as competitive rather than complementary. The impact of endoscopy on contrast studies of the colon has not only resulted in the diminution of positive-contrast studies but also a decreasing recognition of the unique strengths of positive contrast in the evaluation of the colon. At the same time that endoscopy has become prevalent, parallel development of technology in diagnostic imaging has occurred. The current use of computed tomographic scans and sonography in the evaluation of the abdomen have also impacted the traditional role of positive-contrast studies. The more recent development of magnetic resonance scanning will most certainly make significant additions to the evaluation of the abdomen and colon. These developments have not come without cost. High technology is synonymous with high price.

The following comments will be directed toward those areas that should be of use to practicing gastroenterologists, radiologists, and others who are interested in imaging the colon. The colon is contained in the abdomen, and the logical initial examination, in many cases, is a plain film of the abdomen. Films can be taken recumbent as well as erect or in the decubitus position. Plain films of the abdomen can discriminate four densities: soft tissue, fat, gas, and metallic density. Gas is known as "negative" contrast. Use of gas in the abdomen is very useful, especially in the evaluation of the colon. Swallowed gas makes its way to the colon within several hours. The transit time in the colon is variable but much slower. For this reason, a film of the abdomen generally contains a small amount of gas in the stomach and small bowel with a somewhat greater amount in the colon. The anatomic features of the colon that allow for discrimination include not only morphology, which includes the colonic haustral pattern, but also its location. Generally, the right and left colons are immobilized and are invested by the parietal peritoneum, whereas the transverse and sigmoid colons are on a mesentery. Oftentimes, the cecum is on a mesentery as well. Formed feces within the colon generally contain some gas bubbles entrapped within the fecal mass. The characteristic appearance is quite easily discriminated. It should be remembered that gas bubbles in an abscess can be confused with fecal debris. Negative contrast provided by gas is oftentimes all that is necessary to make a definitive diagnosis. Examples of the usefulness of negative contrast include the diagnosis of bowel obstruction, cecal or sigmoid volvulus, toxic megacolon, and occasionally malignancy.

Positive contrast is used when visualization of the colon is necessary for therapeutic and diagnostic reasons. Prior to the advent of double-contrast barium studies of the colon, single-contrast examinations used barium sulfate suspension of 15% to 20% wt/vol. This density of barium was selected in order to allow visualization of intraluminal-filling defects and masses. Higher density (85% wt/vol) contrast is employed when air-contrast barium enemas are used. Single-contrast examinations are generally done with the patient supine using abdominal compression. Air-contrast examinations are done with the patient in a variety of positions including supine, prone, lateral, and erect. For these reasons, an immobile patient is not a good candidate for air-contrast studies. Either examination can be conducted through colostomies. However, the single-contrast examination is easier when the colostomy is being examined. Hartmann pouches and mucus fistulas are generally studied using water-soluble contrast so that the contrast suspension does not inspissate in the bypassed segment of colon. When perforation is suspected or when the examination is to be followed by endoscopy, the selection of water-soluble contrast is advisable. Water-soluble contrast is inadequate for visualization of the mucosa, although the morphologic features are well defined. It is not the intent of this section to describe in detail the technical aspects of positive-contrast studies.

Positive contrast in the lumen of the colon outlines the morphologic appearance of the colon and may surround intraluminal masses such as tumors or polyps. The extraluminal bowel is not seen well unless the process deforms the colon from the external surface. (For the same reason, endoscopy is of little or no value in the evaluation of the extraluminal colon). Computed tomographic scans of the abdomen may be directed primarily at the evaluation of the colon but are most useful in the evaluation of the entire extraluminal abdomen. Both oral and rectal contrast are used to opacify the bowel during computed tomographic scanning. For clinical reasons, it may be unwise to administer an enema in some instances. Of greater importance in the computed tomographic evaluation of the abdomen is the use of intravenous contrast, which is generally described as "contrast-enhanced" scanning. Scans are obtained during the bolus administration of intravenous iodinated contrast. Scans are timed so that the intravascular iodine concentration is high when the scans are taken. Identification of vascular structures using contrast is very useful in the interpretation of computed tomographic scans as well as visualization of abnormalities that enhance or are hypervascular. As intravenous contrast is excreted from the kidneys and ureters and accumulates in the bladder, definition of these structures is much improved. Because one of the major advantages of computed tomographic scanning is the visualization of the extraluminal abdomen, it is becoming much more common to use computed tomographic scans in the evaluation of abnormalities outside of the colon, such as pericolonic abscess related to diverticulitis and other fluid collections, extraluminal tumors, or any other extraluminal pathology. Computed tomographic scans are very accurate in determining the presence of small bowel obstruction and, to a lesser extent, colon obstruction. The retroperitoneum is often the site of abnormalities such as adenopathy or inflammatory disease. Documentation of abnormalities in these areas is within the scope of computed tomographic scanning. Obviously, detection of hepatic abnormalities, *ie*, colon metastases, is best done by computed tomographic scanning.

During computed tomographic scans, a "scout" film or computed radiograph of the abdomen is obtained. Although the resolution on these types of computed radiographs is not as great as standard analog films such as a KUB (kidney, ureter, and bladder) film, they may be very useful in demonstrating pathology such as abnormal gas patterns. Computed tomographic scanning and ultrasound allow guided therapeutic procedures to be performed in and around the colon with great accuracy. One of the most commonly employed interventional procedures in the region of the colon is the drainage of inflammatory fluid collections, including pericolonic abscesses caused by diverticulitis, appendicitis, and Crohn's disease as well as peripancreatic fluid collections such as pancreatic pseudocysts.

The use of magnetic resonance scanning in the abdomen is currently being evaluated. Its major impact initially has been in the pelvis, especially in the evaluation of gynecologic disease. In the liver, magnetic resonance scans are used to evaluate liver masses, both benign and malignant.

Traditional angiography has played a role in defining the site and etiology of colonic hemorrhage and oftentimes has been used for therapeutic control of bleeding vessels. The advent and development of magnetic resonance angiography has added a new dimension to the evaluation of vessels within the abdomen, especially the major arteries and veins.

The luminal viscera can be interrogated with sonography. With the exception of acute appendicitis, the use of ultrasound is generally not an initial examination but rather a confirmatory one to document an abnormality or to follow up a known abnormality such as fluid collection or mass. Endoscopic ultrasound is under investigation and is especially applicable in the anorectal region because of its accessibility.

The following cases have been selected to demonstrate the characteristic appearance of pathology encountered by those of us involved in the day-to-day clinical management of patients with colorectal disease. They have been chosen in a number of instances to emphasize technical and diagnostic considerations as well as some clinical aspects of colorectal disease and are not intended as an exhaustive review of colonic imaging.

NORMAL APPEARANCE OF THE ABDOMEN AND COLON

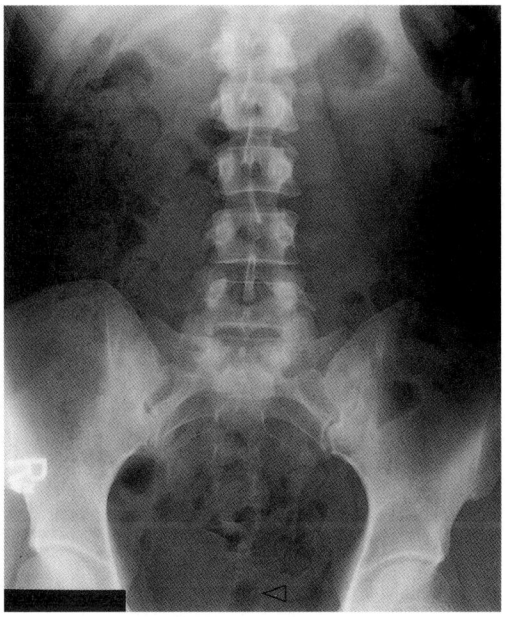

FIGURE 10-1.

Normal appearance of the abdomen and the colon on plain film of the abdomen. The normal appearance of the abdomen on plain film is variable. Fecal debris may be at any level of the colon, and the colon generally contains some gas due to its slow transit time relative to the stomach and small bowel. Notice the appearance of feces in the right colon. Gas trapped in the fecal debris gives it a somewhat bubbly appearance. A tampon is also visible in the pelvis. Gas in the tampon is easily seen on plain films (*arrowhead*).

CARCINOMAS AND POLYPOSIS OF THE COLON

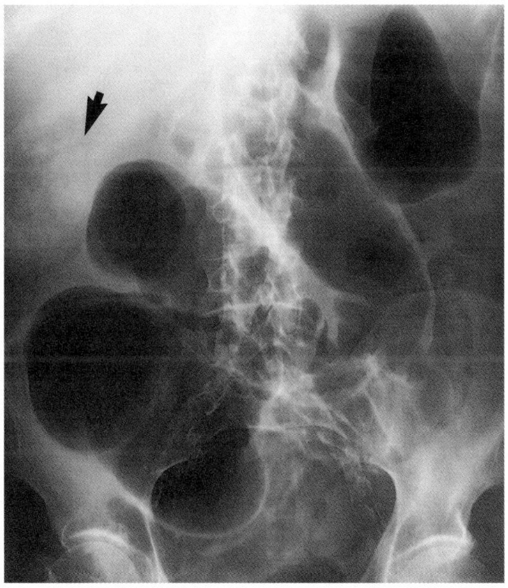

FIGURE 10-2.

Obstructing carcinoma of the left colon with metastatic disease. This elderly patient presented with abdominal distention. This single film of the abdomen allows the physician to make a specific diagnosis. There is evidence of gaseous distention of the colon. The degree of distention is highly suggestive of a partial mechanical obstruction of the colon somewhat distal to the splenic flexure. A hazy calcification is seen in the caudal aspect of the right lobe of the liver (*arrow*). The combination of this type of calcification in the liver in the presence of colon obstruction is very likely caused by malignant disease. A characteristic of mucinous-producing carcinomas of the colon is calcification. Calcific metastases are often seen in computed tomographic scans and occasionally on plain films of the abdomen. It is possible from this single film to make a specific diagnosis of obstructing carcinoma of the colon with metastases to the liver. This diagnosis was confirmed at surgery.

Adenocarcinoma

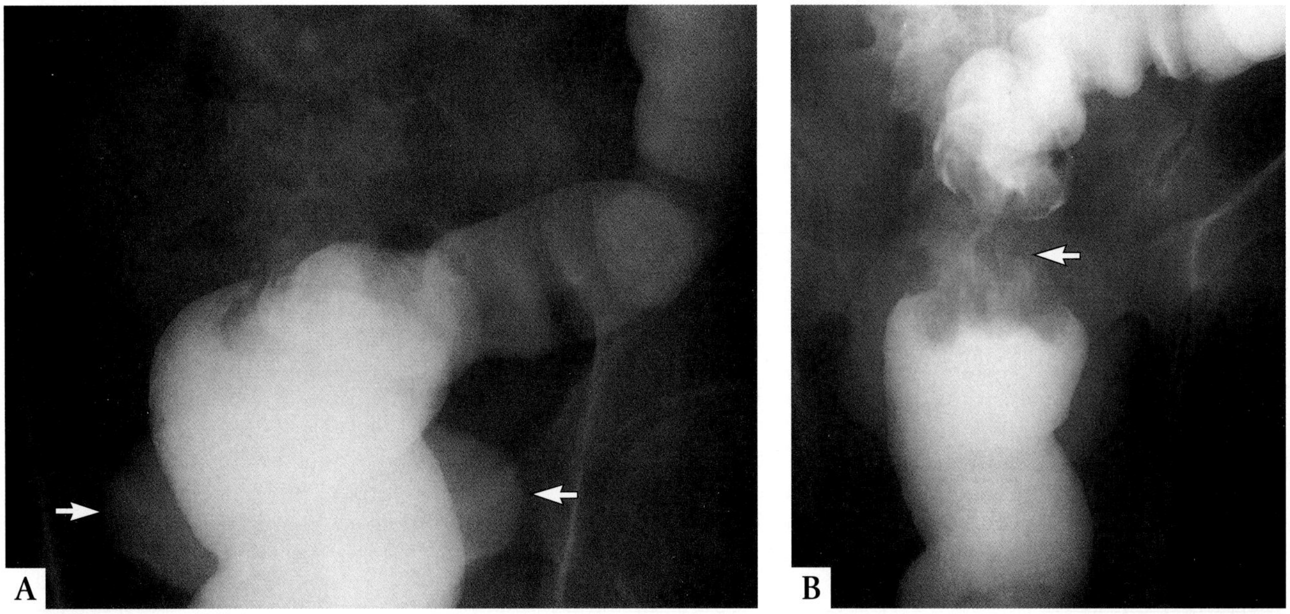

Figure 10-3.

The importance of radiographic techniques is illustrated in this patient who has a circumferential adenocarcinoma of the rectosigmoid junction. **A**, In the anterior-posterior view, the tumor is largely hidden by the redundancy of the bowel on the single-contrast examination. There is also some retained contrast in the bladder from a coexistent excretory urogram (*arrows*). During the performance of positive-contrast examinations, it is important to display redundant portions of the colon so that lesions are identified or excluded. **B**, An angled view of the rectum with the overhead tube angled toward the feet very nicely uncovers the redundant areas and allows much better discrimination of this infiltrating annular carcinoma, which shows the tumor almost obliterating the lumen of the colon (*arrow*). Despite the size and obvious nature of the lesion on this film, it is not nearly as well defined in the projection shown in *A*.

Redundancy of the colon is a problem for the radiologists as well as the endoscopists. Because at least half of the neoplastic lesions encountered will be located somewhere between the rectum and the descending colon, it is important to adequately define this area; this area is the location where redundancy, smooth muscle hypertrophy, and diverticulosis is most common. In order to minimize perceptive or technical misses, it is the radiologist's responsibility to make sure that redundancy is reduced and filming and fluoroscopic examination is adequate to see all areas of the colon.

Sessile adenocarcinoma

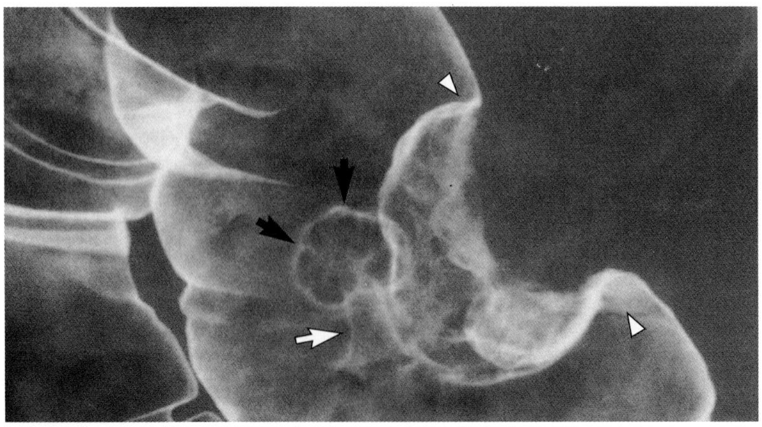

Figure 10-4.

Sessile adenocarcinoma and adjacent pedunculated adenomatous polyp. This single film from an air-contrast examination with malignant lesions as well as benign lesions. The larger sessile polyp originates from the mucosa; it is slightly nodular, and its dimensions are large enough to suspect malignant disease. Although the surface characteristics cannot predict malignancy in the absence of obvious ulceration, the size alone makes this lesion highly likely to be invasive carcinoma, which was present on removal. Notice the undercut margins (*arrowheads*) that support the mucosal origin of this tumor. The second smaller lesion is a very nicely displayed pedunculated polyp on a short stalk (*white arrow*). The head of the polyp is slightly irregular along the surface (*black arrows*). This lesion represents a benign adenomatous polyp and demonstrates the exquisite detail that can be seen on this double-contrast examination in these types of lesions. The coexistence of adenocarcinoma with other neoplastic polyps is common. At least 50% of patients will have additional lesions once the index polyp is identified. It is extremely important to exclude other synchronous lesions whenever a polypoid lesion is found in the colon either endoscopically or radiographically. (*From* Stewart and Dodds [1]; with permission.)

Annular sigmoid carcinoma

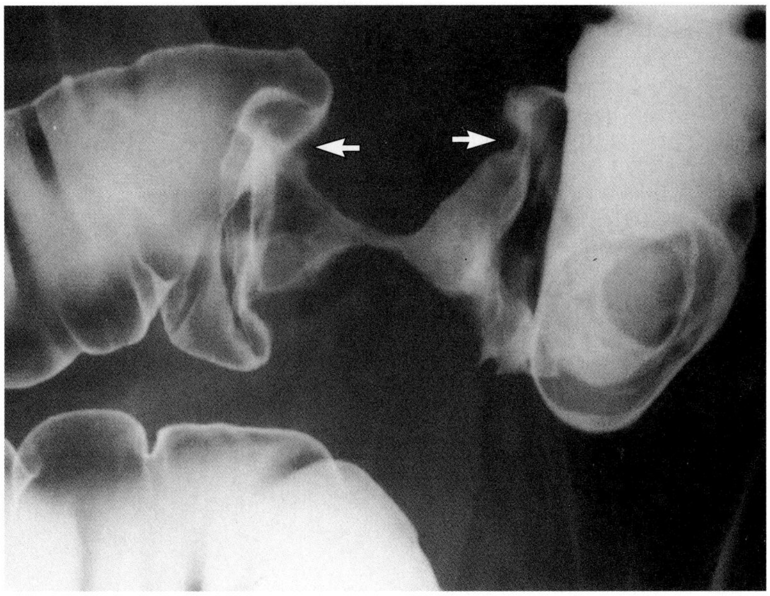

FIGURE 10-5.

As malignancies advance and encompass the lumen of the colon, the annular appearance, often referred to as the *apple core lesion*, may be seen on positive-contrast studies. In this figure, the features of a malignant-circumferential carcinoma are well displayed. Notice the circumferential luminal narrowing of the colon. Sharp margins with overhanging edges are seen on both ends of the lesion (*arrows*). This lesion is probably superficially ulcerated, but this superficial ulceration is not well demonstrated.

Not only does this case graphically demonstrate the morphologic appearance of an infiltrating annular carcinoma, it also demonstrates that it is not likely that an endoscope will pass through the luminal narrowing of this tumor. The remainder of the colon is therefore the domain of the radiologist to exclude synchronous lesions. To remove this lesion without confirming the absence of any other pathology of the colon would be a major error in management. Patients with high-grade colonic obstruction with diverting colostomies must have the proximal colon examined some time during the initial management. (*From* Stewart and Dodds [1]; with permission.)

Scirrhous carcinoma

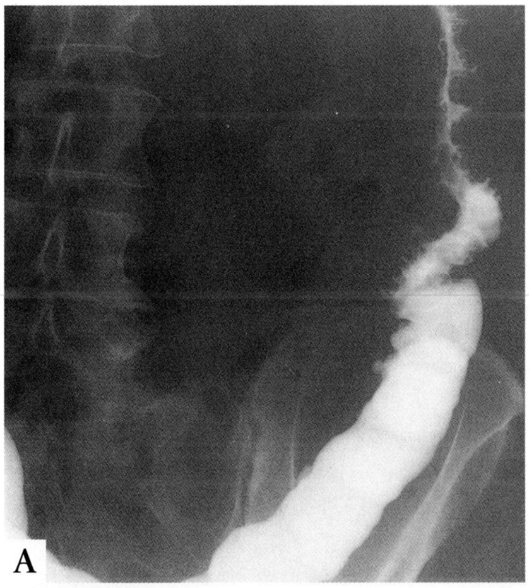

A

FIGURE 10-6.

This patient with vague abdominal symptoms and heme-occult positive stools demonstrates high-grade obstruction in the colon to retrograde flow of barium on a single-contrast examination. **A**, This figure illustrates the appearance of a long, somewhat nodular lesion. **B**, The accompanying computed tomographic scan shows a long, infiltrating lesion affecting the descending colon and the distal transverse colon. There is also edema and infiltration of the mesentery and enlarged lymph nodes around the aorta. Occasionally, adenocarcinoma presents as a scirrhous-infiltrating lesion rather than a polypoid, bulky intraluminal mass. Because of this difference, there is overlap of morphologic features with those of inflammatory disease involving the colon. The morphologic features of this lesion are much better illustrated radiographically than they would be endoscopically. Narrow segments such as this segment are very difficult to see endoscopically. Also notice that despite the severe narrowing of the colon, there is no evidence of proximal colonic obstruction. It is not unusual to have obstruction in the retrograde flow of contrast through narrowed segments, despite the absence of high-grade colonic obstruction in the antegrade direction. This phenomenon is probably caused by prolapse of colonic mucosa into the narrowed portion of the colon preventing retrograde flow of barium. (*From* Stewart and Dodds [1]; with permission.)

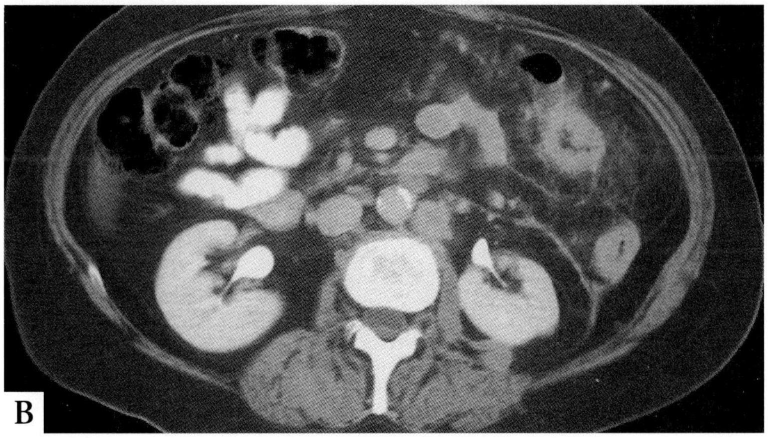

B

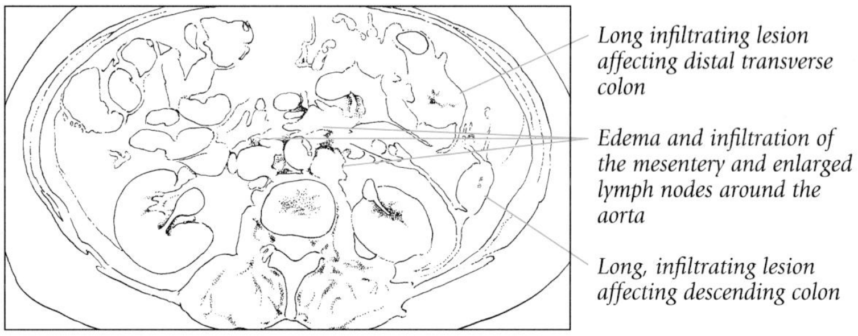

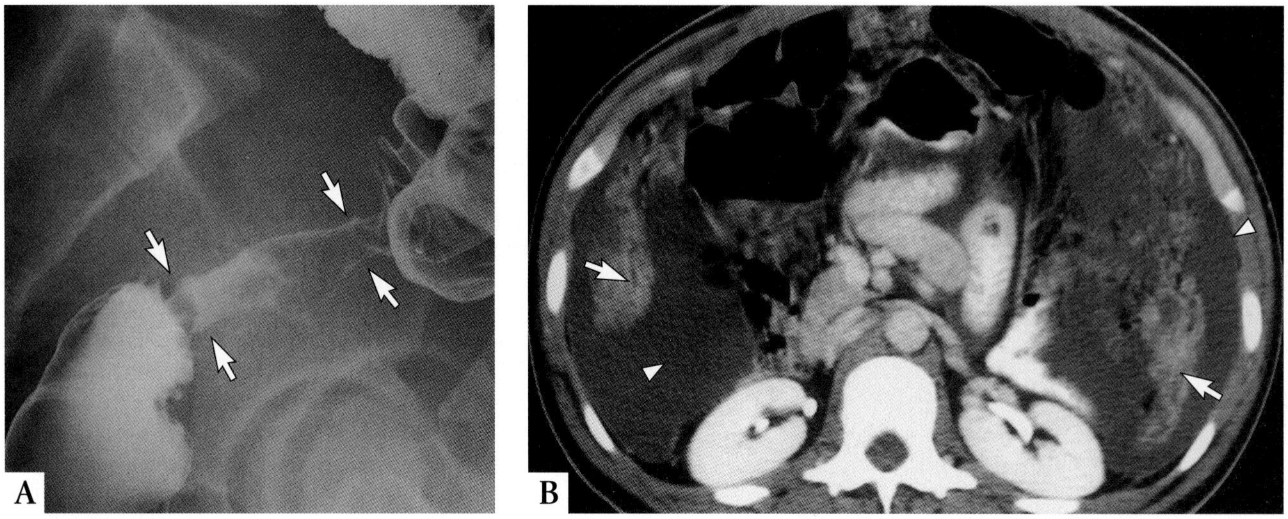

FIGURE 10-7.

A, This figure is a lateral view of an air-contrast examination of the colon. There is a long annular infiltrating neoplastic lesion involving the recto-sigmoid junction (*arrows*). Although there is very little question as to the nature of this lesion being malignant, neither positive-contrast examination of the colon or endoscopy is sufficient to adequately stage these patients. **B**, The computed tomographic scan of the abdomen graphically demonstrates the widespread disease with a great deal of malignant ascites (*arrowheads*) and infiltration of the omentum (*arrows*).

Metastatic spread of adenocarcinoma of the colon to regional nodes, liver, peritoneal cavity, or distant sites is best evaluated with cross-sectional imaging to visualize the extraluminal abdomen. Clinically silent metastatic disease, either at the time of the initial evaluation or in follow-up, may be detected by either computed tomography or ultrasound as well as plain films. Most recurrent disease following resection of colon carcinoma occurs somewhat outside the colon.

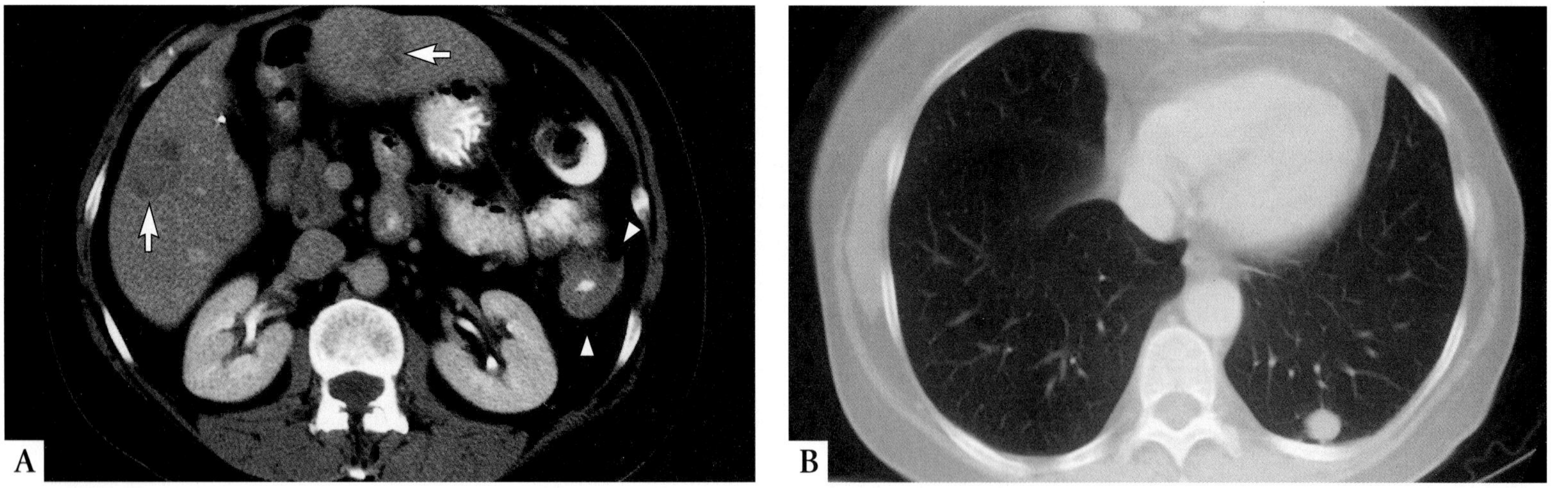

FIGURE 10-8.

Because of vague abdominal symptoms and abnormal liver function, this patient was scheduled for a computed tomographic scan of the abdomen. **A**, This figure is a cross-sectional image of the upper abdomen that demonstrates two well-defined, low-attenuation lesions, one in the right lobe and the other in the left lobe of the liver (*arrows*). The appearance is quite characteristic of metastatic disease. The primary lesion is demonstrated on the computed tomographic scan involving the descending colon (*arrowheads*). In this case, the primary and metastatic disease is seen on a single axial section. The annular nature of the primary lesion is well seen. **B**, This figure is an axial section of the lower lung fields that was included on the abdominal computed tomographic scan and demonstrates another metastatic lesion in the lower left lung field (*arrow*).

The value of cross-sectional imaging in the evaluation of the luminal gut (especially colon) cannot be overemphasized. The amount of information gleaned from this single examination is not only diagnostic but also of great value in staging the disease. This case also demonstrates how the thickness of the bowel wall is much better seen on cross-sectional imaging than with positive-contrast examination or endoscopy.

Gardner's syndrome

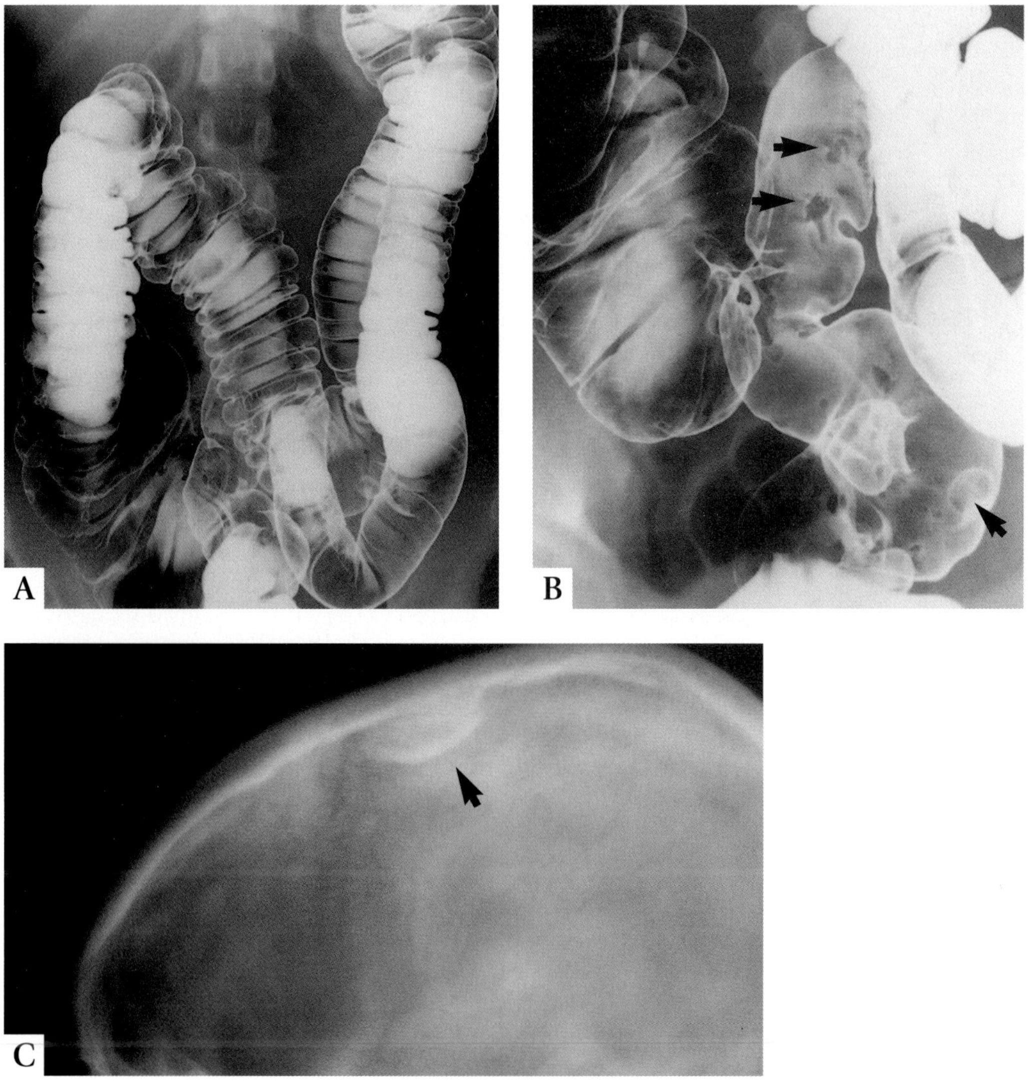

FIGURE 10-9.

Gardner's syndrome. This young female patient initially presented with acute rectal bleeding. The initial examination was an air-contrast examination enema of the colon. **A**, This figure is an overview of the entire colon. A number of adenomatous polyps are seen. **B**, An angled view of the rectum better displays the numerous polyps scattered throughout the colon. Some of the polyps are sessile whereas others are pedunculated (*arrows*). **C**, A lateral view of the skull documents an osteoma involving the vertex of the skull (*arrow*). This patient also had villous adenomas in the duodenum. Subsequently, the patient underwent a total colectomy, and the duodenal adenomas have been resected. The patient is being followed endoscopically. The numerous adenomatous polyps demonstrated on the air-contrast examination of the colon suggest that this patient very likely fits into a syndrome; the skull examination confirms this suggestion by fulfilling the criteria for Gardner's syndrome. The finding of duodenal villous adenomas at the time of endoscopy was initiated by making the diagnosis of Gardner's syndrome.

Multiple familial polyposis

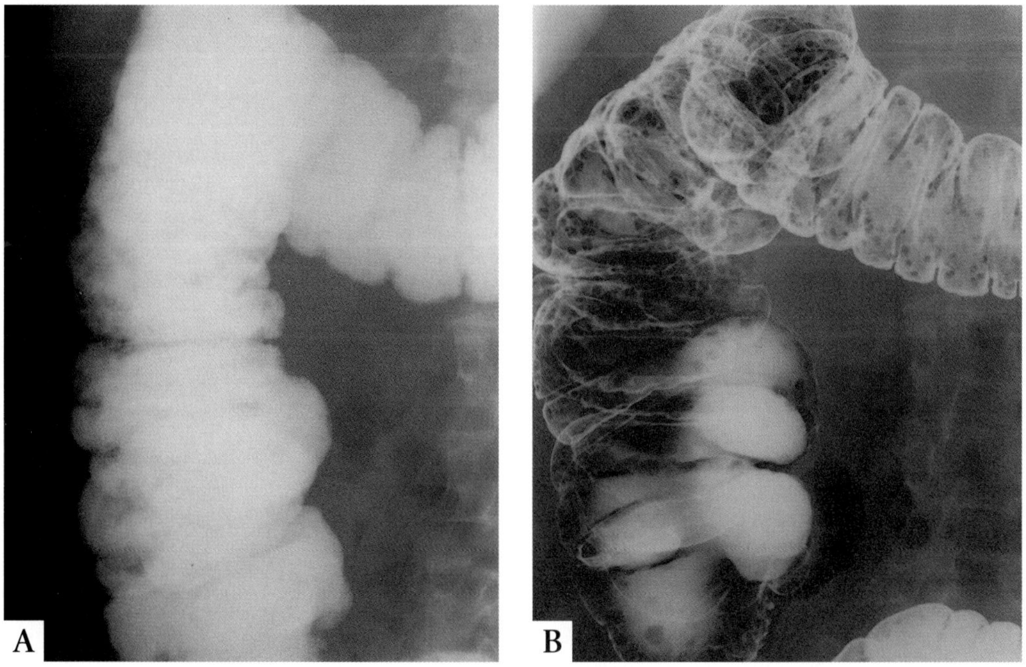

FIGURE 10-10.

Multiple familial adenomatous polyposis. This 40-year-old man initially presented with rectal bleeding. **A**, A single-contrast examination of the colon is shown. Numerous small-filling defects are seen around the margins of the colon but are not well defined. **B**, The air-contrast examination much more graphically demonstrates the multitude of polyps. The polyps, which are too numerous to count, are scattered throughout the colon from the rectum to the cecum. Despite recommendations for colectomy, the patient refused. Three years later he returned with right-sided abdominal pain.

(*Continued on next page*)

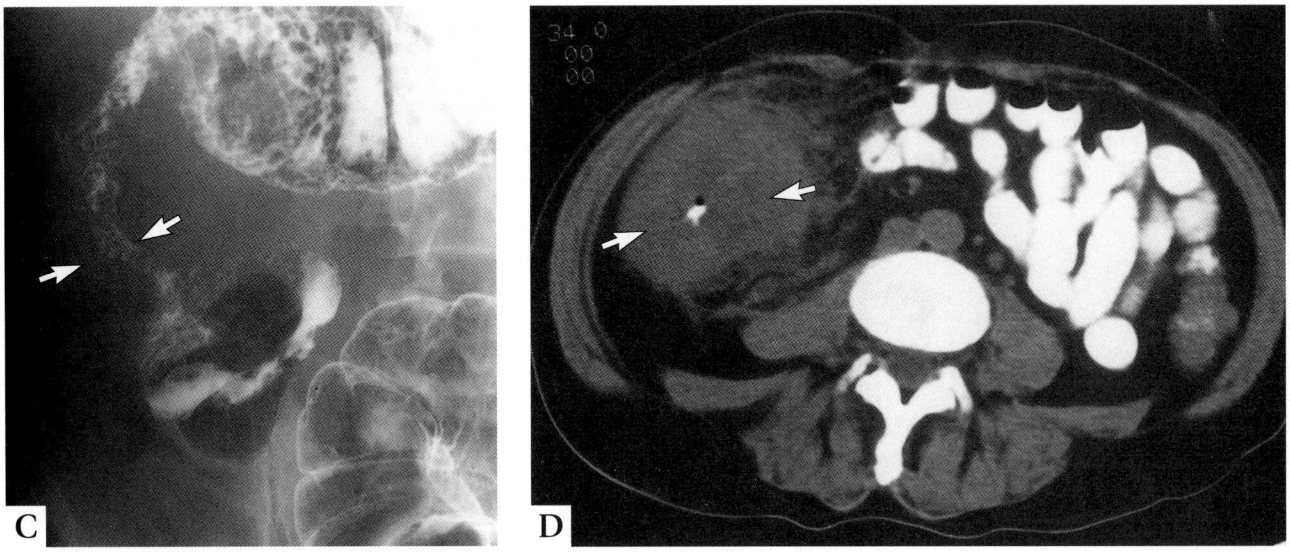

FIGURE 10-10. (*CONTINUED*)

C, A repeat air-contrast examination at that time demonstrates a large infiltrating malignancy in the right colon (*arrows*). **D**, The accompanying computed tomographic scan demonstrates the massive infiltration circumferentially around the ascending colon (*arrows*) by this tumor, which had already metastasized to the liver and to the intra-abdominal nodes.

In most institutions, the air-contrast examination has become the standard examination for the colon. It is advantageous in the detection of early inflammatory disease as well as the demonstration of diminutive polyps. However, single-contrast examinations are still being employed because it may be the best examination for the detection of masses in areas of deformity, such as the colon deformed by sigmoid diverticulosis. Large, bulky tumors and annular tumors may also be better seen on single-contrast examination. The density of barium for single-contrast examination should be in the range of 15% to 20% wt/vol. The density of barium for double-contrast examination of the colon is generally in the range of 80% to 90% wt/vol. (*From* Stewart and Dodds [1]; with permission.)

PSEUDOPOLYPS

Filiform pseudopolyps

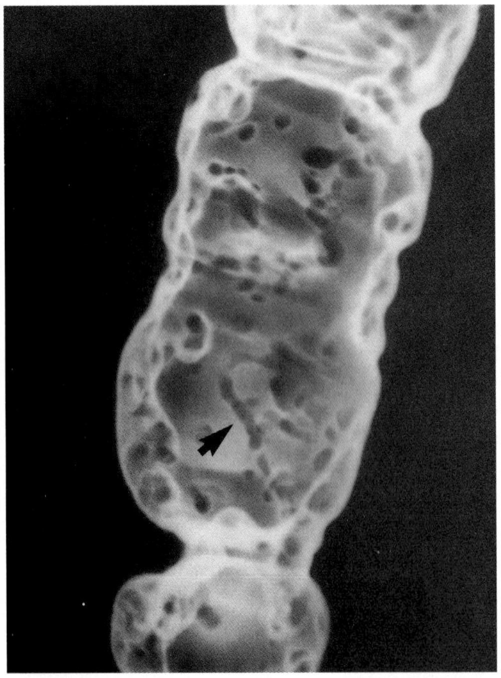

FIGURE 10-11.

Filiform pseudopolyps. This patient with chronic ulcerative colitis is in remission. Filiform pseudopolyps are graphically displayed in these films of this patient. Filiform postinflammatory pseudopolyps may have a characteristic wormlike appearance. They are sometimes confused with multiple adenomatous polyps and might suggest familial adenomatous polyposis. The wormlike appearance as seen in one of the lesions (*arrow*) should allow the strong suspicion that these lesions represent postinflammatory pseudopolyps rather than adenomatous polyps.

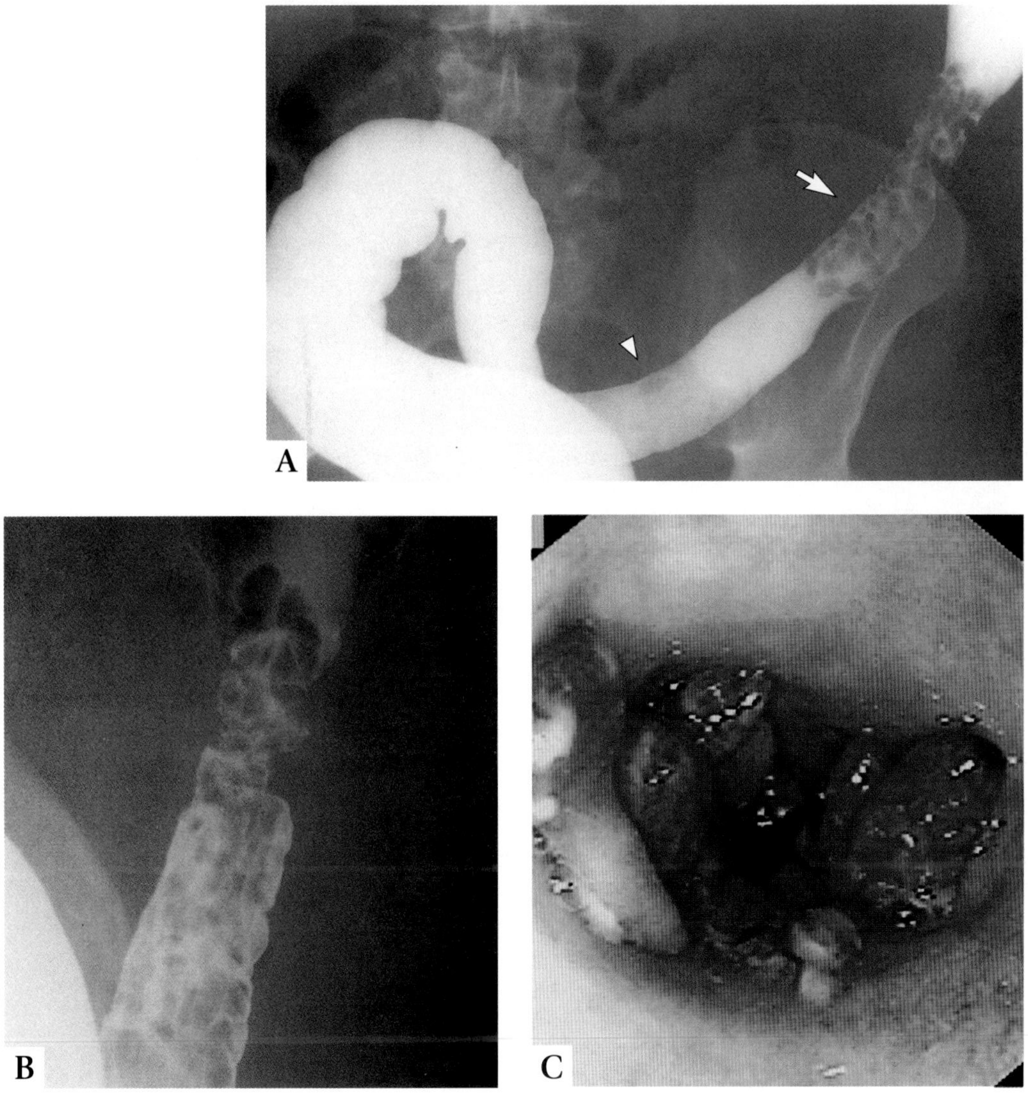

FIGURE 10-12.

Inflammatory pseudopolyps. This patient presented with rectal bleeding. **A**, A single-contrast examination of the colon demonstrates a segment in the descending colon where a long collection of nodular lesions are identified (*arrow*). The colon is moderately narrowed in the same segment. Notice other smaller nodular or polypoid lesions are seen proximal to this area (*arrowhead*). **B**, A more magnified view of the same area shows the nodular appearance of this short segment. **C**, The possibility of a nodular-infiltrating adenocarcinoma was considered in this patient, and endoscopy was performed. The biopsy specimen confirmed that numerous inflammatory pseudopolyps were clustered in the descending colon. When further questioned, the patient admitted to episodes of colitis a number of years before. Postinflammatory pseudopolyps, once present, do not recede in most cases. The focal clustering of pseudopolyps in this patient initiated a search for what was thought to be an infiltrating carcinoma. The atypical presentation of symptoms as well as the atypical presentation of morphologic findings underscore the complementary nature of endoscopic and fluoroscopic examinations and the value of biopsy for confirmation.

DIVERTICULITIS

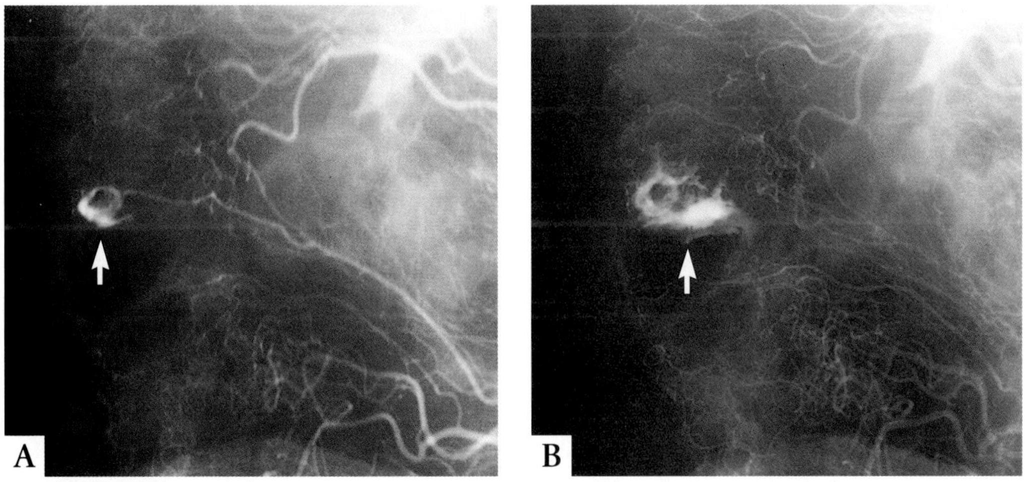

FIGURE 10-13.

Bleeding diverticulitis. Patients with active colonic bleeding are poor candidates for endoscopy as well as for positive-contrast examination of the colon. This limitation is generally caused by the large amount of blood and blood clots. An actively bleeding vessel in the colon is often delineated best at the time of arteriography. **A**, A film during the early arterial phase of an examination of the right colon. This film demonstrates a bleeding vessel in the ascending colon (*arrow*). A few moments later, the rapidity of bleeding is documented in **B**. There has been considerable accumulation of contrast in the lumen of the colon because of the active arterial bleeding (*arrow*). Vessels bleeding at a rate of 1 cm^3/sec are candidates for detection by arteriography.

This study confirms the bleeding source as well as the location in the colon. Either therapeutic application of arteriography by the radiologist or surgical resection can now be directed very accurately. The use of arteriography in the management of patients who are bleeding can reveal either a diagnostic abnormality such as an arteriovenous malformation or may actually demonstrate active bleeding as in this case. This case was a bleeding diverticulum.

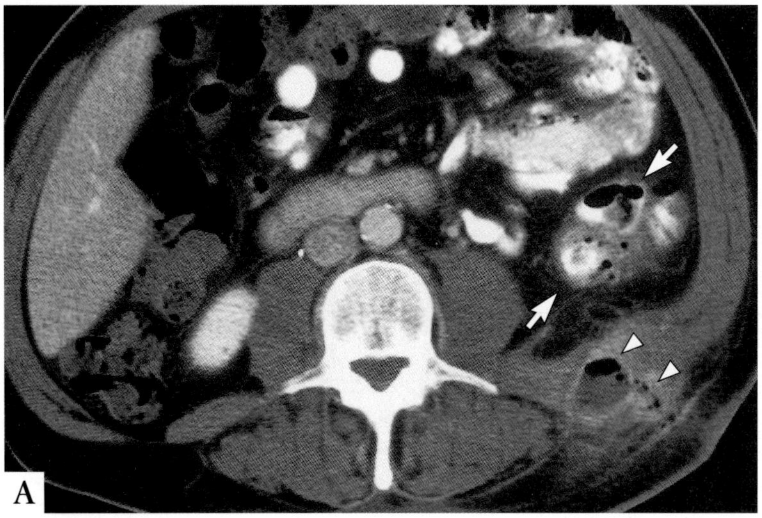

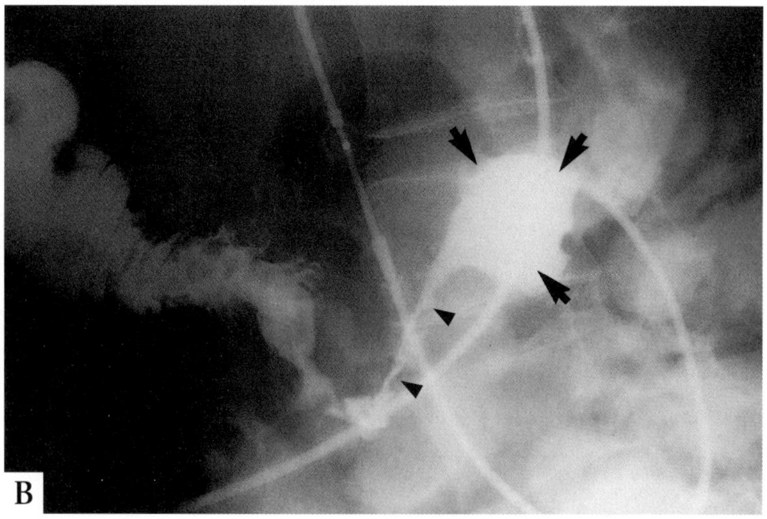

FIGURE 10-14.

Acute diverticulitis with left flank abdominal wall abscess. This elderly male patient with severe obstructive pulmonary disease presented with symptoms suggesting acute diverticulitis. Although historically positive-contrast examinations of the colon were the initial starting point for radiologists in the search for acute diverticulitis, computed tomographic scanning has now become much more commonly used. **A**, The axial section through the abdomen shows the contrast-filled descending colon-sigmoid junction (*arrows*). An abscess in the left posterior abdominal wall contains fluid and gas (*arrowheads*). This patient presented with a flank mass as an initial symptom that corresponded to this abscess cavity. This abscess was drained under computed tomographic guidance with a small pigtail catheter. **B**, Subsequent positive-contrast injection into the catheter opacifies the small abscess cavity in the left flank (*arrows*), which is in direct communication with the colon via a fistulous tract (*arrowheads*).

The advantage of computed tomographic scanning in the presence of acute diverticulitis is the demonstration of the pericolonic abscess, which is always present. Not only will computed tomography show the extraluminal abdomen quite nicely and confirm the diagnosis of diverticulitis, it also allows therapeutic options as in this case, for percutaneous drainage. Obviously, the eventual decision to resect the colon depends on the clinical setting. Complete visualization of the colon either radiographically or endoscopically should be performed before any surgical resection to exclude any synchronous pathology such as colon malignancy elsewhere. It should be noted that a perforated adenocarcinoma of the colon could easily masquerade as acute diverticulitis and could present with similar findings.

INFLAMMATORY BOWEL DISEASES

Ulcerative colitis

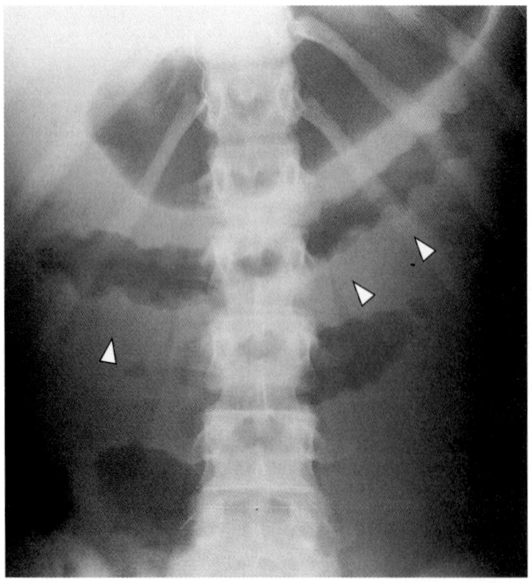

FIGURE 10-15.

Plain film findings of acute ulcerative colitis. This single plain film of the abdomen is taken in a patient with acute ulcerative colitis. Notice the narrowing of the gas-filled transverse colon and the edematous thickening of the wall of the colon (*arrowheads*). A gas-filled loop of small bowel is in the midabdomen as well. The appearance of the gas-filled colon is characteristic of the inflamed colon, which is edematous and not actively contracting; any acute ulcerating colitis could give this appearance. This patient had idiopathic ulcerative colitis. Whether this patient would go on to develop toxic megacolon would be determined by subsequent films and clinical symptoms.

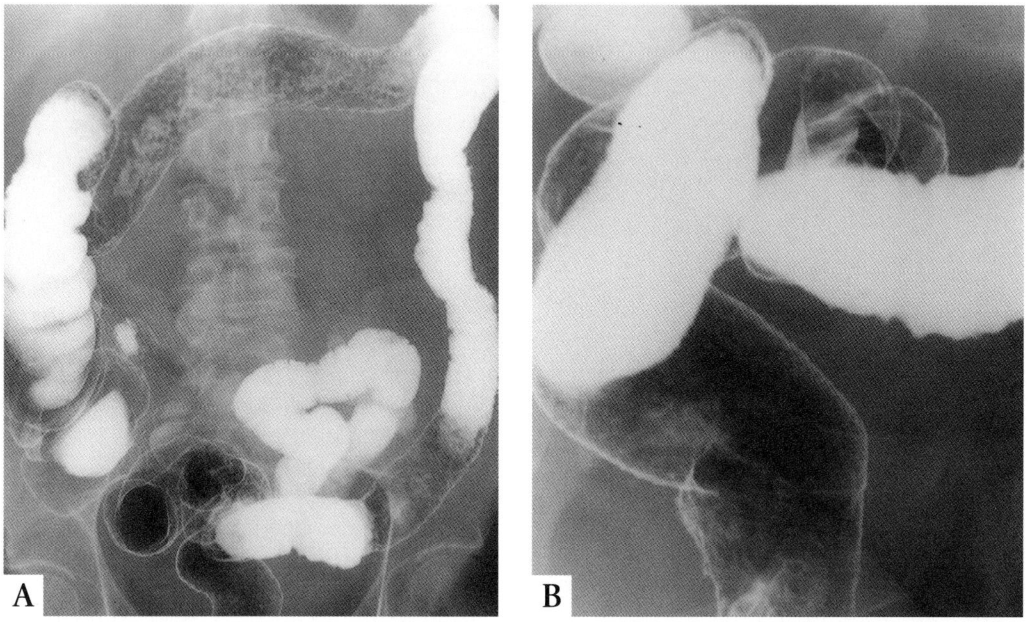

FIGURE 10-16.

Idiopathic ulcerative colitis. **A**, The radiographic features of acute idiopathic ulcerative colitis. The disease characteristically begins in the rectum and extends to the ascending colon. There is diffuse ulceration of the entire colon in this patient. Notice the shortening of the colon and the loss of normal haustral pattern. The terminal ileum is spared and is normal. **B**, A close-up view of the rectosigmoid area. Notice the granular appearance of the mucosa. The earliest radiologic lesion identified in ulcerative colitis is the granular appearance caused by edema and the superficial ulceration in this disease. The air-contrast examination is the most sensitive examination for the early manifestations of inflammatory bowel disease.

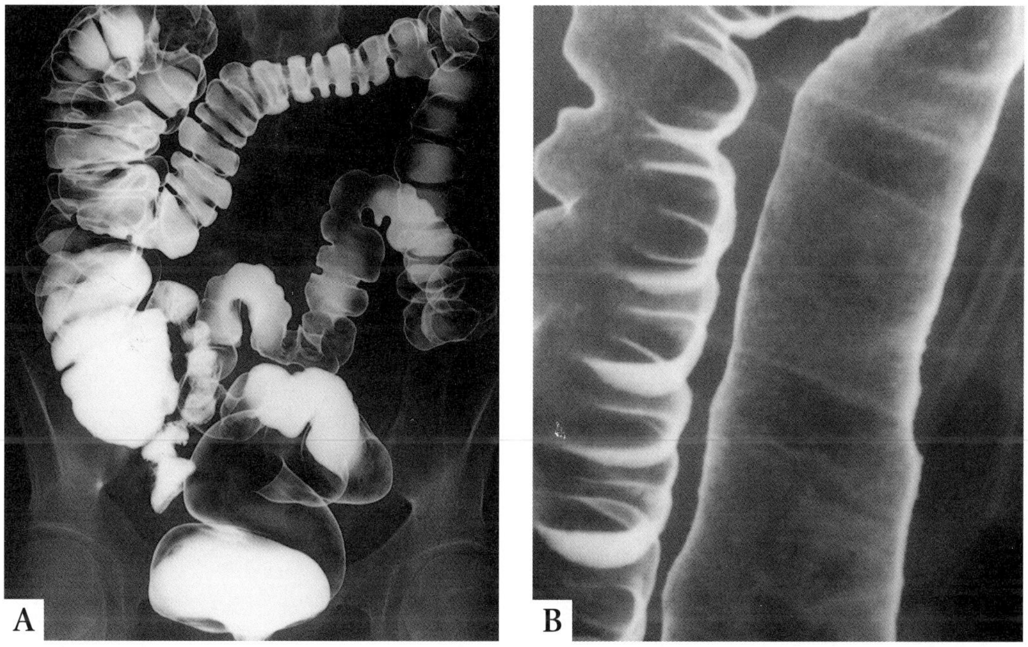

FIGURE 10-17.

Idiopathic ulcerative colitis treated with steroid enemas. This young patient had chronic idiopathic ulcerative colitis and was treated with steroid enemas. **A**, An air-contrast examination of what, at first glance, looks like a relatively normal colon. The haustral pattern is well preserved, and no obvious abnormalities are seen in the mucosa in this overview of the colon. **B**, However, spot films in the region of the splenic flexure demonstrate the typical features of ulcerative colitis. Notice the very fine granular pattern of the barium in the descending colon and transverse colon.

Steroid enemas reverse the changes of acute ulcerative colitis in those areas treated. In this situation, the rectum appears to be essentially normal. It is not until the untreated colon is reached that the findings of inflammatory changes are identified. Meticulous attention to filming and detail of the colonic mucosa is required in order to demonstrate the subtle radiographic features. The value of the air-contrast examination in seeing these subtle findings is very obvious in this case.

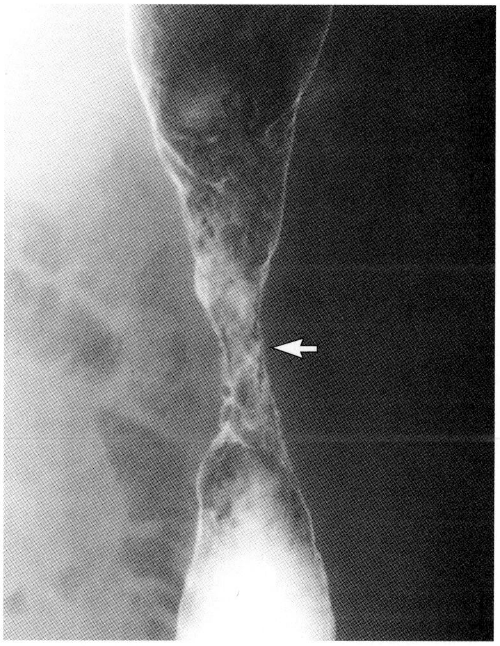

FIGURE 10-18.

Stricture of the colon in a patient with ulcerative colitis. Air-contrast examination of the colon in a patient with ulcerative colitis demonstrates a benign-appearing stricture in the descending colon (*arrow*). In patients with ulcerative colitis, any benign- or malignant-appearing stricture should be considered as malignant until proven otherwise. Infiltrating adenocarcinomas in patients with ulcerative colitis often result in benign-appearing strictures. The role of the radiographic examination is to identify strictures for subsequent colonoscopic surveillance and biopsy. This stricture is focal and markedly narrows the lumen of the colon. The severity of the stricture may not allow passage of the endoscope beyond this area; therefore, the remainder of the colon must be examined by other means, such as an air-contrast examination. The stricture in this case was benign.

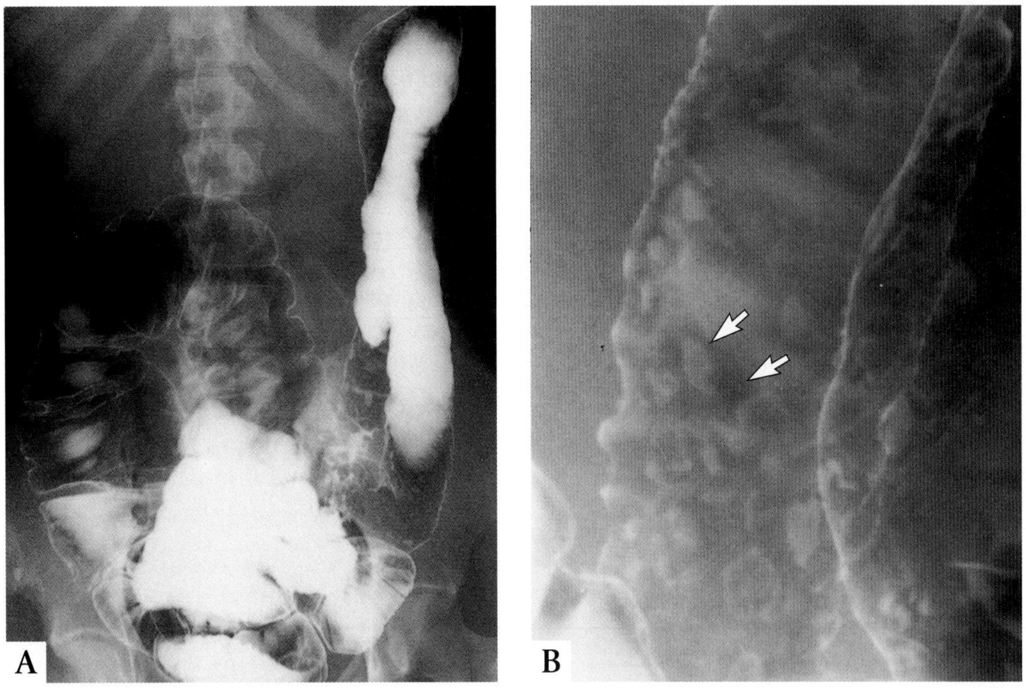

FIGURE 10-19.

Granulomatous colitis. This young patient has symptoms suggesting inflammatory bowel disease. **A**, There are abnormalities of the colon with loss of normal haustral pattern on the left colon and a number of small aphthoid ulcers present throughout the colon, but especially in the right, transverse, and descending colon. **B**, A magnified view of the region of the splenic flexure is depicted. Striking aphthoid ulceration of the transverse and descending colons is much better seen. The large aphthoid ulcers demonstrate the typical changes of this lesion with a rim of edema (*arrows*) and central ulceration. The size of these lesions can vary from small to quite large. The value of the air-contrast examination in showing these ulcerations is demonstrated in this case. The aphthoid ulcer is the earliest diagnostic lesion seen on air-contrast examination in patients with Crohn's disease.

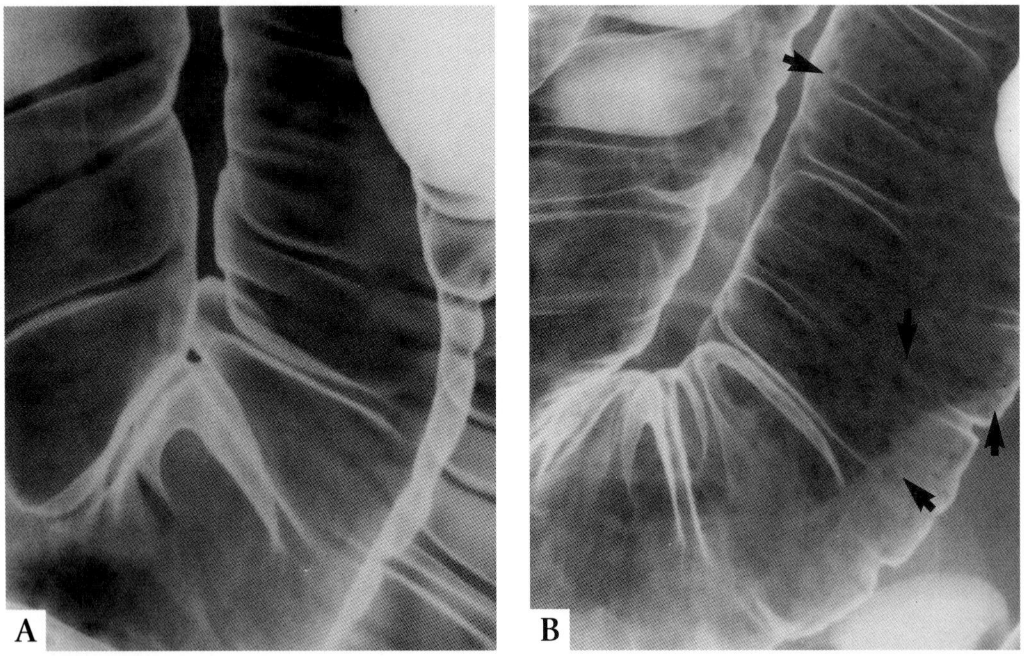

FIGURE 10-20.

A and **B**, Two air-contrast colon examinations in a patient with Crohn's disease are presented. The first examination (*A*) was taken approximately 1 month preceding the second examination (*B*). The colon was normal on the first examination (*A*). Because of persistent symptoms, the second examination (*B*) was performed, and numerous small aphthoid ulcers are now seen in the transverse colon (*arrows*). The rapid development of these tiny lesions is indicative of the rapid progression of the patient's disease. As in this case, the value of considering a repeat examination in a persistently symptomatic individual is emphasized. The sensitivity of the air-contrast examination underscores its use as a primary diagnostic procedure for radiologists in the evaluation of these patients suspected of inflammatory bowel disease.

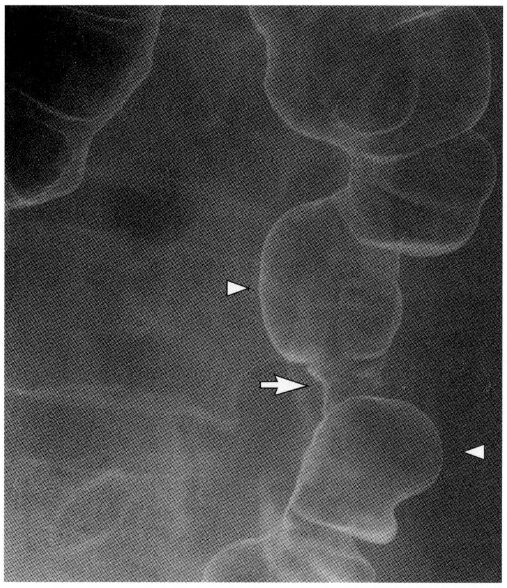

FIGURE 10-21.

This middle-aged man was admitted for evaluation of what was thought to be acute diverticulitis with left abdominal pain. Air-contrast enema of the colon was performed, and a magnified view of the descending colon is shown. In this segment of colon, changes caused by Crohn's disease are quite obvious. Pseudosacculations of the colon (*arrowheads*) and stenotic segments (*arrow*) caused by chronic inflammation are well illustrated.

The features of Crohn's disease involving the colon are displayed in this case. The pseudosacculation formation and alternating areas of narrowing are characteristic of the asymmetric involvement of the colon by granulomatous disease. This asymmetric involvement occurs both circumferentially and longitudinally, producing these changes. Although this patient was over the age of 60, he had never had any colonic symptoms before this time. The value of the positive-contrast examination was to exclude the diagnosis of diverticulitis and make the diagnosis of Crohn's disease involving the colon. The changes are so characteristic that there is little else to consider in the differential. Once again, this case illustrates that many patients initially present with inflammatory bowel disease after age 50.

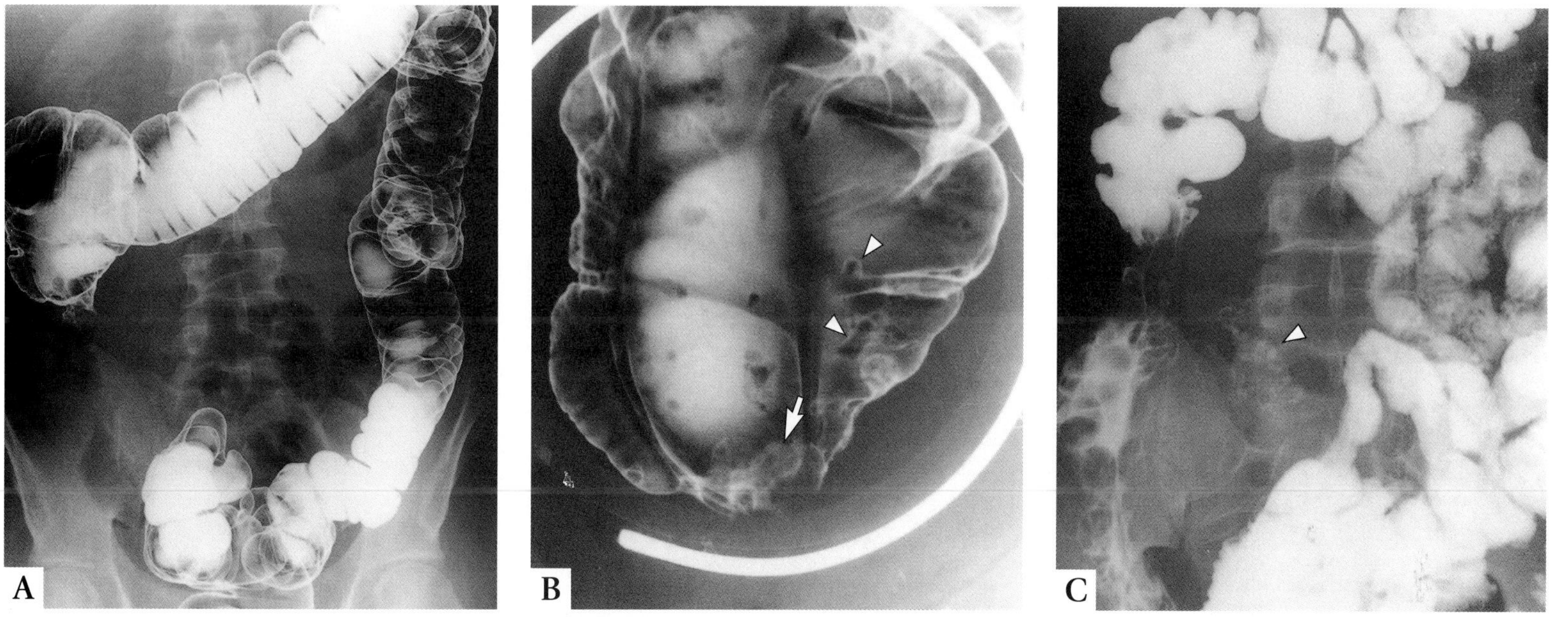

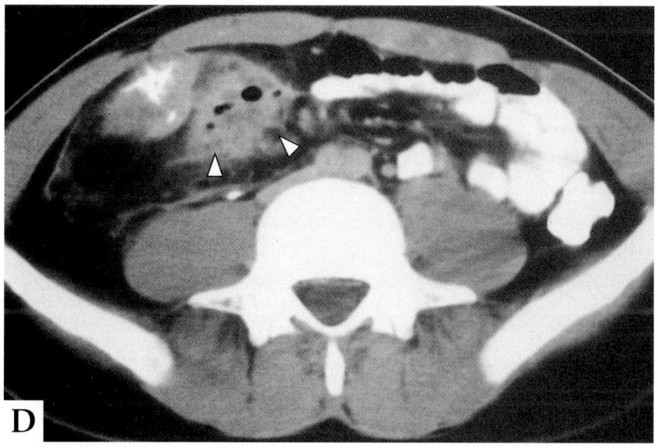

FIGURE 10-22.

This 23-year-old student presented with a palpable, right lower quadrant mass. The patient's discomfort was a new symptom, and he adamantly denied any prior symptoms suggesting inflammatory bowel disease. **A**, The initial examination performed was an air-contrast enema that demonstrates truncation and narrowing of the right colon with failure to demonstrate the cecum and terminal ileum. **B**, Compression and magnification of this area demonstrate numerous polypoid-filling defects that resemble postinflammatory pseudopolyps (*arrowheads*). There is complete obstruction of the ascending colon by a somewhat nodular-appearing abnormality (*arrow*). **C**, A small bowel examination demonstrates the extent of the abnormality. The terminal ileum merges with the right colon. Where the transition between the terminal ileum and the colon occurs is not well defined. The ileocecal valve is not identified. Obviously, this patient has had long-standing, chronic inflammatory bowel disease caused by Crohn's disease. Additionally, there is now an abscess seen lying medial to the right colon (*arrowhead*). Some barium has filled this small communicating abscess. Note the separation of the small bowel from the right colon caused by the inflammatory mass. **D**, A computed tomographic scan of the same area that very graphically demonstrates the inflammatory mass caused by the extracolonic abscess that contains some gas (*arrowheads*).

Once again, the quiescent nature of inflammatory bowel disease is illustrated in this patient who denied any prior symptoms. Obviously, the patient has far advanced inflammatory bowel disease and now presents with a pericolonic abscess that he noticed as a right lower quadrant mass. Additionally, three examinations were required to adequately assess this patient's abdomen. The barium enema followed by the small bowel examination and, ultimately, the computed tomographic scan each contributes significant information to the diagnosis. The logical sequential application of diagnostic procedures is illustrated by these images. Notice the value of the computed tomographic scan in the evaluation of the extraluminal abdomen. This patient was not treated with percutaneous drainage of the abscess. He was treated with antibiotics and ultimately, surgical resection of the right colon and terminal ileum and has done well.

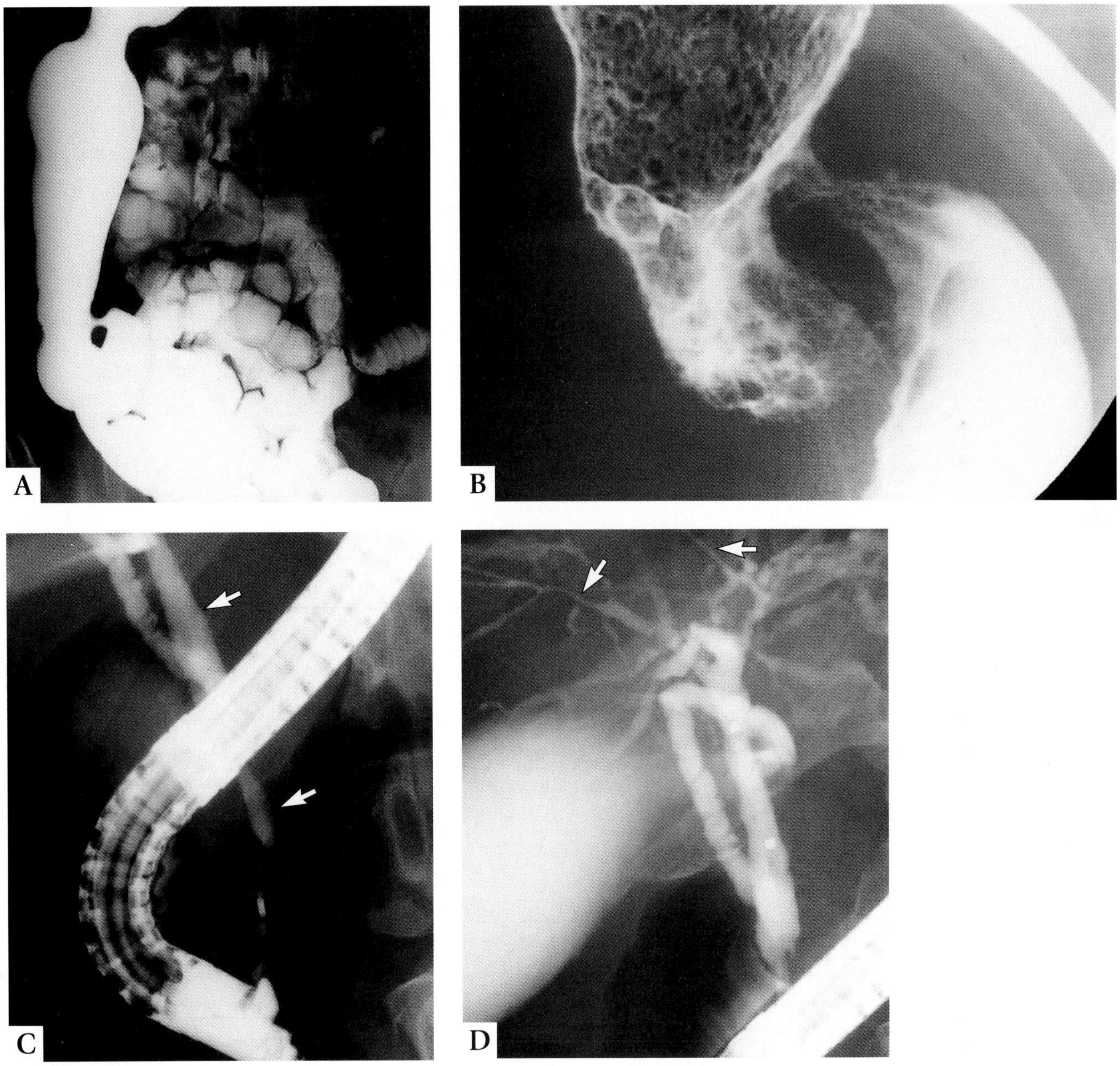

FIGURE 10-23.

Granulomatous colitis and sclerosing cholangitis. This 35-year-old man presented with a 4-year history of vague abdominal pain and abnormal liver function. **A**, This film from a single-column small bowel examination demonstrates an abnormal right colon and a questionable abnormal terminal ileum. The right colon is featureless and without a haustral pattern, and the ileocecal valve appears to be patulous. **B**, After allowing some air to enter, a compression view over the cecum demonstrates a diffusely ulcerated and abnormal cecum and a questionable normal-appearing ileum. This patient clearly has inflammatory bowel disease. Flexible sigmoidoscopy had been normal. Because of abnormal liver function, an endoscopic retrograde cholangiopancreatography (ERCP) was performed. **C** and **D**, Primary sclerosing cholangitis was confirmed. Narrowing of the distal common duct and irregularity of the common hepatic duct (*arrows*) typical of sclerosing cholangitis is shown (*C*). The diffuse abnormalities of the intrahepatic ducts are best seen on *D* with multiple areas of stricture and inflammatory changes involving the intrahepatic ducts (*arrows*).

This patient had granulomatous colitis that obviously was chronic. Initial presentation was with abnormal liver function studies. It is not unusual to "back" into the diagnosis of inflammatory bowel disease in patients with abnormal liver function. In this case, the ERCP was performed after the documentation of the abnormality on the barium study. Oftentimes the diagnosis of primary sclerosing cholangitis is established before the abnormality is documented in the colon or small bowel. Primary sclerosing cholangitis is seen much more commonly in patients with idiopathic ulcerative colitis.

Toxic megacolon

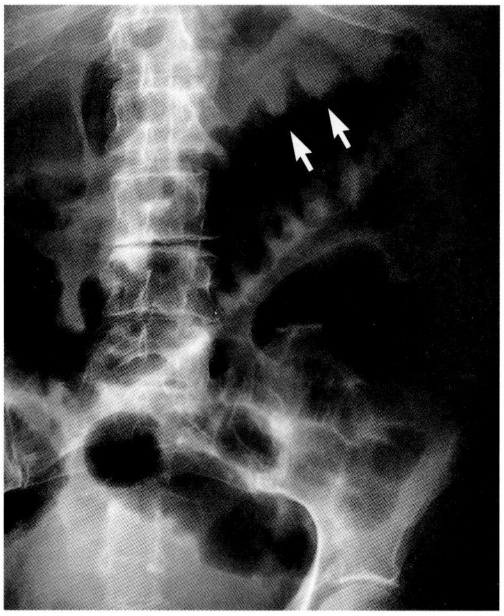

FIGURE 10-24.

This elderly patient presented with symptoms of toxic megacolon. Notice the appearance of the transverse colon which is dilated with markedly thickened haustral folds caused by edema (*arrows*). Oftentimes, inflammatory pseudopolyps can be seen on these plain films as well.

The features of the colon seen on this plain film of the abdomen are often seen in patients presenting with toxic megacolon. Progressive dilatation of the colon may precede perforation. These patients need an immediate therapeutic decision, and oftentimes, colectomy is indicated on an urgent basis. Toxic megacolon is a clinical diagnosis. However, the radiographic features of acute colitis are easily seen and should alert the clinician to a rapid assessment of these patients. Although toxic megacolon is more often seen in acute idiopathic ulcerative colitis, it is occasionally seen in patients with Crohn's disease. This patient had documented granulomatous colitis at resection. It is of interest to note that this patient denied any antecedent symptoms and presented with toxic megacolon as her initial presenting symptom.

Pseudomembranous colitis

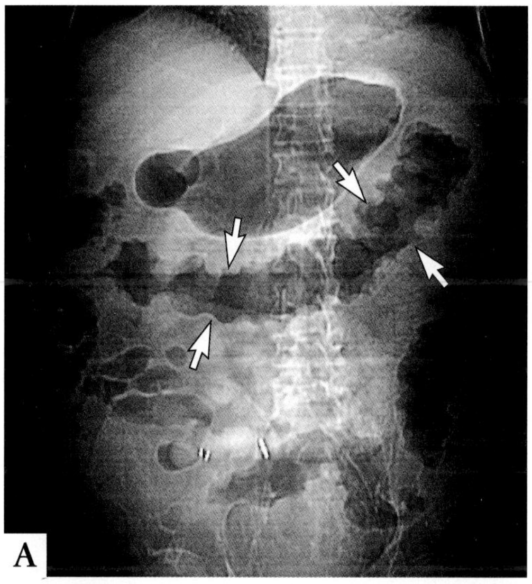
A

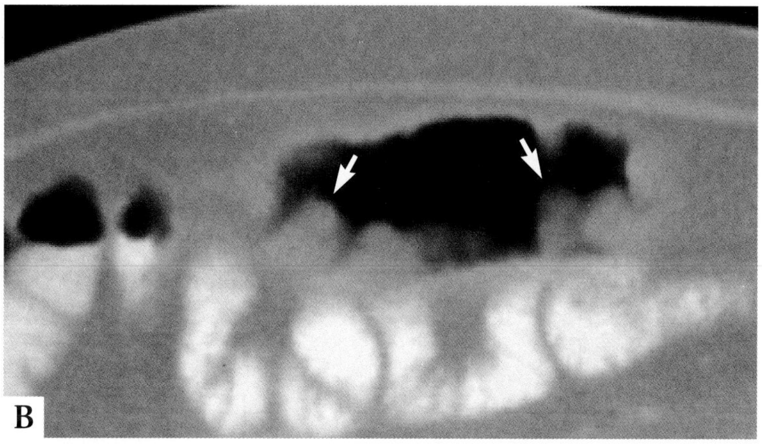
B

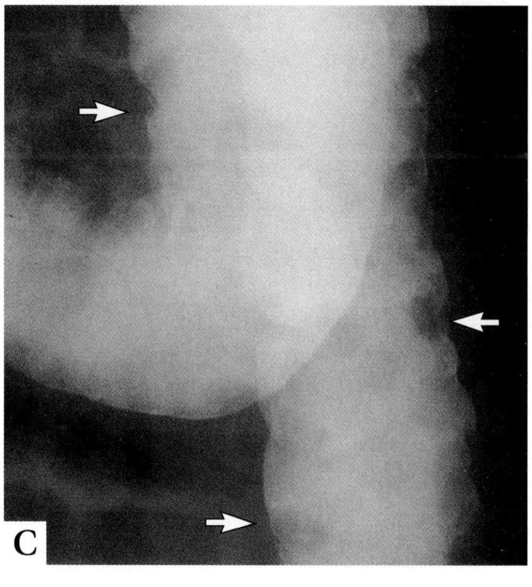
C

FIGURE 10-25.

Clostridium difficile colitis. It is not unusual to identify significant pathology of the colon during computed tomographic scanning. **A**, A computed radiograph obtained at the time of positioning the patient for a computed tomographic scan. The quality of computed radiographs are usually excellent and may be entirely satisfactory to make a diagnosis. In this patient who has a renal transplant, the presence of abdominal pain triggered a search for intra-abdominal disease, and a computed tomographic scan was ordered. Notice the striking abnormality of the gas-filled transverse colon (*arrows*). A markedly thickened nodular appearance of the mucosa of the transverse colon is very evident. Some of the same changes can be seen in the descending and sigmoid colon. **B**, An image from the 1-cm axial section through the transverse colon. Looking at the colonic mucosa is possible using very wide window levels as in this case. Notice the nodular thickening of the wall of the colon (*arrows*). This very abnormal mucosa is nicely demonstrated using this window level. Compare these changes with changes during a single-contrast examination of the colon as shown in **C**. Notice the nodular thickening involving the transverse colon and descending colon (*arrows*).

Both the computed tomographic scan and the positive-contrast examination are sufficient to make a diagnosis of colitis in this clinical setting. Although other forms of colitis cannot be excluded, the presence of a positive *C. difficile* culture confirmed the etiology in this particular case. This case illustrates the value of looking at computed radiographs generated during computed tomographic scans. Oftentimes, abnormalities can direct the physician to either subsequent radiographic or endoscopic visualization of the colon.

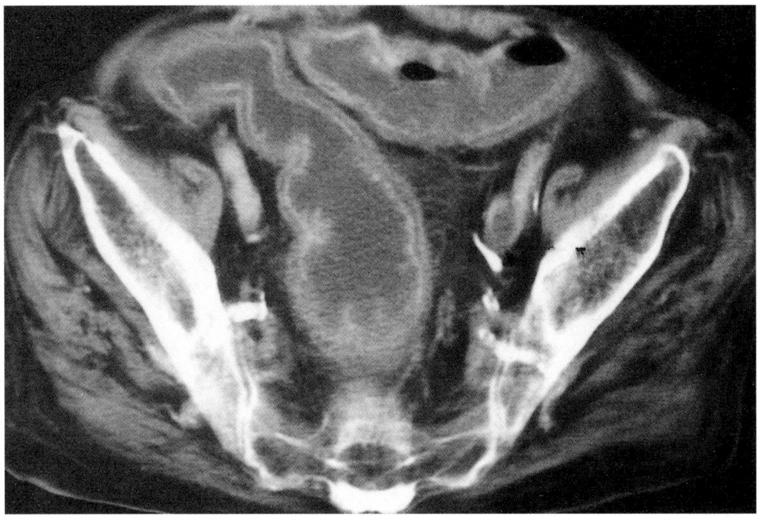

Figure 10-26.

Acute pseudomembranous colitis. A single axial section taken at the time of the computed tomographic scan of the abdomen demonstrates the findings that are often encountered with colitis. There is thickening of the colonic wall and enhancement of the mucosa. This patient's study was done following the administration of intravenous contrast. The fluid-filled diarrheal contents of the colon are also nicely demonstrated. It is not unusual to diagnose pseudomembranous colitis in patients who are being scanned for other reasons in whom the diagnosis has not been previously entertained.

Colitis proximal to obstructing colon cancer

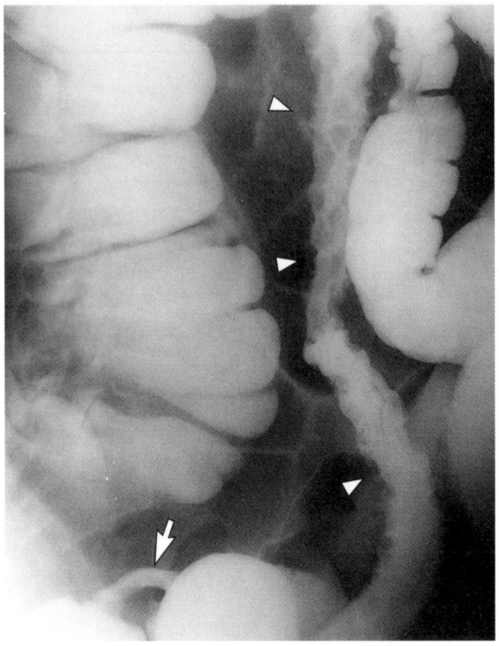

Figure 10-27.

Occasionally, an unusual form of colitis presents proximal to high-grade obstruction. This patient has an obstructing rectosigmoid carcinoma (*arrow*). There is narrowing and nodular thickening of the mucosa of the descending colon above the tumor (*arrowheads*). The differential diagnosis of this form of colitis would be different if the obstructing lesion had not been identified in the rectosigmoid; however, in this setting, it is undoubtedly related to colitis proximal to obstruction. The etiology is unknown but may be vascular in nature. It is very likely that colonoscopy would be unsuccessful in viewing this area because of the malignant stricture. (*From* Stewart and Dodds [1]; with permission.)

PERIANAL FISTULA

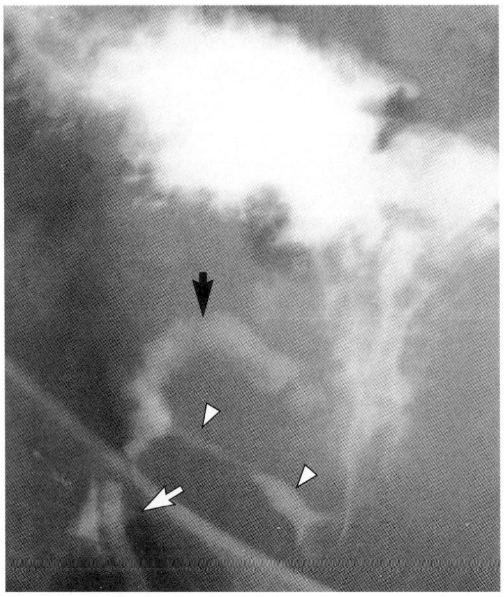

Figure 10-28.

Perianal fistula. This patient has no underlying inflammatory bowel disease and has a spontaneous perianal fistula. The examination of these patients must be done very carefully and repeat examination may be necessary. In this case, there is a Foley balloon that has been distended and held against the orifice of the fistula to the skin (*white arrow*). Water-soluble contrast has been injected, and two fistulous tracts have been identified to the colon. One of these tracts is in the upper anal canal (*black arrow*), and the other tract is in the lower rectum (*arrowhead*). Contrast is filling the rectum and the distal rectosigmoid.

Evaluation of patients with fistulas can be very difficult. Generally, the best way to examine a fistula is to directly inject the opening at the skin rather than to try to fill the colon and the fistula from the inside. Much more pressure can be applied from the outside, and controlled injection of contrast can be performed as well as optimizing positioning for filming. Water-soluble contrast should be employed. A Foley catheter is never distended within a fistulous tract; it is only held against the skin. The most important technical aspect is occluding the external opening so that retrograde instillation of contrast is successful. It should be remembered that fistulas in the perianal area are extremely painful. Patients are very reluctant to have manipulation and may require sedation. Local skin anesthesia is occasionally necessary. Digital radiography has the ability to magnify and is very useful in these procedures as was performed in this case.

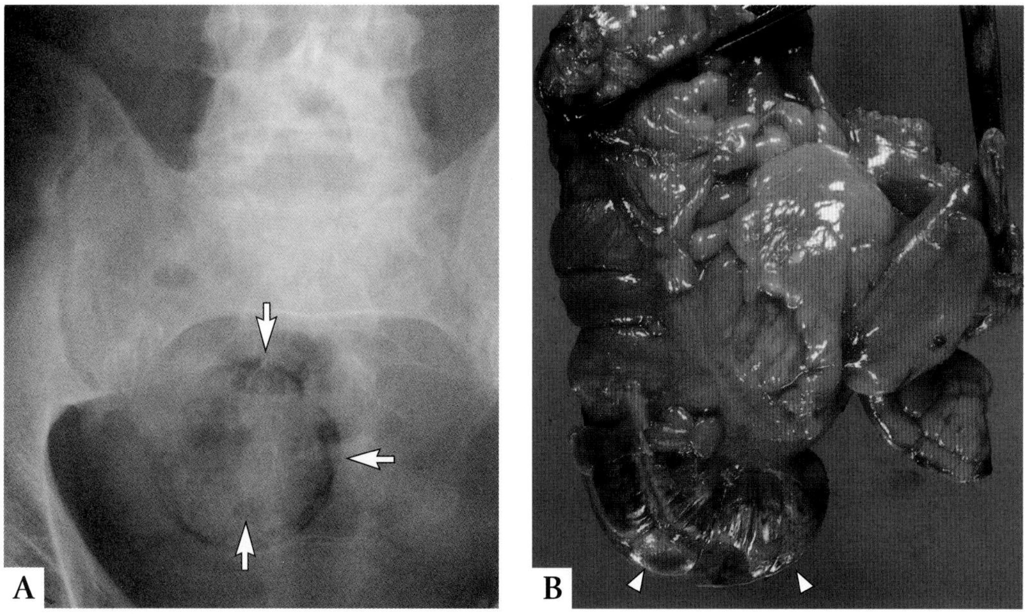

FIGURE 10-29.

Cecal infarction. This 50-year-old man undergoing coronary artery bypass surgery developed right lower quadrant pain 3 days following surgery. **A**, A persistent gas collection (*arrows*) in the right lower quadrant was thought to represent intramural gas rather than gas surrounding stool; its exact location, confirmed by positive-contrast study, was in the cecum. **B**, At surgery, the resected cecum demonstrated transmural infarction of the cecal tip (*arrowheads*). The etiology of the cecal infarction in this patient was thought to be an undetected low flow state sometime during the patient's hospital stay. Intramural gas, in this setting, should raise the suspicion of a significant vascular accident with infarction. Although benign causes of intramural gas and subserosal gas are demonstrated in Figure 10-31, in this setting, gas collection of this type is an abnormal finding. Notice how this collection of gas might go undetected if confused with gas in the rectosigmoid area and stool. If in question, computed tomographic scanning through this area would very nicely confirm the location of gas as being in or out of the bowel wall. Gas within the portal venous system is a very poor prognostic sign when bowel infarction is present.

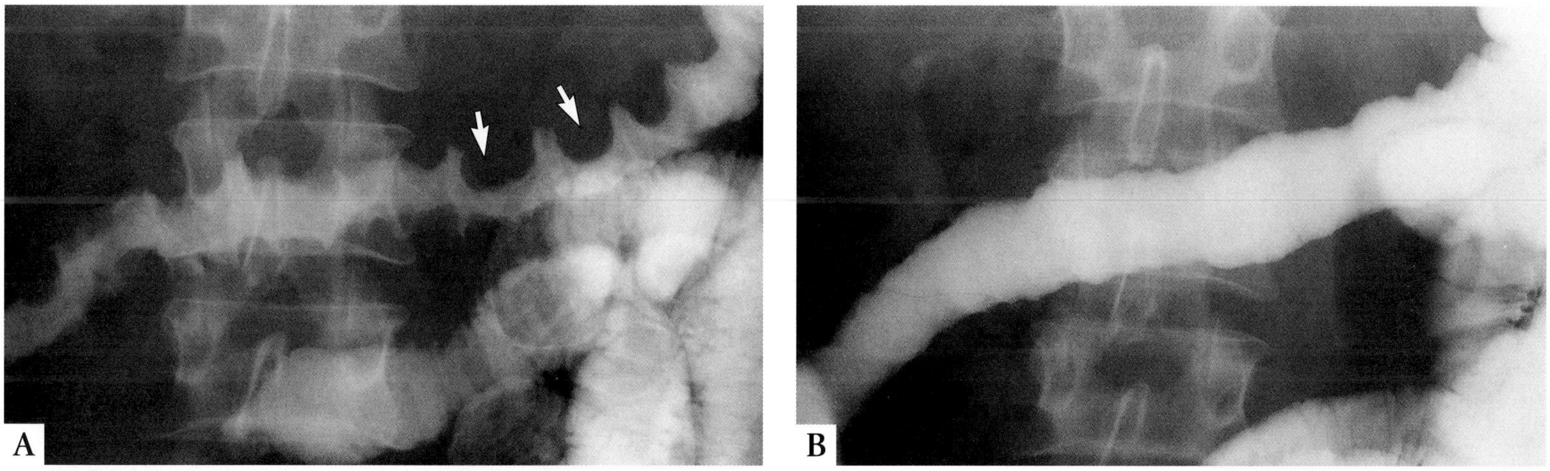

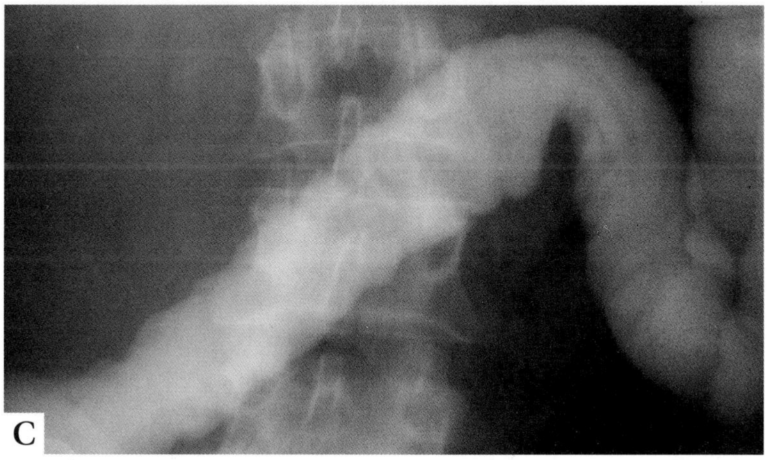

FIGURE 10-30.

Ischemic injury to the colon caused by seat belt injury. This young patient was admitted following abdominal trauma. He was a belted passenger and had a deceleration injury while driving. **A**, This figure depicts the colon using a single-contrast examination. Acute ischemic injury to the colon is caused by severe arterial injury. Notice the intramural hemorrhage and narrowing of the colon secondary to the ischemic injury (*arrows*). Intramural hemorrhage manifests itself as *thumb prints* in the wall of the colon. **B**, Approximately 1 week later, a repeat enema was performed. The intramural hemorrhage has resolved, but there is superficial ulceration of the colonic mucosa with fine-speculated margins seen radiographically. Notice that there continues to be a narrowing of the lumen of the colon. **C**, A third examination approximately 1 week later demonstrates gradual healing of the colon with improved diameter and some continued edema and superficial ulceration of the mucosa. Many of these ischemic injuries completely repair themselves, depending on the degree of collateral circulation that develops; however, a severe stricture can occur. Colonic segments that are put to rest during the healing phase by a diverting colostomy may develop severe strictures caused by the absence of the fecal stream. This case graphically demonstrates the variable appearance of ischemic injury to the colon depending on when the examination is performed.

PNEUMATOSIS INTESTINALIS

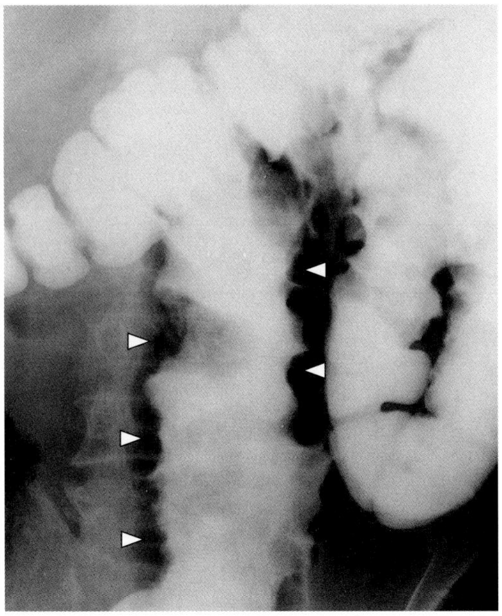

FIGURE 10-31.

Pneumatosis cytoides intestinalis. This elderly nursing home patient chronically carries the diagnosis of pneumatosis cystoides intestinalis; he is asymptomatic. This figure demonstrates a single-contrast examination showing the presence of gas in the wall of the rectosigmoid colon (*arrowheads*). Unless the presence of gas in the wall of the colon is appreciated, these polypoid-filling defects may be misdiagnosed as colonic polyps or, possibly, an intramural hemorrhage. Usually, these gas collections are easily seen on the films of the barium-filled colon. Gas in the bowel wall can be benign or associated with significant disease such as ischemia. The clinical presentation of these patients should allow discrimination as to which patients to follow and which patients require aggressive and possibly surgical management. Gas in the bowel wall accompanied by portal vein gas is an ominous finding suggesting infarction. Prognostically, gas in the portal venous system is accompanied by a very high mortality rate approaching 100%. Benign causes of gas in the portal vein are occasionally encountered because of mucosal disruption, such as following endoscopy and biopsy, and may also be seen in inflammatory conditions, *eg*, acute diverticulitis.

ACUTE PANCREATITIS RESULTING IN COLONIC STRICTURE

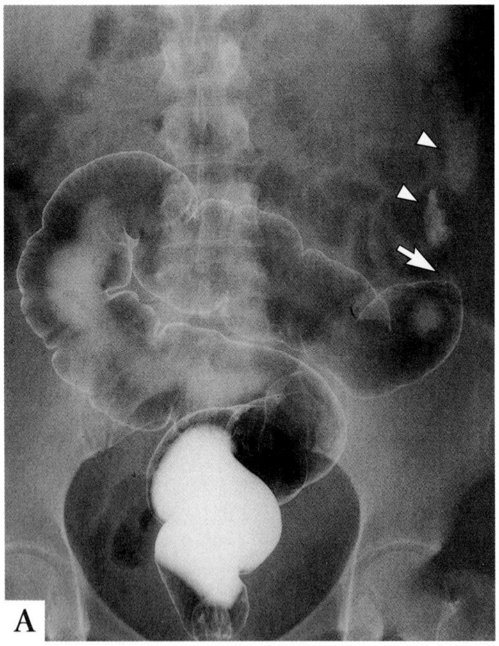

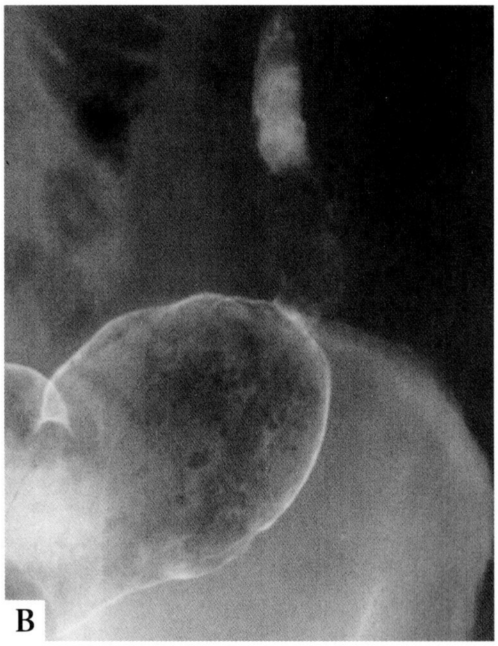

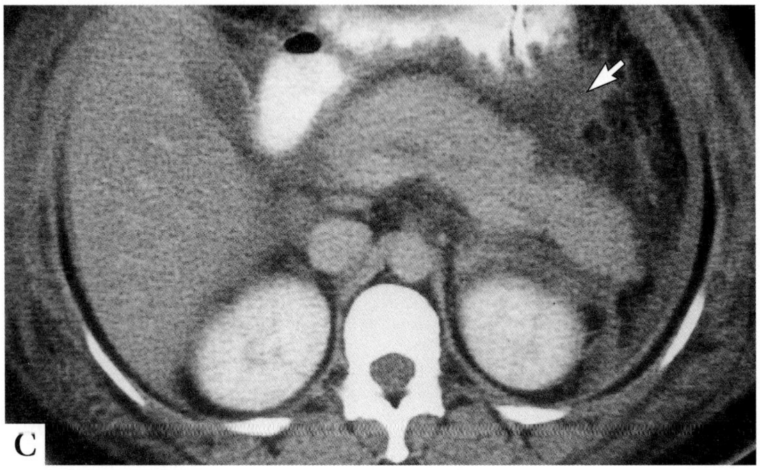

FIGURE 10-32.

A, A pneumocolon in a patient with a history of pancreatitis who now presents with left abdominal pain. There is a rather abrupt narrowing of the descending colon (*arrow*) with a small amount of contrast flowing proximal to the area (*arrowheads*). The gas pattern in the proximal colon and small bowel does not suggest obstruction. **B**, A magnified view of the same area is shown. **C**, Computed tomographic scan of the abdomen taken approximately 1 month before the barium enema displays the typical features of acute pancreatitis. There is enlargement of the pancreas and a great deal of peripancreatic edema (*arrow*). **D**, A follow-up computed tomographic scan was performed approximately 2 weeks later. An image from the midabdomen shows fluid in the left anterior pararenal space (*arrow*) adjacent to the descending colon (*arrowhead*). Notice the thickening of the fascia in the same region caused by the dissecting peripancreatic fluid and edema. **E**, A computed tomographic scan taken several weeks later demonstrates improvement in the anterior pararenal fluid collection (*arrow*). Notice the thick walled strictured segment of the descending colon (*arrowhead*).

This patient has developed an inflammatory stricture of the descending colon because of the adjacent inflammation resulting from the pancreatitis. The evolution of the inflammatory stricture in the colon is beautifully displayed using cross-sectional imaging.

(*Continued on next page*)

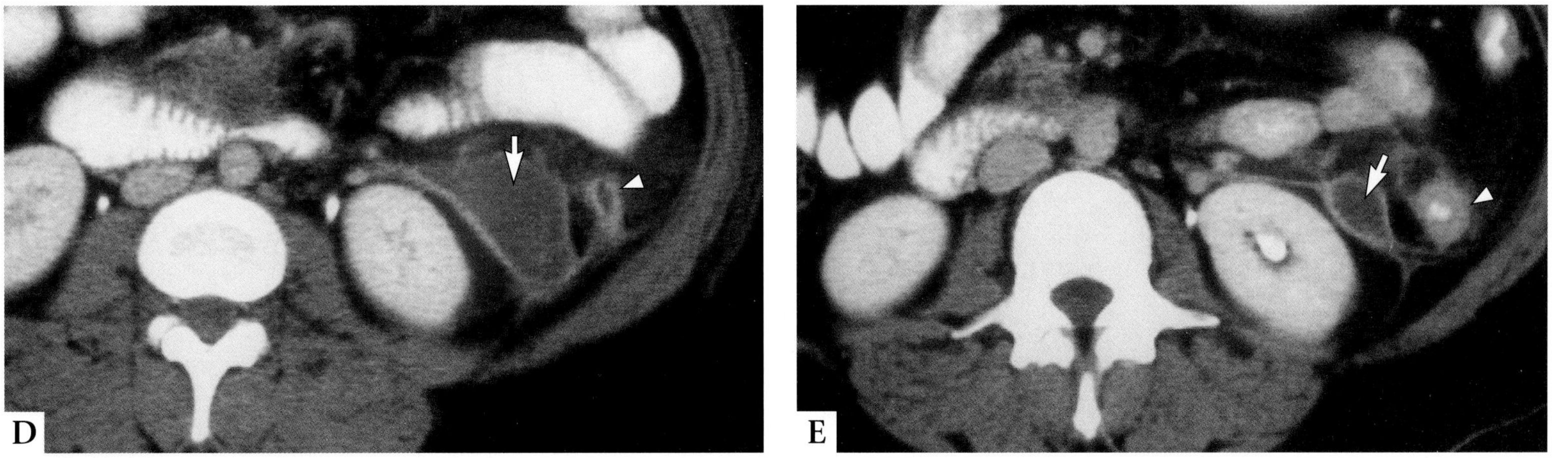

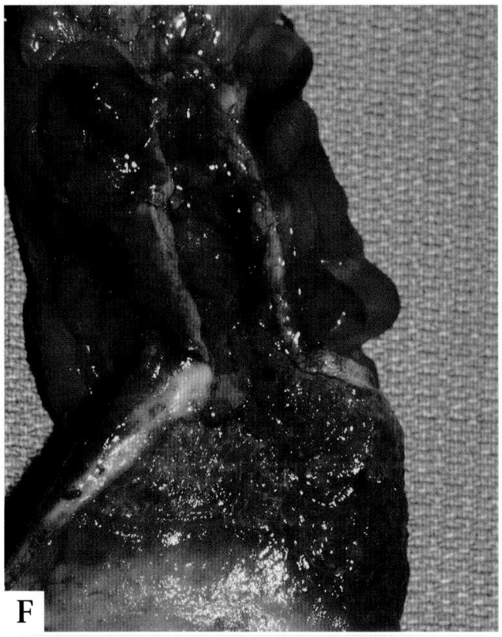

FIGURE 10-32. (*CONTINUED*)

Once again, the value of cross-sectional imaging is in the demonstration of the extraluminal abdominal contents. In this case, no other imaging modality would be better to demonstrate the pathophysiology of this inflammatory process. **F**, Because of the strictured segment, the patient required surgery and resection of the descending colon. Notice the inflammatory narrowing of the colon in the resected specimen.

Peripancreatic fluid collections are seen in computed tomographic scans and can be shown to affect viscera in the abdomen, such as the stomach, duodenum, small bowel, and colon. Spontaneous decompression into the bowel may occasionally occur. Extension of peripancreatic fluid collections outside the abdomen into the chest and groin are not unusual.

ENDOMETRIOSIS

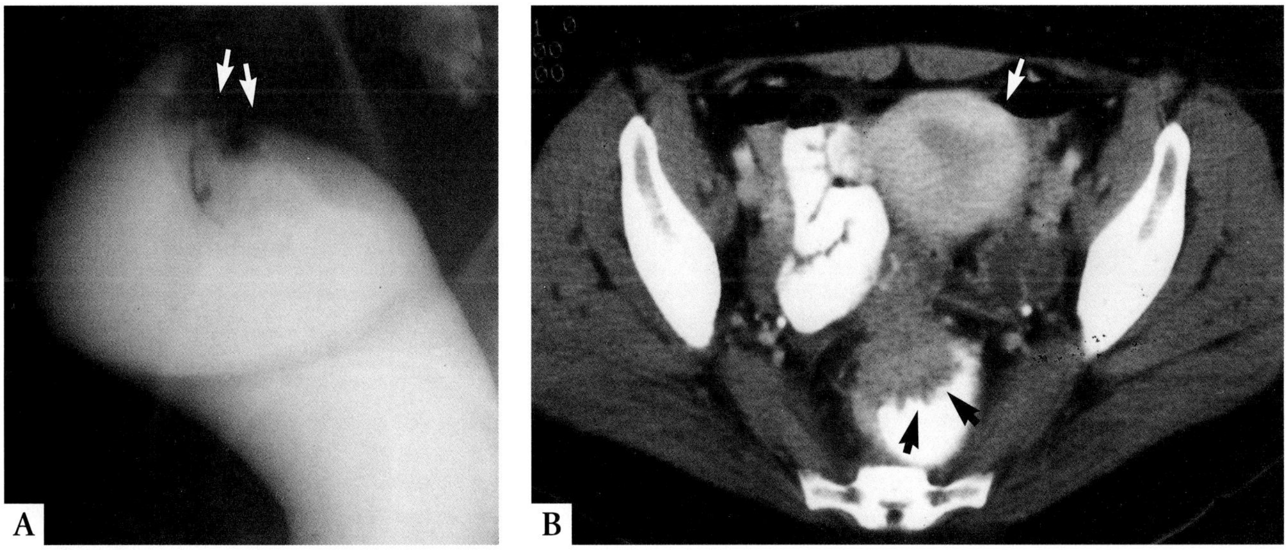

FIGURE 10-33.

Endometriosis. This young female patient was being evaluated for intermittent rectal bleeding and pelvic pain. **A**, A single-contrast barium enema demonstrates a large nodular, partially obstructing lesion in the rectosigmoid junction (*arrows*). **B**, Similar features are seen on the computed tomographic scan. The mass in the cul-de-sac is seen extending into the colon (*black arrows*). Notice the normal uterus (*white arrow*).

(*Continued on next page*)

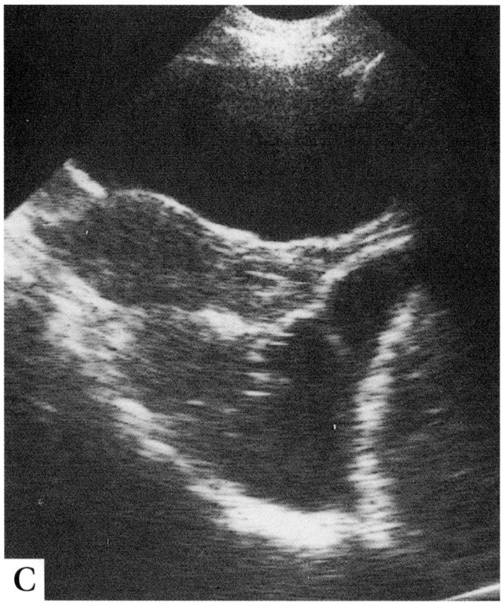

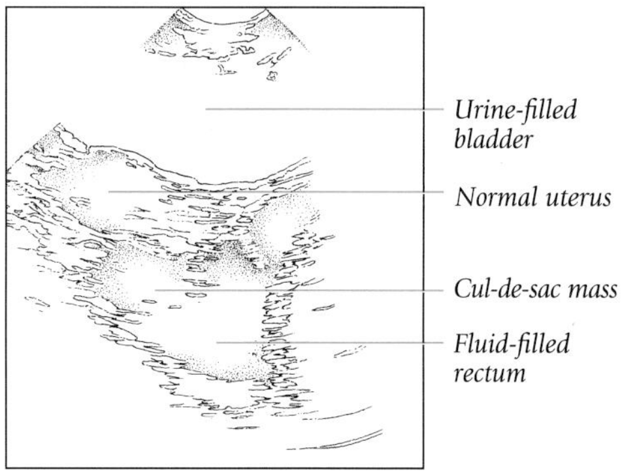

FIGURE 10-33. (CONTINUED)

C, A pelvic ultrasound in the sagittal plane very nicely demonstrates the urine-filled bladder, the normal uterus, the cul-de-sac mass, and the fluid-filled rectum.

Although this patient was initially thought to have adenocarcinoma, a biopsy confirmed that this mass represented a large endometrioma. The cul-de-sac location of the mass is best seen on ultrasound and computed tomography, which complement the positive-contrast examination of the rectum. Endometriomas are most often implanted on the sigmoid colon because of migration to the dependent cul-de-sac. Implantation on the terminal ileum, cecum, and appendix may also occur. Occasionally, an intraluminal nodular mass lesion of substantial proportions is identified as in this case that might be confused with a primary mucosal malignancy. Atypical presentation of endometriosis can occasionally cause puzzling findings for radiologists and gastroenterologists.

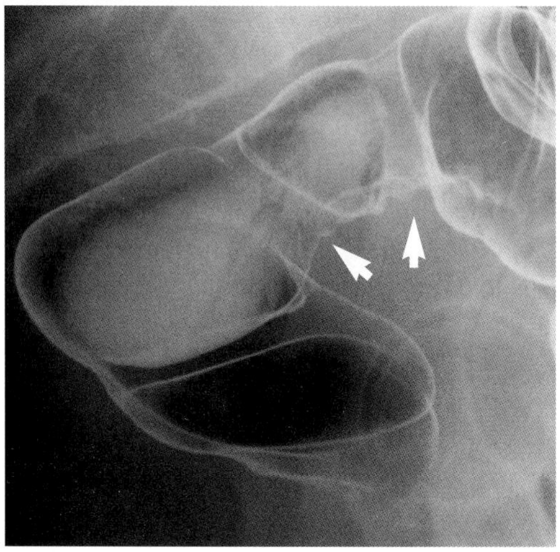

FIGURE 10-34.

This lateral view of the rectum demonstrates the more usual appearance of an endometrioma in the wall of the colon. This particular location, at the rectosigmoid junction, is a favorite site of implantation of endometrial tissue. Notice the somewhat spiculated appearance of the mass in the wall of the colon (*arrows*). In contrast to the patient in Figure 10-33, this lesion is much less dramatic but more typical of the appearance of endometriosis involving the sigmoid colon.

INTRAMURAL HEMORRHAGE OF THE BOWEL

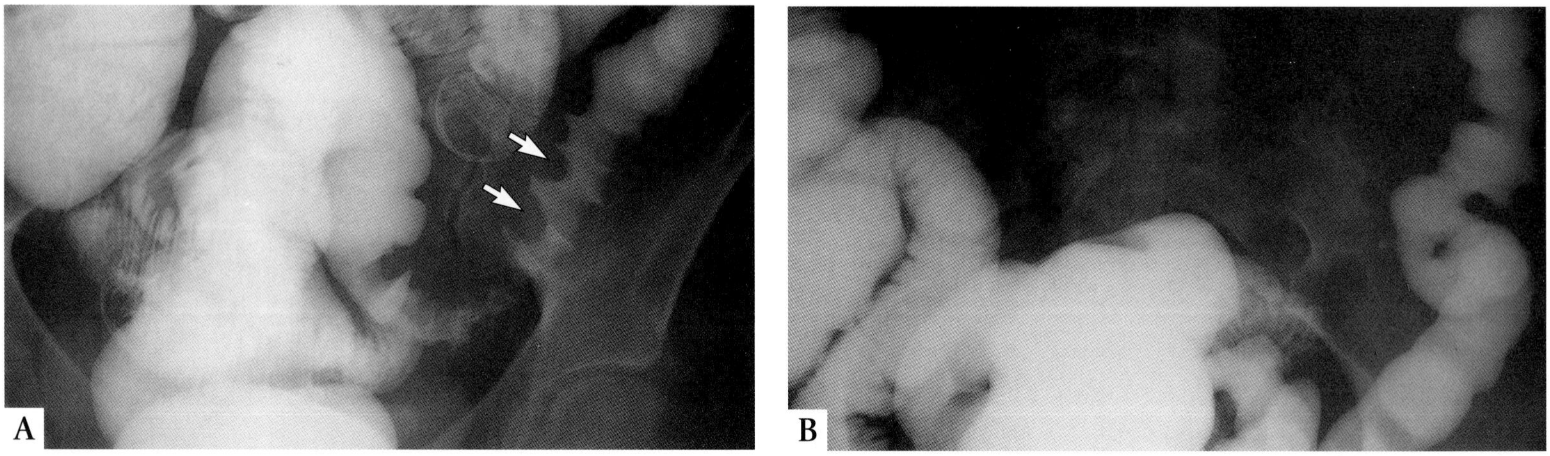

FIGURE 10-35.

Intramural hemorrhage of the bowel. This patient has sustained direct injury from an assault and kicking in the lower left abdomen. Rectal bleeding prompted a positive-contrast examination of the colon. **A**, The appearance of an intramural hemorrhage in the left colon at the junction of the descending and sigmoid colons. Intramural hemorrhage produces what has been called *thumb printing* of the wall of the colon. Thumb printing is seen in a number of areas (*arrows*). **B**, A repeat examination done approximately 2 weeks later demonstrating resolution of the intramural and submucosal hematoma with a return to normal of the morphologic appearance of the colon. Intramural hemorrhage has a similar appearance whether it is caused by trauma or other causes of bleeding, such as ischemia or bleeding diathesis.

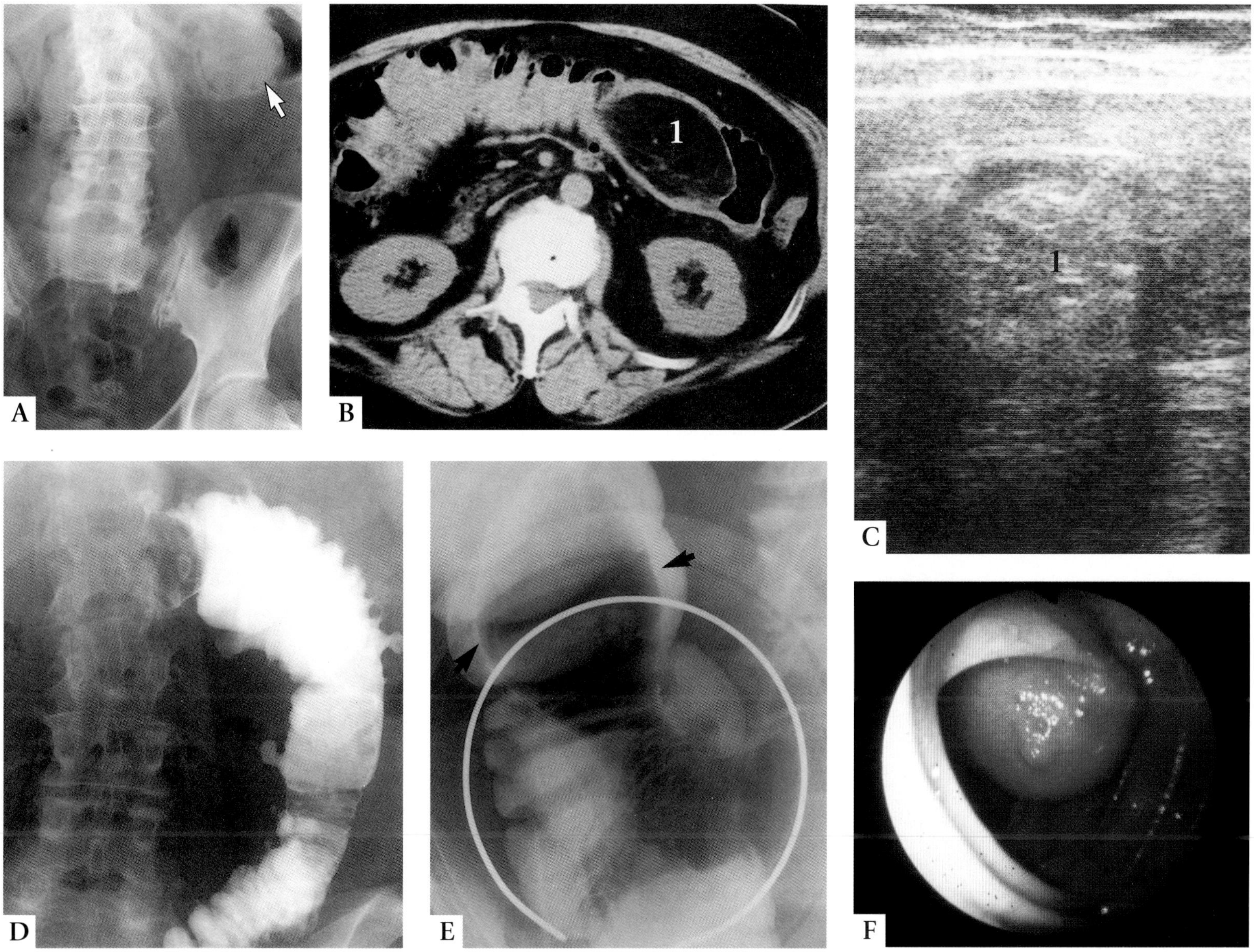

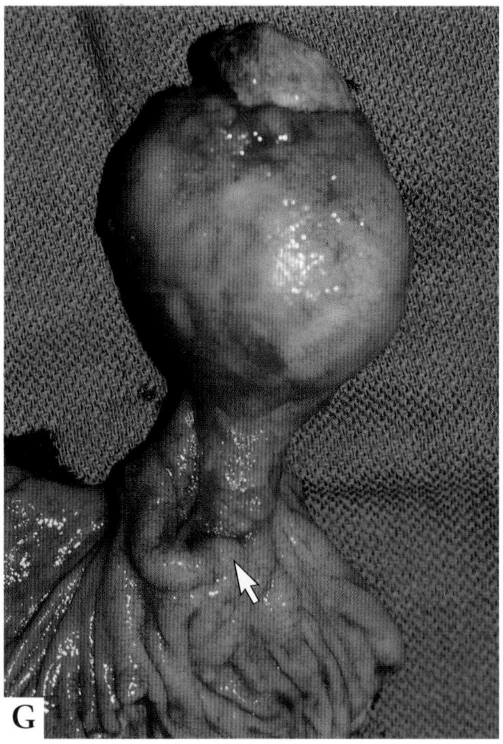

FIGURE 10-36.

Intussuscepting lipoma of the cecum. This patient with recurrent abdominal pain was initially evaluated with plain films of the abdomen. **A**, This figure demonstrates a large soft-tissue density overlying the distal transverse colon (*arrow*). **B**, A subsequent computed tomographic scan through the same area nicely defines a very low attenuation smooth mass lying in the lumen of the distal transverse colon (*1*). The computed tomographic numbers of this lesion are in the range of fat density. Notice the similarity between the omentum and intraperitoneal fat with this lesion. This similarity indicates that the lesion most likely contains a large amount of fat. **C**, An accompanying ultrasound of the same area also shows the lesion to be very hyperechoic, consistent with a fat-containing lesion (*1*). **D**, A barium enema was performed that outlined the head of the lipoma (*arrow*). The large cecal lipoma caused a colo-colo intussusception with the lead point located in the distal transverse colon. The intussusception was easily reduced by increasing the pressure head of the barium column. **E**, The smooth outline of the lipoma is nicely shown (*arrows*). **F**, Endoscopically, the lesion was verified to have features consistent with a lipoma. **G**, This huge lipoma was surgically resected, and the specimen shows a large pedunculated lipoma arising from the ileocecal valve (*arrow*).

In this instance, four radiologic examinations were performed. The plain film examination of the abdomen raised the possibility of a colonic mass. A computed tomographic examination made the diagnosis of a lipoma because of the characteristic computed tomographic numbers. The barium enema was performed to reduce the intussusception, and the ultrasound was done for fun! Each of the major radiologic examinations was useful and contributed to the diagnosis and management of the patient. Although redundancy of examinations is to be avoided, it is not unusual to use a number of diagnostic and therapeutic procedures in the management of patients. It is occasionally possible to make a specific histologic diagnosis using imaging techniques as in this case. (*From* Stewart and Dobbs [1]; with permission.)

CONCLUSION

Radiographic imaging of the colon is best performed when the radiologist and the referring clinician are in direct communication. The selection of the appropriate imaging procedure, interpretation of the images, and the application of therapeutic maneuvers requires an understanding of the pathophysiology as well as the imaging procedures by all those involved in caring for these patients. An appreciation of the unique strengths of plain films, positive-contrast examinations, cross-sectional imaging, and ultrasound by the referring clinician is most important. Conversely, an understanding of the strengths of endoscopy by the radiologist is equally important. Even sophisticated imaging and endoscopy is no substitute for the careful clinical evaluation done by all of the clinicians caring for these patients.

REFERENCE

1. Stewart ET, Dodds WJ: Neoplastic colonic lesions. In *Margulis and Burhenne's Alimentary Tract Radiology*, vol 1, edn 5. Edited by Freeny PC, Stevenson GW. St. Louis: Mosby–Year Book; 1994: 762–800.

Chapter 11

Pathology of the Colon and Rectum

JOEL K. GREENSON

The colon and rectum may be affected by a wide variety of inflammatory, infectious, congenital, or neoplastic processes. Some lesions may represent localized involvement by a systemic disease, whereas other lesions are intrinsic to the colorectum. The majority of this chapter contains examples of common pathologic entities of the colon and rectum. A few examples of rare variants of common lesions are also included. Whenever possible, both gross and microscopic examples of each lesion have been supplied.

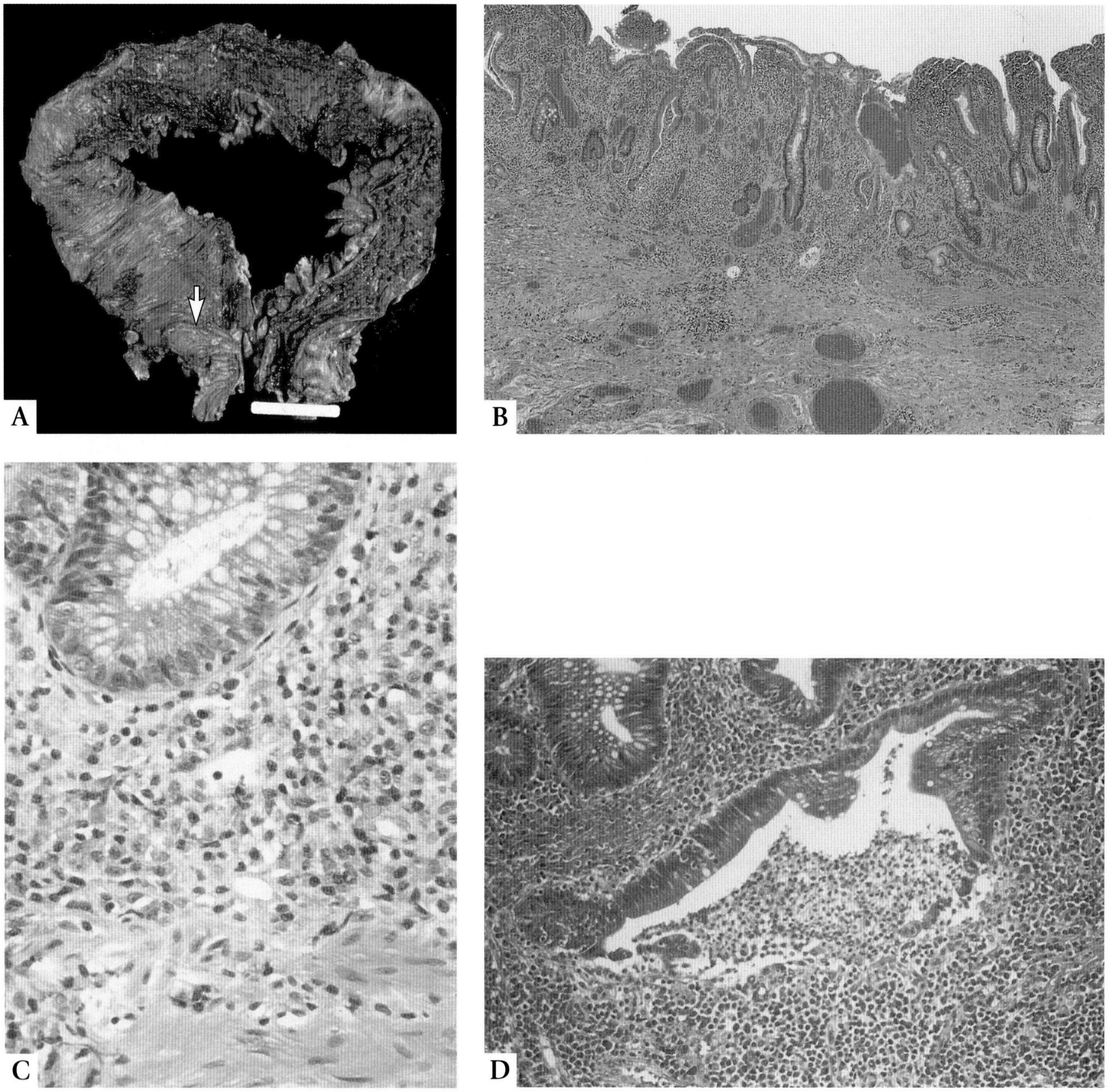

FIGURE 11-1.

Ulcerative colitis. **A**, This total colectomy specimen shows a normal mucosal pattern in the terminal ileum and cecum (*arrow*) with diffuse involvement from the transverse colon to the rectum. The distal mucosa is erythematous and friable with many ulcers and erosions. **B**, This low-power photomicrograph shows diffuse chronic inflammation of the lamina propria with crypt distortion. These two features are important in differentiating ulcerative colitis from acute "self-limited" colitis. **C**, This high-power view depicts the base of a single distorted colonic crypt. There is a large number of "basal" plasma cells between the crypt and the muscularis mucosae. This finding is another important feature that helps differentiate acute from chronic colitis. **D**, This photograph shows a single crypt abscess. The bottom of this distorted crypt has been destroyed by an aggregate of neutrophils. This finding is not specific for ulcerative colitis; Crohn's disease and other active forms of colitis may also have crypt abscesses.

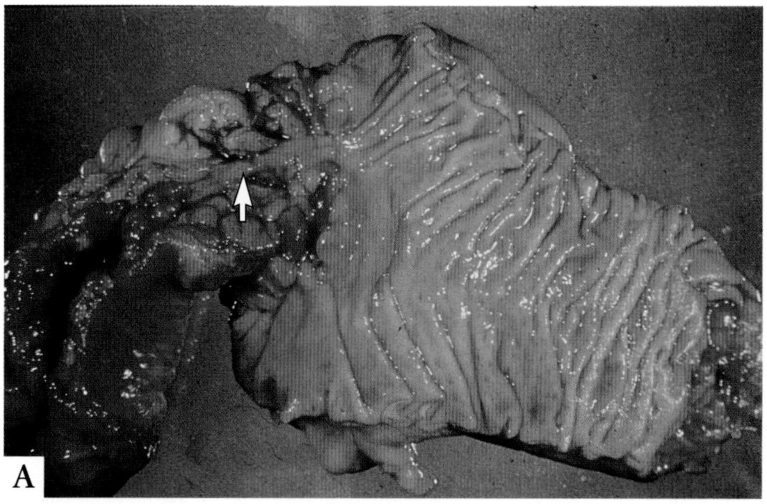

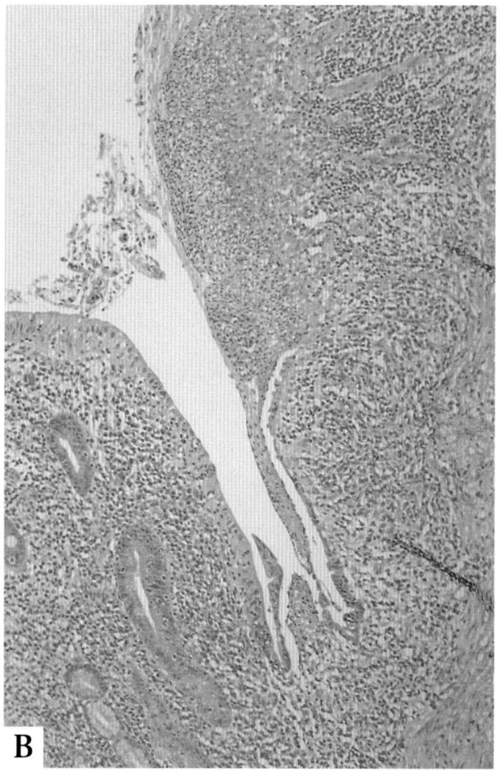

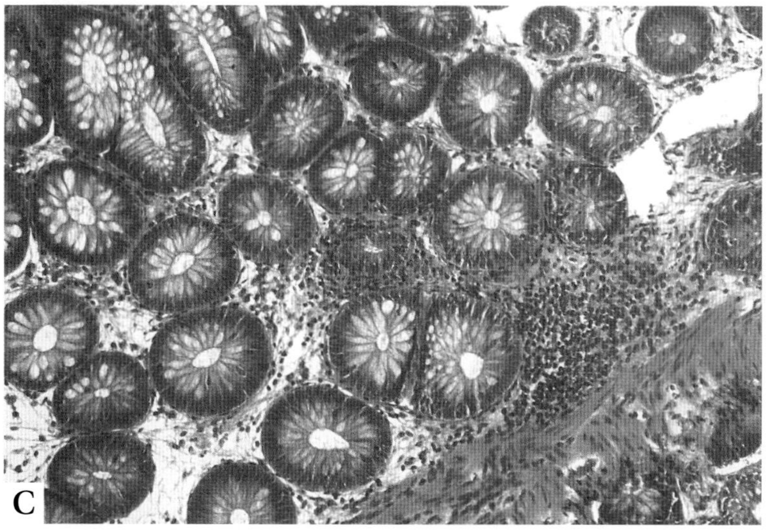

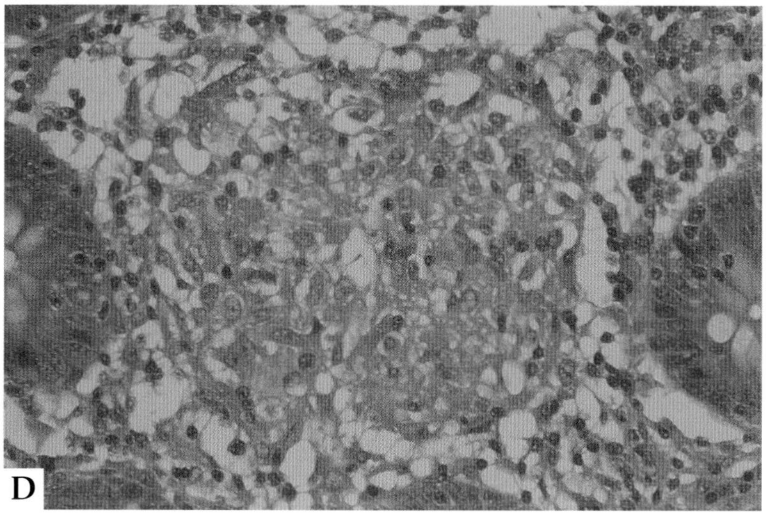

FIGURE 11-2.

Crohn's disease. **A**, This segment of colon shows a stricture in the right colon (*arrow*) with normal appearing mucosa in the distal portion of the specimen. Strictures in the right colon may be seen in both Crohn's disease and ischemic colitis [1]. **B**, Photomicrograph of a fissuring ulcer overlying a lymphoid aggregate (aphthous ulcer) is shown. Aphthous lesions can be seen in Crohn's disease as well as infectious colitis. **C**, This low-power view shows a single inflamed distorted crypt that appears much smaller than the more normal adjacent crypts. Focal lesions such as this lesion are often seen in smoldering Crohn's disease. **D**, An epithelioid granuloma between two colonic crypts is depicted. Although the presence of a granuloma may help establish the diagnosis of Crohn's disease in endoscopic biopsy specimens, serial sections must be examined to be certain that a granuloma is not caused by a ruptured

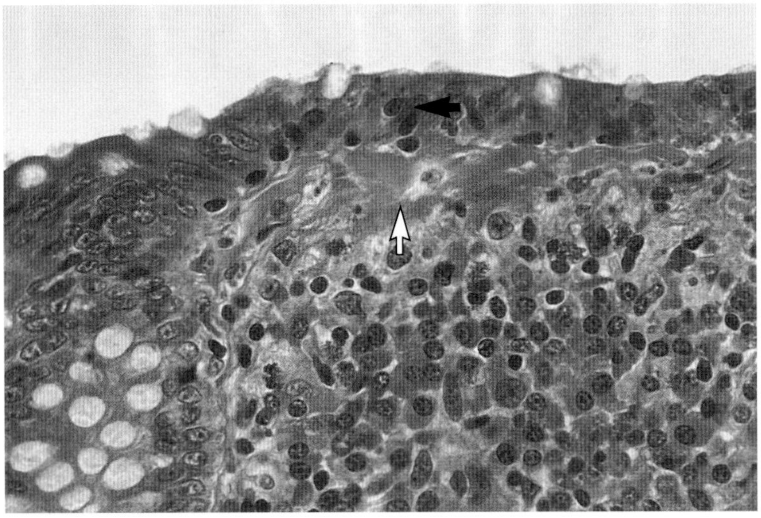

FIGURE 11-3.

Collagenous colitis. A thickened irregular subepithelial collagen table (*open arrow*) with patchy surface epithelial damage is shown. The surface epithelium also contains increased numbers of intraepithelial lymphocytes (*closed arrow*). In addition, there is a superficial plasmacytosis with prominent numbers of eosinophils. Crypt distor-

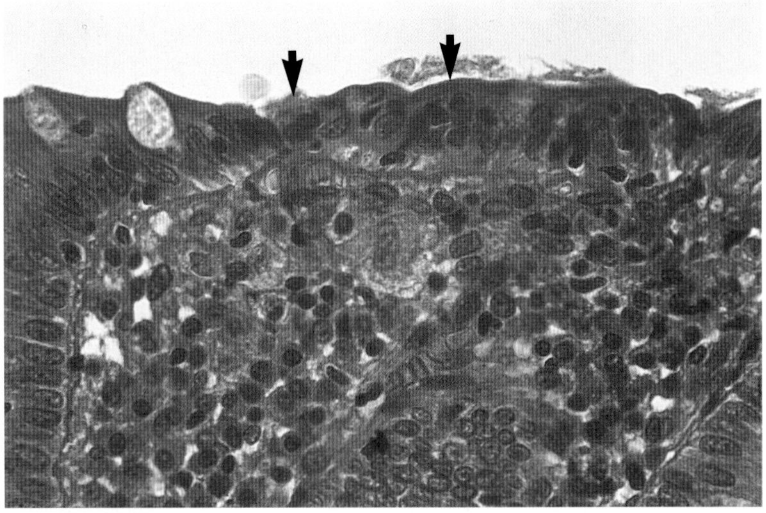

FIGURE 11-4.

Lymphocytic colitis. The *arrows* point to surface epithelial damage with increased numbers of intraepithelial lymphocytes. In addition, there is a superficial plasmacytosis without crypt distortion. Although a few intraepithelial neutrophils may be seen, widespread cryptitis is not a feature of lymphocytic colitis [3].

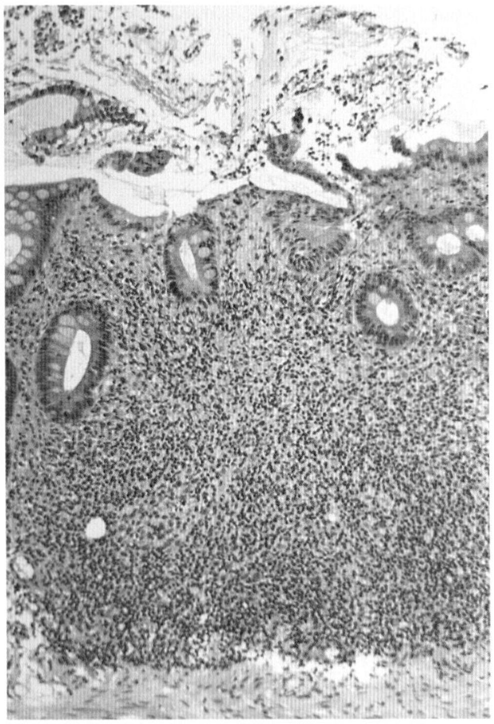

FIGURE 11-5.

Diversion colitis. An expanded lymphoid follicle with patchy cryptitis and an overlying erosion is depicted. A modest increase in lamina propria mononuclear cells is often seen as well. These findings may show overlap with those of smoldering inflammatory bowel disease, but the inflammation resolves once fecal flow is reestablished to the diverted segment [4].

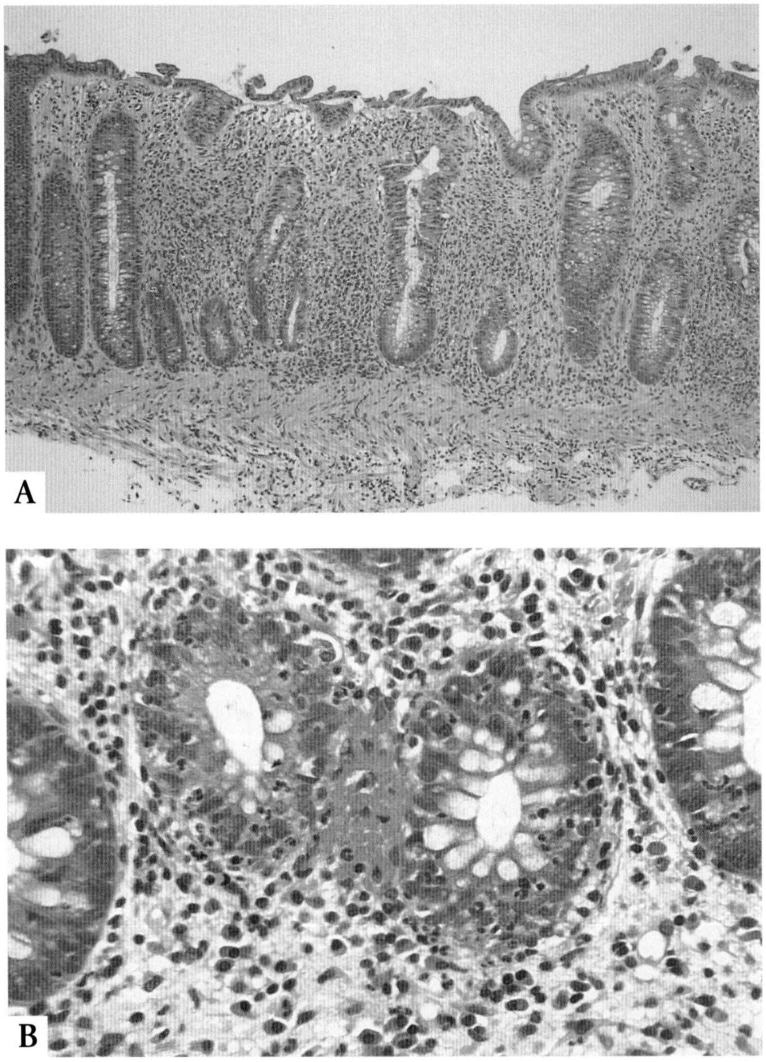

FIGURE 11-6.

Acute self-limited colitis. **A**, This low-power view shows an intact crypt architecture with damaged surface epithelium and a hypercellular lamina propria containing increased neutrophils and lymphocytes. The lack of crypt distortion and the absence of basal plasma cells helps to differentiate this colitis from ulcerative colitis. **B**, A high-power view of colonic crypts infiltrated by many neutrophils (cryptitis).

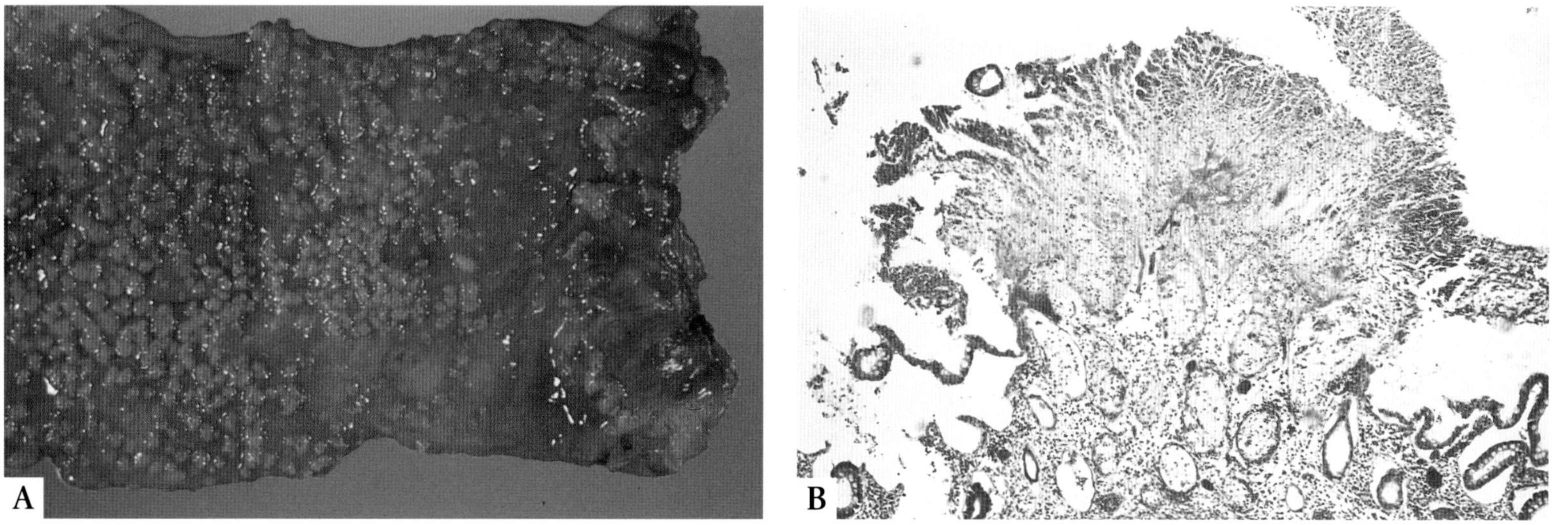

FIGURE 11-7.

Pseudomembranous colitis. **A**, The mucosal surface is dotted with small raised plaques, which in some areas become confluent. This finding is often seen in *Clostridium difficile* colitis, however, *Escherichia coli* O157:H7 and ischemia may cause similar lesions. **B**, This small pseudomembrane is composed of fibrin and inflammatory debris. The underlying mucosa shows superficial necrosis.

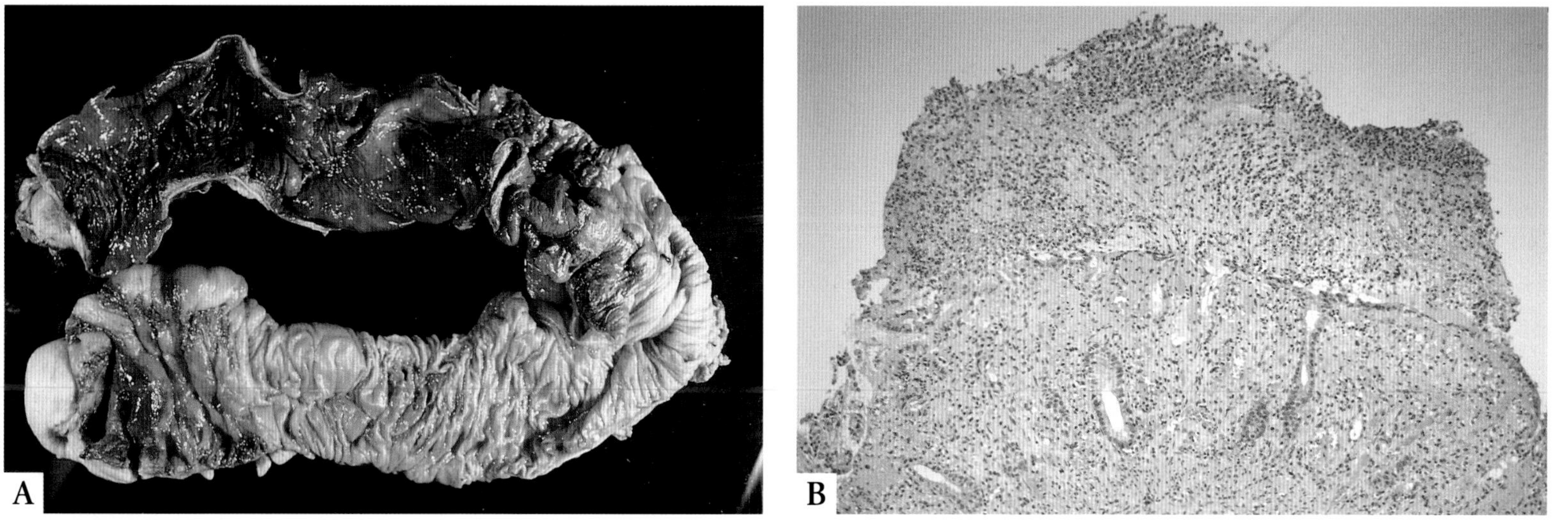

FIGURE 11-8.

Ischemic colitis. **A**, A colectomy specimen that shows a well-demarcated darkened area of hemorrhagic necrosis. The sharp border and diffuse involvement of the affected segment are characteristic of ischemic disease. **B**, This superficial pseudomembrane is identical to that seen in pseudomembranous colitis secondary to *Clostridium difficile* or *Escherichia coli* 0157:H7. The mucosa shows superficial necrosis without much inflammation. The lamina propria often takes on a hyalinized smudgy appearance, and the residual mucosa often shows marked regenerative atypia.

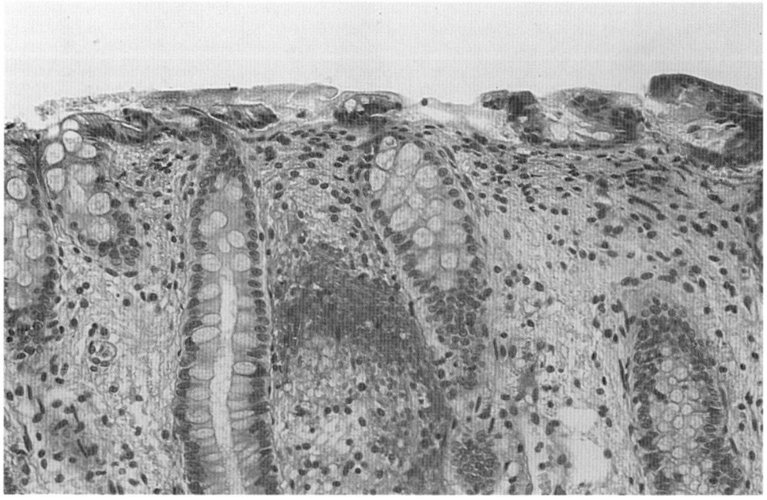

FIGURE 11-9.

Enema effect. This low-power photomicrograph shows the effect of a sodium phosphate enema on the rectal mucosa. Edema of the lamina propria with interstitial hemorrhage, loss and damage of the surface epithelium, and flattening of the mucosal surface are presented. These changes may be misinterpreted as acute colitis or ischemic damage as well as obscure surface damage in lymphocytic colitis [5].

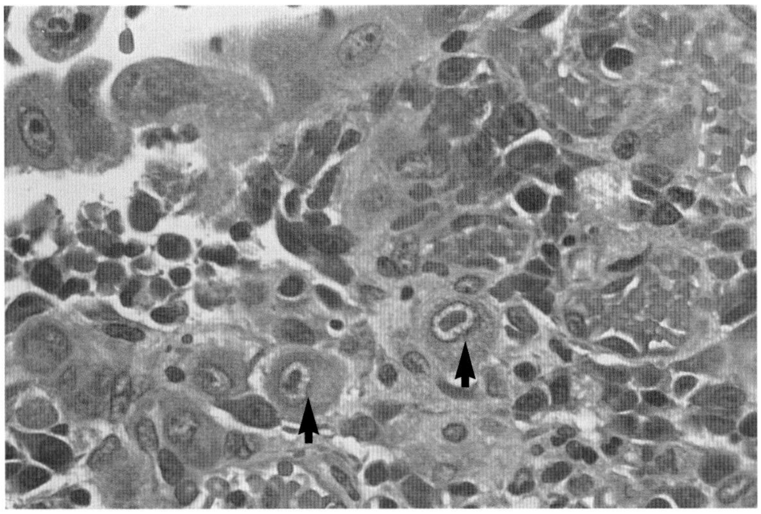

FIGURE 11-10.

Cytomegalovirus. Two classic cytomegalovirus inclusions can be seen (*arrows*) in this focus of granulation tissue. The infected cells are most likely endothelial cells. Cytomegalovirus colitis is usually observed in immunocompromised hosts. Cytomegalovirus can be a secondary pathogen in patients with inflammatory bowel disease who are being treated with steroids.

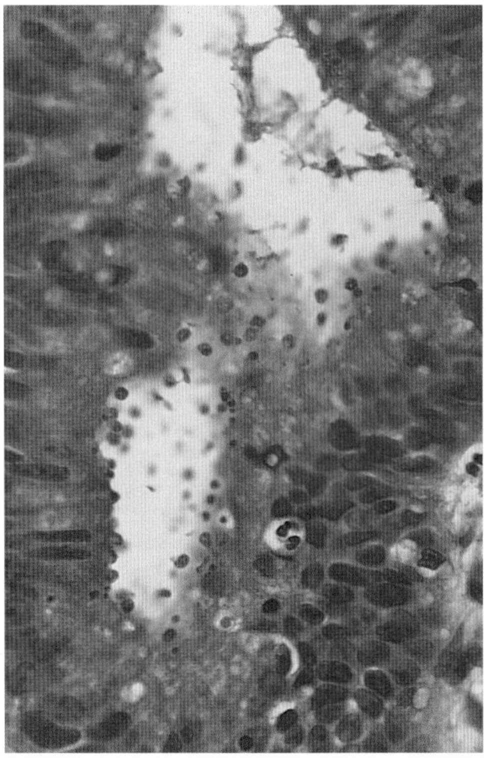

FIGURE 11-11.

Cryptosporidia. The colonic crypt has numerous cryptosporidial organisms lining the surface of the epithelium. The organisms appear as luminal blue dots that vary somewhat in size and shape; some have a visible internal structure.

POLYPS AND NEOPLASMS

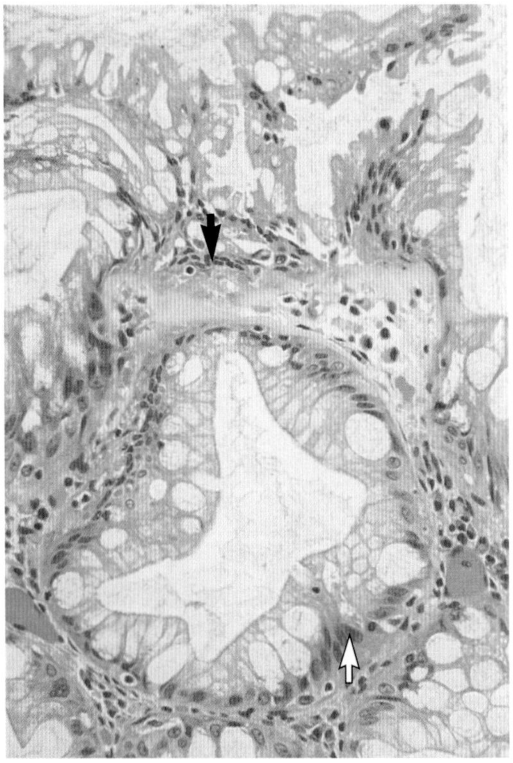

FIGURE 11-12.

Hyperplastic polyp. This high-power view shows a gland with a serrated lumen (*open arrow*) and a thickened subepithelial collagen table (*closed arrow*) [6]. These lesions are fairly common in adults, particularly in the rectum and sigmoid colon. The lesions tend to be smaller than adenomas and do

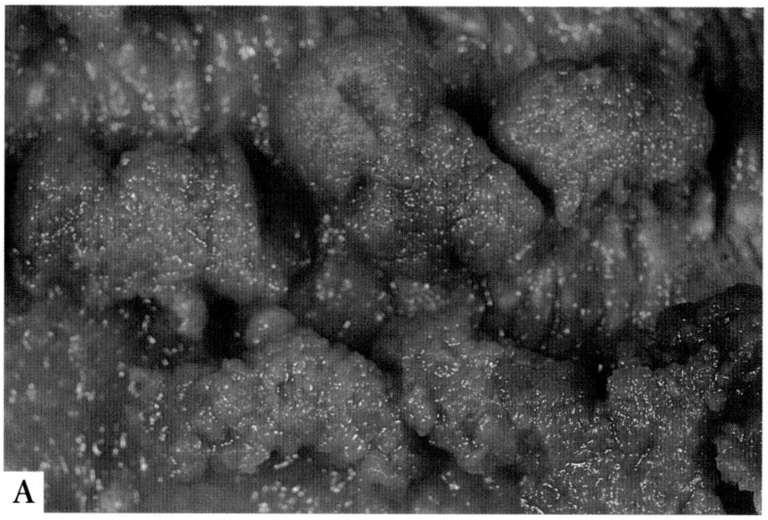

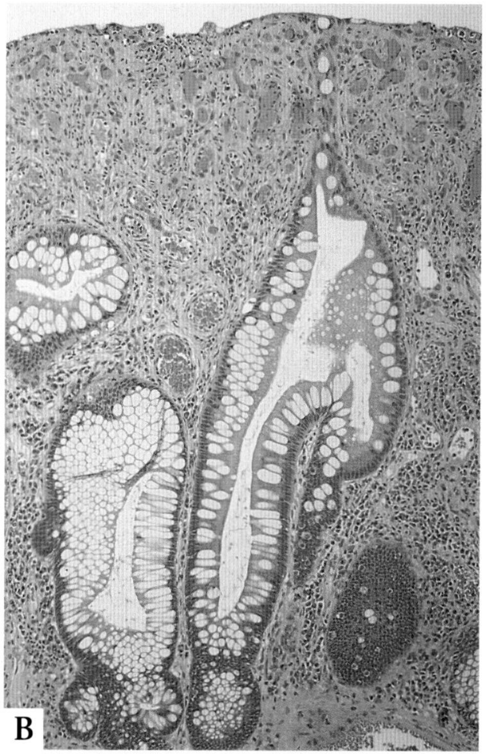

Figure 11-13.

Inflammatory polyps/pseudopolyps. **A**, The colonic mucosa shows numerous inflammatory polyps with intervening areas of ulceration. These lesions develop as by-products of the ulcers that penetrate into the submucosa, leaving islands of adjacent regenerative mucosa. Although most common in ulcerative colitis, inflammatory polyps may also be seen in Crohn's disease, ischemia, and other ulcerative conditions of the colon. **B**, The pseudopolyp has an ulcerated surface lined with granulation tissue. The underlying crypts are distorted and contain regenerative epithelium. The deep lamina propria often contains increased numbers of plasma cells and lymphocytes [9].

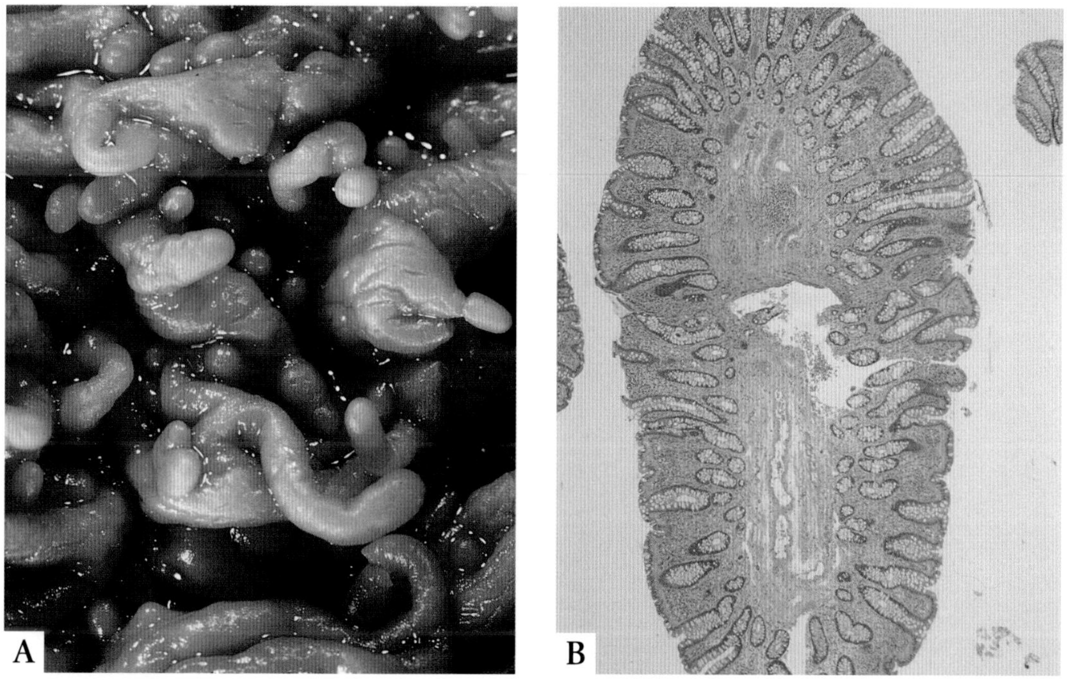

Figure 11-14.

Filiform polyps. **A**, A colectomy specimen with numerous fingerlike projections rising above the mucosa is shown. These mucosal excrescences are often grouped and are typically found in patients with chronic inflammatory bowel disease. These lesions are thought to represent healed inflammatory polyps. **B**, A biopsy specimen shows a finger like portion of colonic mucosa surrounding a fibrovascular core. The epithelium is intact and shows relatively normal architecture [10].

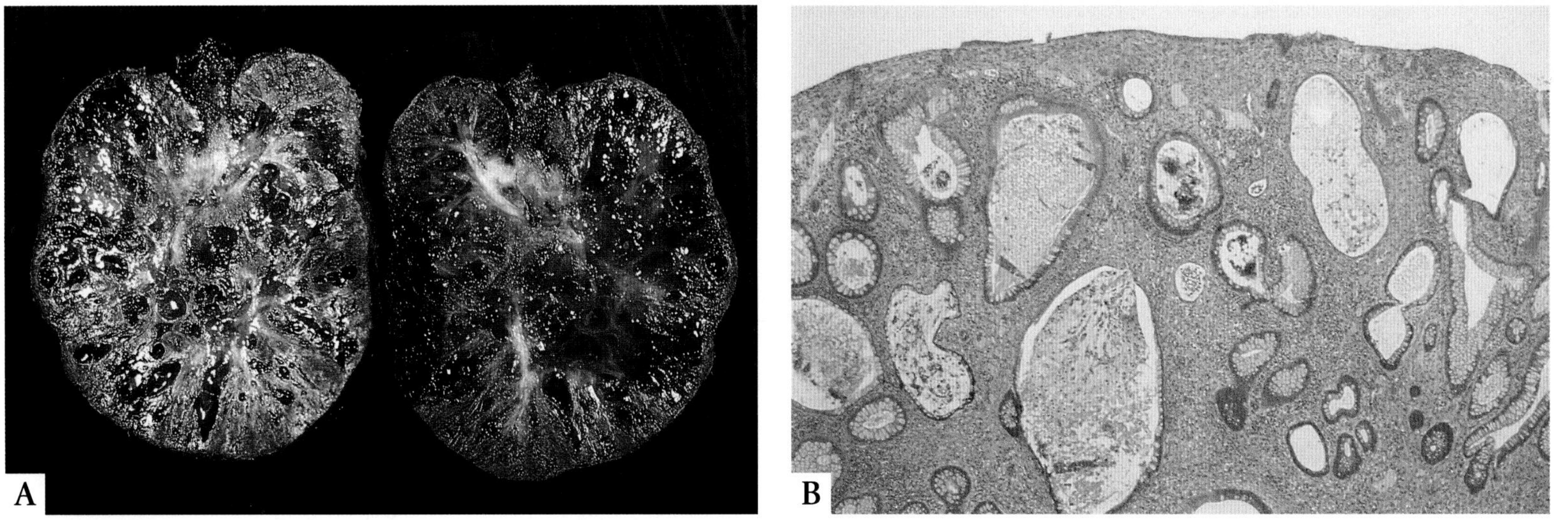

Figure 11-15.

Juvenile or retention polyp. **A**, Bisected juvenile polyp that contains many small cystic spaces and a smooth external surface. Blue ink is present at the stalk margin. These polyps may arise spontaneously as isolated lesions or as part of one of the juvenile polyposis syndromes. **B**, Numerous cystically dilated glands can be seen in this low-power view of a juvenile polyp. In addition, the surface is ulcerated and the lamina propria is chronically inflamed. These polyps share many features with inflammatory polyps, however, the degree of cystic dilatation in juvenile polyps is usually not seen in inflammatory polyps [11–15].

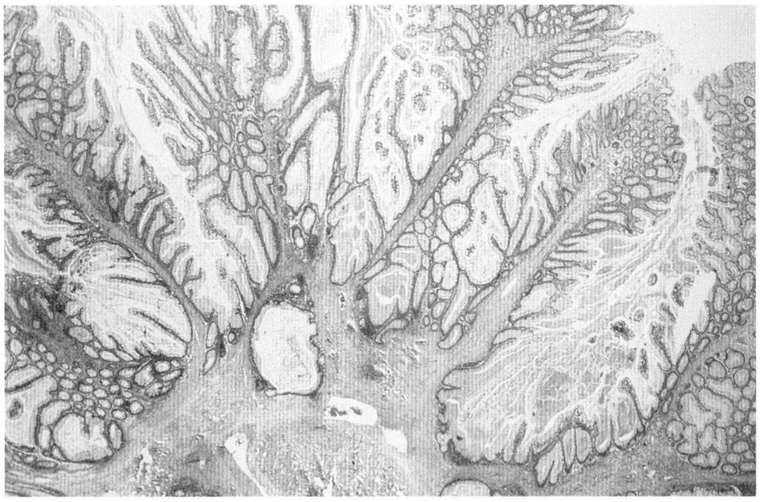

Figure 11-16.

Peutz-Jegher's polyp. A hamartomatous polyp that exhibits arborizing branches of smooth muscle arising from the muscularis mucosae, which are covered by nonneoplastic colonic epithelium. These lesions may be isolated polyps but are usually found scattered throughout the gastrointestinal tract in patients with mucocutaneous pigmentation (Peutz-Jegher's syndrome) [16].

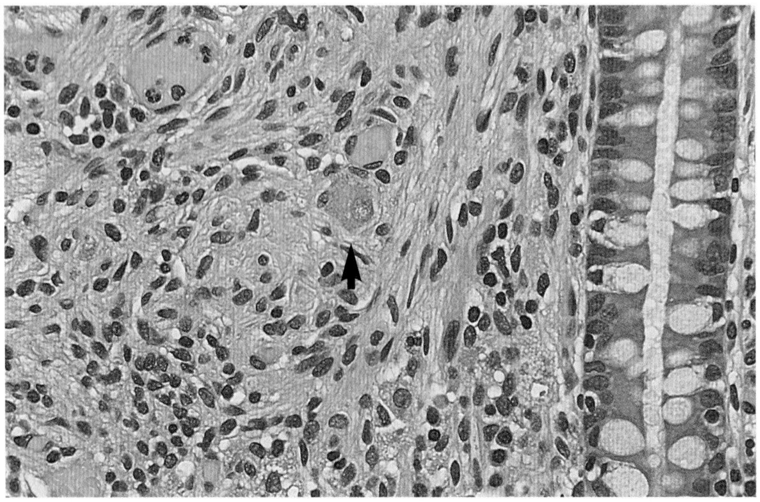

Figure 11-17.

Ganglioneuromatosis. A proliferation of neural tissue within the mucosa is depicted. A ganglion cell is also present (*arrow*). This finding may be seen as an isolated polyp (*eg*, ganglioneuroma) or as a diffuse process throughout the gastrointestinal tract (*eg*, ganglioneuromatosis). The latter is associated with MEN IIb syndrome and von Recklinghausen's disease as well as some polyposis syndromes [17–21].

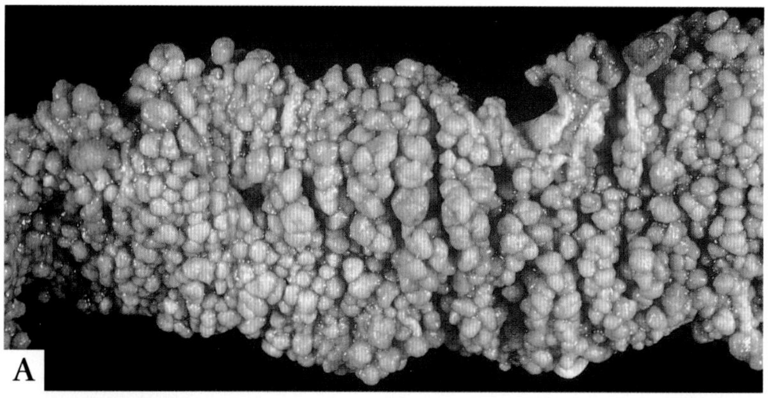

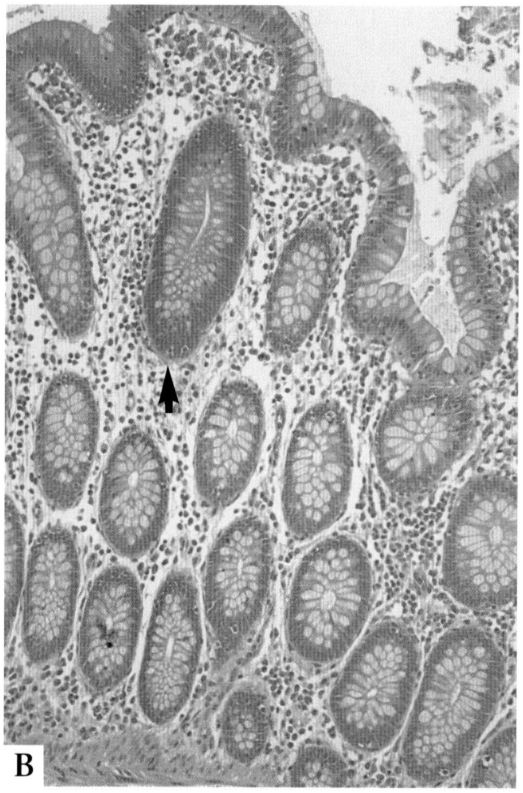

FIGURE 11-18.

Familial adenomatous polyposis. **A**, A portion of a colectomy specimen that shows complete carpeting of the mucosal surface by adenomatous polyps. In general, colons containing more than 100 adenomatous polyps are thought to have this autosomal dominant condition. The genetic defect appears to be caused by mutations or deletions in the *APC* gene located on the long arm of chromosome 5. **B**, A single adenomatous crypt (*arrow*) is present in this section of nonpolypoid mucosa from a patient with familial polyposis. The presence of "unicryptal adenomas" in nonpolypoid mucosa is a diagnostic feature of familial adenomatous polyposis. Identical colonic findings are seen in patients with Gardner's syndrome [22,23].

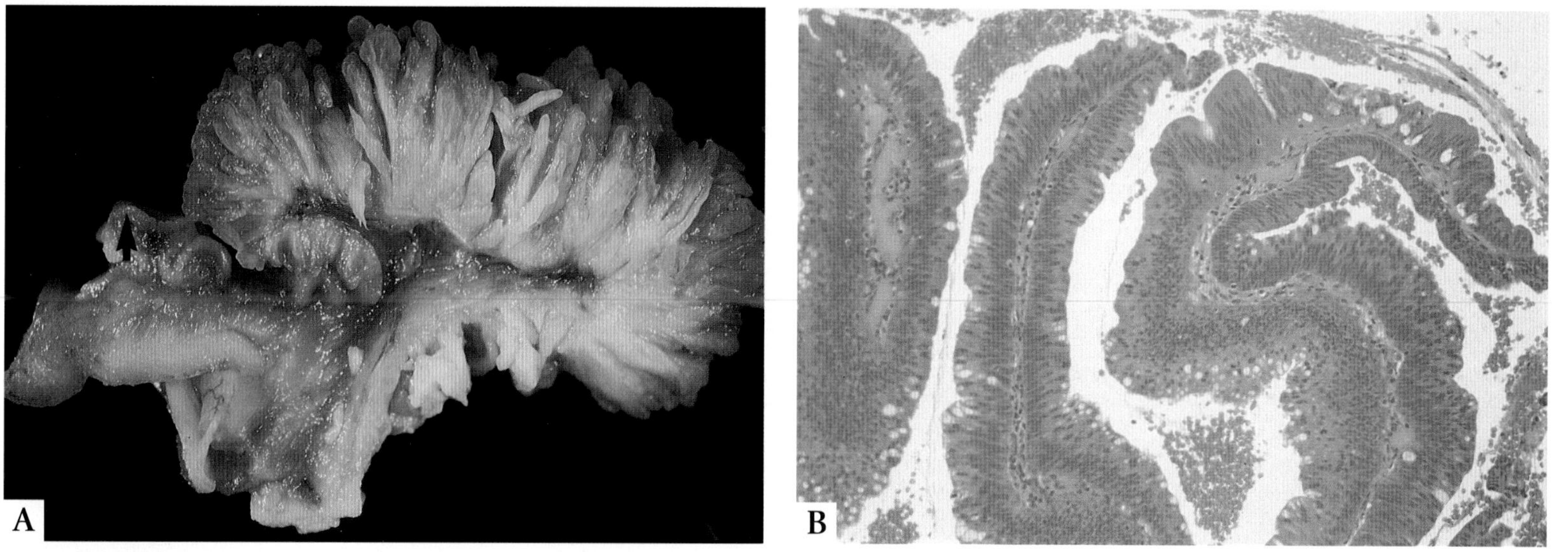

FIGURE 11-19.

Villous adenoma. **A**, This lesion has a sessile configuration with a villiform frondlike surface. The submucosa appears uninvolved by this process. A small amount of normal mucosa is seen at the edge of the specimen (*arrow*). **B**, Three villi lined by dysplastic epithelium-containing hyperchromatic pseudostratified nuclei are seen in this high-power view. The villi correspond to the frondlike surface presented in *A*.

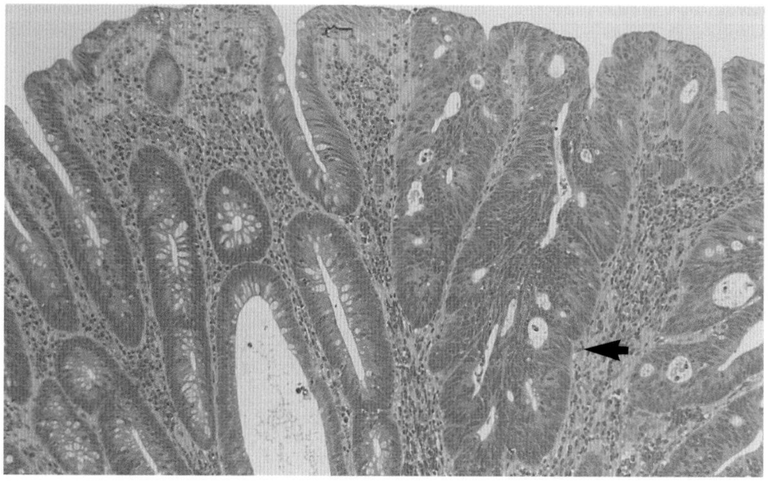

FIGURE 11-20.

Adenoma with high-grade dysplasia (intramucosal carcinoma). This photomicrograph shows an adenoma with a focus of high-grade dysplasia (*arrow*). The focus has a complicated glandular architecture but does not show the desmoplastic stroma seen in invasive carcinomas.

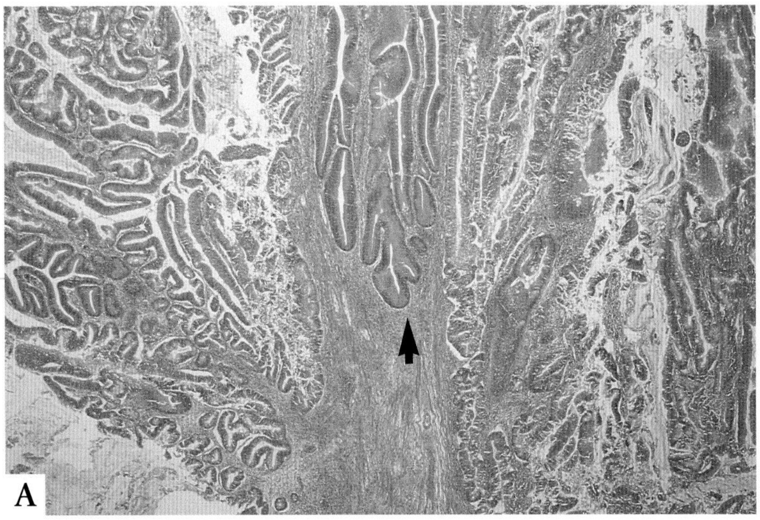

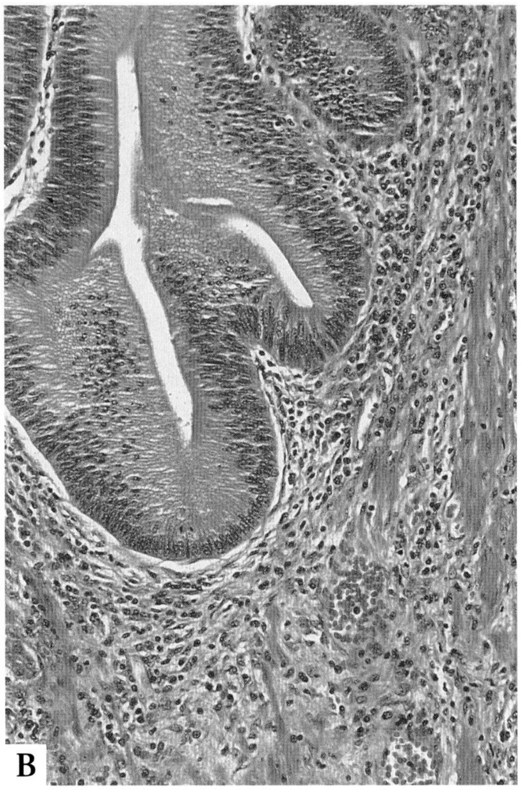

FIGURE 11-21.

Adenoma with pseudoinvasion in the polyp stalk. **A**, A low-power photomicrograph that depicts a tubulovillous adenoma with a focus of glands present within the stalk (*arrow*). **B**, High-power view of the same glands shows that the inflammatory cells of the lamina propria are still surrounding the adenomatous epithelium. In addition, the entrapped glands show only low-grade dysplasia and lack a desmoplastic stroma. These findings are seen in left-sided adenomas and are presumably a result of trauma induced from the solid fecal stream.

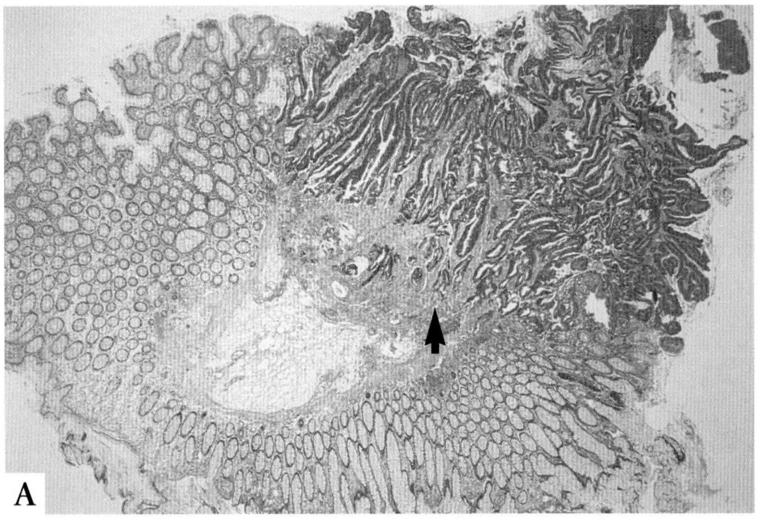

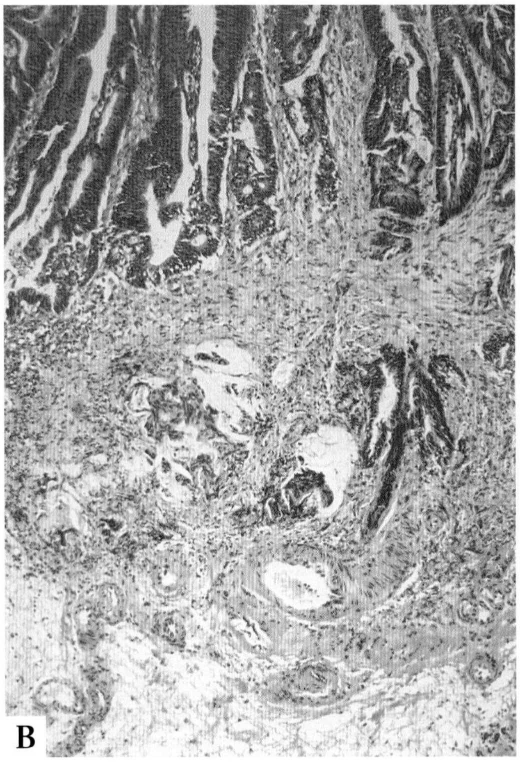

FIGURE 11-22.

Adenoma with invasive carcinoma. **A**, This low-power view shows the stalk of an adenoma that contains a focus of invasive carcinoma (*arrow*). **B**, High-power view of the invasive carcinoma shows desmoplastic stroma separating the carcinomatous tubules. There is also cautery artifact present, indicating that the invasive tumor is present at the endoscopic resection margin.

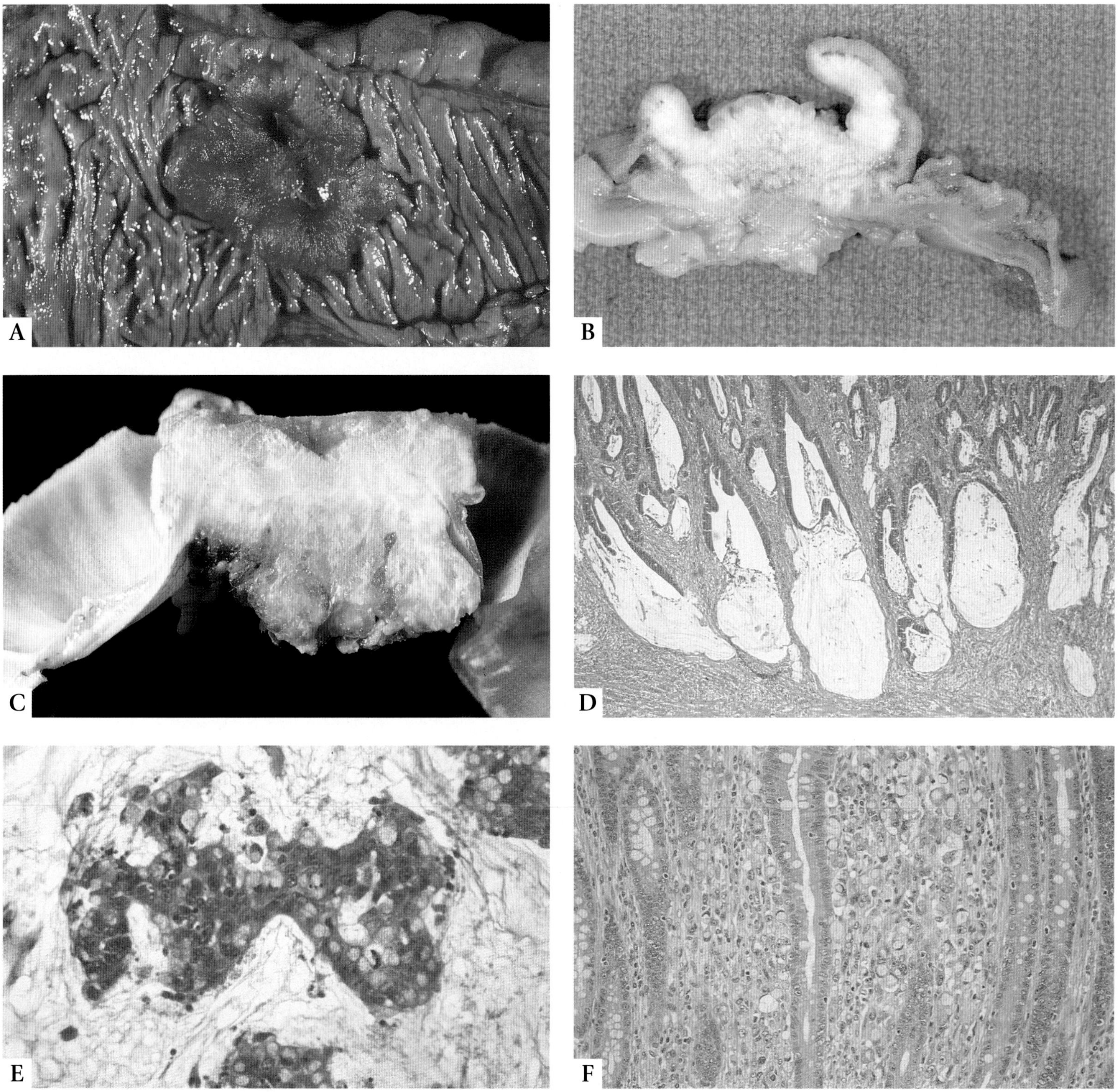

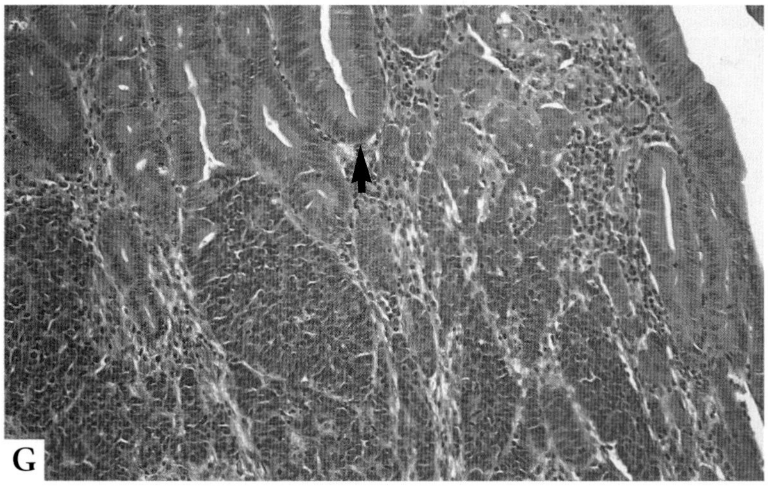

FIGURE 11-23.

Adenocarcinoma of the colon. **A**, This colonic resection specimen shows an erythematous-raised tumor with a central umbilication typical of colon cancer. **B**, A cross-section of a colon cancer that shows transmural invasion of the tumor into the subserosal fat. **C**, A cross-section of a transmurally invasive mucinous carcinoma. Pools of gray mucin can be seen at the deepest point of invasion of the tumor. **D**, Histopathology of mucinous carcinoma shows neoplastic glands producing pools of mucin. **E**, Photomicrograph of neoplastic cells floating in mucin. **F**, Photomicrograph of a rare variant of colon cancer, a primary signet ring cell carcinoma of the colon. **G**, Another rare variant of primary colon cancer, small cell

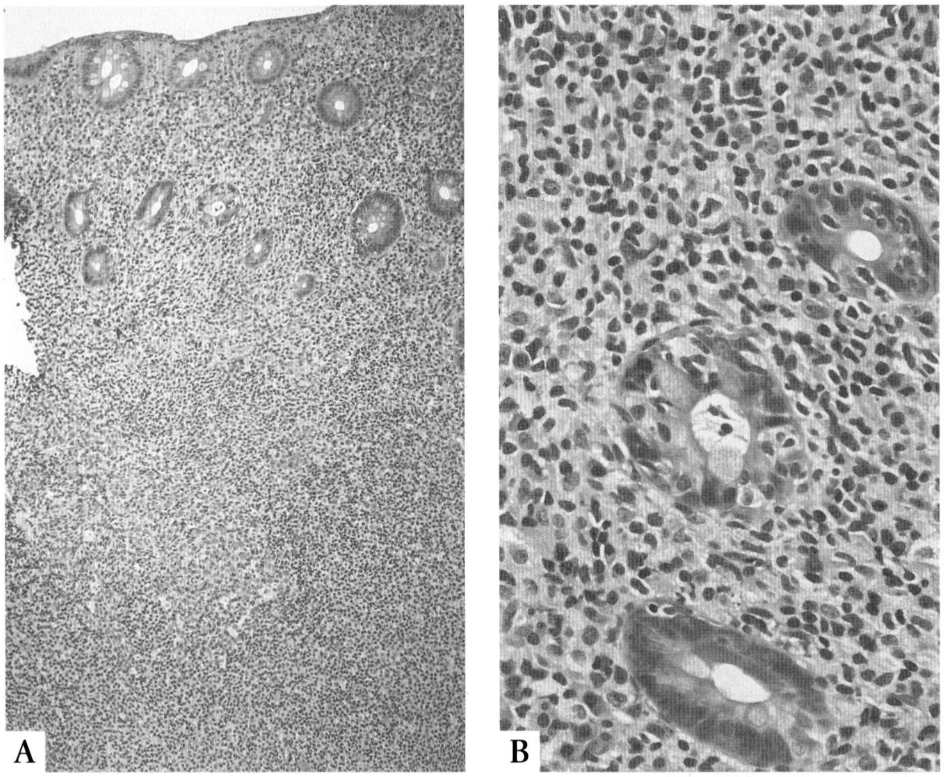

FIGURE 11-24.

Lymphoma of the colon. **A**, A low-power view that shows a diffuse lymphocytic infiltrate effacing the normal colonic architecture. The crypts are spread apart by the monomorphous lymphoid infiltrate, which is quite prominent in the deeper portions of the biopsy specimen. **B**, Histopathology of colonic lymphoma. This high-power view shows small lymphocytes infiltrating the crypt epithelium to form lymphoepithelial lesions. This formation is a characteristic finding of mucosa-associated lymphoid tissue–type lymphomas of the gastrointestinal tract. These lesions are often composed of small centrocytic cells that mark as B cells.

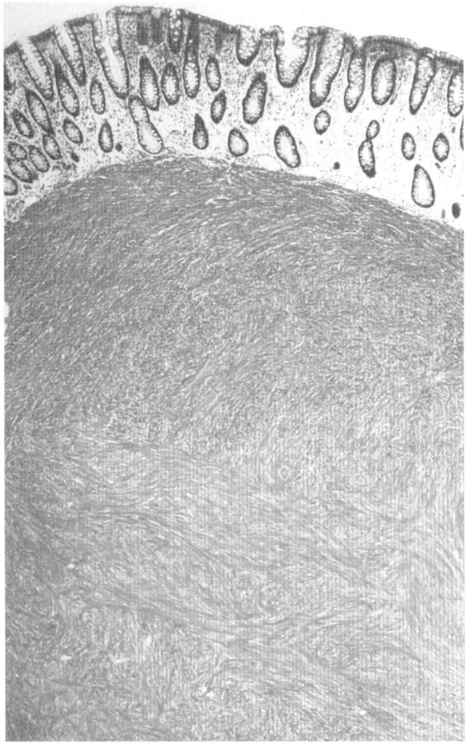

FIGURE 11-25.

Benign gut stromal tumor (leiomyoma). A large area of pink whirling spindle cells is observed directly beneath the mucosa. The lesion has the typical appearance of a leiomyoma, complete with a well-circumscribed smooth border. Recent attempts to identify muscle-specific antigens in these tumors has met with mixed success, hence, the more generic term *benign gut stromal tumor* may be preferred. Malignant gut stromal tumors may also be encountered in the colon.

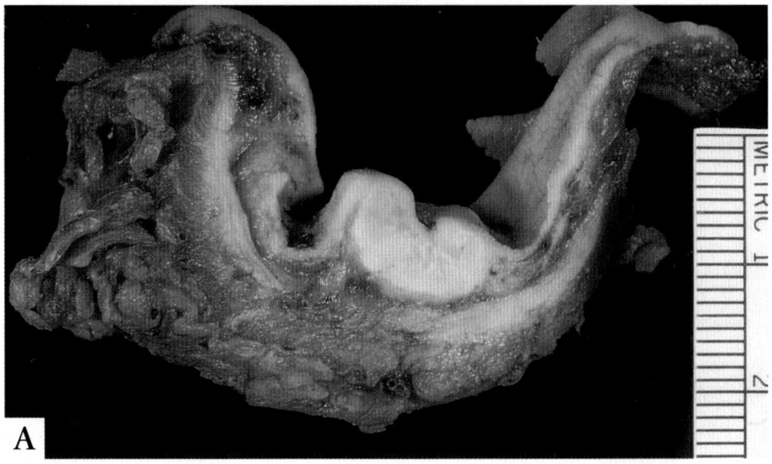

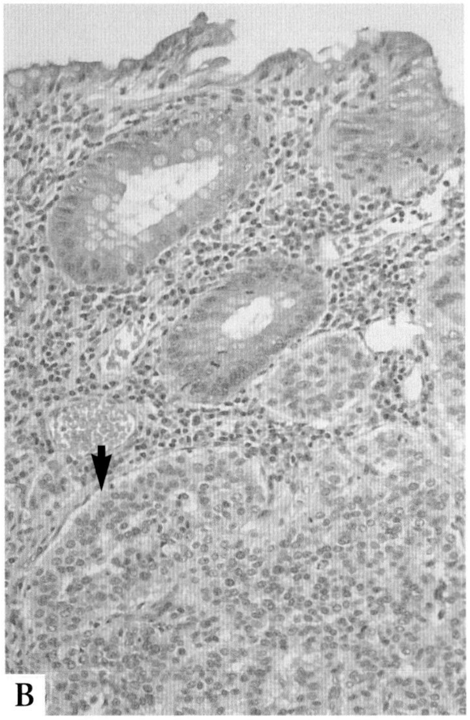

FIGURE 11-26.

Rectal carcinoid tumor. **A**, This specimen shows a cross-section of a carcinoid tumor in the submucosa of the bowel wall. Carcinoid tumors have a typical yellow color and appear to originate within the bowel wall rather than on the surface. **B**, The overlying mucosa is being infiltrated by nests of tumor cells (*arrow*). The tumor cells show the typical features of a neuroendocrine neoplasm with bland nuclei, ample pink cytoplasm, and a nested or trabecular architecture.

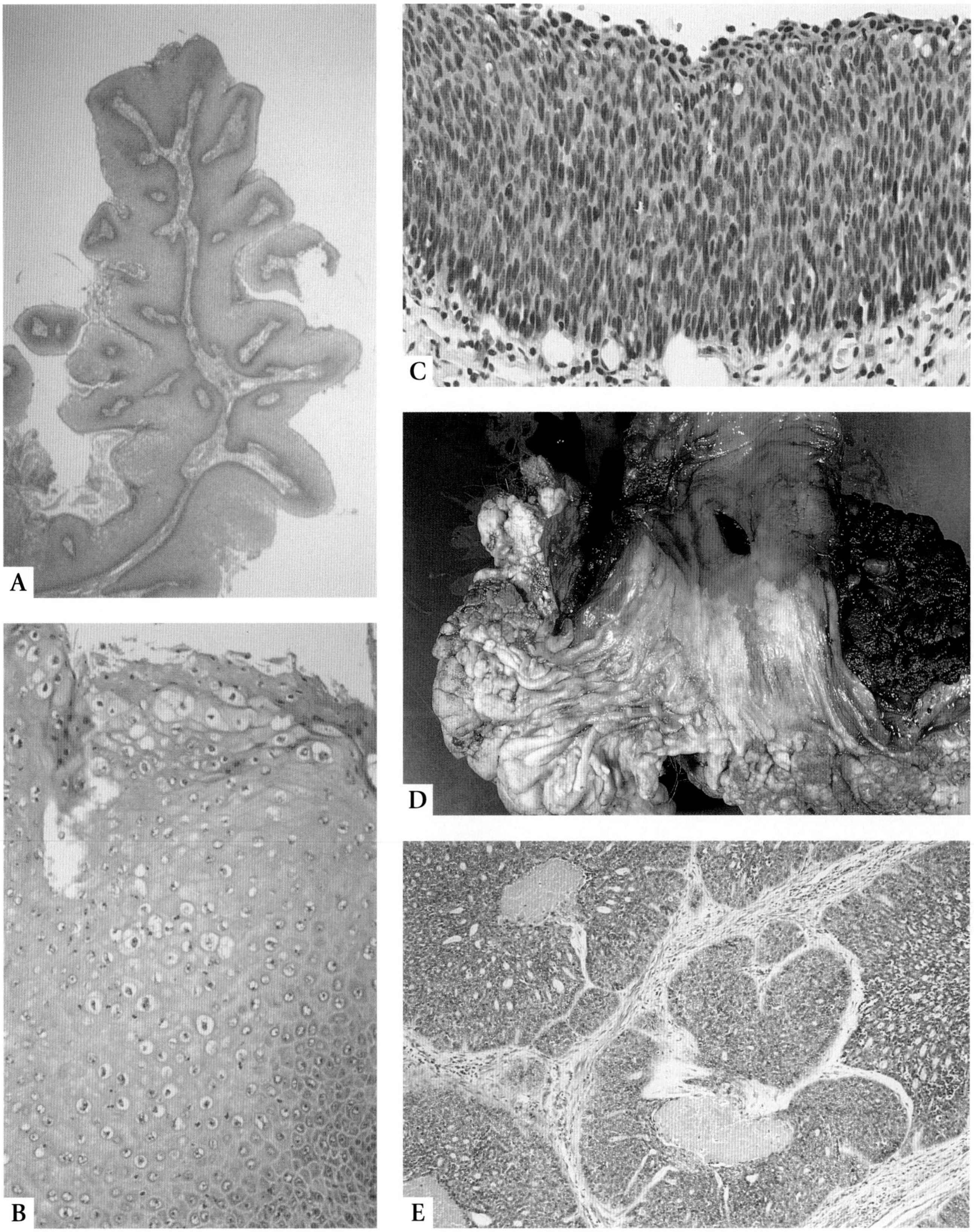

FIGURE 11-27.

Anal condyloma, dysplasia, and carcinoma. **A**, Low-power view of a papillary squamous growth typical of an anal condyloma. **B**, High-power view of a condyloma showing hyperplastic squamous epithelium with several koilocytes (*ie*, squamous cells with atypical nuclei and cytoplasmic clearing). Koilocytes are indicative of human papilloma virus infection. **C**, This high-power view shows high-grade squamous dysplasia (carcinoma *in situ*). Atypical nuclei are oriented in a vertical plane from the base of the epithelium to the surface. **D**, Resection specimen of rectum (*top*) and anus (*bottom*) show a large squamous cell carcinoma arising in anal condylomata. **E**, Low-power view of the basaloid or cloacogenic variant of invasive anal cancer. The tumor is composed of nests of basaloid cells, some of which show central necrosis [24].

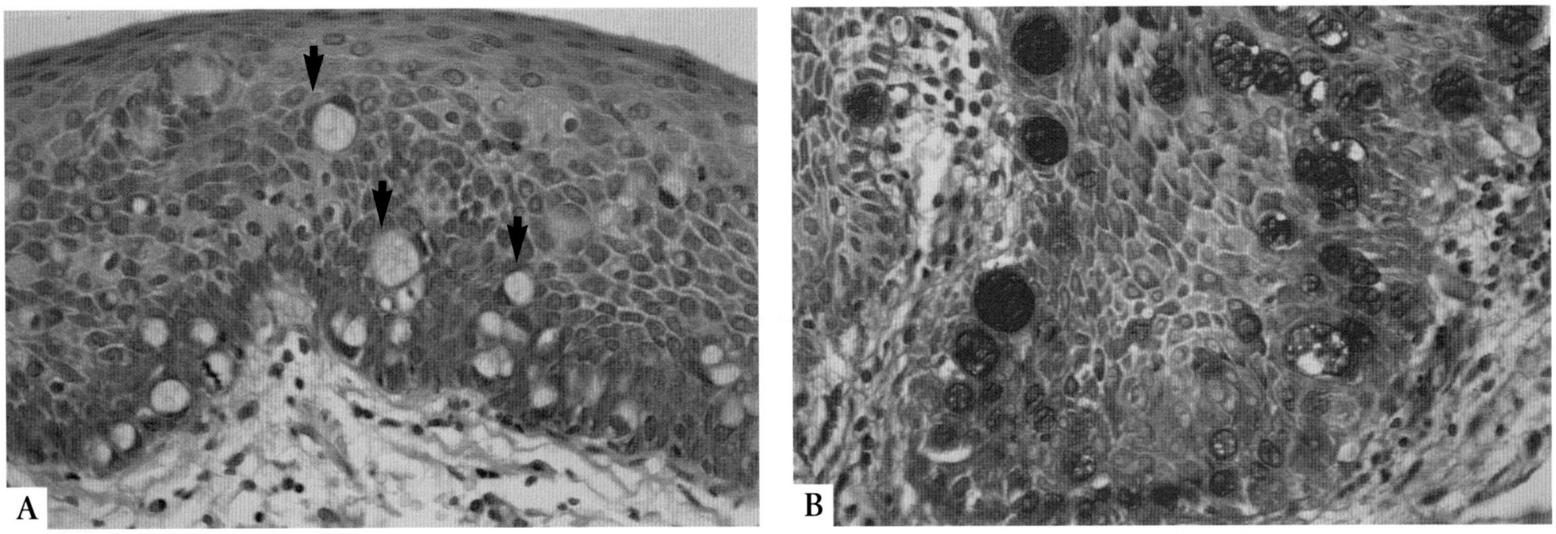

Figure 11-28.

Paget's disease of the anus. **A**, High-power view showing vacuolated signet ring cells scattered throughout the anal mucosa (*arrows*). **B**, A periodic acid Schiff stain showing strong staining of mucin-containing cells. Paget's disease is often associated with an adeno-

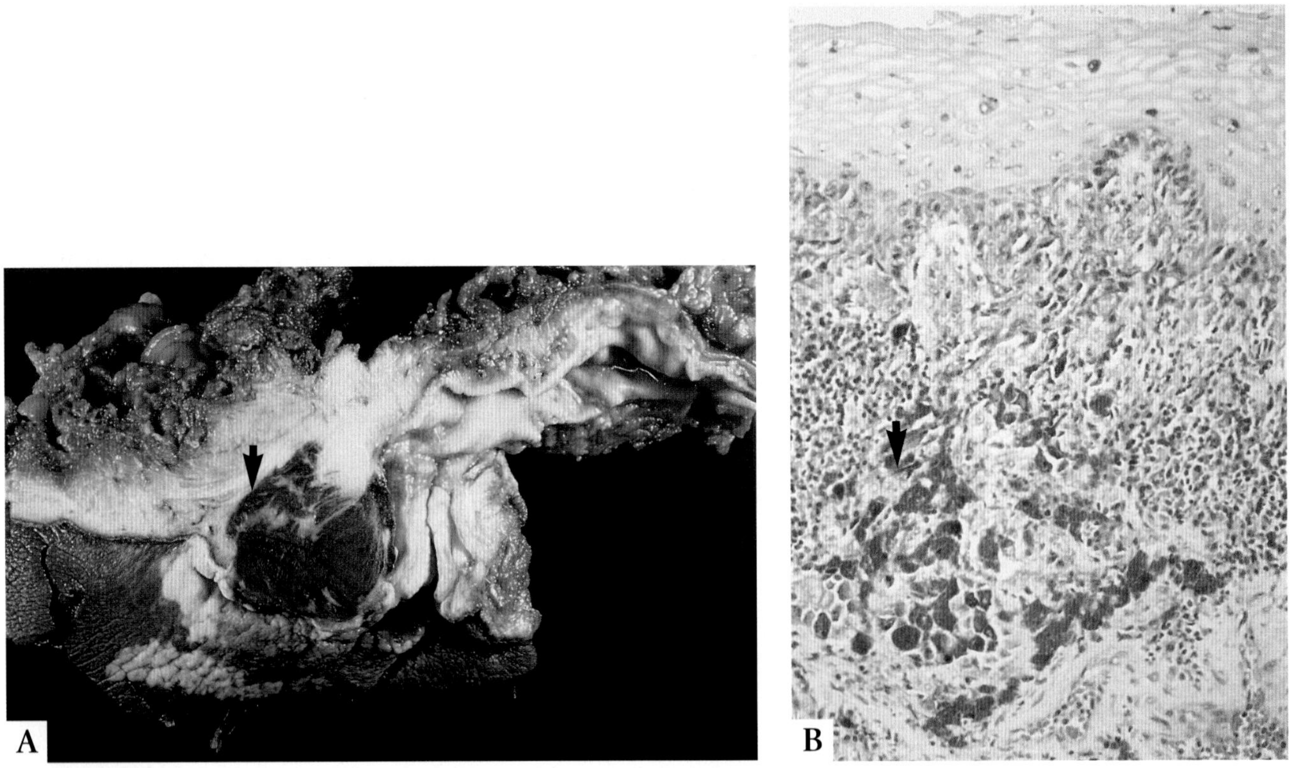

Figure 11-29.

Anal melanoma. **A**, Anal resection specimen shows the cross-section of a black tumor at the anal-rectal junction (*arrow*). The adjacent perianal skin can be seen to the left of the tumor, whereas the rectal mucosa is to the right of the tumor. **B**, Anal mucosa adjacent to the main tumor shows a group of pigmented tumor cells (*arrow*). These cells join the dermal-epidermal junction and show pagetoid spread into the surface epithelium. This finding indicates the tumor arose in this location and is not a metastasis from a distant site. Both the anus and the esophagus may give rise to primary melanomas [25–27].

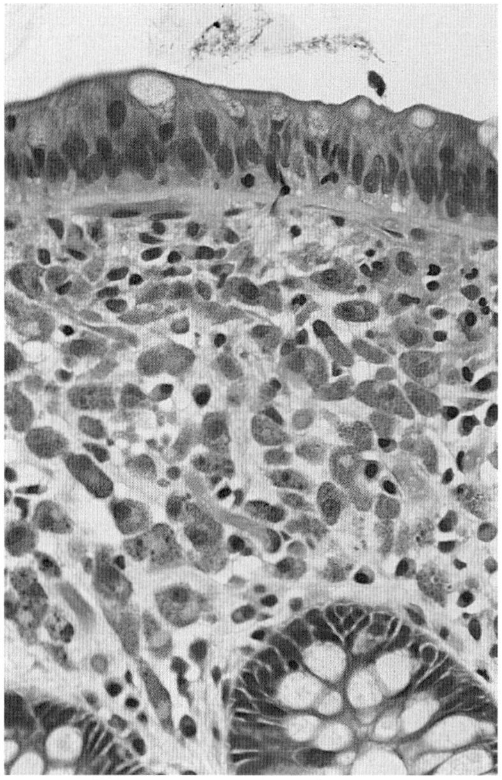

FIGURE 11-30.

Melanosis coli. The superficial lamina propria is filled with macrophages that contain brown granular pigment. These macrophages impart a brown color to the mucosa when present in sufficient quantity. Most cases of melanosis coli are thought to be caused by the use of anthracene-containing laxatives. It should be noted that normal colon biopsy specimens may contain an occasional pigmented macrophage, but not to the degree seen in melanosis coli.

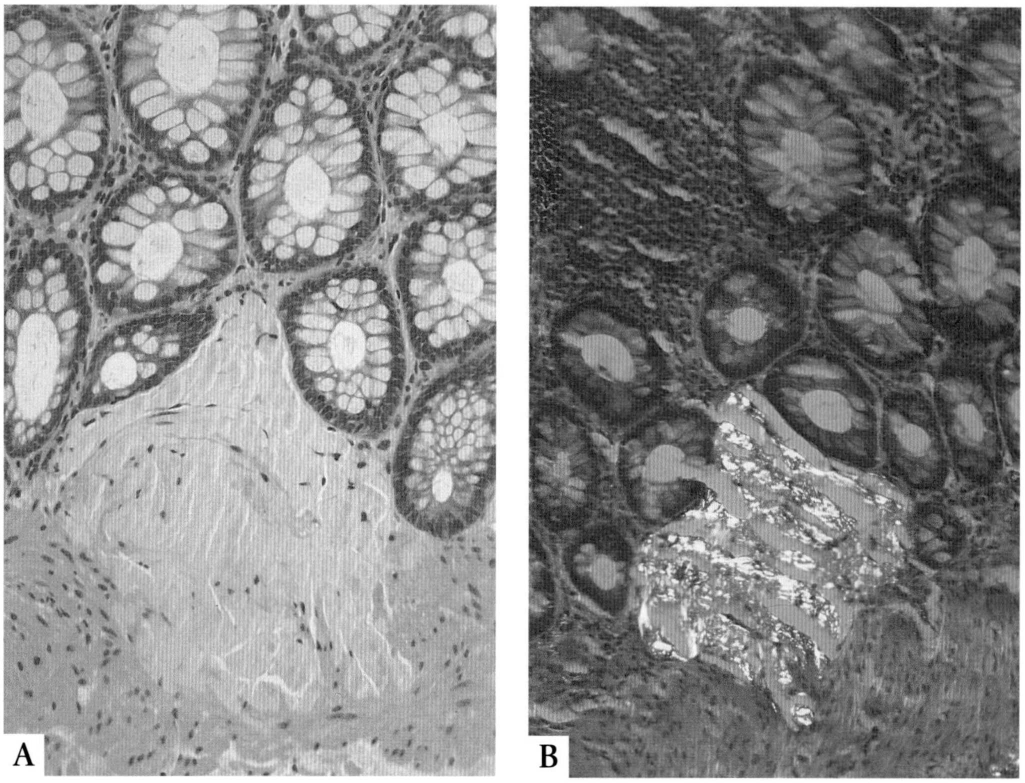

FIGURE 11-31.

Amyloidosis. **A**, The pink amorphous deposit between the base of the crypts and the muscularis mucosae is amyloid. In the gastrointestinal tract, amyloid usually first develops in and around submucosal blood vessels. Thus, to rule out amyloidosis, biopsy specimens must contain an adequate amount of submucosal tissue. **B**, Congo red stain for amyloid. Although the hematoxylin and eosin appearance in *A* is fairly characteristic, confirmatory special stains should always be performed. The congo red stain imparts an apple-green

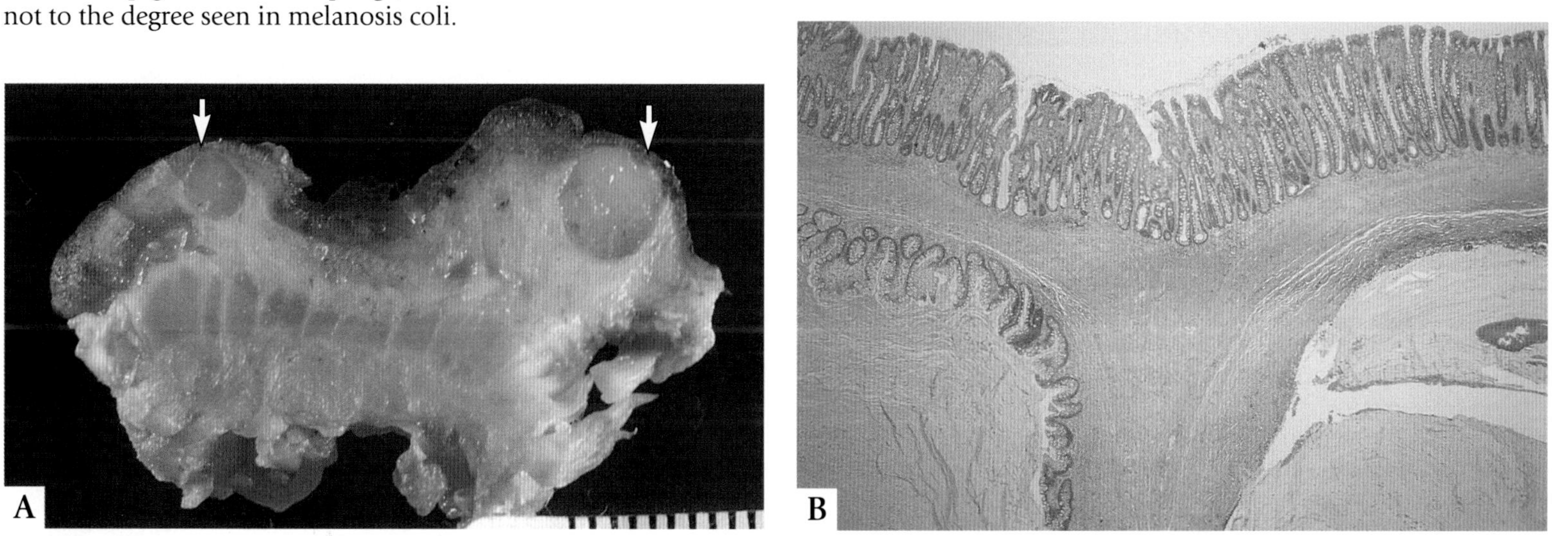

FIGURE 11-32.

Colitis cystica profunda. **A**, Several submucosal cysts are filled with mucinous material (*arrows*). This entity occurs in the setting of chronic inflammatory bowel disease as well as the solitary rectal ulcer syndrome. These lesions have been confused with mucinous carcinomas, which may also be seen in chronic inflammatory bowel disease. **B**, Two mucous-filled cysts are present beneath the surface epithelium. The lining of the cysts is not much different than the overlying epithelium and should not be misinterpreted as being neoplastic. Careful examination of the cells lining the mucinous cysts usually allows for the distinction between carcinoma and colitis cystica profunda, however, this distinction is not always an easy task [28,29].

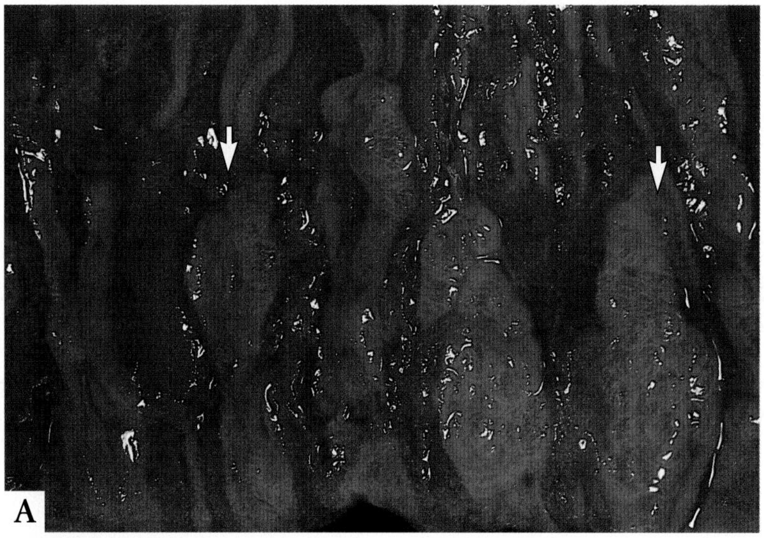

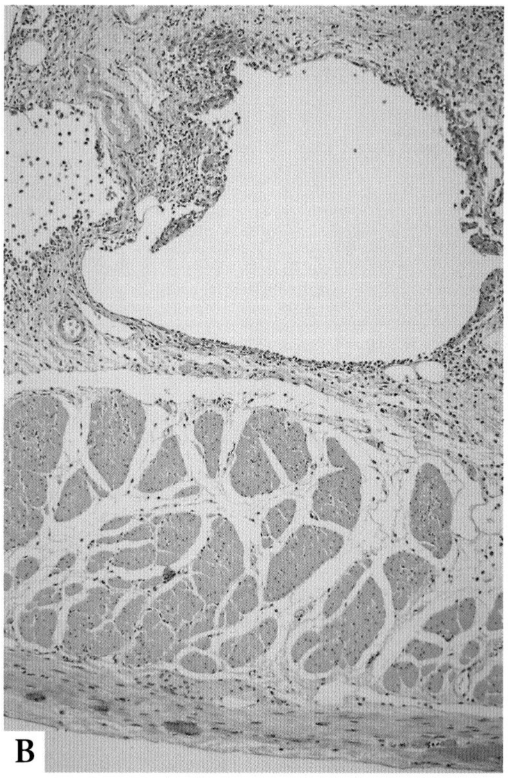

FIGURE 11-33.

Pneumatosis coli. **A**, Numerous gas-filled cysts can be seen in this surface view of the mucosa (*arrows*). These lesions may be seen throughout the small and large intestine owing to several different conditions. Pulmonary emphysema and gastric outlet obstruction may both cause this condition secondary to the escape of air via the retroperitoneum. In the colon, gas-producing bacteria have also been implicated as a possible etiologic agent. **B**, A large gas-filled cyst is seen in the submucosa. These cysts are usually lined by multinucleated giant cells. Cysts may also be present in the subserosa [30–33].

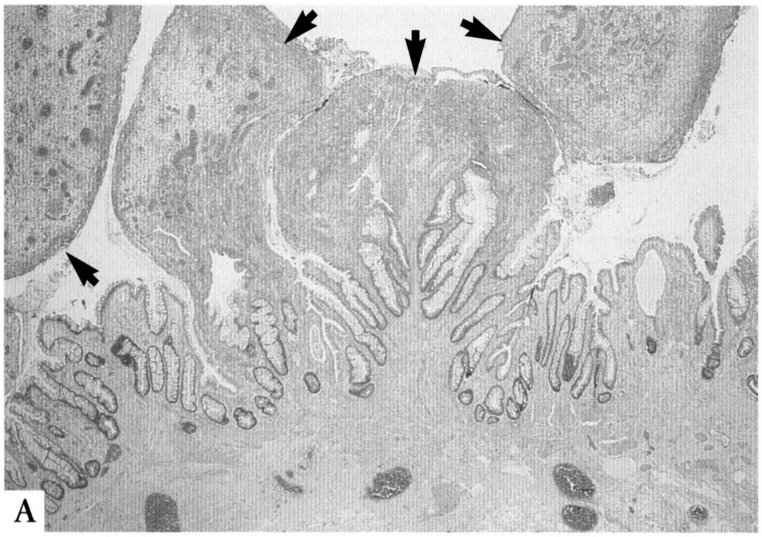

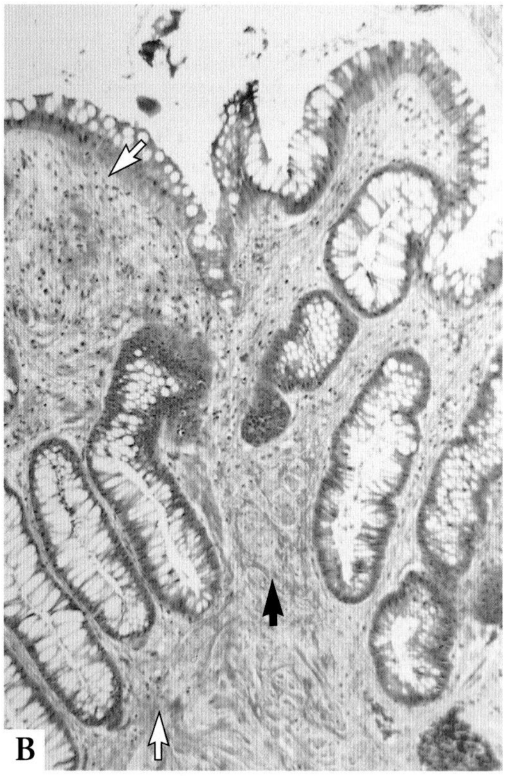

FIGURE 11-34.

Solitary rectal ulcer syndrome or mucosal prolapse. **A**, This low-power view shows distorted villiform rectal mucosa with ulcerated surfaces containing large areas of granulation tissue (*arrows*). Histologically the villiform architecture may resemble a villous adenoma, however, on closer inspection the epithelium shows reactive changes rather than dysplasia. **B**, Trichrome stain of solitary rectal ulcer syndrome shows dense collagen fibers (*open arrows*) within the lamina propria. A few red twigs of proliferating smooth muscle may also be seen (*closed arrow*). This fibromuscular hyperplasia is typical of mucosal prolapse syndromes. These lesions are usually seen on the anterior rectal wall in patients who have difficulty with defecation. Grossly, these lesions may be polypoid or ulcerated such that they simulate malignant neoplasms or Crohn's disease [29,34].

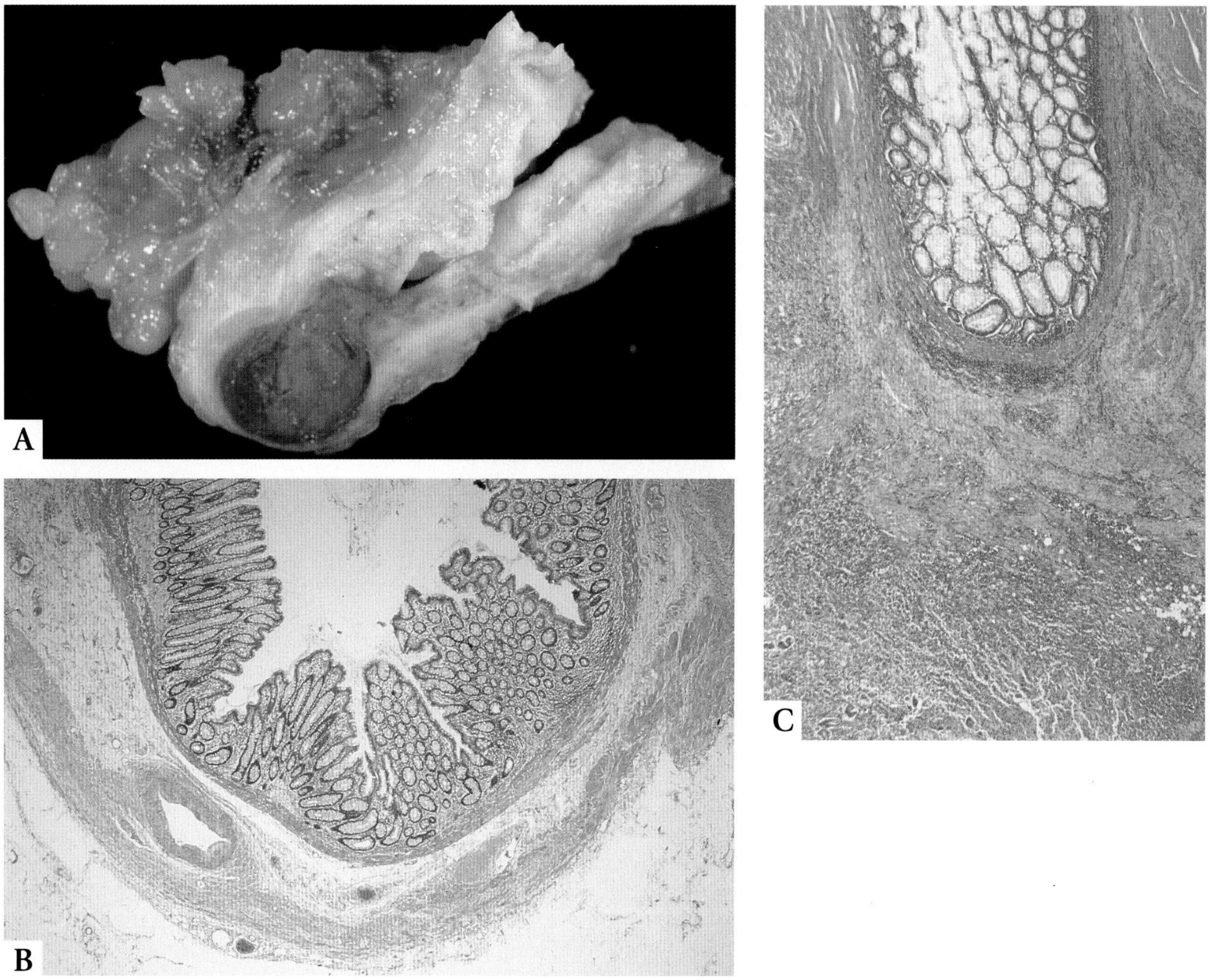

FIGURE 11-35. Diverticular disease. **A**, Cross-section of a diverticulum that shows an impacted fecalith in the distal tip. Fecaliths are thought to contribute to the development of diverticulitis by causing obstruction. **B**, This photomicrograph of the tip of a diverticulum shows just a few strands of attenuated muscularis propria remaining in the bowel wall. A penetrating artery and vein can also be seen. Diverticula often develop at sites where blood vessels enter the muscularis propria, presumably owing to these localized weak spots in the muscle wall. **C**, This low-power view shows the tip of an inflamed diverticulum overlying a diverticular abscess.

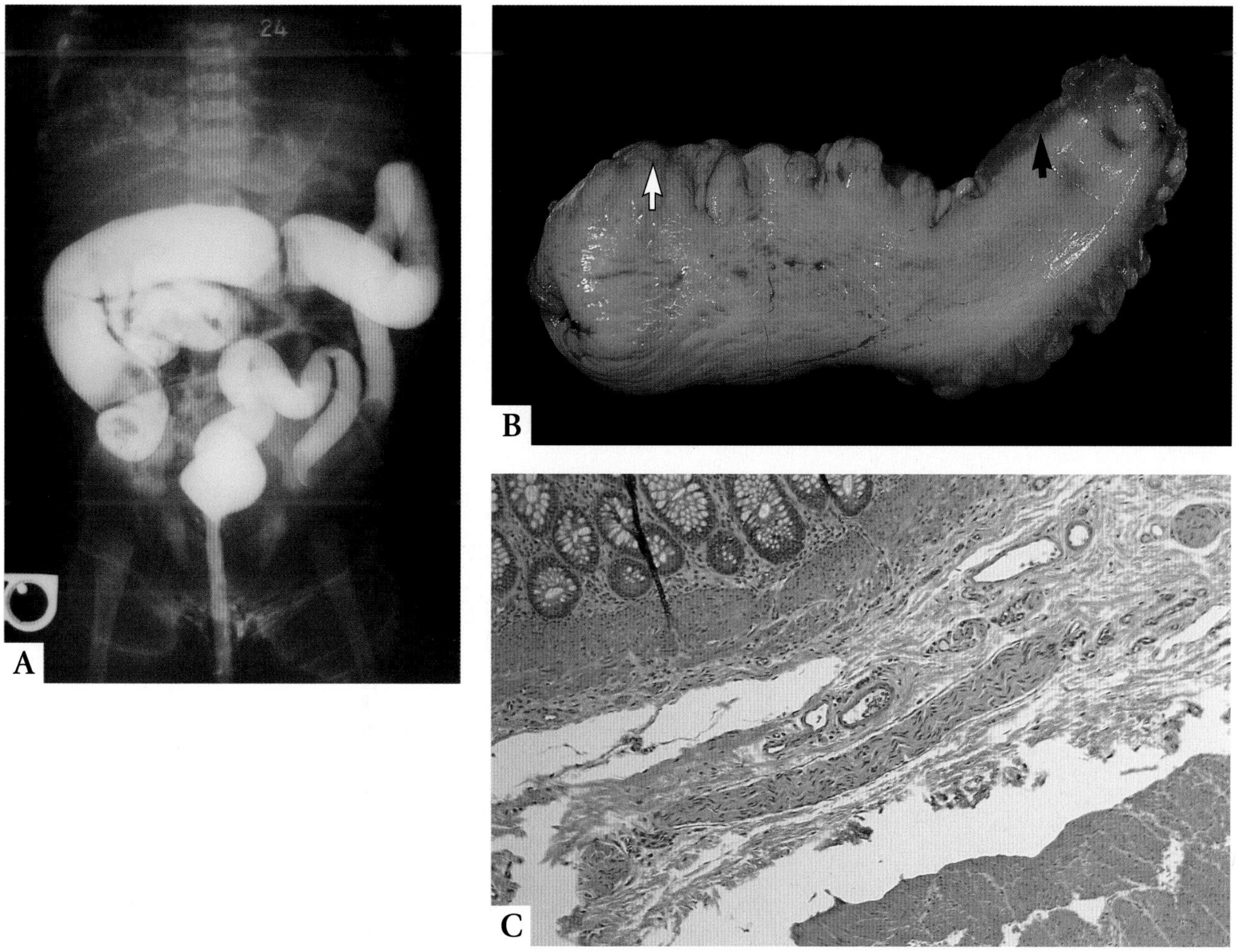

FIGURE 11-36. Hirschsprung's disease (aganglionic megacolon). **A**, This barium study shows a narrowed segment of a sigmoid colon and rectum with marked proximal dilatation of the colon. **B**, This resection specimen shows a dilated proximal segment (*open arrow*) with a narrowed distal margin (*closed arrow*). **C**, Low-power view of the submucosa in Hirschsprung's disease showing an enlarged nerve twig and an absence of ganglion cells.

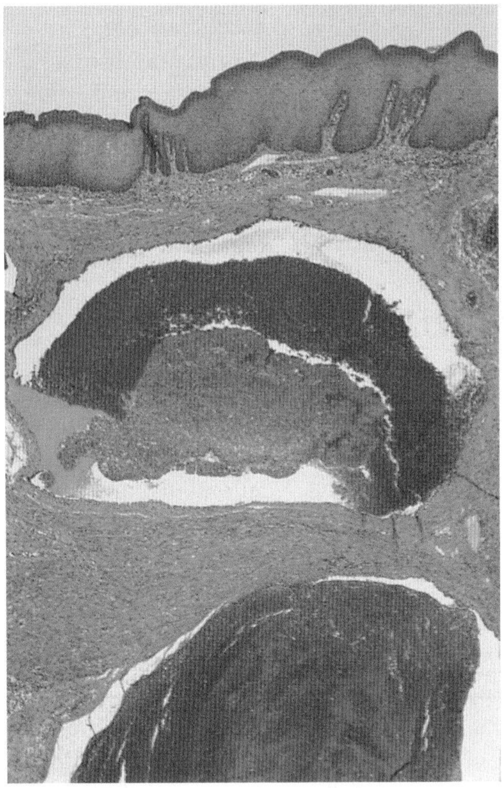

FIGURE 11-37. Hemorrhoids. This photomicrograph shows dilated veins underlying the anal mucosa. An organizing thrombus is within the lumen of the most superficial vein (thrombosed hemorrhoid).

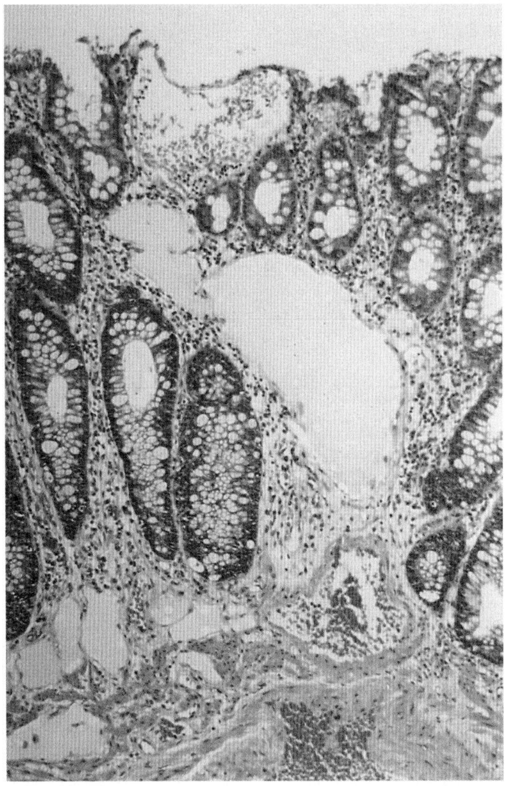

FIGURE 11-38. Vascular ectasias of the colon. The mucosa and submucosa contain several telangiectatic blood vessels. These histologic findings can be seen in vascular tumors, congenital malformations, and acquired lesions such as angiodysplasia and portal colopathy.

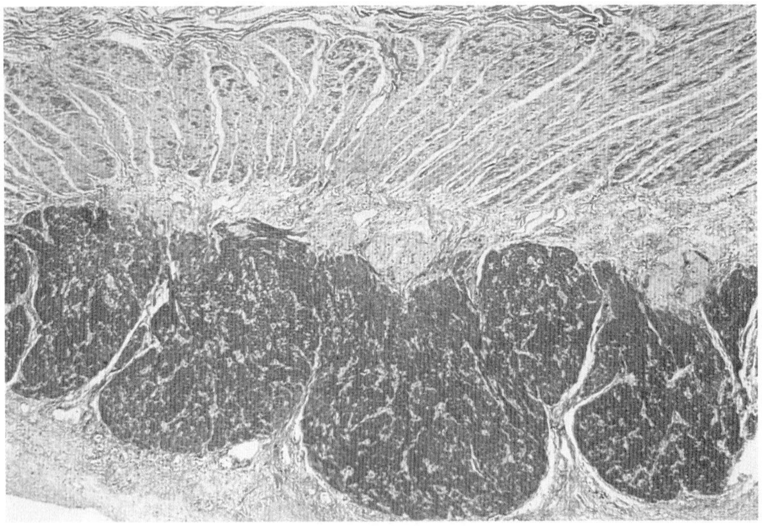

FIGURE 11-39. Progressive systemic sclerosis (scleroderma). This trichrome stain of the bowel wall shows replacement of the inner circular muscle by collagenous scarring. Scleroderma may cause fibrosis of the gut wall at any level along the gastrointestinal tract. Similar changes may be seen in a variety of familial visceral myopathies, however, these cases often show vacuolar degeneration of myocytes and a predilection for destruction of the outer muscle layer [35].

ACKNOWLEDGEMENTS

I would like to thank Dr. Henry D. Appelman and Dr. Katherine P. Heidelberger for contributing photographs and Jann Wesolek, Hannah Wesolek-Greenson, and Sarah Wesolek-Greenson for their continued moral support.

REFERENCES AND RECOMMENDED READING

1. Shepherd NA: Pathological mimics of chronic inflammatory bowel disease [Review]. *J Clin Pathol* 1991, 44:726–733.
2. Jessurun J, Yardley JH, Giardiello FM, *et al.*: Chronic colitis with thickening of the subepithelial collagen layer (collagenous colitis): Histopathologic findings in 15 patients. *Hum Pathol* 1987, 18:839–848.
3. Lazenby AJ, Yardley JH, Giardiello FM, *et al.*: Lymphocytic ("microscopic") colitis: A comparative histopathologic study with particular reference to collagenous colitis. *Hum Pathol* 1989, 20:18–28.
4. Geraghty JM, Charles AK: Aphthoid ulceration in diversion colitis. *Histopathology* 1994, 24:395–397.
5. Sugimura F, Ryoh H, Watanabe T, *et al.*: Comparative studies on the usefulness of phosphate versus glycerin enema in preparation for colon examinations. *Gastroenterologia Japonica* 1990, 25:437–450.
6. Grondin MV, Chang WW, Gaskins RD: Crypt alterations and collagen deposition in hyperplastic polyps of colorectum. *Dig Dis Sci* 1990, 35:12–19.
7. Foutch PG, DiSario JA, Pardy K, *et al.*: The sentinel hyperplastic polyp: A marker for synchronous neoplasia in the proximal colon. *Am J Gastroenterol* 1991, 86:1482–1485.
8. Provenzale D, Garrett JW, Condon SE, Sandler RS: Risk for colon adenomas in patients with rectosigmoid hyperplastic polyps. *Ann Intern Med* 1990, 113:760–763.
9. Buck JL, Dachman AH, Sobin LH: Polypoid and pseudopolypoid manifestations of inflammatory bowel disease [Review]. *Radiographics* 1991, 11:293–304.
10. Rozenbajgier C, Ruck P, Jenss H, Kaiserling E: Filiform polyposis: A case report describing clinical, morphological, and immunohistochemical findings [Review]. *Clin Investig* 1992, 70:520–528.
11. Heiss KF, Schaffner D, Ricketts RR, Winn K: Malignant risk in juvenile polyposis coli: Increasing documentation in the pediatric age group. *J Pediatr Surg* 1993, 28:1188–1193.
12. Longo WE, Touloukian RJ, West AB, *et al.*: Malignant potential of juvenile polyposis coli. Report of a case and review of the literature. Hyperplastic polyps [Review]. *Dis Colon Rectum* 1990, 33:980–984.
13. Nugent KP, Talbot IC, Hodgson SV, Phillips RK: Solitary juvenile polyps: Not a marker for subsequent malignancy. *Gastroenterology* 1993, 105:698–700.
14. O'Riordain DS, O'Dwyer PJ, Cullen AF, *et al.*: Familial juvenile polyposis coli and colorectal cancer. *Cancer* 1991, 68:889–892.
15. Subramony C, Scott-Conner CE, Skelton D, *et al.*: Familial juvenile polyposis. Study of a kindred: Evolution of polyps and relationship to gastrointestinal carcinoma. Hereditary generalized juvenile polyposis: Association with arteriovenous malformations and risk of malignancy. *Am J Clin Pathol* 1994, 102:91–97.
16. Matuchansky C, Babin P, Coutrot S, *et al.*: Peutz-Jeghers syndrome with metastasizing carcinoma arising from a jejunal hamartoma. *Gastroenterology* 1979, 77:1311–1315.
17. Fuller CE, Williams GT: Gastrointestinal manifestations of type 1 neurofibromatosis (von Recklinghausen's disease) [Review]. *Histopathology* 1991, 19:1–11.
18. Lie KA, Lindboe CF, Kolmannskog SK, *et al.*: Giant appendix with diffuse ganglioneuromatosis. An unusual presentation of von Recklinghausen's disease. *Eur J Surg* 1992, 158:127–128.
19. Nasir MA, Yee RW, Piest KL, Reasner CA: Multiple endocrine neoplasia type III. *Cornea* 1991, 10:454–459.
20. Shekitka KM, Sobin LH: Ganglioneuromas of the gastrointestinal tract. Relation to von Recklinghausen disease and other multiple tumor syndromes. *Am J Surg Pathol* 1994, 18:250–257.
21. d'Amore ES, Manivel JC, Pettinato G, *et al.*: Intestinal anglioneuromatosis: Mucosal and transmural types. A clinicopathologic and immunohistochemical study of six cases. *Hum Pathol* 1991, 22:276–286.
22. Bodmer WF, Bailey CJ, Bodmer J, *et al.*: Localization of the gene for familial adenomatous polyposis on chromosome 5. *Nature* 1987, 328:614–619.
23. Roncucci L, Stamp D, Medline A, *et al.*: Identification and quantification of aberrant crypt foci and microadenomas in the human colon. *Hum Pathol* 1991, 22:287–294.
24. Fenger C: Anal neoplasia and its precursors: Facts and controversies [Review]. *Semin Diagn Pathol* 1991, 8:190–201.
25. Clemmensen OJ, Fenger C: Melanocytes in the anal canal epithelium. *Histopathology* 1991, 18:237–241.
26. Gist RS, Waits JO: Malignant melanoma of the anus. *Ala Med* 1990, 59:20–22.
27. Kadivar TF, Vanek VW, Krishnan EU: Primary malignant melanoma of the small bowel: A case study. *Am Surg* 1992, 58:418–422.
28. Kim WH, Choe GY, Kim YI, Kim JP: Localized form of colitis cystica profunda–a case of occurrence in the descending colon. *J Korean Med Sci* 1992, 7:76–78.
29. Vora IM, Sharma J, Joshi AS: Solitary rectal ulcer syndrome and colitis cystica profunda–a clinico-pathological review. *Indian J Pathol Microbiol* 1992, 35:94–102.
30. Chippindale AJ, Desai S: Two unusual cases of pneumatosis coli. *Clin Radiol* 1991, 43:180–182.
31. Johansson K, Lindstrom E: Treatment of obstructive pneumatosis coli with endoscopic sclerotherapy: Report of a case. *Dis Colon Rectum* 1991, 34:94–96.
32. McCollister DL, Hammerman HJ: Air, air, everywhere: Pneumatosis cystoides coli after colonoscopy [Letter]. *Gastrointest Endosc* 1990, 36:75–76.
33. Spigelman AD, Williams CB, Ansell JK, *et al.*: Pneumatosis coli: A source of diagnostic confusion. *Br J Surg* 1990, 77:155.
34. Malik AK, Bhaskar KV, Kochhar R, *et al.*: Solitary ulcer syndrome of the rectum–a histopathologic characterization of 33 biopsies. *Indian J Pathol Microbiol* 1990, 33:216–220.
35. Chokhavatia S, Anuras S: Neuromuscular disease of the gastrointestinal tract [Review]. *Am J Med Sci* 1991, 301:201–214.

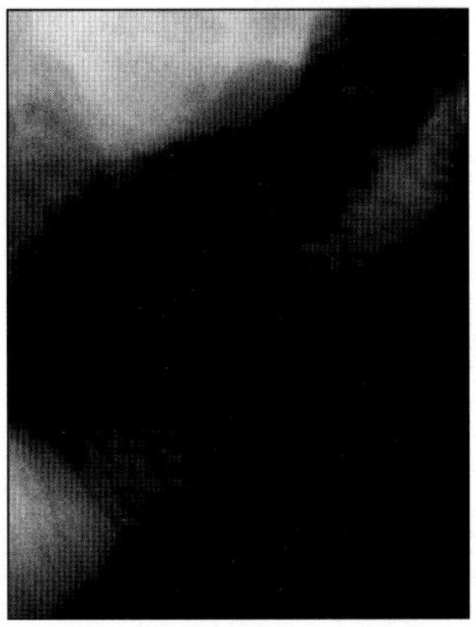

Index

Page numbers followed by *t* or *f* indicate tables or figures, respectively.

B

C

D

E

F

G

H

I

K

L

M

N

O

P

R

S

T

U

V

W

Y